METHODS FOR STUDYING
MONONUCLEAR PHAGOCYTES

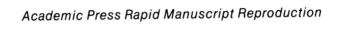
Academic Press Rapid Manuscript Reproduction

METHODS FOR STUDYING MONONUCLEAR PHAGOCYTES

edited by

DOLPH O. ADAMS

Departments of Pathology & Microbiology–Immunology
Duke University Medical Center
Durham, North Carolina

PAUL J. EDELSON

Children's Hospital Medical Center
Harvard University
Boston, Massachusetts

HILLEL S. KOREN

Department of Microbiology–Immunology
Duke University
Durham, North Carolina

ACADEMIC PRESS   1981
A Subsidiary of Harcourt Brace Jovanovich, Publishers
New York   London
Paris   San Diego   San Francisco   São Paulo
Sydney   Tokyo   Toronto

ACADEMIC PRESS, INC.
111 Fifth Avenue, New York, New York 10003

United Kingdom Edition published by
ACADEMIC PRESS, INC. (LONDON) LTD.
24/28 Oval Road, London NW1 7DX

Library of Congress Cataloging in Publication Data
Main entry under title:

Methods for studying mononuclear phagocytes.

Includes index.
1. Monocytes--Research--Methodology. 2. Phagocytes--
Research--Methodology. 3. Cell culture. I. Adams,
Dolph O. II. Edelson, Paul J. III. Koren, Hillel S.
QP95.7.M47   616.07'9   81-20646
ISBN 0-12-044220-5   AACR2

PRINTED IN THE UNITED STATES OF AMERICA

81 82 83 84   9 8 7 6 5 4 3 2 1

To our wives: Jean, Ingrid, and Charlotte.

CONTENTS

Contributors   *xv*

Preface   *xxiii*

I. OBTAINING AND CULTURING MONONUCLEAR PHAGOCYTES

1 The Culture of Mononuclear Phagocytes: A Brief
   Overview   1
   D. O. Adams and P. J. Edelson

2 Murine Mononuclear Phagocytes from Bone Marrow   5
   Carleton C. Stewart

3 Obtaining and Culturing Murine Monocytes   21
   Carleton C. Stewart

4 Obtaining and Culturing Human Monocytes   33
   Steven D. Douglas, Steven H. Zuckerman,
   and Samuel K. Ackerman

5 Isolation of Human Monocytes   43
   Dina G. Fischer and Hillel S. Koren

6 Culture of Human Monocytes in Microplates and
   Enzymatic Assays for Following Their Maturation   49
   Lois B. Epstein, Karen Yu, Lawrence P. Chong,
   and Constance C. Resse

7 Peritoneal Mononuclear Phagocytes from Small Animals   63
   Monte S. Meltzer

8 Obtaining and Culturing Human and Animal Alveolar
   Macrophages   69
   Robert M. Senior, Edward J. Campbell, and Beat Villiger

9   Obtaining Human Mononuclear Phagocytes from
    Colostrum   85
    F. S. Cole

10 Obtaining Adherent Cells from Spleen   89
    Karen S. Hathcock, Alfred Singer, and Richard J. Hodes

11 Obtaining Kupffer Cells   97
    R. Seljelid and B. Smedsrød

12 Obtaining Mononuclear Phagocytes from Disaggregated
    Neoplasms   103
    Stephen W. Russell

13 Obtaining Mononuclear Phagocytes from Granulomas   111
    Robert J. Bonney

    Teflon Film as a Substrate for the Culture of
    Mononuclear Phagocytes   121
    Jos W. M. van der Meer, Joke S. van de Gevel,
    and Ralph van Furth

15 Effects of Husbandry and Mouse Strains on Mononuclear
    Phagocytes   133
    Monte S. Meltzer

16 Endotoxin Contamination and in Vitro
    Monocyte–Macrophage Function: Methods of Detecting,
    Detoxifying, and Eliminating Endotoxin   139
    J. Brice Weinberg

17 Continuous Cell Lines with Properties of Mononuclear
    Phagocytes   155
    Peter Ralph

II. SEPARATION OF MONONUCLEAR PHAGOCYTES
FOR ENRICHMENT OR DEPLETION

18 Separation of Mononuclear Phagocytes for Enrichment
    and for Depletion: An Overview   175
    William S. Walker

19 Separation of Murine Macrophages by Adherence to Solid
    Substrates   179
    Donald E. Mosier

20 Separation of Human Monocytes and Guinea Pig
    Macrophages by Density Gradients of Metrizamide   187
    Barbara A. Sherry, Mathew A. Vadas, and John R. David

21 Separation of Murine Mononuclear Phagocytes by Density
    Gradients of Percoll   195
    Raymond B. Hester and William S. Walker

22 Separation of Human Monocytes by Density Gradients
    of Percoll   201
    R. Seljelid and H. Pertoft

23 Separation of Murine Mononuclear Phagocytes by
    Velocity Sedimentation at Unit Gravity   207
    Louis M. Pelus and Malcolm A. S. Moore

24 Use of Lidocaine for Detachment of Adherent
    Mononuclear Phagocytes   221
    Carl F. Nathan

25 Use of Sephadex Columns to Deplete Mononuclear
    Phagocytes   225
    Robert I. Mishell and Barbara B. Mishell

26 Depletion of Mononuclear Phagocytes: Pitfalls in the Use
    of Carbonyl Iron, Carrageenan, Silica, Trypan Blue, or
    Anti-Mononuclear Phagocytes Serum   231
    Paul A. LeBlanc and Stephan W. Russell

III. IDENTIFICATION OF MONONUCLEAR PHAGOCYTES

27 Identification of Mononuclear Phagocytes: Overview and
    Definitions   243
    R. van Furth

28 Characteristics of Mononuclear Phagocytes from Different
    Tissues   253
    M. M. C. Diesselhoff-den Dulk and R. van Furth

29 Fc and C3 Receptors   273
    Celso Bianco and Bronislaw Pytowski

30 Identification of Mononuclear Phagocytes by Ingestion of
    Particulate Materials, such as Erythrocytes, Carbon,
    Zymosan, or Latex   283
    Steven M. Taffet and Stephen W. Russell

31 Heteroantisera Raised against Mononuclear Phagocytes   295
    Alan M. Kaplan and T. Mohanakumar

32 Monoclonal Antibodies as Tools for the Study of
    Mononuclear Phagocytes   305
    Timothy A. Springer

33   Antisera against Ia Antigens   315
     Carol Cowing

IV. QUANTITATION OF NUMBER OF MONONUCLEAR
                    PHAGOCYTES

34   Quantitation of Adherent Mononuclear Phagocytes by
     Inverted Phase Microscopy   325
     D. O. Adams

35   Quantitation of DNA in Mononuclear Phagocytes   331
     D. O. Adams

36   Lowry and Bradford Assays for Protein   337
     Paul J. Edelson and Robert A. Duncan

V. MORPHOLOGY OF MONONUCLEAR PHAGOCYTES

37   Use of Wright's Stain and Cytocentrifuge Preparations   345
     Monte S. Meltzer

38   Use of Phase Contrast Microscopy   349
     Stanton G. Axline

39   Use of Peroxidase Stain by the Kaplow Method   363
     Monte S. Meltzer

40   Use of Nonspecific Esterase Stain   367
     Glenn A. Miller and Page S. Morahan

41   Histochemical Stains for Macrophages in Cell Smears and
     Tissue Sections: β-Galactosidase, Acid Phosphatase,
     Nonspecific Esterase, Succinic Dehydrogenase,
     and Cytochrome Oxidase   375
     Arthur M. Dannenberg, Jr., and Moritaka Suga

42   Use of Transmission Electron Microscopy   397
     Martha E. Fedorko

43   Preparative Techniques for Scanning Electron Microscopy   403
     Susan R. Walker and John D. Shelburne

44   Use of Ultrastructural Histochemistry   413
     Barbara A. Nichols

VI. BIOCHEMICAL CONSTITUENTS OF MONONUCLEAR PHAGOCYTES

45   Lysosomal Enzymes   433
     Earl H. Harrison and William E. Bowers

46   Microsomal Heme Oxygenase   449
     Diethard Gemsa

47   Histamine *O*-Methyltransferase   455
     Julian Melamed and Harvey R. Colten

48   5'-Nucleotidase Assay   461
     Paul J. Edelson and Robert A. Duncan

49   Alkaline Phosphodiesterase I   469
     Paul J. Edelson and Katherine D. Gass

50   Quantitation of Leucine Aminopeptidase of
     Mononuclear Phagocytes   473
     Page S. Morahan

51   Hexose Monophosphate Shunt Activity and Oxygen
     Uptake   477
     Lawrence R. DeChatelet and J. Wallace Parce

52   Secretion of Superoxide Anion   489
     Richard B. Johnston, Jr.

53   Release of Hydrogen Peroxide   499
     Carl F. Nathan

VII. GENERAL FUNCTIONS OF MONONUCLEAR PHAGOCYTES

54   Antibody–Dependent and Antibody–Independent
     Phagocytosis   511
     Denise R. Shaw and Frank M. Griffin, Jr.

55   Pinocytic Rate Using Horseradish Peroxidase   529
     Paul J. Edelson

56   Chemotaxis of Human and Murine Mononuclear
     Phagocytes   535
     Ralph Snyderman

VIII. SECRETION BY MONONUCLEAR PHAGOCYTES

57 Secretory Functions of Mononuclear Phagocytes:
    Overview and Methods for Preparing Conditioned
    Supernatants   549
    Phillip Davies

58 Characterization and Classification of Macrophage
    Proteinases and Proteinase Inhibitors   561
    Zena Werb

59 Growth of Macrophage on Collagen, Elastin, and
    Glycoprotein–Coated Plates as a Tool for Investigating
    Macrophage Proteinases   577
    Peter A. Jones and Zena Werb

60 Neutral Proteases by ^{3}H-Labeled Casein   593
    D. O. Adams

61 Plasminogen Activators by Use of ^{3}H-Labeled Casein
    Substrate   599
    S. V. Pizzo and J. G. Lewis

62 Elastinolytic Enzymes   603
    Michael J. Banda, H. F. Dovey, and Zena Werb

63 Microtiter Assay for Antiviral Effects of Human and
    Murine Interferon Utilizing a Vertical Light Path
    Photometer for Quantitation   619
    *Lois B. Epstein, Nancy H. McManus, Samuel J. Hebert,
    Judith Woods-Hellman, and Diane G. Oliver*

64 Endogenous Pyrogen   629
    Charles A. Dinarello

65 Prostaglandins   641
    John L. Humes

66 Quantitation of Selected Complement Components   655
    F. Sessions Cole, David J. Gash, and Harvey R. Colten

67 Lysozyme   667
    Lata S. Nerurkar

IX. DESTRUCTION BY MONONUCLEAR PHAGOCYTES

68 Destruction of *Listeria monocytogenes in Vitro*   685
    George L. Spitalny and Robert J. North

69 Ingestion and Destruction of *Candida albicans*   693
    Robert I. Lehrer

70 Quantitation of Destruction of Toxoplasma   709
    Rima McLeod and Jack S. Remington

71 Destruction of Rickettsiae   725
    Carol A. Nacy and Stanley C. Oaks

72 Destruction of Leishmania   745
    Carol A. Nacy and Michael G. Pappas

73 Destruction of Viruses   759
    Stephen S. Morse and Page S. Morahan

74 Cytostasis of Tumor and Nontumor Cells   775
    Alan M. Kaplan

75 Cytolysis of Tumor Cells by Release of [^{3}H-] Thymidine   785
    Monte S. Meltzer

76 Quantification of Cytolysis of Neoplastic Cells by Release
    of Chromium-51   793
    Stephen W. Russell

77 Assessment of Cytolysis of Tumor Cells by Release of
    [^{125}I] Iododeoxyuridine   801
    Ronald B. Herberman

78 Antibody-Dependent Cellular Cytotoxicity (ADCC) of
    Erythroid and Tumor Cells   813
    Hillel S. Koren and Dina G. Fischer

X. MONONUCLEAR PHAGOCYTES AS TOOLS IN CELL BIOLOGY

79 Overview: The Macrophage in Cell Biology   821
    David Vaux and Siamon Gordon

80 Biosynthetic Radiolabeling of Cellular and Secreted
    Proteins of Mononuclear Phagocytes   861
    Zena Werb and Jennie R. Chin

81 Extraction, Identification, and Quantitation of Lipids   873
    Eileen M. Mahoney and William A. Scott

82 Synthesis, Cellular Turnover, and Mass of Cholesterol   893
    Harry W. Chen and Andrew A. Kandutsch

83 Solute Uptake and Membrane Transport by Mononuclear
    Phagocytes   909
    Phyllis R. Strauss

84   Use of Lactoperoxidase for Labeling Membrane Proteins   925
     Helen L. Yin

85   Binding of Synthetic Chemotactic Peptides as a Model of
     Ligand-Receptor Interaction   933
     Edward J. Fudman and Ralph Snyderman

XI. MONONUCLEAR PHAGOCYTES IN VIVO

86   Isolation of Phagosomes from Mouse Peritoneal
     Macrophages   943
     Maja Nowakowski and Celso Bianco

87   Study of Mononuclear Macrophages in Vivo: Overview   951
     D. S. Nelson

88   Quantitation of the Inflammatory Accumulation of
     Mononuclear Phagocytes in Vivo   959
     George J. Cianciolo and Ralph Snyderman

89   Systemic Labeling of Mononuclear Phagocytes   969
     Alvin Volkman and Richard T. Sawyer

90   Labeling of Mononuclear Phagocytes in Granulomas and
     Inflammatory Sites   983
     T. J. Chambers and W. G. Spector

91   Identification of Fc and Complement Receptors
     in Tissue Sections   989
     Jeffrey Cossman and Elaine S. Jaffe

92   Determination of Macrophage-Mediated
     Antibacterial Resistance   1011
     R. J. North and G. L. Spitalny

     Supplement to Table of Contents   1019

     Index   1021

CONTRIBUTORS

Numbers in parentheses indicate the pages on which the authors' contributions begin.

Samuel K. Ackerman (33), *Bureau of Biologics, Division of Biochemistry and Biophysics, Bethesda, Maryland 20014*

Dolph O. Adams (1, 325, 331, 593), *Departments of Pathology and Microbiology–Immunology, Duke University Medical Center, Durham, North Carolina 27710*

Stanton G. Axline (349), *Department of Internal Medicine, Veterans Administration Medical Center, and The Arizona Health Sciences Center, Tucson, Arizona 85724*

Michael J. Banda (603), *Laboratory of Radiobiology, University of California, San Francisco, California 94143*

Celso Bianco (273, 943), *Department of Pathology, State University of New York, Downstate Medical Center, Brooklyn, New York 11203*

Robert J. Bonney (111), *Department of Immunology, Merck Institute for Therapeutic Research, Rahway, New Jersey 07065*

William E. Bowers (433), *The Rockefeller University, New York, New York 10021*

Edward J. Campbell (69), *Pulmonary Disease and Respiratory Care Division, Department of Medicine, Washington University School of Medicine at The Jewish Hospital of St. Louis, St. Louis, Missouri 63110*

T. J. Chambers (983), *Department of Experimental Pathology, St. Bartholomew's Medical College, London EC1, United Kingdom*

Harry W. Chen (893), *The Jackson Laboratory, Bar Harbor, Maine 04609*

Jennie R. Chin (861), *Laboratory of Radiobiology, University of California, San Francisco, California 94143*

Lawrence P. Chong (49), *Cancer Research Institute, and Department of Pediatrics, University of California Medical School, San Francisco, California 94143*

George J. Cianciolo (959), *Howard Hughes Medical Institute, Division of Rheumatic and Genetic Diseases, Duke University Medical Center, Durham, North Carolina 27710*

F. Sessions Cole (85, 655), *Department of Pediatrics, Harvard Medical School, The Division of Cell Biology, The Children's Hospital Medical Center, Boston, Massachusetts 02115*

Harvey R. Colten (455, 655), *Department of Pediatrics, Harvard Medical School, Division of Cell Biology, Children's Hospital Medical Center, Boston, Massachusetts 02115*

Jeffrey Cossman (989), *Hematopathology Section, Laboratory of Pathology, National Cancer Institute, National Institutes of Health, Bethesda, Maryland 20205*

Carol Cowing (315), *Division of Research Immunology, Department of Pathology, University of Pennsylvania, School of Medicine, Philadelphia, Pennsylvania 19104*

Arthur M. Dannenberg, Jr. (375), *Department of Environmental Health Sciences, Department of Epidemiology, School of Hygiene and Public Health, and Department of Pathology, School of Medicine, Johns Hopkins University, Baltimore, Maryland 21205*

John R. David (187), *Department of Medicine, Harvard Medical School, and the Robert B. Brigham Division of Brigham and Women's Hospital, Boston, Massachusetts 02115*

Phillip Davies (549), *Department of Immunology, Merck Institute for Therapeutic Research, Rahway, New Jersey 07065*

Lawrence R. DeChatelet (477), *Department of Biochemistry, Bowman Gray School of Medicine, Winston-Salem, North Carolina 27103*

M. M. C. Diesselhoff-den Dulk (253), *Department of Infectious Diseases, University Hospital, 2333 AA Leiden, The Netherlands*

Charles A. Dinarello (629), *Division of Experimental Medicine, Tufts University School of Medicine, Boston, Massachusetts 02111*

Steven D. Douglas (33), *Departments of Medicine and Microbiology, University of Minnesota School of Medicine, Minneapolis, Minnesota 55455*

H. F. Dovey (603), *Laboratory of Radiobiology, University of California, San Francisco, California 94143*

Robert A. Duncan (337, 461), *Department of Pediatrics, Harvard Medical School, Boston, Massachusetts 02115*

Paul J. Edelson (1, 337, 461, 469, 529), *Department of Pediatrics, Harvard Medical School, Boston, Massachusetts 02115*

Lois B. Epstein (49, 619), *Cancer Research Institute, and Department of Pediatrics, University of California Medical School, San Francisco, California 94143*

Martha E. Fedorko (397), *Kings County Hospital, Brooklyn, New York 11203*

Dina G. Fischer (43, 813), *Department of Microbiology–Immunology, Duke University Medical Center, Durham, North Carolina 27710*

Edward J. Fudman (933), *Howard Hughes Medical Institute, Division of Rheumatic and Genetic Diseases, Duke University Medical Center, Durham, North Carolina 27710*

David J. Gash (655), *Department of Pediatrics, Harvard Medical School, Divi-*

sion of Cell Biology, Children's Hospital Medical Center, Boston, Massachusetts 02115

Katherine D. Gass (469), *Department of Pediatrics, Harvard Medical School, Children's Hospital Medical Center, Boston, Massachusetts 02115*

Diethard Gemsa (449), *Institute of Immunology, University of Heidelberg, D69 Heidelberg, Germany*

Siamon Gordon (821), *Sir William Dunn School of Pathology, University of Oxford, Oxford OX13RE, England*

Frank M. Griffin Jr. (511), *Departments of Microbiology and Medicine, University of Alabama in Birmingham, Birmingham, Alabama 35294*

Earl H. Harrison (433), *The Rockefeller University, New York, New York 10021*

Karen S. Hathcock (89), *Immunology Branch, National Cancer Institute, National Institutes of Health, Bethesda, Maryland 20014*

Samuel J. Hebert (619), *Cancer Research Institute, and Department of Pediatrics, University of California, San Francisco, California 94143*

Ronald B. Herberman (801), *Laboratory of Immunodiagnosis, National Cancer Institute, National Institutes of Health, Bethesda, Mayland 20205*

Raymond B. Hester (195), *Division of Immunology, St. Jude Children's Hospital, Memphis, Tennessee 38101*

Richard J. Hodes (89), *Immunology Branch, National Cancer Institute, National Institutes of Health, Bethesda, Maryland 20014*

John L. Humes (641), *Department of Biochemistry of Inflammation, Merck Institute for Therapeutic Research, Rahway, New Jersey 07065*

Elaine S. Jaffe (989), *Hematopathology Section, Laboratory of Pathology, National Cancer Institute, National Institutes of Health, Bethesda, Maryland 20014*

Richard B. Johnston, Jr. (489), *Department of Pediatrics, National Jewish Hospital and Research Center, and University of Colorado School of Medicine, Denver, Colorado 80206*

Peter A. Jones (577), *Division of Hematology-Oncology, Childrens Hospital of Los Angeles, Los Angeles, California 90027*

Andrew A. Kandutsch (893), *The Jackson Laboratory, Bar Harbor, Maine 04609*

Alan M. Kaplan (295, 775), *Department of Surgery and Microbiology, Medical College of Virginia, MCV/VCU Cancer Center, Richmond, Virginia 23298*

Hillel S. Koren (43, 813), *Departments of Pathology and Microbiology–Immunology, Duke University Medical Center, Durham, North 27710*

Paul A. LeBlanc[1] (231), *Departments of Pathology and Bacteriology/Immunology, and the Cancer Research Center, University of North Carolina School of Medicine, Chapel Hill, North Carolina 27514*

Robert I. Lehrer (693), *Department of Medicine, Center for the Health Sciences, University of California, Los Angeles, California 90024*

[1]Present address: Division of Comparative Pathology, Box J-145, JHMHC, University of Florida, Gainesville, Florida 32610.

J. G. Lewis (599), *Department of Pathology, Duke University Medical Center, Durham, North Carolina 27710*

Eileen M. Mahoney (873), *The Rockefeller University, New York, New York 10021*

Rima McLeod (709), *Division of Infectious Diseases, University of Chicago and Michael Reese Medical Center, Chicago, Illinois 60616*

Nancy H. McManus (619), *Cancer Research Institute, and Department of Pediatrics, University of California Medical School, San Francisco, California 94143*

Julian Melamed (455), *Department of Pediatrics, Harvard Medical School, Division of Cell Biology, Children's Hospital Medical Center,Boston, Massachusetts 02115*

Monte S. Meltzer (63, 133, 345, 363, 785), *Laboratory of Immunobiology, National Cancer Institute, National Institutes of Health, Bethesda, Maryland 20014*

Glenn A. Miller (367), *Department of Microbiology, Medical College of Virginia, Virginia Commonwealth University, Richmond, Virginia 23298*

Barbara B. Mishell (225), *Department of Microbiology and Immunology, University of California–Berkeley, Berkeley, California 94720*

Robert I. Mishell (225), *Department of Microbiology and Immunology, University of California–Berkeley, Berkeley, California 94720*

T. Mohanakumar (295), *Department of Surgery and Microbiology, Medical College of Virginia, MCV/VCU Cancer Center, Richmond, Virginia 23298*

Malcolm A. S. Moore (207), *Laboratories of Developmental Hematopoiesis, Memorial Sloan Kettering Cancer Center, New York, New York 10021*

Page S. Morahan (367, 473, 759), *Department of Microbiology, Medical College of Virginia, Virginia Commonwealth University, Richmond, Virginia 23298*

Stephen S. Morse[2] (759), *Department of Microbiology, Medical College of Virginia, Virginia Commonwealth University, Richmond, Virginia 23298*

Donald E. Mosier (179), *The Institute for Cancer Research, Philadelphia, Pennsylvania 19111*

Carol A. Nacy (725, 745), *Department of Immunology, Walter Reed Army Institute of Research, Washington, D. C. 20012*

Carl F. Nathan (221, 499), *The Rockefeller University, New York, New York 10021*

D. S. Nelson (951), *Kolling Institute of Medical Research, Royal North Shore Hospital of Sydney, St Leonards NSW 2065, Australia*

Lata S. Nerurkar[3] (667), *International Center for Interdisciplinary Studies of Immunology, and the Department of Pediatrics, Georgetown University, Washington, D. C. 20007*

[2]Present address: Department of Microbiology, Rutgers University, Piscataway, New Jersey 08854.

[3]Present address: Infectious Disease Branch, National Institute of Neurological and Communicative Disorders and Stroke, National Institutes of Health, Bethesda, Maryland 20205.

Barbara A. Nichols (413), *Francis I Proctor Foundation for Research in Ophthalmology, University of California, San Francisco, California 94143*

Robert J. North (685, 1011), *Trudeau Institute, Inc., Saranac Lake, New York 12983*

Maja Nowakowski (943), *The Department of Pathology, State University of New York, Downstate Medical Center, Brooklyn, New York 11203*

Stanley C. Oaks[4] (725), *Department of Rickettsial Diseases, Walter Reed Army Institute of Research, Washington, D. C. 20012*

Diane G. Oliver (619), *Comprehensive Health, Inc., San Bruno, California 94060*

Michael G. Pappas (745), *Department of Immunology, Walter Reed Army Institute of Research, Washington, D. C. 20012*

J. Wallace Parce (477), *Department of Biochemistry, Bowman Gray School of Medicine, Winston-Salem, North Carolina 27103*

Louis M. Pelus (207), *Laboratories of Developmental Hematopoiesis, Memorial Sloan Kettering Cancer Center, New York, New York 10021*

H. Pertoft (205), *Institute of Medical and Physiological Chemistry, University of Uppsala, Biomedical Center, S-75123 Uppsala, Sweden*

S. V. Pizzo (599), *Department of Pathology, Duke University Medical Center, Durham, North Carolina 27710*

Bronislaw Pytowski (273), *State University of New York, Downstate Medical Center, Brooklyn, New York 11203*

Peter Ralph (155), *Memorial Sloan Kettering Cancer Center, Rye, New York 10580*

Constance C. Reese (49), *Cancer Research Institute, and Department of Pediatrics, University of California Medical School, San Francisco, California 94143*

Jack S. Remington (709), *Division of Infectious Diseases, Department of Medicine, Stanford University School of Medicine, Stanford, California, and Division of Allergy, Immunology and Infectious Diseases, Palo Alto Medical Research Foundation, Palo Alto, California 94301*

Stephen W. Russell[5] (103, 231, 283, 793), *Departments of Pathology and Bacteriology/Immunology, and Cancer Research Center, University of North Carolina School of Medicine, Chapel Hill, North Carolina 27514*

Richard T. Sawyer (969), *Department of Pathology and Laboratory Medicine, East Carolina University, School of Medicine, Greenville, North Carolina 27834*

William A. Scott (873), *The Rockefeller University, New York, New York 10021*

R. Seljelid (97, 201), *Institute of Medical Biology, University of Tromsø, N-9001 Tromsø, Norway*

Robert M. Senior (69), *Pulmonary Disease and Respiratory Care Division,*

[4]Present address: Department of Microbiology, U.S. Army Medical Research Unit, Institute for Medical Research, Kuala Lumpur 02-14, Malaysia.

[5]Present address: Department of Comparative and Experimental Pathology, College of Veterinary Medicine, Box J-145, JHMHC, University of Florida, Gainesville, Florida 32610.

Department of Medicine, Washington University School of Medicine at The Jewish Hospital of St. Louis, St. Louis, Missouri 63110

Denise R. Shaw (511), Departments of Microbiology and Medicine, University of Alabama in Birmingham, Birmingham, Alabama 35294

John D. Shelburne (403), Department of Pathology, Duke University Medical Center, and V.A. Medical Center, Durham, North Carolina 27710

Barbara A. Sherry (187), Department of Medicine, Harvard Medical School, and the Robert B. Brigham Division of Brigham and Women's Hospital, Boston, Massachusetts 02115

Alfred Singer (89), Immunology Branch, National Cancer Institute, National Institutes of Health, Bethesda, Maryland 20014

B. Smedsrød (97), Simpson Memorial Institute, University of Michigan, Ann Arbor, Michigan 48109

Ralph Snyderman (535, 933, 959), Howard Hughes Medical Institute, Department of Medicine and Department of Microbiology and Immunology, Duke University Medical Center, Durham, North Carolina 27710

W. G. Spector (983), Department of Histopathology, St. Bartholomew's Medical College, London EC1, United Kingdom

George L. Spitalny (685, 1011), Trudeau Institute, Inc., Saranac Lake, New York 12983

Timothy A. Springer (305), Department of Pathology, Harvard Medical School, Boston, Massachusetts 02115

Carleton C. Stewart (5, 21), Section of Cancer Biology, Division of Radiation Oncology, Washington University School of Medicine, St. Louis, Missouri 63110

Phyllis R. Strauss (909), Department of Biology, Northeastern University, Boston, Massachusetts 02115

Moritaka Suga (375), Department of Environmental Health Sciences, School of Hygiene and Public Health, Johns Hopkins University, Baltimore, Maryland 21205

Steven M. Taffet (283), Departments of Pathology and Bacteriology/ Immunology, and the Cancer Research Center, University of North Carolina School of Medicine, Chapel Hill, North Carolina 27514

Mathew A. Vadas[6] (187), Department of Medicine, Harvard Medical School and the Robert B. Brigham Division of Brigham and Women's Hospital, Boston, Massachusetts 02115

Joke S. van de Gevel (121), Department of Infectious Diseases, University Hospital, 2333 AA Leiden, The Netherlands

Jos W. M. van der Meer (121), Department of Infectious Diseases, University Hospital, 2333 AA Leiden, The Netherlands

Ralph van Furth (121, 243, 253), Department of Infectious Diseases, University Hospital, 2333 AA Leiden, The Netherlands

[6]Present address: Walter and Eliza Hall Institute, P. O. Box Royal Melbourne Hospital, Parkville, 3050 Victoria, Australia.

David Vaux (821), *Sir William Dunn School of Pathology, University of Oxford, Oxford OX1 3RE, England*

Beat Villiger[7] (69), *Pulmonary Disease and Respiratory Care Division, Department of Medicine, Washington University School of Medicine at The Jewish Hospital of St. Louis, St. Louis, Missouri 63110*

Alvin Volkman (969), *Department of Pathology and Laboratory Medicine, East Carolina University, School of Medicine, Greenville, North Carolina 27834*

William S. Walker (175, 195), *Division of Immunology, St. Jude Children's Hospital, Memphis, Tennessee 38101*

Susan R. Walker (403), *Department of Pathology, Duke University Medical Center, and V.A. Medical Center, Durham, North Carolina 27710*

J. Brice Weinberg (139), *Division of Hematology-Oncology, Department of Medicine, Duke University Medical Center, and V.A. Medical Center, Durham, North Carolina 27705*

Zena Werb (561, 577, 603, 861), *Laboratory of Radiobiology, and Department of Anatomy, University of California, San Francisco, California 94143*

Judith Woods-Hellman (619), *Comprehensive Health, Inc., San Bruno, California 94060*

Helen L. Yin (925), *Hematology–Oncology Unit, Massachusetts General Hospital, Boston, Massachusetts 02114*

Karen Yu (49), *Cancer Research Institute, and Department of Pediatrics, University of California Medical School, San Francisco, California 94143*

Steven H. Zuckerman[8] (33), *Departments of Medicine and Microbiology, University of Minnesota School of Medicine, Minneapolis, Minnesota 55455*

[7]Present address: Department of Medicine, University Hospital, CH-8091 Zurich, Switzerland.
[8]Present address: Departments of Medical Cell Genetics, Karolinska Institutet, S-10401 Stockholm 60, Sweden.

PREFACE

The study of mononuclear phagocytes has now emerged as a central theme in both immunology and cell biology. The seemingly endless plasticity of these cells has dictated an important strategy for their study: investigators often measure several attributes of mononuclear phagocytes in unison. Indeed, resolution of several of the currently critical issues regarding the mononuclear phagocyte system may depend upon this approach. Such issues include: Does the extravascular development of mononuclear phagocytes represent modulation, differentiation, or a combination of the two? Are there discrete subpopulations of mononuclear phagocytes? How do mononuclear phagocytes activated for heightened microbicidal or tumoricidal capacity mediate their destructive effects? It now appears that panels, comprising several different assays used in conjunction, can be employed to define and, hence, to study selected subpopulations of mononuclear phagocytes. Thus, examination of mononuclear phagocytes with a variety of techniques is becoming increasingly necessary for investigators in this field.

It is the goal of this book to facilitate the study of mononuclear phagocytes by providing, in one collection, protocols of various well-established and useful methods for examining these cells. We have attempted to make the technical protocols detailed, specific, practical, and inclusive of the necessary mystique, so that each can be immediately and directly employed in the laboratory. Some emphasis has been placed on the study of mononuclear phagocytes *in vivo*, because we believe this area to be underdeveloped and ripe for further study. Finally, we are cognizant of at least one significant omission in our selection of topics. Our lack of expertise on the role of mononuclear phagocytes in induction and regulation of the immune response, in the end, precluded consideration of methods on this important topic.

The book is organized according to a sequence of 11 steps that would generally be followed to study a given population of mononuclear phagocytes: (1) methods for obtaining and culturing populations of human and animal mononuclear phagocytes from many sources, including a discussion on use of macrophage-like cell lines; (2) various methods for manipulating populations of leukocytes to enrich or deplete their content of mononuclear phagocytes; (3) criteria and techniques currently judged to be useful for identifying elements of a cellular population as mononuclear phagocytes; (4) methods for quantifying the number of mononuclear phagocytes present; (5) techniques for studying the morphology of these cells, including microscopy, phase microscopy, histology, histochemistry, electron microscopy, scanning electron microscopy, and ultrastructural histochemistry; (6) methods for quantification of selected intracellular and released biochemical constituents such as lysosomal enzymes and oxygen metabolites; (7) methods for quantification of phagocytosis, pinocytosis, and chemotaxis; (8) methods for quantifying many of the defined secretory products of mononuclear phagocytes; (9) procedures for quantifying the destruction of tumor cells and of microorganisms by mononuclear phagocytes; (10) methods for studying the cell biology of mononuclear phagocytes, including assessment of phagolysosomes, membrane transport, secretion of labeled proteins, lipid metabolism, number of receptors, and membrane constituents; (11) techniques useful for studying mononuclear phagocytes *in vivo*, including procedures for estimating their kinetics, accumulation, identification, and microbicidal properties. In our judgment, access to the methods will be most easily gained by scanning the table of contents and its supplementary table, in conjunction with the index.

We most gratefully acknowledge the efforts of our contributors. We deeply appreciate the time our colleagues took to prepare detailed and accurate protocols, their willingness to share their unique expertise, and the zeal they brought to make these protocols uniformly excellent. The strength and utility of this book will ultimately be those of the individual chapters. We are particularly pleased to acknowledge the skill and devoted secretarial assistance of Ms. Lillie Knight, without whose continued efforts this venture would have foundered many times.

D. O. Adams
P. J. Edelson
H. S. Koren

1

THE CULTURE OF MONONUCLEAR PHAGOCYTES: A BRIEF OVERVIEW

D. O. Adams
P. J. Edelson

Cell culture has become a fundamental tool for studying the mononuclear phagocytes, and the basic requirements for culture of these cells have been described (1, 2). Many of the technical details for doing this successfully are described at length in this volume. Techniques for obtaining specific types of mononuclear phagocytes and for separating, counting, and identifying mononuclear phagocytes are presented below. This overview will outline briefly some of the general problems in culturing these cells.

The basic conditions useful for culturing most mononuclear phagocytes are not complex (1 - 3). A variety of basal media including medium 199, Dulbecco's minimum essential medium, and Eagle's minimum essential medium have been successfully employed. In some situations, basal media may be supplemented with nutrients, such as pyruvate, nonessential amino acids, vitamins, and ascorbic acid, or may be replaced by richer media such as MEM-alpha. The pH is usually controlled by the CO_2 - bicarbonate buffer system. Organic buffers such as HEPES may be quite useful for work in room air, but can be toxic. In

general, cultures of mononuclear phagocytes do best at a density where the cells are neither crowded nor sparse
$(2 - 3 \times 10^5$ adherent macrophages/cm^2). The size and shape
of the culture vessel are usually not critical, but the difficulties in removing adherent macrophages generally make it advisable to establish the primary culture in the type of vessel
that will be ultimately employed for each experiment. In the
end, the culture conditions for mononuclear phagocytes that
will prove optimal for a given experiment cannot be completely
determined *a priori* and must be established empirically for
each function.

Cultures of mononuclear phagocytes are generally supplemented with serum (1, 2). Fetal bovine serum, neonatal bovine
serum, or equine serum at 10 - 40% (v/v) are commonly used.
The serum can prove to be a major variable in altering function
of the cultures. The content of endotoxin, of pesticides or
other agricultural chemicals, of hormones, of antimacrophage
antibodies, and perhaps of other as yet unidentified substances
such as trace elements may stimulate or inhibit the function of
macrophages (4, 5). Consequently, it is best to screen each
lot of serum for its suitability in each assay of macrophage
function in which the investigator is interested. Furthermore,
the apparent lability of certain serum constituents may make
special handling of the serum necessary to obtain the desired
results (1). On occasion (e.g., quantification of secreted proteases in the absence of serum inhibitors of proteases such as
α_2-macroglobulin), establishment of cultures of mononuclear phagocytes in the absence of serum is desirable (6). The serumless
medium of Neumann - Tytell is useful for this purpose, as it
will support vigorous cultures of macrophages for several days.

The health and viability of macrophages being cultured
should be established each day by screening the culture plates
with an inverted phase microscope. In healthy cultures, the
macrophages form monolayers of large, plump, stellate, phase-
dense cells (Fig. 1). By contrast, unhealthy cultures contain
sparse accumulations of round, phaselucent, adherent macrophages overlaid by numerous refractile, detached cells.

A major pitfall in study of macrophages *in vitro* is their
physiologic plasticity. Various functions of mononuclear phagocytes, even under apparently optimal culture conditions, may
be reduced or lost after only a few hours of cultivation (7).
Furthermore, subtle alterations in the culture environment can

*Fig. 1. Phase photomicrographs taken with an inverted
phase microscope of cultures of murine peritoneal macrophages
elicited by thioglucollate broth. ×600. (A) Four hours after
explantation. (B) One day after explantation. Note the numerous, prominent vacuoles in the wellspaced macrophages.*

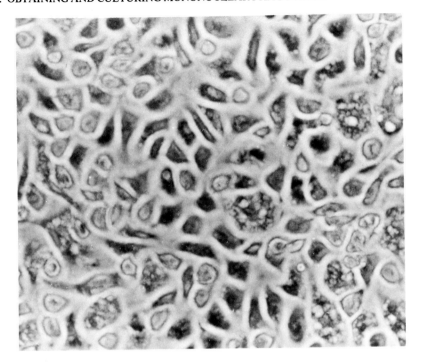

Fig. 1A

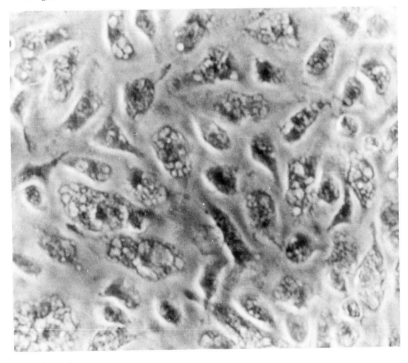

Fig. 1B

strikingly modify certain functions of macrophages. Heparin, a frequent constituent of washout medium, is one of a class of polyanionic substances that are known to stimulate pinocytosis (8). Trace concentrations of endotoxin can strikingly stimulate other functions of macrophages (4). Control of these variables requires, at minimum, meticulous replication of the details of each experimental protocol.

The goal of *in vitro* studies of macrophage function has been to better understand the mechanisms of their function *in vivo*. As we develop better ways of assessing and regulating their behavior in culture, we shall hopefully come closer to understanding their physiology *in situ*.

REFERENCES

1. D. O. Adams. Macrophages. *In* "Methods of Enzymology," Vol. LVIII, Cell Culture (W. Jakoby and I. Pastan, eds.), pp. 495-505. Academic Press, New York, 1979.
2. P. J. Edelson and Z. A. Cohn. *In* "*In Vitro* Methods of Cell-mediated and Tumor Immunity" (B. R. Bloom and J. R. David, eds.), p. 333. Academic Press, New York, 1976.
3. G. D. Wasley and R. John. The cultivation of mammalian macrophages *in vitro*. *In* "Animal Tissue Culture" (G. D. Wasley, ed.), p. 101. Butterworth, London, 1972.
4. J. B. Weinberg, H. A. Chapman, Jr., and J. B. Hibbs, Jr. Characterization of the effects of endotoxin on macrophage tumor cell killing. *J. Immunol. 121*: 72, 1978.
5. Z. A. Cohn and B. Benson. The *in vitro* differentiation of mononuclear phagocytes to the influence of serum on granular formation, hydrolase production, and pinocytosis. *J. Exp. Med. 121*: 836, 1966.
6. D. O. Adams. Effector mechanisms of cytolytically-activated macrophages. I. Secretion of neutral protease as an effect of protease inhibitors. *J. Immunol. 124*: 286, 1980.
7. D. O. Adams and P. A. Marino. Evidence for a multistep mechanism of cytolysis: The interrelationship between capacity for cytolysis, target binding, and secretion of cytolytic factor. *J. Immunol. 126*: 981, 1981.
8. Z. A. Cohn and E. Parks. The regulation of pinocytosis in mouse macrophages. II. Factors inducing vesicle formation. *J. Exp. Med. 125*: 213, 1967.

2

MURINE MONONUCLEAR PHAGOCYTES FROM BONE MARROW

Carleton C. Stewart

I. INTRODUCTION

When bone marrow from mammals, including humans, is cultured in a soft agar medium supplemented with appropriate colony-stimulating factors, discrete colonies of both granulocytes and mononuclear phagocytes will form. Recent studies have suggested the existence of different classes of colony-stimulating factors (1, 2), and one of them, macrophage growth factor (MGF), causes only colonies of mononuclear phagocytes to form (3).

Goud and Van Furth (4, 5) were the first to use extensively medium without agar to grow, in the presence of colony-stimulating factors, bone marrow colonies of mononuclear phagocytes. Buhles (6) has subsequently defined many of these growth kinetics. Liquid culture of bone marrow has several advantages over the agar method: the growth kinetics, functional characteristics, cytochemistry, and receptor analysis can all be easily measured without agar interfering with

the cells. Furthermore, macrophages will continuously phagocytose the agar causing potential functional alteration. On
the other hand, the agar system has a certain advantage: individual colonies can be isolated and removed from culture for
subsequent cloning, either in agar or liquid medium. Since
the least-differentiated progenitor cells are nonadherent,
there is also the possibility that in liquid culture cells can
float to new locations on the dish due to incubator vibration
causing additional colonies other than those produced by the
original progenitor cells to form. This will not occur when
cells are held in the agar matrix.

We shall describe the methodology for obtaining murine
bone marrow and for measuring the growth kinetics and colony-
forming ability of progenitor cells for mononuclear phagocytes. While there are many sources of colony-stimulating activity (1), only that produced by L-929 cells will be considered. The conditioned medium from these cells has predominantly MGF activity, and granulocytes are rarely found after
the third or fourth day of culture. MGF purified from this
conditioned medium results in the formation of only mononuclear
phagocyte colonies in either the liquid or agar culture
systems (3).

II. REAGENTS

A. Animals and L-929 Cells

Mice of any strain may be used. L-929 cells are used to
prepare conditioned medium (LCM) rich in MGF. These cells may
be obtained from the American Type Culture Collection, 12301
Parklawn Drive, Rockville, Maryland 20852. The quality of LCM
varies among different sources of L cells; it may be necessary to test several L-cell lines.

B. Chemicals

The following chemicals are required: Noble agar (Difco,
Detroit, Michigan); pronase Grade B (Calbiochem); hexadecyl-
trimethylammonium bromide (cetrimide) (Fisher Scientific);
methylene blue (Fisher Scientific); formaldehyde (Fisher
Scientific); 0.25% trypsin (GIBCO, Grand Island, New York);
α-MEM (GIBCO, Grand Island, New York); 100 × penicillin
streptomycin solution (GIBCO, Grand Island, New York); 100
glutamine solution (GIBCO, Grand Island, New York); 7.5 sodium
bicarbonate solution (GIBCO, Grand Island, New York);

TABLE I. *Colony Formation by Bone Marrow Cells*

Strain	Cells/femur ($\times 10^6$ cells)	Agar medium	Colonies per 1000 cells		
				Liquid medium	
			Day 7	Day 14	
AKR	14.6 ± 1.8	0.33 ± 0.05	3.9 ± 1.4	18 ± 9.5	
A/J	10 ± 1.6	0.16 ± 0.03	6.2 ± 0.7	–	
C57Bl/6	18.0 ± 5.5	0.10 ± 0.03	1.9 ± 0.11	27.7 ± 5.3	
C57Bl/10	24.0 ± 3.0	0.16 ± 0.02	4.0 ± 0.5	–	
BALB/c	11.9 ± 3.2	0.18 ± 0.03	2.5 ± 0.17	12.2 ± 5.4	
C$_3$Hf/An	12.9 ± 2.0	0.12 ± 0.06	3.4 ± 0.49	29.5 ± 11.9	
C$_3$H/He	12.9 ± 2.1	0.10 ± 0.01	2.7 ± 0.13	28.8 ± 14.7	
DBA	10.1 ± 2.7	0.27 ± 0.06	4.7 ± 0.38	29.6 ± 3.7	

Then add 0.5 ml freshly filtered pronase diluted 1:5 with saline. Mix and incubate the suspension 15 min at 37°C. Add 10 ml of cetrimide counting solution directly to the vial and count the cell suspension using an electronic particle counter. The same procedure is used for hemocytometer counting except that the cells are added to only 1 ml of cetrimide.

While the counter settings used to count erythrocytes can be used as approximate settings for counting nuclei from hematopoietic cells, it is best to determine the exact settings for nuclei. Instructions for this procedure are found in the counter manual.

C. *Colony Formation in Agar Culture*

Prepare cells in growth medium for agar culture at a concentration of about 2×10^5 cells/ml by adding 2×10^6 bone marrow cells to 10 ml agar medium in a 16 × 100 mm plastic culture tube. These cells will also be used in Section D. Add 3 ml of this cell suspension to 3 ml of agar culture medium in a second 16 × 100 mm plastic culture tube, mix, and immediately pipette 1 ml into four 35-mm culture dishes. Place these dishes in two humidity chambers and incubate them for 7 days. Count the number of colonies that have formed, using a dissecting microscope.

It is possible to fix the colonies *in situ* by adding 1.0 ml of 1.5% glutaraldehyde to the cultures. Refrigerate cultures and read them as soon as possible before they become dehydrated. Individual colonies can be removed for cytology using a Pasteur transfer pipette and dissecting microscope. We disperse the colony in 0.3 ml of α-10 by repeated passage through a 27-gauge needle attached to a tuberculin syringe and then prepare slides using a cytocentrifuge (Shandon Southern Instrument, Inc.,

Sewickley, Pennsylvania 15143). These preparations can then
be stained with Wright or Giemsa blood stains.

D. Growth Curve and Colony Formation in Liquid Culture

Add 2.5 ml of the cell suspension prepared above to
2.5 ml of α-0 in a 50-ml conical centrifuge tube. Then add
45 ml of growth medium for liquid culture. This will result
in 50 ml of bone marrow cells at a concentration of 10,000
cells/ml. Pipette 3 ml (30,000 cells) into 14 35-mm culture
dishes. Place them into seven humidity chambers prepared
above and place these in the CO_2 incubator.

To prepare cultures for colonies, add 0.7 ml of the suspension to 6.3 ml growth medium for liquid culture (1000
cells/ml) and plate 3 ml into two 35-mm culture dishes. Place
these dishes into the humidity chambers and incubate them for
7 days. (Plates may be stained directly with methylene blue
or, just prior to staining, the adherent cells can be pulsed
with yeast. First, rinse the cultures to remove nonadherent
cells. Cytocentrifuge preparations may be made of the nonadherent cells. Add 1 ml of medium containing 10% fetal bovine
serum and 1% freshly reconstituted (with distilled water, do
not use restoring solution as it contains sodium azide) guinea
pig complement to the adherent cells. Add 50 μl of yeast and
mix. Incubate cells for 30 min at $37°C$. Remove plates, rinse
plate three times with 3 ml saline and add 2 ml methylene
blue solution. After 20 min, discard stain, rinse with running tap water, and air dry.

It was noted above that extra cells were prepared in
growth medium for agar culture for the purpose of determining
the initial number of adherent and nonadherent cells. Add
3.5 ml of these cells to 3.5 ml of α-0. Plate 3 ml (3×10^5
cells) of this suspension directly in two 35-ml culture dishes.
Incubate these cells for 1 hr.

Determine the number of adherent and nonadherent cells on
two cultures at 1 hr and every day for 7 days. For the 1-hr
determination, use the culture prepared above containing
3×10^5 cells and, for the subsequent days, use the cultures
prepared at 3×10^4 cells. To count cells, resuspend the nonadherent cells in the growth medium and transfer it to a 7-dram
vial. Rinse the plates with 2 ml of α-0 and pool it with nonadherent cells. Immediately add (so it will not dry) 1 ml of
pronase diluted 1:10 with α-0 to the culture dish containing
the adherent cells. Then add 0.5 ml undiluted pronase to the
vial containing the nonadherent cells. (A portion of the nonadherent fraction may be processed for cytology as described
for agar colonies.)

Incubate vials and dishes at 37°C for 15 min. Add 10 ml of cetrimide to the vial of nonadherent cells and count them (or count directly with a hemocytometer). Rinse off adherent cells as follows: Transfer diluted pronase in culture dish to a 7-dram counting vial. Add 2 ml of cetrimide solution and systematically rinse the plate using a transfer pipette. We generally rinse the dish in a clockwise fashion, beginning at 1:00, proceeding around the plate to 12:00, and then ending up in the center of the dish. Be careful not to create air bubbles by keeping the pipette tip submerged. This systematic rinse is important, because macrophages are extremely adherent and they will not be quantitatively removed unless this procedure is strictly followed. It takes about 1 min per plate. If a large number of plates are going to be treated, they should be processed in batches of ten so that none of the plates are incubated longer than 25 min with pronase. For electronic particle counting, transfer the 2 ml of nuclei to 8 ml of cetrimide. For hemocytometer counting, count directly without further dilution. On days 1 - 3 counts will be low due to cell death.

Extra cultures can be prepared for specific mononuclear phagocyte marker or functional studies. Bone marrow-derived mononuclear phagocyte colonies contain all forms of mononuclear phagocytes from the monoblast to the mature macrophage in varying proportions.

IV. CONCLUDING REMARKS

The expected yield of cells and the frequency of colony-forming cells for bone marrow obtained from several mouse strains is shown in Table I. When cells are grown in liquid medium, large colonies with an average diameter of 2.7 ± 0.7 mm have formed by day 7; there is, however, a tenfold increase (29 ± 1.2) in the number of colonies on the culture dish by day 14. These latter colonies are nearly all small colonies whose average diameter is 1.1 ± 0.1 mm. Thus, two populations of bone marrow progenitor cells for mononuclear phagocytes are found: One is nonadherent and characterized by a short lag period and extensive proliferation. The other population of cells is adherent and is characterized by a longer lag period before proliferation begins (4 - 6 days). This offers a convenient means of separating the less mature nonadherent progenitor cells from the more mature adherent cells of the mononuclear phagocyte series for studying proliferative and functional potential. Colonies of bone marrow cells that have formed on day 7 are shown in Fig. 1.

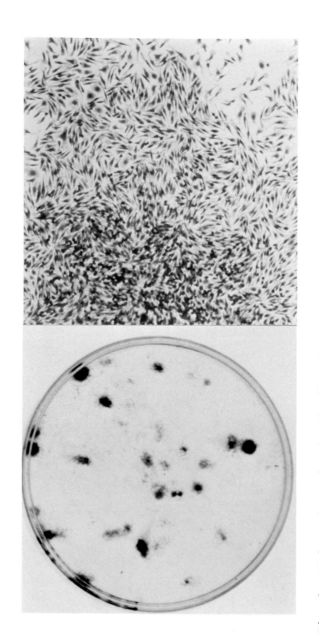

Fig. 1. Colony formation in liquid culture. Bone marrow cells from C₃Hf/An mice were plated in 35-mm culture dishes at 10⁴ cells/culture in 3 ml of growth medium for liquid culture. Cells were fixed and stained with methylene blue. The gross appearance of the colonies is shown on the left, and a photomicrograph (×100) of the edge of a colony is shown on the right.

When the number of colonies formed in liquid culture is used as an index of progenitor cells within the population, it is possible that some of the colonies formed are derived from nonadherent progenitor cells that have floated to a distant location where a new colony is produced. Thus, a single progenitor cell could produce two or more colonies. One way to determine if this problem exists is to culture serially diluted cells. As shown in Fig. 2, a greater deviation from linearity occurs as the cell number is increased, when colony formation is plotted against cells plated. While this problem does not occur when agar is used because the cells are held in a matrix,

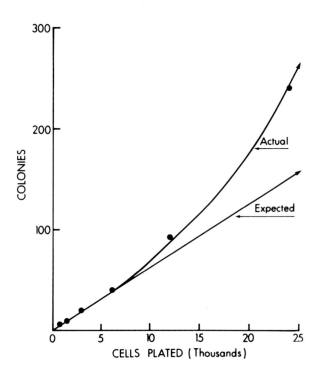

Fig. 2. *Nonlinear colony formation in liquid culture: Bone marrow cells from C₃Hf/An mice were serially diluted 1:2 in growth medium for liquid culture and 3 ml was plated on 35-mm culture dishes. After 7 days incubation, the cultures were stained with methylene blue and colonies were counted. Colony formation was linear with plated cells up to 6000 cells/culture. As cell number was further increased, a continuing deviation from linearity occurred. Cultures established at 48,000 cells were completely confluent.*

the number of colonies formed in agar is one-third to one-tenth
as many as in liquid culture medium (Table I). This difference
is not due to the above described progenitor cell flotation.
The reasons for the difference, however, are not known. Indeed,
the difference between the two culture systems is generally not
recognized as most investigators only use the agar system and
have never compared the two.

It has been shown that the addition of hemolysate to agar
medium (7-9) will result in a two- to fivefold increase in the
number of colonies which form. Similar increases have been reported when cells are cultured in low oxygen tension (10). In
both situations, however, the number of colonies that form do
not exceed the number that normally form in liquid medium. We
have never been able to find an increase in plating efficiency
due to oxygen or hemolysate when cells are cultured in liquid
medium. It would appear, therefore, that the presence of agar
compromises the colony-forming ability of some potential
colony-forming cells and that colony formation in the agar system reflects only a portion of them.

The single most important variable is medium pH. For good
growth, it is absolutely essential that cells not be subjected
to a fluctuating pH as might be encountered if the incubator
door is frequently opened. We cannot emphasize enough the importance of this variable. If an incubator must be used that
is frequently opened so air mixes with the internal atmosphere,
then cultures should be placed in a closed container inside the
incubator, which can be independently supplied with the humidified CO_2 and air atmosphere. (These containers are available
from Streck Laboratories, Inc., Box 6036, Omaha, Nebraska 68106
or Bellco Glass, Inc., 340 Edrudo Road, Vineland, New Jersey
98360.)

It is advisable to prescreen fetal bovine serum to select
a batch that is not toxic to cells and that will promote good
growth. For most of our experience in culturing bone marrow
cells, we have used fetal bovine serum as the supplement. We
recently found that bovine newborn or calf serum can also be
used. Results from one series of tests are shown in Table II.
It may be necessary to heat inactivate the sera at 56°C for a
full 30 min to detoxify the serum before it is used.

The growth of kinetics bone marrow mononuclear phagocytes
is shown in Fig. 3. Cells (3×10^4) were initially plated and,
as a function of time, the nonadherent and adherent cells were
separately counted. Adherent cells proliferated exponentially
with a doubling time of about 24 hr, while a relatively constant
recovery of nonadherent cells was obtained during the first week
of culture. Thereafter, the nonadherent cells also exponentially increased. Note that cells stop proliferating exponentially about day 10, when the cultures have been depleted of essential factors. Proliferation can be maintained for longer

TABLE II. *Colony Formation in Different Batches of Serum*

Type of bovine serum	Batch	Heat inactivated	Colonies/10^4 cells[a]
Newborn	141	–	61 ± 21
		+	25
	331	–	52 ± 19
		+	52 ± 11
Calf	714	–	3 ± 1
		+	27 ± 8
	002	–	44 ± 10
		+	28 ± 14
Fetal	308	–	30 ± 9
		+	8

[a]*Results from three experiments.*

periods if more growth medium is added. We find that each milliliter of growth medium will support the growth of bone marrow cells to a maximum number of 2×10^5 cells. If 2×10^6 cells are desired, 10 ml of growth medium would be required. There is a simple calculation to determine how long it will take an initial number of cells to reach a desired number of cells. The time (t) to reach this number (e.g., 2×10^6 cells) from any starting number (e.g., 10^4) of bone marrow cells (N_0) with a known fraction ($f = 0.1$) of progenitor cells and a known doubling time (e.g., $T_D = 24$ hr) is given by

$$t = (T_D/0.693)\ln(N/fN_0)$$

For the example above,

$$t = \frac{24}{0.693} \ln \frac{2 \times 10^6}{0.01 \times 10^4} = 343 \text{ hr or } 14 \text{ days}$$

It is possible to passage these nonadherent progenitor cells and establish new cultures. As shown in Fig. 4, when the nonadherent cells are sequentially passed every 3 or 4 days (usually Mondays and Fridays), they will give rise to new cultures of adherent cells. The adherent cells will proliferate exponentially, and the nonadherent cells will renew themselves for the next passage. The simplest interpretation of this data is that, on the average, each nonadherent cell gives rise to two daughters, one of which remains nonadherent and one of which becomes adherent.

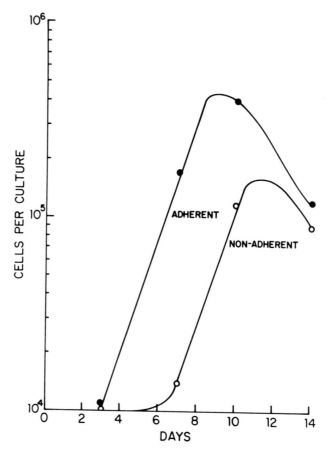

Fig. 3. Proliferation of bone marrow cells. Bone marrow cells from C₃Hf/An mice were plated in 35-mm culture dishes at 3 × 10⁴ cells/culture in 3 ml of growth medium for liquid culture. On days 3, 7, 10, and 14, the nonadherent cells were removed from two plates and put in separate 7 dram vials. Both the adherent (●) and nonadherent cells (○) were treated with pronase for 15 min and then counted with cetrimide using an electronic particle counter as described in Section II. A. The doubling time of each population during exponential growth is 24 hr.

The passages cannot be maintained indefinitely, however, and by day 30 no nonadherent cells can be recovered from the cultures. We calculate that a single progenitor cell can give rise to approximately 10^9 progeny. This can provide a sufficient number of cells for functional studies. In fact, if every progenitor cell from a single mouse femur were cultured,

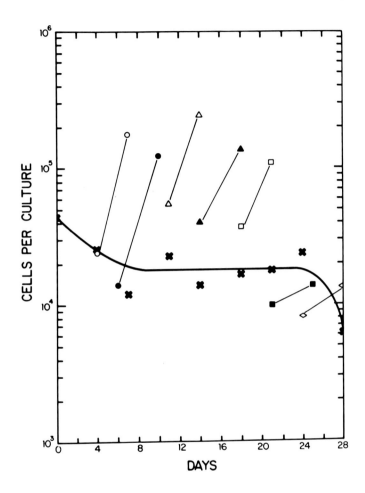

Fig. 4. Maintenance of nonadherent cell proliferation.
Bone marrow cells from C₃Hf/An mice were plated in 35-mm cul-
ture dishes at 3 × 10⁴ cells/culture in 3 ml of growth medium
for liquid culture. Every 3 or 4 days the nonadherent cells
(x) were removed, pooled, and counted. These cells were then
replated (3 ml) into new culture dishes. Fresh growth medium
was added to the adherent cells (○ , ● , △ , ▲ , □ , ■) and they
were counted a week later.

one could obtain between 10^{13} and 10^{14} cells. Since these
cells are absolutely dependent on MGF for growth, one would
require 10^4 liters of growth medium to accomplish this. Only

1 liter would be required, however, to obtain 10^9 ($\sim$1 gm) mononuclear phagocytes, and this would take about 14 days if all the cells from a single femur were cultured.

REFERENCES

1. C. C. Stewart and H-s. Lin. Macrophage growth factor and its relationship to colony stimulating factor. *J. Reticuloendothel. Soc. 23*: 269-285, 1978.

2. E. R. Stanley. Colony-stimulating factor (CSF) radioimmunoassay: Detection of CSF subclass stimulating macrophage production. *Proc. Nat. Acad. Sci. 76*: 2969-2973, 1979.

3. E. R. Stanley and C. J. Guilbert. Regulation of macrophage production by a colony-stimulating factor. *In* "Mononuclear Phagocytes - Functional Aspects" (R. van Furth, ed.), pp. 417-433. Nijhoff, Boston, 1980.

4. Th. J. L. M. Goud and R. van Furth. Identification and characterization of the monoblast in mononuclear phagocytes colonies grown *in vitro*. *J. Exp. Med. 142*: 1180-1199, 1975.

5. Th. J. L. M. Goud and R. van Furth. Proliferative characteristics of monoblasts grown *in vitro*. *J. Exp. Med. 142*: 1200-1217, 1975.

6. W. C. Buhles. Studies on mononuclear phagocyte progenitor cells: Morphology of cells and colonies in liquid culture of mouse bone marrow. *J. Reticuloendothel. Soc. 25*: 363-378, 1979.

7. T. R. Bradley, P. A. Telfer, and P. Fry. The effect of Erythrocytes on mouse bone marrow colony development *in vitro*. *Blood 38*: 353-360, 1971.

8. J. Rothmann, C. F. Hertogs, and O. H. Pluznik. Replacement of serum by hemolysate as groth promoter for murine leukemic and normal hemopoietic progenitor cells in culture. *Exp. Hematol. 5*: 117-124, 1977.

9. K. Tsuneoka, Y. Takagi, K. Hirashima, and M. Shihita. Enhancement of the action of colony stimulating factor (CSF) by soluble components of erythrocytes in mouse bone marrow cell cultures. *Exp. Hematol. 6*: 445-450, 1978.

10. T. R. Bradley, G. S. Hodgson, and M. Rosendal. The effect of oxygen tension on hemapoietic and fibroblast cell proliferation *in vitro*. *J. Cell. Physiol. 97*: 417-522, 1978.

3

OBTAINING AND CULTURING MURINE MONOCYTES

Carleton C. Stewart

I. INTRODUCTION

Murine monocytes, like other sources of mononuclear phagocytes, will proliferate and form colonies when they are grown
in medium containing fetal calf serum and L-cell conditioned
medium (1,2), a potent source of macrophage growth factor (3).
Monocytes are probably the immediate precursor to the tissue
macrophage (4). The colony-forming cells found in the tissues
are also the most likely descendants of monocytes.

Due to the small quantity of blood that can de derived
from mice, we have tried to optimize our procedures for the
greatest yield of mononuclear cells. We shall describe the
methodology for isolating and culturing murine blood monocytes.

Copyright © 1981 by Academic Press, Inc.
ISBN 0-12-044220-5

II. REAGENTS

All the reagents used to culture bone marrow cells will be used to culture monocytes. Refer to Chapter 2 for their preparation. In addition to those reagents it is necessary to prepare other solutions for separating peripheral blood mononuclear cells.

A. *Ficoll-Hypaque*

Prepare 100 ml of stock Ficoll solution by dissolving 9 gm Ficoll (Sigma Chemical Co., St. Louis, Missouri) in 100 ml distilled water. Heat to 40°C with stirring to dissolve. Sterilize by passing through 0.45 μm micropore filter. To prepare the gradient, mix together 7 ml of Ficoll, 2 ml of 50% sodium hypaque (Winthrop Laboratories, New York) and 1 ml of distilled water. Shake the solution vigorously to make sure the ingredients are well mixed.

B. *αMOPS Preparation Medium*

The organic buffer, 2-N-morpholinopropane sulfonic acid (MOPS), is used for the manipulative procedures so that the pH of the medium remains stable in an air atmosphere. This medium must not be used in a CO_2-containing atmosphere. It is our experience that cell survival is exquisitely dependent on a stable pH within the physiologic range of 7.0-7.4.

Mix 1 gm αMEM powder without sodium bicarbonate with 0.4 gm MOPS, 0.04 gm NaCl, 0.27 ml of 5 N NaOH, 2 ml 100× penicillin-streptomycin solution (GIBCO) and 98 ml distilled water. Filter and sterilize the medium by passing it through a 0.22 μm micropore filter. The additional sodium chloride is required to produce a final osmolality of 300±5 Mosm and the NaOH is necessary to produce a pH 7.2-7.4.

C. *Removing Adherent Monocytes*

(a) Lidocaine solution (12 mM)
Mix together 1.7 ml of 2% lidocaine-HCl (Astra Pharmaceutical Products, Inc., Framingham, Massachusetts), 1 ml fetal or newborn bovine serum and 7.3 ml αMOPS.

(b) Ethylenediaminetetraacetic acid solution (m0 mM)
Mix together 0.37 gm EDTA (disodium), 0.85 gm NaCl, and 100 ml distilled H_2O. Adjust the pH to 7.2 with 1 N NaOH.

(c) Sodium Pyrophosphate (10 mM)
Mix together 0.45 gm tetrasodium pyrophosphate (Sigma T-6379)
and dissolve in 100 ml phosphate-buffered saline. Adjust pH
to 7.2 with about 1 ml of 1 N HCl.

Filter sterilize all solutions by passage through a 0.22 μm
micropore filter.

III. PROCEDURES

A. *Humidity Chambers:* See Chapter 2.

B. *Obtaining Blood Mononuclear Cells*

First read all the procedures listed below. Assuming a
recovery of 0.5 ml of whole blood per mouse, add a volume of
αMOPS, containing 20 U heparin/ml, equal to the amount of
blood desired. We usually put no more than 7 ml heparinized
αMOPS and 7 ml blood per 15 ml conical centrifuge tube. For
example, if 8 ml of blood are required from 16 mice, we would
add 4 ml heparinized αMOPS to two tubes and put 4 ml blood in
each.
Anesthetize the mouse using ether, pin it supine to a
board, and wash thoroughly with 70% EtOH, maintain anesthesia
by placing an etherized gauze pad in a 50-ml beaker over its
nose. Cut a midline incision in the chest wall and expose the
heart and lungs. Insert a 26-gauge needle on a 1-ml syringe
into the left ventricle and aspirate the blood. When aspirating the blood from the heart, use gentle suction so as not to
collapse the heart. Put blood in the heparinized αMOPS (at
room temperature).
In these separation procedures we shall account for all
cells to determine the actual recovery of monocytes. After
collecting all the blood, pool it and obtain a cell count (use
the pronase cetrimide procedure outlined in Chapter 2 for
counting cells). Also prepare two or more slides (using a
cytocentrifuge, if possible. Shandon Southern Instruments,
Inc., 515 Broad St., Bewickley, Pennsylvania 15143). The cells
will be stained later for esterase activity. Overlay up to
10 ml of the cell suspension over 5 ml Ficoll-Hypaque gradient
solution in a 15-ml conical centrifuge tube. Make sure all
solutions remain at room temperature. Centrifuge cells at
1200 g for 10 min. This procedure is different than the standard procedure originally described by Boyum (5), but we have
found it satisfactory for separation of murine mononuclear
cells. If difficulty is encountered, more or less, water may
be added to the 7 parts of Ficoll and 2 parts of Hypaque to

change the density of the solution. After centrifugation, a
band of mononuclear cells and platelets should be found with
little erythrocyte contamination. Withdraw the medium/plasma
layer to within 1 cm of the gradient mixture and discard.
Withdraw the gradient solution containing the mononuclear cells
to within 1 cm of the erythrocyte layer and put it in a 50-ml
conical centrifuge tube (Falcon No. 2070). Pool up to four
gradients into one centrifuge tube and then bring the volume
to 50 ml with αMOPS. Mix thoroughly to eliminate any possibility of reforming a gradient. Centrifuge cells at 200 g for
10 min at 4°C. Withdraw supernatant to 0.1 cm of the pellet.
Resuspend pellets and pool all samples into one, bring to 50 ml
with αMOPS and centrifuge again. Now resuspend the pellet in
αMOPS using a volume of 1 ml times the number of mice used.
At this point obtain another cell count and prepare two more
slides using the cytocentrifuge. All slides should be stained
using the esterase staining procedure outlined in Morahan's
Chapter.

C. *Colony Formation of Monocytes in Agar Culture*

The method for separating monocytes from lymphocytes will
be described later. Prepare a 24-ml stock solution of 2×10^5
mononuclear cells/ml in Agar Growth Medium. Add 3 ml of this
suspension to 3 ml of Agar Medium, mix and plate 1 ml into
4-35 mm culture dishes. Place in two humidity chambers and
incubate. On days 21 and 28, count the number of colonies
that have formed using a dissecting microscope. Since the
lymphocytes do not proliferate in the growth medium, their
presence can be ignored and the total mononuclear cell fraction
can be used.

Colonies may be fixed *in situ* from two cultures each time
by adding 1 ml of 3% glutaraldehyde. Colonies may also be removed using a Pasteur pipette and, after preparing a cytocentrifuge preparation, cells may be processed for cytological identification.

D. *Colony Formation in Liquid Culture*

Colony formation by the total mononuclear cell population
or by the adherent and nonadherent fractions may be obtained
as follows: Make a 1/100 dilution of the suspension prepared
in Section III. C by adding 0.15 ml of cells to 15 ml liquid
growth medium. Mix thoroughly and plate 3 ml of cells into
4-35 mm culture dishes, label two dishes "TOTAL" and place
them in a humidity chamber. Incubate all dishes at 37°C for
1 hr. Remove the two unlabeled dishes, resuspend the cells in

the overlying medium and transfer them to new 35-mm dishes
labeled "nonadherent cells." Immediately add 3 ml liquid
growth medium to the empty dish. Label it "adherent cells."
Keep dishes paired by designating them A and B. Put each pair
in a humidity chamber and incubate them all for 14 days.

Plates may be stained directly with methylene blue, Wrights
blood stain, or giemsa stain. The phagocytic activity of the
adherent cells can also be determined prior to staining. First,
rinse the cultures to remove nonadherent cells. Cytocentrifuge
preparations may be made of these nonadherent cells. Add 1 ml
medium containing 10% fetal or newborn bovine serum and 1%
freshly reconstituted (with distilled water, do not use restoring solution as it contains sodium azide) guinea pig complement to the adherent cells. Add 50 µl of autoclaved bakers
(Chapter 2) yeast and mix. Incubate the cells for 30 min at
37°C. Remove the cultures, rinse them three times with 3 ml
saline each time and add 2 ml methylene blue solution, Chapter 2. After 20 min, discard stain, rinse with running tap
water, and air dry.

E. Growth of Mononuclear Cells in Liquid Culture

Dilute the cells prepared in Section III.C by adding 18 ml
of α-O to 18 ml of the cell suspension in a 50-ml conical centrifuge tube; these cells are now at a concentration of 10^5
cells/ml. Then add 3 ml of this suspension to 27 ml of liquid
growth medium; these cells are now at a concentration of 10^4
cells/ml.

Pipette 3 ml of cells at 10^5 cells/ml into 6-35 mm culture
dishes labeled 10^5; pipette 3 ml of cells at 10^4 cells/ml into
12-35 mm dishes labeled 10^4. Place cultures into humidity
chambers and incubate them. The adherent and nonadherent cell
count can be made every two days using two cultures each day.
For days 0, 2, 4, 6, and 8 use dishes plated with 3×10^5 cells
(labeled 10^5) and, for days 8, 10, 12, 14, use dishes plated
with the lower cell concentration. Since both concentrations
are counted on day 8, a comparison of the growth kinetics of
the two groups can be made. To count cells, resuspend the nonadherent cells in the growth medium and transfer them to a
7-dram vial. Rinse the plates with 2 ml of αMOPS and pool it
with the nonadherent cells. Immediately add (so it will not
dry) to the culture dish containing the adherent cells 1 ml
pronase diluted 1 to 10 with αMOPS. Then add 0.5 ml undiluted
pronase to the vial containing the 5 ml of nonadherent cells.

Incubate vials and dishes at 37°C for 15 min. Add 10 ml
cetrimide to the vial of nonadherent cells and count them (or
count directly with hemocytometer). Rinse off adherent cells
as follows: Transfer diluted pronase in culture dish to a

7-dram counting vial. Add 2 ml of cetrimide solution and systematically rinse the plate using a transfer pipette. We
generally rinse the dish in a clockwise fashion beginning at
1:00 and proceed around the plate to 12:00 and then end up in
the center of the dish. Be careful not to create air bubbles
by always keeping the pipette tip submerged. This systematic
rinse is important because macrophages are extremely adherent
and they will not be quantitatively removed unless this procedure is strictly followed. Do not scrape bottom of dish
with pipette tip to avoid plastic particles. This procedure
takes about 1 min/plate, therefore, if a large number of
plates are going to be treated, they should be processed in
batches of ten so that none of the plates are incubated longer
than 25 min with pronase. For electronic particle counting,
transfer the 2 ml of nuclei to 8 ml of cetrimide. For hemocytometer counting, count directly without further dilution.
On days 1-6 counts will be low due to cell death. Extra cultures can be prepared for specific mononuclear phagocyte marker or functional studies.

F. Separation of Monocytes from Lymphocytes

The procedure we have developed for isolating monocytes
from lymphocytes utilizes the adherence properties of both
cell types. It has the advantage that all cells can be accounted for even if they are lost. The procedure has the disadvantage that monocytes, once adherent, must be removed and
most methods for removing them do not always give good viable
cell recoveries.

There are two populations of adherent monocytes: One
population will adhere in the presence of serum and the second
population will adhere only in the absence of serum. Lymphocytes will adhere under either of these conditions and the
monocyte preparations are contaminated by them. In the following procedure it is possible to obtain a highly enriched population of monocytes.

After counting the cells in Section III.B, adjust them in
αMOPS, so that NO MORE than 10^5 cells/cm^2 will be plated.
This is important because a subconfluent monolayer of cells is
required if all monocytes are to be recovered. The wells of a
24-well cluster plate (Costar No. 3524) have a surface area of
2 cm^2 (diameter = 16 mm). This plate will be used to obtain
the monocytes. The procedure outlined is designed to account
for all the mononuclear cells and their purity as well as to
obtain monocytes for the desired experiments.

Place 12-mm round coverslips (Belco Glass Co., Vineland, New Jersey) into the four wells Al through Dl of the cluster plate. Coverslips may be sterilized by quickly passing them through a flame.

Prepare a 50 ml mononuclear cell suspension at 10^5/ml and plate 2 ml in each well (10^5 cells/cm^2). Use about eight mice for this number of mononuclear cells.

Incubate the cells for 1 hr at 37°C. Rinse the nonadherent cells from each well and pool them as follows: Resuspend the nonadherent cells in overlying medium doing one well at a time; after removing cells, immediately add 1 ml αMOPS containing 10% newborn bovine serum to each well so the adherent cells do not become dry. Pool all nonadherent cells. At this point, most monocytes have adhered but so have a significant number of lymphocytes.

Remove the coverslips from wells Al and Bl. Mount the coverslips *cell side up* on the end of a microscope slide using permount and fix them. Also remove the adherent cells from wells A2 and B2 using cetrimide (Section III.E) to determine the actual number of cells that have adhered. Incubate the plate at 37°C in humidified air overnight. Do not use a CO_2 incubator.

Prepare two cytocentrifuge preparations of the nonadherent cells and count 2 ml of the suspension (Section III.E) to determine the actual number that were removed. These nonadherent cells can be used to determine if any will form colonies (see Section III.D for details). To do this, centrifuge 200 g for 10 min and resuspend pellet in liquid growth medium to give 7 ml at 10^4 and 7 ml at 10^3 cells/ml. Plate 3 ml into two 35-mm dishes each, place them in humidity chambers and incubate for 14 days. Stain and count colonies. Correlate esterase positive cells in the original sample of nonadherent cells with the number of colonies formed.

Stain all slides and mounted coverslips for nonspecific esterase using the procedures outlined in Morahans Chapter. Determine the number of esterase positive cells in each fraction: Number of esterase positive cells = fraction positive × number of cells/well.

After overnight incubation, rerinse each well with αMOPS pooling the nonadherent cells as before. Add αMOPS immediately after rinsing so the monolayer does not dry out. Remove coverslips from wells Cl and Dl mount and fix them and count the number of adherent cells in wells C2 and D2 as before. Prepare cytocentrifuge preparations and count the cells in the nonadherent fraction. Determine nonadherent cells that will form colonies as described above. The remaining 16 wells containing monocytes can be used for functional studies.

We have found no procedure for removing all monocytes in a viable state. We have, however, used lidocaine, EDTA, or sodium pyrophosphate with varying degrees of success using the following procedure:

Remove the medium overlying the adherent cells, discard, and add 0.5 ml of either lidocaine, EDTA, or sodium pyrophosphate. Do not treat any more wells than can be processed in 5 min. Incubate these cells for 10 min and then add 1.0 ml αMOPS containing 10% newborn bovine serum (α10MOPS) and rinse the surface of the wells systematically and pool them. After removal of cells, put 0.5 ml of the suspension in 10 ml cetrimide for a cell count and then dilute the rest of the cells threefold in α10MOPS to further reduce the drug concentration. Centrifuge the cells for 10 min at 150 g at 40°C.

Rinse two of the treated wells with cetrimide and, along with 0.5 ml of the sample of removed cells, count them to determine the recovery: Fraction recovery = cells removed/(cells removed + cells still adherent).

After centrifuging the cells, resuspend them to the desired concentration. We usually replate two wells with 10^5 cells to determine the number that will readhere after overnight culture. The number that will form colonies can also be determined using 10^4, 10^3, and 10^2 cells/ml and plating 3 ml into 35-mm culture dishes. These two parameters, readherence and colony formation, provide stringent assessments of the recovered cell viability.

IV. CONCLUDING REMARKS

We have described how to isolate monocytes, how to account for all the cells, and how to culture them. A typical accountability chart is shown in Table I for C_3H mice. The actual

TABLE I. *Isolation of Mononuclear Cells from Murine Blood*

Cell fraction	Cells/ml blood[a] (millions)
Peripheral blood	9.75 ± 0.88
Mononuclear cells	2.87 ± 0.82
Erythrocyte pellet	1.90 ± 0.32
Total cells	4.77 ± 11.13
Recovery (%)	49.0 ± 16.0

[a]*Number of cells per milliliter of the original blood that were recovered in each fraction (± standard error, four experiments).*

number of cells recovered after each step from the original number of cells per milliliter of blood is shown. The cumulative recovery is shown by the last number. In our experience about half the cells are lost during isolation.

The distribution of adherent cells is shown in Table II. When serum was absent, 41% of the mononuclear cells adhered and 38% of the adherent cells were monocytes (esterase positive). This represents virtually all the monocytes as none were found in the nonadherent fraction. Thus 15% of the mononuclear cells in the suspension were monocytes (41% × 0.38). It should be pointed out, however, that if the number of cells plated greatly exceeds 10^5 cells/cm^2, an increasing number of monocytes will be found in the nonadherent fraction because there are too many cells plated for the amount of surface area available for them to adhere. Nonadherent cells as well as platelets in the mononuclear cell fraction will compete for space interfering with monocyte adherence.

When serum is present, adherence falls to about 9% of the mononuclear cell fraction. While two-thirds of the adherent cells are monocytes, only about 40% of the monocytes were adherent, i.e., 60% of them were found in the nonadherent fraction. Because fewer lymphocytes also adhered, the monocyte purity was much better.

It is possible to remove the adherent lymphocytes. By adding medium with serum to the cultures after the initial 1-hr incubation in serum-free medium, culturing overnight and rerinsing, virtually all lymphocytes can be removed leaving a highly purified monocyte preparation.

With regard to adherence properties, it follows that there are two monocyte populations, those which adhere in serum and those which do not. These two populations can be separated from one another by first adhering the cells in serum-containing medium to give the serum-adherent monocyte population. The nonadherent cells derived from the cultures are then washed, resuspended, and replated in serum-free medium. After an addi-

TABLE II. *Adherence of Mononuclear Cells*

Serum (%)	Adherent (%)	Monocytes (%)	Percentage of monocytes	
			Adherent	Nonadherent
0	41	38	>99	<1
1	9	69	40	60
10	9	58	33	67

tional hour of incubation, the serum-nonadherent monocyte population can be obtained. To remove adherent lymphocytes, both adherent cell populations are incubated overnight with αMOPS containing 3% serum, the plates are rerinsed to remove lymphocytes, and fresh medium is added.

The formation of colonies in the different fractions are shown in Table III for C_3H mouse cells. The appearance of colonies is shown in Fig. 1. Colony formation by monocytes is a very sensitive indicator of monocyte contamination because they do form colonies. For the experiment shown, 10^4 mononuclear cells produced one colony in the nonadherent and 72 in the adherent fraction. However, monocytes clearly went through the Ficoll-Hypaque into the erythrocyte fraction during separation as 45 colonies/10^4 nucleated cells were found in that fraction.

We attempt to plate the density of mononuclear cells that will give the desired number of monocytes so they will not have to be removed. This is because the recovery of viable monocytes, once they have attached, is not predictable and usually only about half the cells recovered are viable. While the viability of a freshly isolated preparation is often greater than 90% initially, it has been our experience that by the next day many of the previously viable cells have died; this is likely due to the fact that it takes time for cells to die once they have acquired lethal damage.

TABLE III. *Colony Formation by Murine Monocytes*

	Colonies per 10^4 cells
1 Hour	
Nonadherent mononuclear cells	*1*
Adherent mononuclear cells	*72*
Erythrocyte fraction	*45*
24 Hours	
Nonadherent mononuclear cells	*2*
Adherent mononuclear cells	*22*

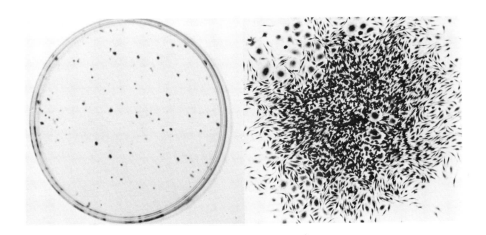

Fig. 1. Colony formation by murine peripheral blood mono-
nuclear cells. 10^4 Peripheral blood mononuclear cells were
cultured 14 days in 3-ml liquid growth medium. Colonies as
they appear on the culture dish after staining with methylene
blue are shown on the left and a photomicrograph of one of the
colonies is shown on the right. Note the larger polyhedral
like cells particularly in the upper left corner. The majori-
ty of cells, however, have an ameboid like morphology.

REFERENCES

1. H. Lin. Colony formation *in vitro* by mouse blood mono-
    cytes. *Blood 49*:593-598, 1977.
2. C. C. Stewart. Formation of colonies by mononuclear
    phagocytes outside the bone marrow. *In* "Mononuclear
    Phagocytes: Functional Aspects" (R. van Furth, ed.),
    pp. 377-413. Martinus Nijhoff, Boston, 1980.
3. C. C. Stewart and H. -S. Lin. Macrophage growth factor
    and its relationship to colony-stimulating factor.
    J. Reticuloendothel. Soc. 23:269-285, 1978.
4. R. van Furth. Cells of mononuclear phagocyte system.
    Nomenclature in terms of sites and conditions. *In* "Mono-
    nuclear Phagocytes: Functional Aspects" (R. van Furth, ed.),
    pp. 1-31. Martinus Nijhoff, Boston, 1980.

5. A. Boyum. Isolation of mononuclear cells and granulocytes from human blood. *Scand. J. Clin. Lab. Invest. 21 (Suppl. 97)*:77, 1968.

4

OBTAINING AND CULTURING HUMAN MONOCYTES

Steven D. Douglas
Steven H. Zuckerman
and
Samuel K. Ackerman

I. GENERAL INTRODUCTION

Since tissue sources are not routinely available, the
blood monocyte is an obvious choice for studying human mononuclear phagocytes. Peripheral blood is easily obtained in
sufficient quantities for investigations. There are, however,
numerous technical difficulties that complicate study of the
human monocyte. It is the purpose of this chapter to describe
methods for the isolation (1) and *in vitro* maintenance
(2) of human blood monocytes, which have been reliable and
reproducible in our laboratory. Sanderson *et al.* (3) have
reported a method for preparation of monocytes in suspension
using countercurrent centrifugation that is not universally
available. The methods have been designed to produce a pure
population of blood monocytes in suspension form derived from
between 10 and 100 ml of blood and to allow culture of the
cells for periods up to 4 months. This isolation technique is
valuable for the investigation of the blood monocyte per se,

33

and the culture technique should allow in depth analysis of the changes that occur during *in vitro* maturation of monocytes to macrophages.

II. METHOD FOR MONOCYTE ISOLATION ON MICROEXUDATE-COATED SURFACES

A. *Introduction*

Our method for purification of human monocytes relies on the fact that these cells adhere to, and are easily releasable from, plastic surfaces that have been previously coated with the microexudate of an adherent fibroblast cell line. That mononuclear phagocytes adhere to many surfaces has been known for decades, and in fact this property serves as a characteristic and identifying feature of these cells. However, unlike other adherent cells, mononuclear phagocytes are extremely difficult to detach from the substratum once they have attached. Consequently, purification techniques based on adherence have not been extensively employed for preparation of monocytes if the cells are required to be in suspension. Although chelators of divalent cations *tend* to detach them from glass or plastic surfaces, this effect is neither complete nor reproducible enough for use as a preparative method. In our technique, interface cells from Ficoll-Hypaque gradients (a mixture of lymphocytes, monocytes, and platelets) are applied to a plastic surface from which a confluent growth of fibroblasts has been removed. Monocytes adhere to this surface and, in contrast to their behavior on uncoated surfaces, can be easily and completely removed with EDTA after the nonadherent cells have been poured from the flask. Cells thus obtained are in suspension and easily adaptable to a variety of experimental protocols. An added advantage of using the "coated" flasks is that platelets do not adhere to them, whereas platelets do adhere to uncoated surfaces, and thus platelet contamination is much reduced.

B. *Reagents*

Eagle's minimum essential medium, or other standard
   tissue culture medium (MEM)
MEM containing 10% horse, human, or fetal calf serum
   (Mem/HS)
EDTA solution, 0.01 M in phosphate-buffered saline, pH 7.4
   (check pH after EDTA is added)

Ficoll-hypaque solution: 24 parts of 9% Ficoll to 10
  parts 33% hypaque
Microexudate-coated flasks (BHK flasks), prepared as
  described below

C. METHOD

1 Preparation of "BHK" Flasks. For preparation of
microexudate-coated flasks, we utilize BHK-21 fibroblasts
(clone 13) obtained from the American-type culture collection.
These are grown to confluence in Falcon plastic T-75 flasks.
We have used basal minimal Eagle's medium with 10% fetal calf
serum, 10% tryptose phosphate broth, and antibiotics, although
other media to which the cells were accommodated would be
satisfactory. After the cells reach confluence, incubation is
continued 2 days more, with daily changes into fresh medium,
to allow the cells to reach "superconfluence." Medium is then
poured off and EDTA [0.01 M in phosphate-buffered saline (PBS)]
is added. Flasks are left at room temperature for 10-15 min,
by which time the fibroblasts should be completely detached.
Fibroblasts are removed from the flasks and set aside to be
passed. Ten milliliters of fresh EDTA solution are added to
the "empty" flask and shaken vigorously to remove all fragments of fibroblasts but leaving the microexudate. Shaking is
repeated with 10 ml of fresh EDTA solution, and the flask
rinsed with 5 ml MEM to remove EDTA. If the flask is not to
be used immediately, it may be stored at 4°C with 5 ml of the
EDTA solution and then rinsed with MEM immediately prior to
use.

2 Preparation of Monocytes. Twenty milliliters of
heparinized blood is mixed with 15 ml of MEM, underlaid with
15 ml of Ficoll-hypaque, and centrifuged at 400 g for 45 min.
The interface cells are removed in a total volume of 7-8 ml
and diluted to 36 ml with MEM with fetal calf serum (FCS).
(If it is desired to remove cells immediately from the remaining Ficoll-hypaque, they may be spun at 400 g for 15 min
after dilution to 36 ml and then resuspended to 36 ml. Cells
should be spun at 4°C to minimize clumping of monocytes. However, some compromise of yield usually accompanies any extra
manipulation of monocytes.) Each of three BHK flasks receives
12 ml of the cell suspension and are incubated for 45 min at
37°C in a CO_2 incubator. The flasks are gently agitated after
20 min to promote maximal exposure of all monocytes to the
surface of the flasks. Precise control of pH during this step
is critical for good yield of monocytes (see earlier). Following incubation and agitation, the nonadherent cells and platelets are decanted. Each flask is then rinsed with two to
three changes of MEM (*prewarmed to 37°C* each time) with gentle

agitation. Prewarming the MEM is necessary to maximize monocyte yields. At this point, the flask should be examined with
an inverted microscope: Only monocytes should be adherent and
no round cells or platelets should be seen between the monocytes. If platelets or lymphocytes are adherent, either the
flask had not been grown to full confluence or BHK cell fragments remain. A few platelets may, however, remain attached
to the adherent monocytes as a rosette. If necessary these
may be eliminated as indicated below. Following the final
rinse with warm MEM, monocytes are detached by introducing
into the flasks 5 ml of a 1:1 mixture of PBS-EDTA and MEM-10%
FCS. This mixture was chosen for convenience, and other combinations may be used that contain EDTA (in excess of divalent
cations) and 10% serum. Serum is not required for detachment,
and is included to prevent sticking of the monocytes to the
side of the tube during subsequent centrifugation.

Flasks containing the EDTA-serum mixture are incubated at
37°C for 15 min and then examined with the inverted microscope
to verify complete detachment. The 5 ml of fluid is removed
from the flask, placed in a 12 × 75 mm plastic tube and centrifuged at 200 g for 15 min at 4° or 22°C. Both EDTA and serum
are required during centrifugation to prevent irreversible
sticking of the monocytes to each other and to the side of the
tube. Following centrifugation, the monocytes should be in a
loose button at the bottom of the tube and may be resuspended
in the medium of choice. However, as soon as the EDTA is removed, the cells become extremely sticky. We therefore make
every attempt to keep them at 4°C and use them as rapidly as
possible. Also, centrifugation following removal of EDTA may
clump the cells, and we are therefore careful to resuspend the
cells in a smaller volume than will be needed. Following
counting, the cells may then be diluted (not spun) to the
correct final concentration. If extensive washing of the
cells is necessary, this can ordinarily be easily done while
the cells remain attached to the BHK flasks.

D. *Critical Comments*

We have had only limited experience with fibroblasts other
than BHK cells, but we believe that other lines would also be
satisfactory, including normal fibroblasts from explanted
tissue. We believe that the most important aspect of the
preparation of the flask is growth of the cells to excessive
confluence with frequent changes of medium.

Adequate control of pH is critical during both attachment
and detachment. In general, low pH favors attachment. We
keep the pH at 7.3-7.5 throughout the entire procedure, which
seems to give optimal yields. Incomplete detachment of mono-

cytes may result from too low a pH during either step of
the procedure.

If many platelets rosette around the monocytes during
attachment, these may be eliminated from the final monocyte
preparation by a 30 sec exposure at 22°C of the rinsed monocyte monolayer to the EDTA-serum mixture. The attachment of
platelets to the monocytes is reversed virtually instantaneous-
ly upon exposure to the EDTA, and the platelets can be poured
from the flask before the monocytes have detached. Five milliliters of fresh EDTA-serum are then added to the flask and
monocyte detachment continued at 37°C as usual.

Normal yields of monocytes are 2-7 x 10^6 monocytes from
20 ml of blood, but there is considerable donor-to-donor
variability. Purity is generally 95% as judged by staining
for nonspecific esterase, phagocytosis of antibody-coated red
cells, and cytoplasmic spreading (1) (Figs. 1 and 2). Poor
purity usually reflects inadequate rinsing of the flasks following adherence.

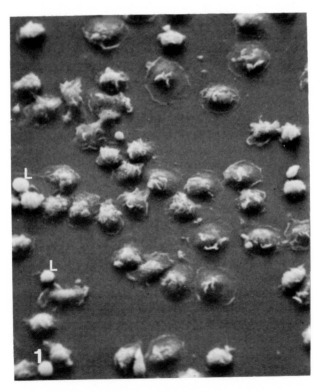

Fig. 1. Scanning electron micrograph of freshly isolated
monocyte undergoing cytoplasmic spreading. Most cells are
monocytes, although two lymphocytes (L) are also seen. × 625.

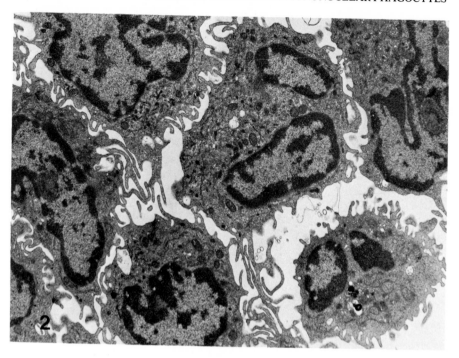

Fig. 2. Transmission electron micrograph of freshly isolated monocytes. × 6000.

III. CULTURE OF ISOLATED HUMAN BLOOD MONOCYTES

A. *Introduction*

We have recently developed a method for prolonged *in vitro* culture of the purified human monocytes. Although reports of techniques for culturing monocytes have appeared in the literature (4-10), none of these procedures in our hands has been consistently capable of establishing successful cultures. Interestingly, each of the published methods are significantly different. Hence, we believe that small variations in tissue culture technique from laboratory to laboratory may have dramatic effects on the success of culturing these notoriously fastidious cells. We have developed a technique that results in successful establishment of primary monocyte cultures with virtually every attempt. In addition, the technique has been utilized in other institutions with comparable results.

5

ISOLATION OF HUMAN MONOCYTES

Dina G. Fischer
Hillel S. Koren

I. INTRODUCTION

Investigations on and availability of human macrophages
are limited. The most available source of these cells is
peripheral blood, from which the mononuclear cells can be
easily isolated. Separating the monocytes from the lymphocytes involves numerous technical difficulties. Techniques
for monocyte isolation in suspension use gradients (1, 2) or
countercurrent centrifugation (3). The method most commonly
used to obtain monocytes utilizes their property of adhering
to surfaces. Adherent monocytes are difficult to detach, and
therefore investigators commonly plate the cells in the actual assay vessel, then wash off the nonadherent cells. The
method of Ackerman and Douglas (4) enables one to overcome the
difficulty in detaching monocytes, by precoating plastic surfaces with microexudate of an adherent fibroblast cell line.
Using any of the described methods, only 50% or less of
the monocytes can be recovered with high purity, thus the

METHODS FOR STUDYING
MONONUCLEAR PHAGOCYTES

43

purification procedures also involve selection of populations on the basis of particular biophysical properties that distinguish them from the lymphocytes. It is very likely that the cell populations obtained differ with the isolation procedure used. The choice of a particular monocyte isolation technique may depend on the requirements of the investigator and the nature of the functions studied.

In our technique (5), we have used EDTA-reversible attachment of monocytes to autologous serum-coated plastic surface. Use of autologous serum minimized introduction of foreign proteins, and eliminated the necessity of maintaining adherent cell lines for coating the flasks, thus saving effort and time in the coating procedure. The monocytes obtained are mostly viable and contain <2% lymphocytes, and up to 70% of the monocytes can be recovered from the mononuclear cell suspension.

II. REAGENTS

RPMI-1640
Ficoll - Hypaque (LSM, Litton Bionetics, Kensington, Maryland)
Versene (1 : 5000 Gibco Laboratories, Grand Island, New York)
Fetal calf serum (FCS), heat inactivated 30 min at 56°C
Autologous serum: not heat inactivated. The serum can be stored at -20°C until the same donor is bled for cell isolation
Plastic tissue culture plates (60 mm Falcon Plastics, Oxnard, California, No. 3002)
Phosphate-buffered saline (PBS) pH 7.2
Conical tubes, 50 ml

III. PROCEDURES

A. Coating of Plates

Plastic tissue culture plates (60 mm) are overlayed with 2 ml autologous serum and incubated at 37°C in a humidified incubator for 15 min. The plates can be left with the serum until the mononuclear cells are ready for plating. The serum is removed, and the plates are immediately used.

B. *Mononuclear Cell Isolation*

Heparinized blood (20 U/ml) is diluted in PBS 1:1. Each 35 ml is underlaid with 15 ml Ficoll - Hypaque (which is pre-warmed to room temperature) in 50-ml conical tubes and centri-fuged at room temperature at 400 g for 25 min. The interface cells are diluted in excess PBS and centrifuged at 500 g for 10 min, then twice at 100 g for 12 min to remove platelets (3). All centrifugations are done at 4°C.

C. *Preparation of Monocytes*

The mononuclear cells are adjusted to 3 - 4 × 10^6 cells/ml in RPMI supplemented with 10% autologous serum or 10% FCS de-pending on the individual needs of the investigator (see below Section IV. A). Each precoated plate receives 5 ml of the cell suspension and is incubated 1 hr at 37°C in a humidified CO_2 incubator. After incubation, 3 ml of the medium is removed from the plates and the nonadherent cells are resuspended by gently squirting the remaining 2 ml of medium in and out with a Pasteur pipette (rinsing the plate several times). The sus-pended nonadherent cells, containing variable numbers of mono-cytes, are removed and can be used for lymphocytes preparation. The plates are rapidly rinsed with several changes of RPM1 prewarmed to 37°C, and examined under an inverted microscope to determine if all the nonadherent cells were removed. The medium is then replaced by 4 ml of Versene. After 15 min in-cubation at room temperature, variable number of monocytes are released from the plastic, and the remaining monocytes are loosely adherent. (Following the initial 1 hr incubation at 37°C, the monocytes are spread on the surface, but the cells round up after the incubation in Versene.) One milliliter of serum is added to the Versene, and the loosely adherent mono-cytes are scraped off with a rubber policeman. Scraping the monocytes in the presence of serum improves the viability and decreases clumping during centrifugation. Monocytes from several plates can be pooled, centrifuged at 400 g for 10 min, and resuspended in the medium required for further procedures. The cells are kept at 4°C, counted, diluted, and used imme-diately to prevent clumping and sticking to the tube. If the monocytes cannot be further processed immediately, they should be kept pelleted in the tube on ice until ready to use.

IV. CRITICAL COMMENTS

A. *Use of Serum for Isolation*

Coating the plates with autologous serum rather than FCS
improves the yield and purity of the monocytes recovered.
Supplementing the cell suspension during the plating, with
either 10% autologous serum or 10% FCS, results in similar recovery and purity. However, we have found that the cells differ in their activity. Monocytes recovered from FCS-supple-
mented suspensions were more effective in tumor cell-killing
assays (5). The difference might be due to either the effect
of the serum combination or to selection of different cell
populations. Thus, the serum combination used depends on the
type of studies to be done with the monocytes. Pooled human
AB serum can replace autologous serum, but the introduction of
foreign proteins should be considered. The autologous serum
used is not heat inactivated, since heat-inactivated serum can
cause clumping of the monocytes (6).

B. *Purity*

To determine the percentage of monocytes in different cell
preparations before and after fractionation, slides are prepared from each suspension using a cytocentrifuge (Cytospin,
Shandon Southern). The cells can be stained with Wright
stain, nonspecific esterase (7), or a peroxidase stain (8).
Contamination by less than 1% lymphocytes can be reproducibly
achieved by our procedure.

C. *Yield*

Fifty to 70% of the monocytes present in the mononuclear
cell preparation can be recovered after the adherence. The
number of monocytes in the mononuclear cell suspension varies
with different donors. Thus, the number of monocytes recovered can vary between 1 to 5 × 10^5 monocytes from each
milliliter of blood.

D. *Using the Monocytes as Effector Cells*

The monocytes suspended by EDTA readhere easily when the
EDTA is removed. The cells can be plated in any vessel if
used immediately, and most investigators use flat bottom wells
or cover slips. However, when *in vitro* manipulations precede

the assay, various number of monocytes may detach and result in a selected adherent population of cells different from the original population. For example, incubating the monocytes overnight in RPMI supplemented with 10% FCS results in detachment of a high proportion of the cells while very few are lost after incubation in medium supplemented with autologous serum. To overcome this difficulty, the highly purified monocytes can be plated in V-shaped wells and centrifuged before the medium is aspirated. This is especially advantageous when the assay itself involves several changes of medium.

Acknowledgment

The authors thank Ms. Linda Nash for her excellent secretarial assistance. This work was supported by a grant from the National Institutes of Health CA 23354. HSK is a recipient of a Research Career Development Award CA 00581.

REFERENCES

1. W. E. Bennett and Z. A. Cohn. The isolation and selected properties of blood monocytes. *J. Exp. Med. 123*: 145-159, 1966.
2. F. Gmelig-Meyling and T. A. Waldmann. Separation of human blood monocytes and lymphocytes on a continuous percol gradient. *J. Immunol. Methods 33*: 1-9, 1980.
3. R. J. Sanderson, F. T. Sheppardson, A. E. Vatter, and D. W. Talmage. Isolation and enumeration of peripheral blood monocytes. *J. Immunol. 118*: 1409-1414, 1977.
4. S. K. Ackerman and S. D. Douglas. Purification of human monocytes on microexudate coated surfaces. *J. Immunol. 120*: 1372-1374, 1978.
5. D. G. Fischer, W. J. Hubbard, and H. S. Koren. Tumor cell killing by freshly isolated peripheral blood monocytes. *Cell. Immunol. 58*, 426-435, 1981.
6. W. D. Johnson, Jr., B. Mei, and Z. A. Cohn. The separation, long-term cultivation, and maturation of the human monocytes. *J. Exp. Med. 146*: 1613-1626, 1977.
7. S. B. Tucker, R. B. Pierre, and R. E. Jordon. Rapid identification of monocytes in a mixed mononuclear cell preparation. *J. Immunol. Methods 14*: 267-269, 1977.
8. L. S. Kaplow. Simplified myeloperoxidase stain using benzidine dihydrochloride. *Blood 26*: 215-219, 1965.

6

CULTURE OF HUMAN MONOCYTES IN MICROPLATES
AND ENZYMATIC ASSAYS FOR FOLLOWING THEIR MATURATION

Lois B. Epstein
Karen Yu
Lawrence P. Chong
Constance C. Reese

I. INTRODUCTION

Over the past several years, we cultured human macrophages
on a large scale in Leighton tubes. We obtain these cells by
maturation *in vitro* from human monocytes obtained from
peripheral blood. Such macrophage cultures are very versatile
and have readily lent themselves for study in three distinct
areas of research in our laboratory: (a) as a model system
for the investigation of enzyme replacement and other modes of
therapy for patients with lysosomal storage diseases (1);
(b) in studies to determine the cellular origin and the nature
of cellular interactions involved when interferon is produced
by leukocytes in response to mitogens or specific antigens (for
review, see 2 - 5); and (c) for exploration on the many non-
antiviral actions of interferon (6 - 9). However, the Leighton
tube macrophage culture system we employed was very costly, not
only in terms of medium and serum but also in requiring large
donations of blood. Thus, this chapter will detail our new

micromethod for the preparation of human monocyte-derived
macrophage cultures (10) and a recently developed fluorometric
micromethod for monitoring the maturation of monocytes to macrophages by following the specific activity of two lysosomal
enzymes, β-galactosidase and β-N-acetylglucosaminidase.

II. REAGENTS

A. Reagents for Preparation of Macrophage Cultures

1. McCoy's 5a medium (Grand Island Biological Co.
[Gibco], Santa Clara, California) is prepared with 100 U penicillin and 100 μg streptomycin/ml, respectively, and is used
throughout the procedure. For diluting plasma, McCoy's medium
containing 5 U/ml phenol-free sodium heparin (Lipo-Hepin,
Riker Laboratories, Northridge, California) is prepared. For
washing the macrophages, McCoy's medium is supplemented with
10% AB positive serum, and, for the culture of macrophages, the
medium is supplemented with 30% AB positive serum.
2. Dextran (MW 500,000, Sigma Chemical Co., St. Louis,
Missouri) is prepared as a 4.5% solution in pH 7.4 phosphate-
buffered saline and is used for sedimenting erythrocytes to
obtain leukocyte-rich plasma.
3. NH$_4$Cl - Tris solution is prepared by combining 9 ml of
0.83% NH$_4$Cl with 1 ml of Tris buffer (pH 7.65). This solution
is used to free leukocyte-rich plasma of any residual erythrocytes remaining after dextran sedimentation.

B. Reagents for Lysosomal Enzyme Assays

Distilled water is used throughout.

1. Buffers for Enzyme Assays

(a) Sodium acetate buffer (0.1 M, pH 4.5) is used in the
assay of β-galactosidase. Prepare a 1 M acetic acid solution
by combining 5.75 ml glacial acetic acid with 94.25 ml water.
Prepare a 1 M solution of sodium acetate by combining 13.61 gm
(0.1 mole) sodium acetate with 100 ml water. To prepare the
buffer, combine in a beaker 6.25 ml of 1 M acetic acid and
3.7 ml of 1 M sodium acetate. Add 90.05 ml water. Using a pH
meter, add glacial acetic acid dropwise until pH 4.5 is reached.
To sterilize the buffer, filter it through a Millipore filter
(pore size 0.22 μm) into a sterile 100-ml bottle. Store at
room temperature.

(b) Citrate phosphate buffer (1 M, pH 4.6) is used in the assay of β-N-acetylglucosaminidase. Prepare a 0.2 M solution of Na_2PO_4 by combining 14.198 gm Na_2PO_4 and 500 ml water. Prepare a 0.2 M citric acid solution by combining 21.015 gm citric acid and 500 ml water. Prepare a 2 M KCl solution by combining 37.28 gm KCl and 250 ml water. To prepare the buffer combine in a beaker 49.3 ml of the 0.2 M Na_2PO_4 with 25.5 ml of the 0.2 M citric acid and 13.3 ml 2 M KCl. Add water to a total volume of 100 ml. To sterilize the buffer, filter it through a Millipore filter (pore size 0.22 μm) into a sterile 100-ml bottle. Check pH of aliquot. Store at room temperature.

(c) Glycine - NaOH buffer (0.4 M, pH 10.3) is used to terminate the enzymatic reactions and to enhance the fluorescence of the liberated product, 4-methylumbelliferone (see below for details of enzymatic reactions). Dissolve 30.028 gm glycine (MW 75.07) in 900 ml sterile deionized double-distilled water. Add 13 gm NaOH. Check pH on pH meter and add extra NaOH pellets if necessary. Store at room temperature.

2. *Substrate Buffer Solutions*

Substrates obtained from Sigma Chemical Co., St. Louis, Missouri.

(a) 4-Methylumbelliferyl-β-D-galactopyranoside is the substrate for the assay of β-galactosidase. Weigh out 16.9 mg and dissolve in 100 ml sodium acetate buffer, pH 4.5, in a volumetric flask. Transfer this volume to a 250-ml Erlenmeyer flask and heat the solution until the substrate dissolves. Aliquot the solution to 4-ml sterile disposable Pyrex tubes and store the tubes at -70°C. Thaw tubes on the day of assay in the amount desired, and heat gently to dissolve substrate if necessary.

(b) 4-Methylumbelliferyl-2-acetamido-2-deoxy-β-N-acetyl-glucopyranoside is the substrate for the assay of β-N-acetyl-glucosaminidase. Weigh out 18.95 mg and dissolve in 100 ml citrate - phosphate buffer, pH 4.6. This solution is light sensitive and so must be kept in the dark. Aliquot the solution into aluminum foil-wrapped, 4 ml, sterile - capped, plastic test tubes. Store the tubes at -70°C. Thaw tubes on the day of assay in the amount desired.

(c) 4-Methylumbelliferone Standard Solution (4-MUSS). This solution is used to generate data for a standard curve against which is compared the enzyme-induced hydrolysis of substrates. The molecular weight of 4-methylumbelliferone is 176.2. Weigh out 2.643 mg of the crystalline substance and dissolve by adding absolute ethanol drop by drop. Add to the solution 0.01 N H_2SO_4 until the final volume equals 100 ml, and the solution is 0.15 mM. Store the solution in a dark bottle, as it is light sensitive.

To obtain the data for the standard curve, prepare the dilutions on the day of the assay in semidarkness as follows.

Make a 1/50 dilution to be used as a stock solution by combining 2 ml of the 0.15 mM solution with 98 ml sterile twice-distilled water. Make all subsequent dilutions in a 0.4 M glycine - NaOH, pH 10.3 in Pyrex glass dilution tubes as shown in the tabulation below.

Dilutions	Preparation 4-MUSS (ml) + Buffer (ml)	Final concentration (nm/ml)
1/50	2 of 0.15 mM + 98	3
1/100	1 of 1/50 + 1	1.5
1/200	1 of 1/100 + 1	0.75
1/500	0.05 of 1/50 + 0.45	0.30
1/1000	0.1 of 1/50 + 1.9	0.15
1/5000	0.1 of 1/1000 + 0.4	0.03
1/7500	0.1 of 1/1000 + 0.65	0.02
1/10,000	0.1 of 1/1000 + 0.9	0.15
1/20,000	0.1 of 1/10000 + 0.1	0.0075

Cover the tubes with a Parafilm and put them in the dark until they are read in the spectrophotometer.

C. *Reagents for Protein Determinations on Cell Lysates*

  1. Stock solutions
    2% NaCO$_3$ in 0.1 N NaOH
    0.5% CuSO$_4$
    1% Na tartarate
    Folin - Ciocalteau phenol reagent (Harleco, Gibbs-town, New Jersey), dilute with equal volume of dis-tilled water on day of assay
    Bovine serum albumin (BSA) (Sigma Chemical Co., St. Louis, Missouri)
    0.1% Triton in 0.85% saline
  2. Preparation of BSA standard dilutions. The concentration of our original stock of BSA is 50 mg/ml. The concentration of our working stock is 1 mg/ml, made in distilled water (see tabulation below).

Solution designation	Preparation BSA (ml) + distilled H_2O (ml)	Final Concentration (mg/ml)
a	1 of original stock + 49	1
b	0.75 of a + 0.25	0.75
c	0.75 of a + 0.75	0.5
d	0.5 of b + 0.5	0.375
e	0.85 of c + 0.85	0.25
f	0.8 of e + 0.2	0.20
g	0.5 of d + 0.5	0.188
h	0.5 of e + 0.5	0.125
i	0.5 of f + 0.5	0.100
j	0.5 of h + 0.5	0.0625
k	0.5 of i + 0.5	0.0469
l	0.5 of j + 0.5	0.0313
m	0.5 of l + 0.5	0.0156

III. PROCEDURE

A. *Preparation of Macrophage Microcultures*

Withdraw venous blood into plastic syringes previously
heparinized with Lipo-Hepin (100 U/10 ml blood) and transfer
10 ml aliquots to 16 × 150 mm round bottomed, plastic, screw-
topped tubes that contain 4 ml 4.5% dextran in PBS. Incubate
the dextran - blood mixture for 21 min at 37°C and transfer
the leukocyte-rich plasma to 50 ml plastic centrifuge tubes to
which an equal volume of plain McCoy's medium has been added.
Centrifuge the diluted, leukocyte-rich plasma at 1000 rpm for
10 min and discard the supernatant fluid. Resuspend the pellet in 10 ml wash medium, recentrifuge as above, and discard
the supernatant wash medium. Lyse the erythrocytes that did
not settle during the dextran treatment by an 8-min exposure
to NH_4Cl in Tris buffer at 37°C. Remove the erythrocyte ghosts
by centrifugation at 1000 rpm for 5 min. Discard the supernatant and resuspend the pellet in 10 mg of culture medium and
mix well. Perform a leukocyte count and make a Wright's
stained cytocentrifuge preparation (Shandon-Elliott cytocentrifuge, London, England). Adjust the cell concentration to
10×10^6 cells/ml with the culture medium.
Perform cell suspension transfers with a Minitek pipetter
(BBL Microbiology Systems, Becton, Dickinson and Co., Cockeysville, Maryland). Prepare the appropriate number of Nunclon
Micro Test Plates (Nunc Products, Irvine Scientific Sales Co.,
Irvine, California) according to the design of the experimental

protocol. If the cells are to be used to prepare cell lysates for enzyme activity measurements, allow one plate for each day of harvest (i.e., 3 plates, one to be harvested at day 3, one at day 5, one at day 7) and place 0.2-ml aliquots of the cell suspension containing 2×10^6 leukocytes in the desired number of wells in alternate rows on each plate. Allow replicate wells for each enzyme assay, i.e., four to five or more.

Incubate the microplates for 2 - 2.5 hr at 37°C in a humidified 5% CO_2 atmosphere. To remove nonadherent cells, aspirate the supernatant fluids with a finely tapered Pasteur pipette with the tip bent at a 90° angle. Wash each well with 0.05 ml of wash medium, using gentle application of the Minitek pipetter. Aspirate the wash medium and refeed the cells with 0.15 ml culture medium. Incubate the microplates for 3 days at 37°C in a humidified 5% CO_2 atmosphere. Wash all the plates to be harvested at day 5 or day 7 on day 3, and refeed with fresh culture medium. The preparation of cell lysates at the time of harvest is detailed below.

B. Preparation of Cell Lysates

The following procedure is used to prepare lysates from cells harvested at 3, 5, and 7 days after initiation of cultures. Aspirate the culture medium from each well on the plates to be harvested with bent-tip Pasteur pipettes. Wash the cells to be harvested that day twice with wash medium, using a Pasteur pipette. Wash another two times with PBS, using Pasteur pipettes. Aspirate the PBS. Examine the wells with an inverted microscope and grade each well from 1 to 6, to have a record of the relative density of cells and degree of maturation. This information is useful later to help explain infrequent single samples with spurious enzyme results. Add 0.05 ml of 0.1% Triton in 0.85% saline to each well with the Minitek gun. Freeze-thaw the cells by putting culture plates on the flat surface of a piece of Dry Ice. Once completely frozen, remove from Dry Ice. Let the frozen pellet thaw and immediately return plate to Dry Ice. Repeat the freeze-thaw procedure six times. Transfer with a Finn pipette thawed cell lysates into 0.5 ml microtubes (Brinkman 2236430-8), which are labeled with the day of harvest, donor, and well number. Store cell lysates at -70°C until the day of assay.

C. Enzyme Assay

Prepare 0.5 ml Brinkman microtubes for the assay by labeling them with regard to enzyme to be assessed, well number, and a, b, or c for triplicate determinations on a given well. For example, tubes for assay of β-galactosidase would be labeled β-Gal-1-a, β-Gal-1-b, β-Gal-1-c, and assay of the same enzyme from well No. 2 would be labeled β-Gal-2-a, β-Gal-2-b, β-Gal-2-c. Also label additional tubes as reagent controls for each enzyme to be assayed. Nunclon plates serve as excellent tube holders.

Meanwhile, thaw substrate buffer reagents, i.e., the 4-methylumbelliferyl-β-D-galactopyranoside in sodium acetate buffer, pH 4.5, and the 4-methylumbelliferyl-2-acetamido-2-deoxy-β-D-glucopyranoside in citrate - phosphate buffer, pH 4.6. Warm the former slightly to dissolve the substrate. Equilibrate the substrate buffers in a stable 37°C water bath.

In addition, as described in Section II.B.2.c, prepare the dilutions of the 4-methylumbelliferone for use in obtaining the standard and keep tubes in the dark until read with the spectrofluorometer.

Thaw out cell lysates from five wells from the 3-, 5-, or 7-day harvest and place the tubes in an ice bath. If necessary, centrifuge at 4°C at 1700 rpm for 10 min to pellet any debris. Prepare a solution of 1 mg/ml BSA in 0.85% saline with which to dilute the cell lysates. The presence of BSA stabilizes the enzymatic reaction. Dilute a given lysate either 1/5, 1/10, or 1/20 with the BSA - saline solution (where enzyme activities are expected to be high, i.e., at 7 days, we usually use the 1/10 or 1/20 dilutions).

Using a P_{200} Pipetman (Rainin Instruments Co., Inc., Emeryville, California), pipette 40 μl of each substrate buffer into the appropriate reaction microtubes. Set an automatic timer for 60 min. Immediately, using the P_{20} Pipetman, add 10 μl of the first tube of diluted cell lysate into the first set of reaction tubes (e.g., all of those from well No. 1). Do not add cell lysates to the control reagent tubes until later (see below). Vortex the first set of reaction tubes and put in rack in 37°C bath.

Record the time and add the second diluted cell lysate to the second set of reaction tubes, vortex, put in 37°C bath, and record the time. Continue until all sets of the cell lysates are added. Incubate the reaction tubes for 60 min.

During this incubation period, it is convenient to read the 4-methylumbelliferone standard solution (MUSS) dilutions from which the standard curve will be generated.

When the 60 min is up, add 200 μl 0.4 M glycine - NaOH buffer to the reaction tubes to terminate the reaction. Add this in the same order as the cell lysate dilutions and with the same amount of time between each cell lysate addition and vortex.

At this time, add 10 μl of the appropriately diluted cell lysates to the controls, which contain 40 μl of enzyme substrate and 200 μl of 0.4 M glycine - NaOH buffer.

Fluorescence is measured with a model SPF 125 spectrofluorometer (American Instrument Co., Silver Springs, Maryland) with
excitation and emission wavelengths set at 368 and 448 nm, respectively. Microcuvettes are employed and the machine is
zeroed with 0.4 M glycine - NaOH buffer. Between samples the
cuvettes are rinsed with twice-distilled deionized water. Enzyme activity is expressed as nanomoles of 4-methylumbelli-
ferone released per hour per milligram of protein.

D. Assay of Protein in Cell Lysates

This technique is a micro modification of the method originally described by Lowry et al. (11). Prepare fresh on the
day of the assay a solution that contains 0.1 ml of 0.5%
$CuSO_4$, 0.1 ml of 1% Na tartarate, and 10 ml of 2% $NaCO_3$ in
0.1 N NaOH (reagent A). Also prepare fresh a solution that
contains 5 ml of Folin-Ciocalteau phenol reagent and 5 ml
distilled H_2O (reagent B).

Then set up 0.5-ml Brinkman microtubes for reaction, allowing one blank tube for distilled water, as a blank for the
BSA dilutions employed for the protein standard curve, and
another blank tube for 0.1% Triton in 0.85% saline, which
serves as a blank for the cell lysates.

With a Pipetman, add 20 µl of original cell lysates to
microtubes. Add 20 µl distilled water to the tube designated
as BSA blank and 20 µl Triton in saline to the tube designated
as blank for cell lysates. In separate reagent tubes, add
20 µl BSA standard dilutions (see Section II.C.2). With the
Pipetman, add 200 µl of reagent A to each microtube; vortex
and let stand at room temperature for 10 min. Add 20 µl of
reagent B to each microtube; Vortex and let stand at room temperature for 30 min. Centrifuge out the green precipitate in
the cell lysate sample tubes and their blanks by centrifuging
the tubes at 1000 rpm for 5 min.

Read the samples within the next 2 hr on a Gilford spectrophotometer with visible light source at 750 nm. Clean the cuvettes with distilled water, alcohol, and acetone between
samples.

IV. CALCULATION OF DATA

Construct a BSA standard linear curve by plotting concentration of BSA in milligrams per milliliter on the abscissa and
optical density readings at 750 nm on the ordinate. Use this
curve to determine the concentration of protein in the various

cell lysates in milligrams per milliliters. Prepare another
graph by plotting the values for n moles per milliliter
4-methylumbelliferone standard solution on the abscissa and
values for optical density obtained from the Aminco fluorometer on the ordinate. From this graph, the values for n moles
per milliliter of 4-methylumbelliferone (reaction product)
liberated can be obtained. Then, correct for the fact that in
the reaction mixture (glycine - NaOH) there is only 0.25 ml
instead of 1 ml and for the fact that only 10 µl of cell lysate
was used at a dilution of either 1/5, 1/10, or 1/20 of the
original cell lysate. The resultant value can be expressed as
nanomoles product per hour per milligram of protein.

V.   CRITICAL COMMENTS

    For clarity, the procedures described above are shown
below.

    (a) Preparation of Cell Lysate

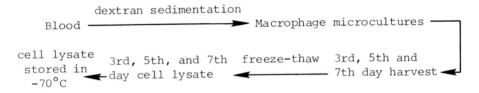

    (b) Enzyme Assay

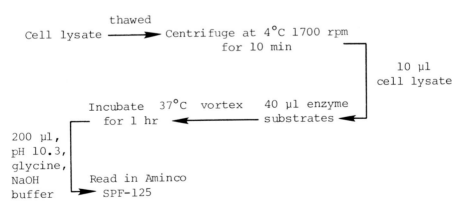

(c) Micro Lowry Protein Assay

A. Dilution of BAS Standard

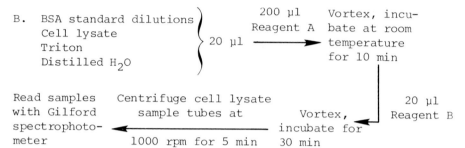

B. BSA standard dilutions
    Cell lysate
    Triton
    Distilled H$_2$O

    20 µl — Reagent A 200 µl → Vortex, incubate at room temperature for 10 min

    20 µl Reagent B

    Vortex, incubate for 30 min

    Centrifuge cell lysate sample tubes at 1000 rpm for 5 min

    Read samples with Gilford spectrophotometer

Table I summarizes the results of our microassay for
β-galactosidase on the monocyte cultures prepared from the
blood of 13 normal donors. Each value in the table represents
the mean ± S.E. of the results of 4 or 5 wells studied per
donor at a given time point.

Table II summarizes the results of our microassay for
β-N-acetylglucosaminidase obtained in a similar manner. Both
sets of data indicate an increase in lysosomal enzyme activity
from 3 to 7 days, and illustrate that this assay can be used
as a biochemical parameter of the maturation of human monocytes to macrophages *in vitro*.

Table III compares the results of the data obtained with
our enzyme microassays with that previously published for our
macro culture system and enzyme macro assays (6). They are in
excellent agreement.

The success of these techniques depends on several factors.
Careful aspiration and addition of culture medium is essential
for obtaining optimal macrophage cultures that are >99% pure
as indicated by their phagocytic capacity (10). It is important to wash away nonadherent cells without disturbing macrophage adherence. Wells with >50% of their surface area covered
with cells are suitable for use, although it is important to
note that the results expressed are independent of cell number
or cell size, but are related instead to milligrams of protein.

In preparing standard curves for BSA dilutions or MUSS dilutions, it is important to include dilutions that span the
entire range of lowest and highest readings obtained for either
protein concentration data or enzyme activity data from the
cell lysates.

These micromethods are far more versatile than the macro-
methods previously employed in our laboratory. In addition
they are more economical, and as only 5 - 10 ml blood are

TABLE I. Change in β-Galactosidase Activity[a] During Monocyte Maturation

Donor	Day 3	Day 5	Day 7
JM	259 ± 10	805 ± 57	413 ± 81
JA	93 ± 13	243 ± 20	247 ± 17
JB	225 ± 13	338 ± 22	330 ± 13
TD	191 ± 20	262 ± 19	254 ± 25
JS	148 ± 24	378 ± 50	365 ± 37
EW	164 ± 20	391 ± 10	502 ± 100
NL	194 ± 19	401 ± 55	1484 ± 63
TK	154 ± 19	527 ± 35	791 ± 122
KS	143 ± 9	316 ± 18	565 ± 33
JS	233 ± 44	362 ± 34	1889 ± 238
WH	220 ± 68	503 ± 58	352 ± 40
SB	215 ± 10	433 ± 9	497 ± 8
MK	198 ± 5	420 ± 45	360 ± 6
Mean SE	187 ± 13	414 ± 40	619 ± 139

[a] Activity in nmol/hr/mg protein.

TABLE II. Change in β-N-Acetylglucosaminidase Activity[a] During Monocyte Maturation

Donor	Day 3	Day 5	Day 7
JM	1920 ± 93	ND[b]	4188 ± 725
JA	1113 ± 213	2001 ± 102	2376 ± 120
JB	1894 ± 149	2248 ± 241	3102 ± 124
TD	1738 ± 191	1969 ± 159	2264 ± 219
JS	1178 ± 207	2959 ± 324	2761 ± 246
EW	1384 ± 134	2854 ± 115	5132 ± 1001
NL	1843 ± 254	3048 ± 600	9093 ± 717
TK	1864 ± 211	5808 ± 436	5452 ± 424
KS	1830 ± 114	3196 ± 247	4874 ± 388
JS	2308 ± 255	2765 ± 281	11,273 ± 1526
WH	1894 ± 374	5335 ± 620	4032 ± 276
SB	1970 ± 66	5041 ± 190	4277 ± 829
MK	1792 ± 88	4604 ± 636	2658 ± 136
Mean	1748 ± 92	3486 ± 389	4729 ± 742

[a] Activity in nmol/hr/mg protein.
[b] ND, not done.

TABLE III. *Comparison of Results of Macro–[a] and Microassays of Monocyte + Macrophage Lysosomal Enzyme Activities[b]*

Enzyme	Day 3		Day 5		Day 7	
	Macro	Micro	Macro	Micro	Macro	Micro
β-Galactosidase	142 ± 16	187 ± 13	312 ± 24	414 ± 40	402 ± 65	619 ± 139
β-N-Acetylglucosaminidase	1503 ± 304	1748 ± 92	3604 ± 420	3486 ± 389	5093 ± 747	4729 ± 742

[a]Data previously published in reference (6).
[b]Activity in nmol/hr/mg protein.

required per patient, these techniques can now be applied to the study of monocyte function in a wide variety of disease states.

Acknowledgments

This work was supported by NIH Grant CA 27903 and Grant 6-126 from the March of Dimes Birth Defects Foundation. The authors wish to thank Dr. Charles Epstein and Ms. Georgianne Tucker for their advice and helpful suggestions concerning microenzyme assays, Nancy McManus for editorial assistance, and Mary Evelyn Rose for typing the manuscript.

REFERENCES

1. S. Yatsiv, L. B. Epstein, and C. J. Epstein. Monocyte-derived macrophages: An *in vitro* system for studying hereditary lysosomal storage diseases. *Pediatr. Res. 12*: 939-944, 1978.
2. L. B. Epstein. Mitogen and antigen induction of interferon *in vitro* and *in vivo*. *Tex. Rep. Biol. Med. 35*: 43-56, 1978.
3. L. B. Epstein. The ability of macrophages to augment *in vitro* mitogen- and antigen-stimulated production of interferon and other mediators of cellular immunity by lymphocytes. *In* "Immunobiology of the Macrophage" (D. S. Nelson, ed.), pp. 201-234. Academic Press, New York, 1976.
4. L. B. Epstein and A. J. Ammann. Evaluation of T lymphocyte effector function in immunodeficiency diseases: Abnormality in mitogen stimulated interferon in patients with selective IgA deficiency. *J. Immunol. 112*: 617-626, 1974.
5. L. B. Epstein and M. J. Cline. Chronic lymphocyte leukemia: Studies on mitogen-stimulated interferon as a new technique for assessing T lymphocyte effector function. *Clin. Exp. Immunol. 16*: 553-563, 1974.
6. S. H. S. Lee and L. B. Epstein. Reversible inhibition by interferon of the maturation of human peripheral blood monocytes to macrophages. *Cell. Immunol. 50*: 177-190, 1980.
7. L. B. Epstein, S. H. S. Lee, and C. J. Epstein. Enhanced sensitivity of trisomy 21 monocytes to the maturation-inhibiting effect of interferon. *Cell. Immunol. 50*: 191-194, 1980.
8. J. Weil, L. B. Epstein, and C. J. Epstein. Synthesis of

interferon-induced polypeptides in normal and chromosome 21-aneuploid human fibroblasts: Relationship to relative sensitivities in antiviral assay. *J. Interferon Res. 1*: 111-124, 1980.

9.   L. B. Epstein and C. J. Epstein. T lymphocyte function and sensitivity to interferon in trisomy 21. *Cell. Immunol. 51*: 303-318, 1980.

10. D. Goldblatt, N. H. McManus, and L. B. Epstein. A micromethod for preparation of human macrophage cultures for the study of lymphocyte-macrophage interaction in immune interferon production and blastogenesis. *Immunopharmacology 1*: 13-20, 1978.

11. O. H. Lowry, W. J. Rosebrough, A. L. Farr, and R. J. Randall. Protein measurement with the Folin phenol reagent. *J. Biol. Chem. 193*: 265-275, 1971.

PERITONEAL MONONUCLEAR PHAGOCYTES FROM SMALL ANIMALS

Monte S. Meltzer

I. INTRODUCTION

Peritoneal cavities of rodents offer a convenient source
for collection of mononuclear phagocytes. Mature tissue macrophages, the resident peritoneal macrophage, can be easily recovered. The untreated peritoneal cavity, in fact, is probably
the most convenient site for recovery of mature macrophages:
cells can be obtained without complicated tissue disaggregation
or enzymatic digestion, and the level of contamination by other
cells is low. The yield of peritoneal cells from unmanipulated
mice, rats, or guinea pigs is about $3 - 5 \times 10^6$/animal. Cellular composition is about 40 - 60% macrophages, 40 - 60% lymphocytes, 1 - 5% mast cells, and rare neutrophilic granulocytes.
Neutrophilic or eosinophilic granulocyte contamination above
1 - 2% usually indicate inapparent infection among experimental
animals.
Macrophages can also be isolated from inflammatory exudates
induced in the peritoneal cavity by any of several sterile irri-

tants. These inflammatory macrophages are <u>not</u> the equivalent
of mature resident peritoneal cells but rather are mononuclear
phagocytes recently derived from peripheral blood. It should
be emphasized that while these inflammatory macrophages may be
immature, many enzymatic and functional activities of mononuclear phagocytes are found <u>only</u> in these young cells. For a
detailed comparison of many characteristics of inflammatory and
resident peritoneal macrophages of mice, see reference (1).
Macrophages that stain positively for peroxidase activity (a
cytochemical index of macrophage maturation) can be detected
among peroxidase-negative resident cells by 4 - 6 hr after irritant treatment. By 16 - 20 hr, 70 - 90% of peritoneal macrophages are peroxidase positive. These immature cells decrease to about 5 - 10% by 3 - 4 days. An influx of neutrophilic granulocytes is coincident with the immigration of inflammatory macrophages, but these cells are usually gone by
2 - 3 days (1).

    The yield of inflammatory macrophages is dependent upon the
irritant injected and the time elapsed after treatment. Peritoneal cell yield and composition for several treatments in
mice is shown in Table I. Cell yields can be up to tenfold
higher in guinea pigs. Two additional points should be emphasized: (a) It is necessary to determine the time course of appearance and yield of peritoneal cell types after irritant injection in one's own laboratory and animal system. There may,
for example, be great variation among mouse strains in responses
to peritoneal irritants. (b) In general, cells harvested 4 - 7
days after injection of poorly digestible substances (e.g.,
mineral oil, starch, and thioglycollate) have the largest macrophage yields. However, high yields must be balanced against the
fact that these substances remain within cells at harvest and
persist in culture. Moreover, macrophages may release these irritants into culture fluids through exocytosis, and they may act
as continuing pinocytic and phagocytic stimuli.

II.   REAGENTS AND EQUIPMENT

    Tissue culture medium: Dulbecco's modified Eagle's minimal
essential medium with 4.5 gm/liter glucose and 2.0 gm/liter
NaHCO$_3$ supplemented with 10% (v/v) heat-inactivated fetal bovine
serum and 10 U/ml sodium heparin (Panheprin, Abbott Laboratories).
    1 pair 8 - 10 inch paper scissors
    2 pairs 6 inch rat-toothed forceps
    Syringe (10 - 35 ml) with 20-gauge needle
    Polypropylene centrifuge tubes (15, 50, or 250 ml) (Corning
Plastics)

TABLE I. *Peritoneal Cell Yield and Composition after Intraperitoneal Injection of Sterile Irritants into C3H/HeN Mice*

Treatment[a]	Days after treatment	Cell yield $(\times 10^{-6})$	Peritoneal cell composition (%) Macrophages	Lymphocytes	Granulocytes
Nothing	–	4.0	60 0^{b}	40	0
PBS	1	4.0	50 80	40	10
Starch	1	8.0	20 90	20	60
	3	15.0	60 40	30	10
	5	20.0	80 10	20	0
Thioglycollate	7	30.0	90 10	10	0
Mineral oil	3	20.0	60 50	20	20
Latex beads	5	20.0	80 10	20	0

[a]Reagents: (1) 1 ml 0.02 M phosphate-buffered saline (PBS), pH 7.4; (2) 1 ml 2.0% starch (Connaught Medical Research Laboratories) in water; (3) 1 ml 3.0% Brewer's thioglycollate broth (Difco Laboratories); (4) 3 ml mineral oil (Drakeol 6VR, Penreco, Butler, Pa.); (5) 1 ml 1/1000 latex bead (1 μm polystyrene beads, Dow Chemical Co.) in water.

[b]Percentage of peroxidase-positive macrophages is shown in parenthesis.

III. PROCEDURE

(1) Food should be removed from mice 12 - 16 hr prior to peritoneal cell collection. Reduced volumes of stomach and intestine reduce chances of accidental puncture of gut.

(2) Mice are exsanguinated by decapitation with paper scissors. Decapitation avoids possible artifacts associated with anesthetic agents or the acidosis of CO_2 narcosis. Exsanguination reduces chances of intraperitoneal bleeding and contamination of peritoneal cells with blood cells.

(3) Flood skin over abdomen with 70% ethanol. Alcohol is used as a wetting agent to dampen fur, not as a disinfectant.

(4) Grasp skin over abdomen with two pairs of rat-toothed forceps. Lift skin up and away from abdominal wall. Pull forceps cranially and caudally to expose abdominal muscles. Retract skin to above shoulder girdles and below knees. Take care not to tear abdominal wall.

(5) Inject 10 ml of medium through needle along midanterior line. Medium should be expressed just before entry into peritoneal cavity to avoid puncture of gut. Fluid should be rapidly and forcefully injected.

(6) Position needle tip bevel down just below xyphoid process. Elevate mouse with needle and tent peritoneal wall.
Slowly withdraw peritoneal fluid. About 8 - 9 ml can be recovered without moving needle.

(7) Remove needle from syringe and place peritoneal fluids
into polypropylene centrifuge tubes on ice. More than 90% of
recoverable cells can be obtained in the first 10 ml harvest.
Repeat injections are inefficient and only increase probability
of puncture of gut.

(8) Cells from syngeneic mice can be pooled. Remove an aliquot of cell suspension for total and differential cell counts.

(9) Centrifuge tubes at 300 - 500 g for 10 min at 4°C.
Discard supernatant fluid and resuspend cell pellet in small
volume (1 - 2 ml) of medium (omit heparin). Adjust volume to
desired cell concentration.

IV. GENERAL COMMENTS ON THE CULTURE OF MOUSE PERITONEAL MONO-
     NUCLEAR PHAGOCYTES

(1) Mouse peritoneal macrophages are relatively easy to
maintain in short-term culture (macrophages will not replicate
in culture except under special circumstances). We have not
seen obvious differences between several media in ability to
support these short-term cultures. Dulbecco's modified Eagle's
minimal essential medium with 4.5 gm/liter glucose, 2.0 gm/liter
NaHCO₃ supplemented with 10% (v/v) heat-inactivated fetal bovine
serum and 50 µg/ml gentamicin has been used in our laboratory
for a variety of short-term assays (up to 72 hr) of macrophage
function.

(2) In contrast to our experience with various tissue culture media, changes in serum supplements can markedly affect
macrophage function. (a) Adult sera and fetal sera are not in-
terchangable. These sera differ widely in at least antibody,
hormone, and lipid content, each of which can profoundly affect
macrophage function. (b) Batch lots of fetal bovine serum can
vary with respect to contamination by bacterial endotoxic lipopolysaccharide or to content of nonspecific "growth" or "toxic"
factors. Whenever possible, several lots of serum should be
screened for the assay in question. (c) Protein hydrolysates,
often used as a serum substitute, are very stimulatory to mononuclear phagocytes. Protein hydrolysates may contain endotoxin
or peptides that are chemotactic for macrophages, which increase
cell spreading on plastic substrates and which increase phagocytic responses.

(3) About 30 - 50% of resident peritoneal macrophages and
50 - 70% of inflammatory macrophages will adhere to plastic

culture substrates in 2 - 4 hr. While adherence can be useful for macrophage enrichment in mixed populations by washing away nonadherent cells, it can also present problems: detachment of macrophages unharmed from plastic or glass surfaces is exceedingly difficult, if not impossible. Yields of viable cells by enzymatic or mechanical detachment procedures are often less than 50%; detached cells sustain membrane damage or loss. One should, therefore, plan to use these cells where they are initially cultured. There are, however, two methods that avoid cell detachment: (a) Macrophages can be cultured on glass coverslips. The entire coverslip with attached cells can be transferred for further manipulation. (b) Macrophages can also be cultured for days in a mixed cell population as a pellet in polypropylene centrifuge tubes. Aliquots of cells can be recovered over time by resuspension of the cell pellet in the supernatant fluid (2).

(4) Macrophages, as scavenger cells, are very responsive to environmental changes. Cell culture on plastic in medium with fetal bovine serum is not their normal environment. Macrophages endocytose serum components and attempt to endocytose plastic culture surfaces. The longer these cells are in culture, the less they resemble their *in vivo* counterparts. Working with these responsive cells in effect is a race, a race against time and continuing culture-induced morphologic, functional, and biochemical changes.

REFERENCES

1. P. S. Morahan. Macrophage nomenclature: Where are we going? *J. Reticuloendothel. Soc.* 27: 223-245, 1980.
2. L. P. Ruco and M. S. Meltzer. Macrophage activation for tumor cytotoxicity: Increased lymphokine responsiveness of peritoneal macrophages during acute inflammation. *J. Immunol.* 120: 1054-1059, 1978.

8

OBTAINING AND CULTURING HUMAN AND ANIMAL ALVEOLAR MACROPHAGES

Robert M. Senior
Edward J. Campbell
Beat Villiger

I. GENERAL INFORMATION

Alveolar macrophages have been studied extensively in recent years. The high level of interest has been promoted by two factors: (a) recognition that alveolar macrophages have an important role in lung biology, and (b) the ease with which a nearly pure population of these cells can be obtained for immediate study or culture. Except for long-term cultivation of monocytes wherein the cells assume some macrophage-like characteristics, alveolar macrophages are the only macrophages that can be recovered from human volunteers (1, 2). Current knowledge about alveolar macrophages has been reviewed in depth (3, 4).

Two techniques, bronchoalveolar lavage and lung tissue mincing, have been used to harvest alveolar macrophages. Lavage is the most widely applied method. First described in a classic article by Myrvik *et al.* as a procedure for obtaining alveolar macrophages from rabbits, lavage is now used

widely in animals and humans (5). Interest in the procedure
has extended beyond its use for obtaining alveolar macrophages,
as other cells in the lavage fluid and the supernatant fluid
itself have become the subject of investigation. Bronchoalveolar lavage is even beginning to be clinically useful (6).

Lavage involves instilling fluid into the lungs through
an airway and then promptly removing it by suction. Cells in
the airways, mainly alveolar macrophages and lymphocytes, are
dislodged by the lavage fluid and are recovered when the fluid
is aspirated. In humans and large animals, only a portion of
one lung is lavaged (7). In small experimental animals, both
lungs are lavaged promptly after the animal is killed.

Compared to whole-lung lavage, a much larger number of
alveolar macrophages can be obtained from minces of lungs (8).
Macrophages are recovered from 1 - 3 mm minces of tissue by
vigorous shaking, followed by filtration through nylon cloth
and low-speed centrifugation.

Macrophages collected from minces differ qualitatively
from macrophages obtained by lavage, having a higher oxygen
consumption and greater resistance to ionizing radiation and
chemicals that produce oxygen radicals (9-11). There are probably other differences. These findings suggest the need for
caution in generalizing about alveolar macrophages from observations limited to cells recovered by lavage.

This chapter describes details of performing bronchoalveolar lavage and culturing the macrophages obtained by
lavage.

III. OBTAINING HUMAN ALVEOLAR MACROPHAGES

A. *Introduction*

Large numbers of viable alveolar macrophages can be
lavaged from autopsy material or from surgically removed lungs
having an intact visceral pleura and a patent bronchus.
Lavage of healthy volunteers is preferred, however, because
the cells are obtained from normal tissue, the lavaged airways
are free of infection, and the procedure can be scheduled at
the investigator's convenience (12).

B. *Materials*

1. *Equipment*

Fiberoptic bronchoscope (Olympus BF-Type5B2)
Resuscitation equipment
Electrocardiographic monitoring equipment
Oxygen supply and nasal cannula
Swinging-bucket, refrigerated centrifuge (International
   PR-2)
Cytocentrifuge (Cytospin, Shandon Southern)
Cell counting apparatus (particle counter or upright
   microscope and hemocytometer)
Laminar-flow hood

2. *Supplies for One Lavage*

Medications: Lidocaine HCl for topical anesthesia
   (xylocaine 50 mg/ml and Jelly 2%, Astra Pharmaceutical
   Products); atropine sulfate 0.4 mg/ml, 1.0-ml vial;
   diazepam, 5.0 mg/ml, 2-ml vial (Valium, Roche Labora-
   tories)
Apparatus for intravenous infusion: Sterile 5% dextrose
   in water (500 ml); IV tubing; 19 gauge scalp vein
   needle (catalog No. V 1100, McGaw Laboratories); alco-
   hol swabs; adhesive tape
Sterile, nonbacteriostatic, saline [0.9% (w/v)] for ir-
   rigation, warmed to 37°C, 500 ml.
Sterile iv extension tubing (k50L, Pharmaseal)
Conical centrifuge tubes, 50 ml, 5 (Falcon Plastics)
Siliconized glass syringes, 50 ml, Luer-lok, 5 (Becton
   Dickinson)
Ice bucket, with ice
Microscope slides, 2
Dif-Quik stain
Sterile, plugged 10 ml pipettes
Medium: 250 ml, Dulbecco's modified Eagle medium or
   RPMI 1640 (GIBCO)

C. *Procedures*

   The volunteer should be questioned and examined. Volunteers with cardiac disease, pulmonary disease (particularly
asthma), or drug sensitivities, especially to local anesthetics,
must be excluded to reduce the risk of serious reaction. Prior
to lavage, the volunteer must be informed as to the details of
the procedure and give written consent on the forms for human

experimentation applicable to the investigator's institution.
Along with the consent form, it is useful to include a separate brief description of the procedure for the volunteer to
initial after reading. A sample statement follows:

The procedure for which I am volunteering has been explained to me in detail. I understand I will have a flexible
tube (bronchoscope) placed through my nose and into my trachea
(windpipe and bronchial tubes) for the purpose of obtaining
lung cells and lung fluid for laboratory studies. Before the
tube is passed, a local anesthetic will be sprayed in my nose
and throat. After the tip of the tube is in place in my
bronchial tube, several volumes (the total to be about 250 ml
or one-half pint) of sterile salt solution will be placed
through the tube and immediately recovered by suction. When
the liquid has been recovered, the tube will be removed and
the procedure terminated.

In a bronchoscopy procedure room, the volunteer is connected to electrocardiographic monitoring equipment, an intravenous infusion of 5% dextrose in water is begun, atropine
(0.01 mg/kg of body weight up to 1 mg) is given intravenously,
and nasal oxygen is administered at 3 liters/min. Local
anesthesia of the nasopharynx and oropharynx is achieved with
lidocaine spray and intranasal lidocaine jelly.

The bronchoscope is passed transnasally by an investigator familiar with the technique. As an effective lavage is
not possible in the presence of persistent coughing, adequate
anesthesia of the larynx must be achieved by lidocaine delivered onto the vocal cords through the bronchoscope. The
tip of the bronchoscope is wedged in a segmental or subse-
quental bronchus, most often in the lateral basal segment of
the right lower lobe, although some investigators prefer to
use the middle lobe. The positioning of the instrument is important because the instilled fluid can only be recovered if
the bronchoscope completely blocks the bronchus where the
fluid enters. A wedged position is assured when respiratory
motion of the airways is no longer observed. Once the bronchoscope is wedged, the bronchoscopist holds the instrument
steady while an assistant performs the lavage. The suction
attachment of the bronchoscope is replaced by a Luer-lok
("cleaning") attachment, then 50-ml aliquots of warmed
sterile saline in sterile siliconized glass syringes (which
has been filled by drawing saline via sterile extension tubing
from the sterile saline bottle) are instilled and aspirated
through the bronchoscope.

Hydrostatic pressure alone is sufficient to instill the
fluid, and traction on the plunger of the syringe while drawing the fluid back must be gentle to avoid distal bronchial
collapse. If air or large bubbles return, the bronchoscope

is not wedged and it must be repositioned. A maximum of five
aliquots of 50 ml each are instilled and aspirated. The fluid
return averages 60% of the amount instilled. The harvested
fluid is immediately transferred to 50-ml sterile conical centrifuge tubes that are then capped and chilled in an ice
bucket.

In a laminar-flow hood, bronchial mucus is removed from
the lavage fluid by filtration through two layers of gauze (a
sterile 4 × 4 gauze pad without cotton absorbent backing that
has been unfolded using sterile technique). The cells are
sedimented by centrifugation at 200 g for 10 min at 4°C, then
resuspended in 20 ml of serumless culture medium and washed
two more times with 20-ml aliquots of medium. The first supernatant may be saved for biochemical studies. After the cells
are counted, a differential count is performed on a button of
10^5 cells that has been deposited on a glass slide by the cytocentrifuge and stained with Dif-Quik or Wright's stain. No
effort is made to lyse the few red cells that may be present.

D. Critical Comments

Bronchoalveolar lavage has proved remarkably safe and
free of complications. In several hundred volunteers the
authors have encountered only four problems. One volunteer,
who had not received atropine, had momentary unconsciousness
associated with sudden slowing of the heart rate as the bronchoscope passed between the vocal cords, probably due to a
vasovagal reaction. Three others developed fever and pleuritic
chest pain within 24 hr after the procedure that disappeared
over 1 - 2 days coincident with a brief course of oral antibiotics. Lavage can cause transient, minor abnormalities of
lung function, but these are preventable by warming the saline
used for the lavage (13). Of note, repetitive lavages in
large animals do not appear to lead to functional or morphologic changes in the lungs (14).

Five 50-ml aliquots is a safe maximum volume of instilled
saline. The procedure may be modified by installation of
fewer, or smaller (20-ml) aliquots, with slightly smaller cell
recoveries.

Lavage of healthy nonsmokers yields $1 - 2 \times 10^7$ macrophages. The cell yield from smokers is highly variable, but
averages five times the number obtained from nonsmokers. In
lavage fluid from nonsmokers, alveolar macrophages comprise
about 80% of the cells, with the balance being lymphocytes.
The percentage of macrophages is higher in fluid from smokers,
and the fluid may also contain a small number of neutrophils.
The increased yield of alveolar macrophages from cigarette
smokers is counterbalanced by the observation that their cells

display a number of differences from cells harvested from
nonsmokers (15). As noted above, lavage is becoming useful
as a clinical procedure. Preliminary studies indicate that
the types of cells and the fluid composition give information
as to diagnosis and activity of various diseases (6).

III. OBTAINING ANIMAL ALVEOLAR MACROPHAGES

A. *Introduction*

The authors have performed bronchoalveolar lavage in
mice, rats, hamsters, guinea pigs, and rabbits. The procedure
can be accomplished quickly and with relative ease.

B. *Materials*

  1. *Equipment (see Section II.B.1)*

  2. *Supplies (first six items in Section II.B.1 and the*
     following):

  Small-animal board and pins or rubber bands
  Ring stand with clamp
  Pentobarbital sodium, 50 mg/ml (Nembutal, Abbott
    Laboratories)
  Turberculin syringe with 25 gauge needle for injecting
    anesthesia
  iv solution administration set with 250 ml, sterile
    saline [0.9% (w/v)]
  Sterile three-way stopcock
  Sterile 18 gauge catheter placement unit (Cathlon IV,
    Jelco Laboratories)
  Sterile disposable syringe 10 ml (60 ml for use with
    rabbits)
  Suture silk, 4-0 (umbilical tape for use with rabbits)
  Surgical scissors and scalpel with sterile blade (shaver
    also for use with rabbits)

C. *Procedure*

The animal is lightly anesthetized, using 0.15 - 0.30 ml
pentobarbital sodium intraperitoneally for mice and rats,
respectively, and 2 - 5 ml intravenously, by ear vein, for
rabbits. After the animal is supine on the animal board, the

abdomen is opened using a lower midline incision extending
from the xyphoid of the sternum to the symphysis pubis. The
intestines are retracted and the vena cava is exposed. To
prevent red blood cell contamination of the lavage fluid, the
vena cava is cut and the animal is allowed to exsanguinate.
The diaphragm is exposed, and a small incision is carefully
made through it on both sides to allow the entry of air.
After the lungs have collapsed, the anterior half of the rib
cage is removed, widely exposing the lungs. The lavage is
performed with the lungs *in situ* to minimize the chances of
tearing the pleura and causing leaks. A small midline incision in the neck is made and the trachea is exposed. The
trachea is cannulated with catheter, and the catheter is secured distally and proximally with suture. One arm of a
three-way stopcock is attached to the end of the indwelling
catheter, and a second arm is joined to tubing connected to
a bottle of saline supported on the ring stand. Saline, at
room temperature, is then allowed to run into the lungs by
gravity from a height of about 25 cm above the open thorax.
Care must be taken to avoid overdistending the lungs. In a
mouse, for example, the lungs fill with about 1 ml. Once the
lungs are expanded, the fluid is withdrawn using gentle suction on a 10 ml syringe (for small animals) that is attached
to the third arm of the three-way stopcock. Fluid installation and aspiration is repeated ten to twelve times, and the
recovered fluid is pooled and chilled on ice. With rabbits,
the lungs are filled and emptied only three times with aliquots of 50 ml.

D. Critical Comments

The number of alveolar macrophages recovered by lavage
is influenced by the composition and temperature of the lavage
fluid and by whether or not the lungs are massaged when the
fluid is instilled. If precise quantification of the cells
recovered by lavage is part of the study, the lavage conditions must be rigorously controlled and control animals must
be included with each experiment (16).

The optimal fluid for lavage is not settled, but it is
clear that divalent cations should be omitted; otherwise, the
cell yields will be poor (17). The authors have not tried to
verify the recent observation that the yields of viable macrophages from small animals are increased severalfold by including 12 mM lidocaine in the lavage solution (18). Isotonic
saline, delivered by the procedure described above, is simple
and reasonably efficient for obtaining viable macrophages. In
typical-sized animals, approximate numbers of macrophages recovered are as follows: mouse 5×10^5; rat 3×10^6; hamster

TABLE I. *Examples of Experimentally Induced Increases of Alveolar Macrophage Populations*

Animal	Manipulation	Interval after manipulation	Quantification of macrophages	Increase	Reference
	Cigarette smoke inhalation, repeated	Several weeks	Lavage in situ Microscopy	3x	20 21
Hamster	Fe_2O_3 aerosol, 3 hr	3 – 11 days	Lavage	15%	22
Rat	PbO in saline intracheal, once	7 – 40 days	Lavage	Up to 20x	23
Rabbit	BCG intravenous, once	21 days	Lavage	Up to 20x	24

8×10^6; guinea pig 2×10^7; rabbit 6×10^7. With guinea pigs, bronchospasm can prevent successful lavage. This difficulty is avoided by lavaging promptly after exsanguination, or by giving diphenhydramine hydrochloride intraperitoneally 30 min before lavage (19).

Apart from the details of the lavage procedure and the size of the animal, the yield of macrophages obtained by lavage depends upon whether the animal has had manipulations to influence the alveolar macrophage population. Experimentally, alveolar macrophage populations can be boosted markedly in a number of ways (Table I). In some experimental models the increased population appears to be due mainly to recruitment of cells from the bone marrow, rather than division of resident macrophages, while in other models, both mechanisms are operative (25, 26).

IV. CULTURING ALVEOLAR MACROPHAGES

A. Introduction

Human and animal macrophages obtained by lavage as described in Sections II.C and III.C remain viable in long-term culture (12, 20). In general, the technical details for culture are similar to those for culturing peritoneal or bone marrow macrophages.

B. Materials

1. Equipment

Laminar-flow hood
Inverted phase-contrast microscope
Cell-counting apparatus (particle counter or upright
  microscope and hemocytomer)

2. Supplies

Sterile plugged pipettes
Sterile transfer pipettes
Culture vessels (see below)
Medium: Human cells: Dulbecco's modified Eagle medium
  or RPMI-1640 (Catalog No. 320-1885 and 320-1875, GIBCO),
  containing 10% (v/v) human serum or fetal calf serum,
  penicillin 100 U/ml fungizone, 0.25 μg/ml/streptomycin
  100 μg/ml (Antibiotic-Antimycotic Solution, Catalog

No. 600-5240, GIBCO)
Animal cells: α-MEM (Flow Laboratories, Inc.) containing
   10% fetal calf serum and 5% horse serum

C. Procedure

In a laminar flow hood, macrophages are suspended in
sterile medium at a concentration of 2×10^6 cells/ml. The
cell suspension is transferred to sterile culture vessels.
Representative culture vessels, minimum medium volumes, and
number of macrophages are listed in Table II. If confluent
cultures are not desired (as, for example, in experiments involving macrophage proliferation), the cell concentration in
the final suspension before plating is decreased, keeping
constant the volume of medium per culture vessel. After addition of the cell suspension, the culture vessel is gently
swirled to distribute the cells over the entire surface, and
then it is placed in a water-jacketed CO_2 incubator. To
eliminate nonviable cells, neutrophils, red blood cells, and
the majority of lymphocytes, at 1 hr the medium is removed
with a sterile transfer pipette and the plate is washed with
warm, sterile saline. Warm, fresh medium is then added immediately and the culture vessel is returned to the incubator. When confluent cell layers are maintained in the volumes
of medium described, the medium is spent rapidly and must be
replaced with fresh, warm medium at least every 2 - 3 days (or
when the indicator begins to turn yellow).

D. Critical Comments

Human alveolar macrophages survive well in medium supplemented with fetal calf serum or adult human serum (Fig. 1)
(12, 27). Dulbecco's modified Eagle medium, RPMI-1640, or
other media, such as McCoys or 199, may be used with little

TABLE II. Preparation of Confluent Cultures of Alveolar
Macrophages

Culture/Vessel	Medium (ml)	Cells ($\times 10^{-6}$)
35-mm dish	1	2
60-mm dish	5	10
100-mm dish	10	20
25-cm^2 T flask	3	6
75-cm^2 T flask	10	20
150-cm^2 T flask	20	40

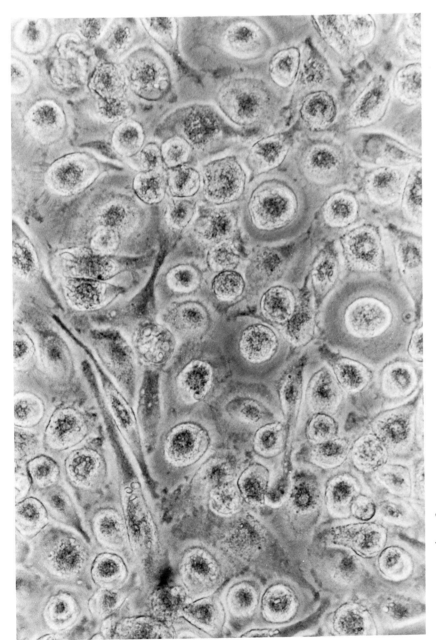

Fig. 1a

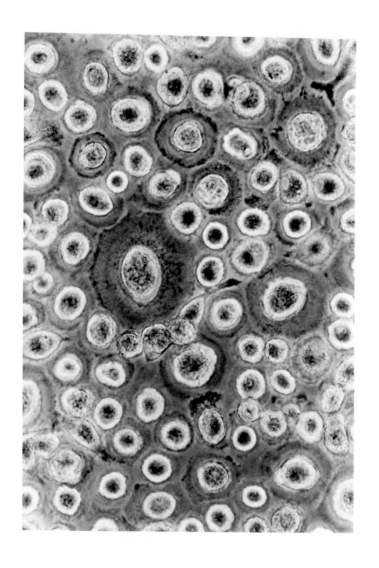

Fig. 1b

Fig. 1. Seven-day-old culture of human alveolar macrophages obtained from a smoker. The cells were plated at 3 × 10⁵/cm² in DMEM containing 10% fetal calf serum (a) or 10% human serum (b).

influence on cell survival. Irrespective of the type of medium, however, the cells have rapidly deteriorating viability after 3 - 4 days in serumless medium, even when it is enriched with lactalbumin hydrolysate, transferrin, and insulin. RPMI-1640 appears to be the medium of choice for human alveolar macrophages in serum-free conditions.

We do not use antibiotics when rodent alveolar macrophages are cultured. However, because of the inherent lack of sterility associated with bronchoscopy, we routinely include antibiotics in cultures of human alveolar macrophages.

To avoid variations in pH of the medium, it is wise to minimize the frequency of observation of the cells and even to avoid repeated opening of the incubator. Handling of 35-mm culture dishes is facilitated, and their gaseous environment stabilized, by keeping the dishes within larger culture dishes, several per container.

The success in maintaining human alveolar macrophages in culture has not extended to efforts at growing them. In contrast to rodent alveolar macrophages, techniques have not been developed for promoting cell growth and colony formation of human alveolar macrophages (28, 29).

Acknowledgment

The authors thank Dr. R. Russell Martin for advice regarding bronchopulmonary lavage in human volunteers. This work was supported by USPHS Grants HL 16118 and 24265 and by the American Lung Association of Eastern Missouri.

REFERENCES

1. J. J. Rinehart, M. Orser, and M. E. Kaplan. Human monocyte and macrophage modulation of lymphocyte proliferation. *Cellular Immunol.* *44*: 131-143, 1979.
2. K. Alitalo, T. Hovi, and A. Vaheri. Fibronectin is produced by human macrophages. *J. Exp. Med.* *151*: 602-613, 1980.
3. Unit five: The role of pulmonary macrophages. *In* "Respiratory Defense Mechanisms," Part II, Volume 5, Lung Biology in Health and Disease (J. D. Brain, D. F. Proctor, and L. M. Reid, eds.), pp. 709-1102. Marcel Dekker, New York, 1977.
4. W. G. Hocking and D. W. Golde. The pulmonary-alveolar macrophage. *N. Engl. J. Med.* *301*: 580-587, 639-645, 1979.

5. Q. N. Myrvik, E. S. Leake, and B. Fariss. Studies on pulmonary alveolar macrophages from the normal rabbit: A technique to procure them in a high state of purity. *J. Immunol.* *86*: 128-132, 1961.

6. G. W. Hunninghake, J. E. Gadek, W. Kawanami, V. J. Ferrans, and R. G. Crystal. Inflammatory and immune processes in the human lung in health and disease: Evaluation by bronchoalveolar lavage. *Am. J. Pathol.* *97*: 149-206, 1979.

7. A. G. Harmsen, J. R. Birmingham, R. L. Engen, and E. L. Jeska. A method for obtaining swine alveolar macrophages by segmental pulmonary lavage. *J. Immunol. Methods 27*: 199-202, 1979.

8. Y. Kikkawa and K. Yoneda. The type II epithelial cell of the lung. I. Method of isolation. *Lab. Invest. 30*: 76-84, 1974.

9. M. Hoffman and A. P. Autor, personal communication.

10. G. McLennon, K. B. Wallace, and A. P. Autor, personal communication.

11. A. W. Fox and A. P. Autor, personal communication.

12. A. B. Cohen and M. J. Cline. The human alveolar macrophage: Isolation, cultivation *in vitro*, and studies of morphologic and functional characteristics. *J. Clin. Invest. 50*: 1390-1398, 1971.

13. D. Barus, D. Shure, R. Francoz, M. Kalafer, V. Sgroi, T. Hartman, A. Catanzato, J. Harrell, and K. M. Moser. Physiologic sequences of lobar lavage in normal human adults. *Chest 76*: 347 (abstract), 1979.

14. B. A. Muggenburg, J. L. Mauderly, W. H. Halliwell, and D. O. Slauson. Cardiopulmonary function and morphologic changes in beagle dogs after multiple lung lavages. *Arch. Environ. Health 35*: 85-91, 1980.

15. R. R. Martin and G. A. Warr. Cigarette smoking and human pulmonary macrophages. *Hospital Practice 12*: 97-104, 1977.

16. J. D. Brain, J. J. Godleski, and S. P. Sorokin. Quantification, origin, and fate of pulmonary macrophages. *In* "Respiratory Defense Mechanisms," Part II (J. D. Brain, D. F. Proctor, and L. M. Reid, eds.), pp. 849-892. Marcel Dekker, New York, 1977.

17. J. D. Brain and N. R. Frank. Alveolar macrophage adhesion: Wash electrolyte composition and free cell yield. *J. Appl. Physiol. 34*: 75-80, 1973.

18. P. G. Holt. Alveolar macrophages. 1. A simple technique for the preparation of high numbers of viable alveolar macrophages from small laboratory animals. *J. Immunol. Methods 27*: 189-198, 1979.

19. M. E. Whitcomb, V. J. Merluzzi, and S. R. Cooperband. The effect of levamisole on human mediator production

in vitro. *Cell. Immunol.* *21*: 272–277, 1976.

20. R. White, J. White, and A. Janoff. Effects of cigarette smoke on elastase secretion by murine macrophages. *J. Lab. Clin. Med.* *94*: 489–499, 1979.

21. D. H. Matulionis and H. H. Traurig. *"in situ"* response of lung macrophages and hydrolase activities to cigarette smoke. *Lab. Invest.* *37*: 314–326, 1977.

22. R. I. Kavet, J. D. Brain, and D. J. Levens. Characteristics of pulmonary macrophages lavaged from hamsters exposed to iron-oxide aerosols. *Lab. Invest.* *38*: 312–319, 1978.

23. E. J. Kaminski, C. A. Fischer, G. L. Kennedy, Jr., and J. C. Calandra. Response of pulmonary macrophages to lead. *Br. J. Exp. Pathol.* *58*: 9–12, 1977.

24. Q. N. Myrvik, E. S. Leake, and S. Oshima. A study of macrophages and epithelioid-like cells from granulomatous (BCG-induced) lungs of rabbits. *J. Immunol.* *89*: 745–751, 1962.

25. D. H. Matulionis. Reaction of macrophages to cigarette smoke. II. Immigration of macrophages to the lungs. *Arch. Environ. Health* *34*: 298–301, 1979.

26. D. H. Bowden and I. Y. R. Adamson. Adaptive responses of the pulmonary macrophagic system. 1. Kinetic studies. *Lab. Invest.* *38*: 422–429, 1978.

27. M. R. Green, J. S. Lin, L. B. Berman, M. M. Osman, J. M. Cerreta, I. Mandl, and G. M. Turino. Elastolytic activity of alveolar macrophages in normal dogs and human subjects. *J. Lab. Clin. Med.* *94*: 549–562, 1979.

28. Y. Naum. Growth of pulmonary alveolar macrophages *"in vitro"*: Responses to media conditioned by lung cell lines. *Cytobios.* *14*: 211–220, 1975.

29. H. Lin, C. Kuhn, and T. Kuo. Clonal growth of hamster free alveolar cells in soft agar. *J. Exp. Med.* *142*: 877–886, 1975.

9

OBTAINING HUMAN MONONUCLEAR PHAGOCYTES FROM COLOSTRUM

F. S. Cole

I. INTRODUCTION

The cellular content of human colostrum was first recognized by Alexander Donne in 1839 (1). The corpuscles of Donne
were identified as cells in 1868 after stained preparations
were examined (2). Since the mid-1960s, considerable interest
has been generated in the characterization, origin, and function of these cells (3 - 10). By histologic staining and
membrane characteristics, lymphocytes, polymorphonuclear leukocytes, and macrophages have been identified in human colostrum
(11, 12). While the regulation of the cellular composition of
human colostrum is not well understood, peripheral blood monocytes are presumably the cellular precursors of colostral
mononuclear phagocytes. Human colostrum represents a readily
available source of human tissue mononuclear phagocytes.

A population of mononuclear phagocytes can be obtained from
human colostrum with the methods described below. The surface
membrane characteristics, morphologic features, and synthetic

85

capacities of these cells *in vitro* have been investigated.
Receptors for C3b and for the Fc portion of the IgG molecule
as assessed by immune rosetting have been demonstrated (12).
The cells are positive when stained for nonspecific esterase
activity, but have no demonstrable peroxidase positive
granules by electron microscopy even early in culture (13).
Within the first 3 days in culture, colostral macrophages
synthesize and secrete hemolytically active C2 and factor B
as well as immunochemically identifiable C3 protein (13).

In this procedure, adherence of macrophages to glass surfaces and repeated applications of colostral cell suspensions
to coverslips allow separation of mononuclear phagocytes from
lymphocytes and neutrophils. Application of colostral macrophages to transferable glass coverslips permits convenient
variation in the cellular environment. This procedure has
been adapted from methods described for establishing long-term
human monocyte cultures (14).

II. REAGENTS

Medium 199 (M 199) - Microbiological Associates, Bethesda,
    Maryland (store at 4°C)
Heat-inactivated (56°C for 2 hr) fetal bovine serum (HIFBS)
    - Microbiological Associates, Bethesda, Maryland (store
    at -20°C)
Penicillin and streptomycin (final concentration 100 U/ml
    and 10 µg/ml, respectively) (P/S) - Microbiological
    Associates, Bethesda, Maryland (store at -20°C)
Heat-inactivated (56°C for 2 hr) autologous serum (HIAS)
    (store at 4°C)
Circular glass coverslips - 15 mm diameter, No. 2, SGA
    Scientific, Inc., Bloomfield, New Jersey - the coverslips
    are thoroughly washed by dropping each of approximately
    80 slips into a solution of about 9 g of soap (Ivory
    Snow, Procter and Gamble, Cincinnati, Ohio) in 600 ml of
    deionized water. To facilitate uniform washing, allun-
    dum boiling chips (Fisher Scientific Co., Pittsburgh,
    Pennsylvania) are placed in the water bath and the mix-
    ture boiled for 4 hr. The slips are then rinsed 20
    times with deionized water and boiled for an additional
    4 hr in deionized water. After ten additional rinses in
    deionized water, the slips are individually dried by
    placing them on Whatman filter paper and then autoclaved.
    This washing procedure is essential for preparation of
    macrophage cultures with a high degree of plating ef-
    ficiency.

III. PROCEDURE

Human colostrum is expressed by hand or by breast pump into 50-ml plastic tubes (Falcon Plastics, Oxnard, California) within the first 7 days postpartum. Thirty milliliters of colostrum usually contain 5×10^6 to 50×10^6 total cells (mean, 15×10^6), approximately 75% of which are macrophages by morphology, histochemical staining for nonspecific esterase activity, and presence of IgG - Fc surface receptors. Within 3 hr of collection, the colostrum is diluted 1:1 with M 199 plus P/S and centrifuged at 120 g for 20 min. Milk collected after the first postpartum week does not yield adequate numbers of cells. Increasing fat ingestion by colostral macrophages may account for these difficulties in obtaining cells. The supernatant is discarded, and the cell pellet washed three times with M 199 with P/S. After the final wash, the cell pellet is resuspended in approximately 2.5 ml of M 199 with P/S, and the cells counted. The cell suspension may then be employed as needed. To establish macrophage monolayers, the cell suspension is divided into three aliquots. At 2-hr intervals, each aliquot is centrifuged and resuspended in M 199 10% HIAS at a concentration of 6×10^6 cells/ml, and then applied to glass coverslips in 0.2 ml aliquots. During adherence, monolayers are incubated at 37 C°in a 5% CO_2/95% air atmosphere. After three applications, monolayers are washed and transferred to appropriate medium.

IV. Critical Comments

The cells isolated by this procedure are macrophages by the criteria of membrane receptors, nonspecific esterase staining, secretion of complement proteins, and adherence properties. However, morphologically, a variety of cell types can be recognized in each monolayer. Some cells appear irregularly round with large nuclei, while some assume a spindle-shaped, elongated appearance. This morphologic heterogeneity may reflect differences in cellular function and must be considered when evaluating synthetic capacities and other characteristics of these monolayers.

This procedure permits isolation of human tissue macrophages that may be used to study the role of mononuclear phagocytes in local host defenses as well as questions of cellular differentiation.

REFERENCES

1. A. S. Goldman. Immunological factors and leukocytes in human milk. *In* "Selected Aspects of Perinatal Gastroenterology" (Mead Johnson Symposium on Perinatal and Developmental Medicine, No. 11, R. S. Bloom, J. C. Sinclair, and J. B. Warshaw, eds.), p. 49. Mead Johnson & Co., Evansville, Indiana, 1977.

2. G. Mayer and M. Klein. Histology and cytology of the mammary gland. *In* "Milk: The Mammary Gland and Its Secretions" (S. K. Kon and A. T. Crowie, eds.), p. 363. Academic Press, New York, 1961.

3. C. W. Smith and A. S. Goldman. The cells of human colostrum. I. *In vitro* studies of morphology and functions. *Pediatr. Res.* 2: 103-109, 1970.

4. G. J. Murillo and A. S. Goldman. The cells of human colostrum. II. Synthesis of IgA and β1C. *Pediatr. Res.* 4: 71-75, 1970.

5. A. K. Lascelles, B. W. Gurner, and R. R. A. Coombs. Some properties of human colostral cells. *Aust. J. Exp. Biol. Med. Sci.* 47: 349-360, 1969.

6. J. A. Mohr, R. Leu, and W. Mabry. Colostral leukocytes. *J. Surg. Oncol.* 2: 163-167, 1970.

7. A. S. Goldman and C. W. Smith. Host resistance factors in human milk. *J. Pediatr.* 82: 1082-1090, 1973.

8. W. B. Pittard, S. H. Polmar, and A. A. Fanaroff. The breast milk macrophage: A potential vehicle for immunoglobulin transport. *J. Reticuloendothel. Soc.* 22: 597-603, 1977.

9. M. H. Parmely, A. Beer, and R. Billingham. *In vitro* studies on the T lymphocyte population on human milk. *J. Exp. Med.* 144: 358-370, 1976.

10. R. Goldblum, S. Ahlstedt, B. Carlsson, L. A. Hanson, U. Jodal, G. Lidin-Jason, and A. Sohl-Akerlund. Antibody-forming cells in human colostrum after oral immunisation. *Nature* 257: 797-798, 1975.

11. W. B. Pittard. Breast milk immunology. *Am. J. Dis. Child.* 133: 83-87, 1979.

12. J. Pitt. The milk mononuclear phagocyte. *Pediatrics* 64 (Suppl.): 745-749, 1979.

13. F. S. Cole, D. Beatty, A. E. Davis, and H. R. Colten. Complement synthesis by human breast milk macrophages and blood monocytes. *Fed. Proc.*, April, 1980.

14. L. P. Einstein, E. E. Schneeberger, and H. R. Colten. Synthesis of the second component of complement by long-term primary cultures of human monocytes. *J. Exp. Med.* 143: 114-120, 1976.

10

OBTAINING ADHERENT CELLS FROM SPLEEN

Karen S. Hathcock
Alfred Singer
Richard J. Hodes

I. INTRODUCTION

The functional significance of adherent, phagocyte-
enriched cell populations has been demonstrated for a number
of different immune responses. In general, these cells are
required for the successful generation of immune responses,
but are not themselves the responding cell population. While
such populations have been isolated from a number of anatomic
sites, further enrichment procedures have generally been based
upon such properties as glass adherence, phagocytosis, and
radiation resistance. The functions performed by such cell
populations have included both "accessory" and antigen-
presenting functions in humoral and cell-mediated responses
(1 - 14), as well as in T cell proliferation to concanavalin A
(Con A) and phytohemagglutinin (PHA) (15 - 17). This chapter
describes a technique to obtain a non-T, non-B, radio-resistant,
glass-adherent cell population from mouse spleen cells. This
splenic adherent cell (SAC) population fulfills both the ac-

ISBN 0-12-044220-5

cessory cell and antigen-presenting cell requirements of primary and secondary *in vitro* antibody responses (2 - 5, 11),
permitting the study of cell interactions involving both "self"
recognition and Ir gene expression. In addition, SAC populations have been employed in the analysis of T cell-mediated
responses to alloantigens and "modified self" specificities
(12, 13). Thus, SAC populations isolated by the technique
presented are appropriate cell populations for the study of
adherent or macrophagelike cells participating in a variety
of immune response systems.

II. REAGENTS

A. *Preparation of Media and Cells*
    Eagles minimal essential medium (MEM)
    Fetal calf serum (FCS) (inactivated at 56°C for 30 min)
    3% *L*-glutamine
    Penicillin - streptomycin
    HEPES buffer solution (1 *M*)
    Ammonium chloride - K buffer (ACK)
    Osmotic lysing buffer (18)

B. *Cell Adherence and Harvesting*
    100-mm glass petri dishes (autoclaved for sterility)
    Plastic pipettes
    Versene 1:5000 (GIBCO, Grand Island, New York)
    50-ml polyethylene tubes (Falcon 2070)
    37°C humidified incubator with 5% CO_2

C. *Further Enrichment of Adherent Cells*
    T cell-specific rabbit anti-mouse brain antisera (RαMB)
      (19) or anti-Thy 1.2 serum (Litton Bionetics, Kensing-
      ton, Maryland) (2)
    Complement (lyophilized guinea pig complement, Grand
      Island Biological, Grand Island, New York)
    Irradiation source: X ray or cesium (Isomedix, Inc.,
      Parsippany, New Jersey)
    37°C water bath
    Roller drum

III. PROCEDURE

A. *Media and Cell Preparation*

1. *Media Preparation*
(a) Prepare a washing buffer of MEM containing 20 mM HEPES, 2 mM L-glutamine, 100 U/ml penicillin, 100 µg/ml streptomycin, and 5% FCS (MEM-5).
(b) Prepare an incubation buffer of MEM containing 20 mM HEPES, 2 mM L-glutamine, 100 U/ml penicillin, 100 µg/ml streptomycin, and 20% FCS (MEM-20).

2. *Cell Preparation*
(a) Using reagents at $4°C$, prepare a single cell suspension of mouse spleen cells and osmotically lyse the erythrocytes. Maintain reagents at $4°C$ unless directions specify otherwise.
(b) Resuspend spleen cells in MEM-20 at 1 spleen : 10 ml MEM-20 (approximately 10^7 cells/ml).

B. *Cell Adherence and Harvesting*

(1) Add 5 ml of spleen cell suspension to each 100-mm glass petri dish; swirl each plate gently to spread cell suspension evenly over bottom surface. Incubate dishes for 1 hr at $37°C$ in a humidified incubator maintained with a 5% CO_2 atmosphere.
(2) At the completion of this first incubation period, remove dishes from the incubator and wash to remove nonadherent or loosely adherent contaminating cells by gently swirling, removing incubation medium and adding an additional 5 ml of MEM-20 (prewarmed to $37°C$). Incubate dishes for an additional 1 hr at $37°C$.
(3) At the completion of this second incubation period, remove dishes from the incubator and gently swirl to resuspend any nonadherent or loosely adherent contaminating cells. After discarding the incubation medium, gently add 4 ml of MEM-5 (prewarned at $37°C$). Repeat washing procedure twice.
(4) Versene harvest of adherent cells. (a) After removing wash medium (MEM-5) from the final wash step, add 5 ml of Versene (prewarmed to $37°C$) to each dish and incubate for 15 min at $37°C$. (b) Harvest the adherent cells by repeatedly pipetting ten times Versene over the entire plating surface of the petri dish. Collect and pool the Versene - cell suspensions in 50-ml conical tubes containing 10 ml MEM-5 on ice. Centrifuge cell suspensions at 250 g for 10 min in a refrigerated centrifuge ($4°C$) and resuspend cells in MEM-5 to count.

C. Further Enrichment Procedures

(1) To remove contaminating T cells, resuspend the adherent cells in either RαMB or anti-Thy 1.2 and incubate on ice for 30 min. Wash by centrifugation in MEM-5 and expose to complement for 30 min at 37°C. Wash twice by centrifugation and count, and resuspend at a final cell concentration of 1×10^7 viable cells/ml in MEM-20.

(2) Irradiate cell suspension with 1000R (x ray or cesium source).

(3) Incubate cells overnight (12 - 18 hr) at 37° in plastic or siliconized glass tubes on a roller drum.

(4) Centrifuge cell suspension, resuspend for culture, and maintain on ice until used. Viable cell recovery is approximately 1% of the initial spleen cell population.

IV. CRITICAL COMMENTS

An essential requirement for the function of a non-T, non-B adherent cell population has been demonstrated in a number of immune response systems. This chapter describes a technique that isolates adherent accessory or macrophagelike cells (SAC) from mouse spleen cells on the basis of their radio-resistance and adherence properties. This procedure is easily adapted to sterile culture systems and consistently yields a functional subpopulation of adherent cells which are predominantly (75%) mononuclear phagocytes.

Viable cell recovery of the adherent, radio-resistant, T cell-depleted SAC populations after overnight incubation is approximately 1% of the initial spleen cell population. The SAC population is itself composed of three identifiable cell subpopulations: (a) 50 - 80% latex-phagocytic cells (macrophages); (b) 8 - 15% nonphagocytic sIg⁺ cells (B cells), and (c) 15 - 25% nonphagocytic sIg⁻, RαMB⁻ cells ("null" cells) (20). In addition, it has been demonstrated that MHC determinants encoded in the I-A and the I-E/C subregions are expressed on 40 - 50% of the phagocytic SAC population (21).

Extensive characterization of the functional activities of the SAC population has been carried out for *in vitro* primary and secondary antibody responses to soluble (2 - 5, 11) and erythrocyte antigens (unpublished data) and for T cell proliferative responses to soluble antigen (12). In each of these systems, responses were abrogated or significantly reduced by the removal of adherent or phagocytic cells from the cultured spleen population. Furthermore, in each case, these responses were completely restored by the addition of small numbers of SAC, demonstrating that the SAC population provides a source of functional accessory cells. The accessory cell activity of SAC populations for both humoral and proliferative responses has been shown to be mediated by the Ig^-, Ia^+ phagocytic cells in the SAC populations (3,4). It has also been demonstrated that SAC are highly enriched in the ability to stimulate allogeneic T cell responses in MLR (12), and that they are functional accessory cells in T cell-mediated CML responses to "modified self" determinants (13).

The cell fractionation procedure described in this chapter is consistently successful in isolating the non-T, non-B radio-resistant, adherent cell population present in mouse spleen cells that provides accessory cell function in a number of immune response systems. During the standardization of the conditions necessary to obtain maximal viable cell recovery, critical variables and potential modifications were investigated. Since it has been demonstrated that cell adherence properties vary substantially with temperature, incubation and reagent temperatures have been carefully controlled. Specifically, to maximize viable cell recovery plate adherence, complement incubation and overnight suspension cultures are carried out at 37°C, while all other cell treatments are performed at 4°C. MEM-20 (20% FCS) can be successfully used throughout this procedure, but this concentration of FCS has only been shown to be important during the plate adherence incubations and the overnight suspension cultures. For all other steps in this procedure, MEM-5 (5% FCS) can be used without changing the SAC recovery.

REFERENCES

1. D. E. Mosier. A requirement for two cell types for antibody formation *in vitro*. *Science 158*: 1573-1575, 1967.
2. R. J. Hodes and A. Singer. Cellular and genetic control of antibody responses *in vitro*. I. Cellular requirements for the generation of genetically controlled primary IgM responses to soluble antigens. *Eur. J. Immunol.* 7: 892-897, 1977.
3. R. J. Hodes, G. B. Ahmann, K. S. Hathcock, H. B. Dickler, and A. Singer. Cellular and genetic control of antibody responses *in vitro*. IV. Expression of Ia antigens on accessory cells required for responses to soluble antigens including a response under Ir gene control. *J. Immunol.* 121: 1501-1509, 1978.
4. A. Singer, C. Cowing, K. S. Hathcock, H. B. Dickler, and R. J. Hodes. Cellular and genetic control of antibody

response *in vitro*. III. Immune response gene regulation of accessory cell function on non-T, non-B spleen adherent cells. *J. Exp. Med. 147*: 1611-1620, 1978.

5. H. B. Dickler, C. Cowing, G. B. Ahmann, K. S. Hathcock, S. O. Sharrow, R. J. Hodes, and A. Singer. Characterization of the accessory cells required in T lymphocyte-dependent antigen-specific immune responses. *In* "Regulatory Role of Mononuclear Phagocytes in Immunity" (A. Rosenthal and E. Unanue, eds.), pp. 265-275. Academic Press, New York, 1979.

6. T. M. Chused, S. S. Kassen, and D. E. Mosier. Macrophage requirement for the *in vitro* response to TNP-Ficoll: A thymic independent antigen. *J. Immunol. 116:* 1579-1581, 1976.

7. C. W. Pierce, J. A. Kapp, D. D. Wood, and B. Benecerraf. Immune responses *in vitro*. X. Functions of macrophages. *J. Immunol. 112*: 1181-1189, 1974.

8. P. Erb and M. Feldmann. The role of macrophages in the generation of T-helper cells. I. The requirement for macrophages in helper cell induction and characteristics of the macrophage - T cell interaction. *Cell. Immunol. 19*: 356-367, 1975.

9. A. S. Rosenthal and E. M. Shevach. Function of macrophages in antigen recognition by guinea pig T lymphocytes. I. Requirement for histocompatibile macrophages and lymphocytes. *J. Exp. Med. 138*: 1194-1212, 1973.

10. C. Cowing, S. H. Pincus, D. H. Sachs, and H. B. Dickler. A subpopulation of adherent accessory cells bearing both I-A and I-E or C subregion antigens is required for antigen-specific murine T lymphocyte proliferation. *J. Immunol. 121*: 1680-1686, 1978.

11. A. Singer, K. S. Hathcock, and R. J. Hodes. Cellular and genetic control of antibody responses. V. Helper T-cell recognition of H-2 determinants on accessory cells but not B cells. *J. Exp. Med. 149*: 1208-1226, 1979.

12. G. B. Ahmann, P. I. Nadler, A. Birnkrant, and R. J. Hodes. T cell recognition in the mixed lymphocyte response. I. Non-T, radiation-resistant splenic adherent cells are the predominant stimulators in the murine mixed lymphocyte reaction. *J. Immunol. 123*: 909-909, 1979.

13. C. B. Pettinelli, A.-M. Schmitt-Verhulst, and G. M. Shearer. Cell types required for H-2-restricted cytotoxic responses generated by trinitrobenzene sulfonate-modified syngeneic cells or trinitrophenyl-conjugated proteins. *J. Immunol. 122*: 847-854, 1979.

14. J. G. Woodward, P. A. Fernandez, and R. A. Daynes. Cell-mediated immune response to syngeneic UV-induced tumors. III. Requirement for an Ia$^+$ macrophage in the *in vitro* differentiation of cytotoxic T lymphocytes. *J. Immunol.*

122: 1196-1202, 1979.

15.   S. Habu and M. C. Raff.   Accessory cell dependence of lectin-induced proliferation of mouse T lymphocytes. *Eur. J. Immunol.* 7: 451-457, 1977.

16.   D. L. Rosenstreich, J. J. Farrar, and S. Dougherty.   Absolute macrophage dependency of T lymphocyte activation by mitogens.   *J. Immunol.* *116*: 131-139, 1976.

17.   P. E. Lipsky, J. J. Ellner, and A. S. Rosenthal.   Phytohemagglutinin-induced proliferation of guinea pig thymus-derived lymphocytes. I. Accessory cell dependence.   *J. Immunol.* *116*: 868-875, 1975.

18.   R. J. Hodes and W. D. Terry.   Comparison of irradiated and mitomycin-treated mouse spleen cells as stimulating cells in mixed lymphocyte cultures and *in vitro* sensitization.   *J. Immunol.* *113*: 39-44, 1974.

19.   R. J. Hodes, B. S. Handwerger, and W. D. Terry.   Synergy between subpopulations of mouse spleen cells in the *in vitro* generation of cell-mediated cytotoxicity.   *J. Exp. Med.* *140*: 1646-1659, 1974.

20.   R. J. Hodes, G. B. Ahmann, C. Cowing, K. Hathcock, H. B. Dickler, D. H. Sachs, and A. Singer.   Expression of I region products on accessory cell populations.   *In* "Immunobiology and Immunotherapy of Cancer" (W. D. Terry and Y. Yamamura, eds.), pp. 33-49.   Elsevier North-Holland, New York, 1979.

21.   P. I. Nadler, R. J. Klingenstein, and R. J. Hodes.   Ontogeny of murine accessory cells: Ia antigen expression and accessory cell function in *in vitro* primary antibody responses.   *J. Immunol.* *125*: 914-920, 1980.

11

OBTAINING KUPFFER CELLS

R. Seljelid
B. Smedsrød*

I. GENERAL INFORMATION

To be able to separate Kupffer cells from the liver, one
must first disperse the organ, either by perfusion of the
liver with enzymes or by immersion of liver pieces. The enzymes generally used to disperse the liver are collagenase
and/or pronase. Here we describe the use of collagenase for
dispersions with subsequent incubation with pronase to destroy
parenchymal cells (1). One can obtain similar results by incubation or perfusion with only pronase as far as isolation of
Kupffer cells is concerned. Collagenase perfusion or immersion is, however, of more general use since it is then possible
to preserve parenchymal cells at an intermediate stage of the

*Present address: The Univeristy of Michigan, The Thomas
Henry Simpson Memorial Institute for Medical Research, 102 Ob-
servatory, Ann Arbor, Michigan 48109, USA.

METHODS FOR STUDYING
MONONUCLEAR PHAGOCYTES

process. It should be noted that the following description is
really concerned with the production of nonparenchymal cells,
i.e. Kupffer cells, endothelial cells, fibroblasts, and some
biliary epithelial cells. To produce pure Kupffer cells, one
has to follow the separation of nonparenchymal cells by a
short-term incubation *in vitro* to select adherent cells or perform another kind of separation of the various other cell
types. The best results in this latter regard are undoubtedly
produced by countercurrent centrifugation (2).

II. SEPARATION BY PERFUSION

A. *Introduction*

In short, the liver is perfused via the portal vein with
calcium-free buffer and subsequently with a collagenase solution. The liver is then teased apart and a single cell suspension is produced by shaking or gently pipetting. The
parenchymal cells are then destroyed by incubation in pronase.

B. *Reagents*

1. Perfusion Buffer
NaCl, 8.3 g
KCl, 0.5 g
HEPES, 2.4 g
NaOH, 1 M 6.0 ml
H_2O add 1000 ml
The pH is adjusted to 7.5 at 37°C.

2. Collagenase Buffer
NaCl, 4.0 gm
KCl, 0.5 gm
HEPES, 24.0 gm
$CaCl_2 \cdot 2\ H_2O$, 0.7 gm
NaOH, 1 M 66 ml
Collagenase, 0.5 gm (Sigma Chemical Corp. St. Louis,
    Missouri)
H_2O add 1000 ml
The pH is adjusted to 7.5 at 37°C.

3. Suspension Buffer
NaCl, 4.0 gm
KCl, 0.4 gm
KH_2PO_4, 0.15 gm

Na$_2$SO$_4$, 0.10 gm
HEPES (N-2-Hydroxyethylpiper-azine-N'-2-ethane-sulfonic
  acid, 7.08 gm
TES [N-Tris(hydroxymethyl)methyl-2-aminoethanesulfonic
  acid], 6.90 gm
Tricine [N-Tris(hydroxymethyl)methylglycine], 6.50 gm
NaOH, 2.1 gm
MgCl$_2$·6 H$_2$O, 0.13 gm
CaCl$_2$·2 H$_2$O, 0.18 gm
H$_2$O add 1000 ml
The pH is adjusted to 7.5 at 37°C.

4. Pronase Solution
Suspension buffer with 0.45% (v/v) pronase (B-grade,
Calbiochem AG, Lucern, Switzerland) is to be diluted with sus-
pension buffer to a final concentration of 0.15% (see Section
II.C.5).

5. Washing Buffer
NaCl, 8.3 gm
KCl, 0.5 gm
HEPES, 2.4 gm
NaOH (1 M), 6.0 gm
CaCl$_2$·2H$_2$O, 0.18 gm
H$_2$O add 1000 ml
The pH is adjusted to 7.5 at 37°C. All buffers are
  sterilized by filtration (0.22 µm) before use.

C. Procedures

1. The equipment needed is a peristaltic pump that can
be adjusted from a few drops per minute to about 50 - 75 ml/
min. Soft plastic tubing leads from a reservoir of the solutions to be used during perfusion through a water bath, set
at 37°C, and ends in a cannula about 1 mm in diameter to be
inserted into the portal vein. As reservoir, we use a 500-ml
measuring cylinder. To prevent the cannula from slipping out
of the portal vein, we put 4 mm of a tight-fitting plastic
tube over the tip of the cannula. The tubing is sterilized
by perfusion with 96% ethanol. The ethanol is thereafter
carefully washed out with sterile water. The end of the
tubing is then immersed in the reservoir containing about 500
ml of perfusion buffer. Perfusion buffer is passed through
the system until all air bubbles are removed from the tubing.
It is well to have a small air-bubble trap as close to the
cannula as possible. If parenchymal cells are to be used after perfusion, oxygen must continuously bubble through the
perfusion buffers, and all subsequent buffers before they are

pumped into the system. The description of the perfusion is here adjusted to the perfusion of rat livers. With small modifications, the same procedure can be performed with other animals (e.g., mouse and guinea pig).

2. A rat is anesthesized with ether, and the abdomen is opened. The intestines are carefully moved over to the left side to expose the portal vein. A strong medium thickness of thread is positioned around the portal vein, and a loose knot is made.

3. The perfusion pump is regulated down to minimum speed (a few drops per minute) to force out small amounts of air at the very tip of the cannula. Then the portal vein is opened with a pair of scissors, and the cannula inserted. The knot around the portal vein (and the cannula) is tightened and the portal vein behind the cannula is cut. To let out the perfusate the inferior vena cava below the liver is cut, and the speed of the perfusion pump is increased to about 50 ml/min.

4. The liver is now removed with the help of a pair of scissors, taking care not to sever the intestines. The liver with the cannula positioned in the portal vein is transferred to a petri dish or preferably to a small sterile metal screen in a funnel. When almost all of the perfusion buffer has passed into the tubing (i.e., after about 10 min) 50 ml of buffer with collagenase is poured into the reservoir (also a measuring cylinder). When the rest of the perfusion buffer is estimated to have been pumped out of the system, the funnel with the metal screen and the liver is transferred to the top of the reservoir. In this way, the collagenase buffer will recirculate.

5. When the collagenase buffer has passed through the liver for about 10 min, the perfusion is stopped and the liver is placed in a petri dish with about 50 ml of suspension buffer at 4°C. At this stage, if the perfusion has been successful, the liver should be completely bleached and very soft. The liver capsule is now opened with a pair of scissors and the liver cells can easily be dispersed by simply moving the tissue about with the help of a forceps. In some cases one may find that a steel comb, where every second tooth has been removed, can be useful to facilitate the dispersion.

6. The cell suspension with remnants of tissue and the liver capsule is now filtered through a double layer of sterilized gauze. The parenchymal cells may now be collected by a low-speed centrifugation or destroyed by a subsequent pronase incubation. Optimal condition for pronase incubation is $2 - 2.2 \times 10^6$ viable parenchymal cells per milliliter (as judged by trypan blue exclusion) and a final pronase concentration of 0.15% (w/v). Pronase incubation is performed with shaking at 39°C. Total disintegration of parenchymal cells is usually

accomplished in about 2 hr.

7. When all the parenchymal cells are disintegrated, the pronase incubation is completed by shaking on ice for 5 min. The cell suspension is then filtered through a layer of sterile nylon cloth (mesh 60 µm). The cells are washed four times by centrifugation at 300 g at 4°C for 5 min in washing buffer.

D. Calculation of Data

A successful perfusion of a rat liver of ordinary size will usually produce around 600 - 800 × 10^6 parenchymal cells before pronase incubation. The number of nonparenchymal cells at this stage will be around 300 - 350 × 10^6. This figure is not changed significantly by pronase treatment. About 40% of the nonparenchymal cells are Kupffer cells as judged by the presence of intracellular particles taken up by the liver phagocytes *in vivo* before perfusion.

E. Critical Comments

To produce a final suspension of viable and comparatively pure nonparenchymal cells, it is essential to have all the parenchymal cells destroyed by pronase and to perform a careful washing. As mentioned in the introduction, the method produces a 40% Kupffer cell suspension. To purify this further, one must either perform a centrifugation or select the Kupffer cell by an overnight incubation to allow the Kupffer cells to attach to a tissue culture dish. This is performed at ordinary tissue culture conditions, with any conventional tissue culture medium, and 20 - 40% fetal calf serum.

Kupffer cells tolerate well the rather extensive enzyme treatment. It must not be forgotten, however, that cell surfaces have been subjected to both collagenase and pronase, and this might have effects on chemical properties of the cell surface as well as some biological properties. Of course, the elucidation of possible unwanted effects must await the establishment of an alternative method for the separation of liver cells.

III. THE ROCK-AND-ROLL METHOD (DISPERSION BY IMMERSION)

A. *Introduction*

This method is less time-consuming and can be used with liver pieces rather than whole livers (which, e.g., allows the preparation of Kupffer cells from human liver), but the yield of nonparenchymal cells as well as Kupffer cells is only about 20% of what is usually obtained by perfusion.

B. *Reagents*

If possible, an isotonic solution (0.15 M NaCl) is injected into the portal vein to remove intrahepatic blood.

C. *Procedures*

Liver tissue about the amount of a rat liver is cut in small pieces and is incubated for about 1 hr at 37°C in about 100 ml of collagenase buffer.

The suspension with single cells and small pieces of tissue is cooled down to 4°C with shaking and is thereafter filtered through one layer of nylon cloth (mesh around 100 μm); the filtrate is centrifuged at 300 g, 4°C for 10 min.

The pellet is resuspended in ice-cold pronase buffer. Further preparation is as in Section II.

REFERENCES

1. A. C. Munthe-Kaas, T. Berg, P. O. Seglen, and R. Seljelid. Mass isolation and culture of rat Kupffer cells. *J. Exp. Med. 141*: 1-10, 1975.
2. D. L. Knook and E. Ch. Sleyster. Separation of Kupffer and endothelial cells of the rat liver by centrifugal elutriation. *Exp. Cell Res. 99*: 444-449, 1976.

12

OBTAINING MONONUCLEAR PHAGOCYTES FROM
DISAGGREGATED NEOPLASMS

Stephen W. Russell

I. INTRODUCTION

Since Robert Evans first conclusively demonstrated the
presence of macrophages in animal neoplasms (1), investigators
in many other laboratories have confirmed that most tumors,
including those of man, contain substantial numbers of mononuclear phagocytes. Isolation and functional characterization
are now key to determining what roles these cells have in the
biology of neoplasia. The approach described here (2) is one
that has permitted isolation of mononuclear phagocytes from a
variety of tumors for the purpose of assaying cytotoxic activity (3,4), prostaglandin production (5), membrane perturbation associated with exposure to lipopolysaccharide (6), and
their effects on the *in vitro* development of cytolytic activity by T lymphocytes (7). The principal advantage of the method is that it will provide good recoveries of highly enriched
populations of functional mononuclear phagocytes.

II. REAGENTS AND MATERIALS

A. Enzymes

Generally, a combination of trypsin (e.g., trypsin solution, 2.5%, Flow Laboratories, Rockville, Maryland), collagenase (e.g., CLS II, Worthington Biochemicals, Freehold, New Jersey) and deoxyribonuclease (e.g., DNase 1, Calbiochem, La Jolla, California) has proved most effective. The most efficacious combination can be chosen by means that have been described previously (2). The concentrations of trypsin and collagenase that we have found most useful are 100 µg/ml each, and for DNase 25 µg/ml. For each system, the appropriate combination of enzymes and the minimum effective concentration of each should be determined experimentally, however. Crude enzymes often work better than those that are highly purified, presumably because of the synergistic effects of other enzymatic activities that contaminate these preparations. Supplier-to-supplier variation, as well as batch-to-batch variation from the same vendor, should be expected if relatively crudely purified enzymes are used. We have found it most convenient to prepare and store each enzyme frozen in a concentrated (100-1000×) stock solution. The working enzyme mixture is prepared just before it is needed by thawing and mixing the stock solutions, after which the mixture is diluted appropriately with tissue culture medium.

B. Medium

1. Tissue Culture Medium
We have used either Eagle's minimun essential tissue culture medium (MEM) or Hank's balanced salt solution. In either case, it has proved helpful to buffer with 15 mM HEPES.

2. Fetal Bovine Serum
This reagent is used both to stop proteolytic activity and for the maintenance of cells after they have been isolated.

C. Equipment

1. Scalpel blade -- used for mincing tumor tissue. Preferred type is No. 11, sterile.
2. Dental wax -- sheets of this material, sterilized by storage for 24 hr or more in 70% ethanol, are ideal as a surface on which to mince tumor fragments. Little dulling of the scalpel blade is produced. One source is No. 10 wax; 5 lb; Kerr Laboratory Products Division, Sybron Corporation, Emeryville, California.

3. Digestion flask -- a 100 ml Berzelius beaker (looks like a standard beaker, but without the pouring spout; Scientific Products, McGaw Park, Illinois) with a magnetic bar suspended from a stopper that seals the beaker completely, should be used. We have used the stopper (No. 10), impeller assembly and glass shaft from a spinner culture flask (Bellco, Vineland, New Jersey; catalogue numbers 1969-80050, 1969-30050, and 1969-70050, respectively).

4. Stirring apparatus -- a nonheating magnetic stirrer, or a standard magnetic stirrer with several pieces of insulation (as asbestos) between stirrer and digestion flask can be used. We routinely employ a 9-place stirrer of the type that is used for spinner flasks (Bellco).

5. Tissue culture plate with 16-mm diameter wells (e.g., tissue culture cluster 24, No. 3524, Costar, Cambridge, Massachusetts or Bellco).

6. Mechanical pipetting device, for example, "Pipet-Aid" (Drummond Scientific, Broomald, Pennsylvania or Bellco).

III. PROCEDURE

A. Harvest of Tumor

The tumor or tumors should be excised aseptically into ice-cold medium. Representative material should be taken for histologic examination. Obviously necrotic areas should be removed. To ensure representative sampling for disaggregation, as much of the viable tumor or tumors should be processed as is practicable.

B. Mincing of Tumor Tissue

Excessive mincing should be avoided, as this tends to increase mechanical injury. Fragments 2-3 mm in their greatest dimension have provided us with the best cell recoveries. Tumors should be minced with a scalpel blade rather than a razor blade, as the latter dulls more rapidly and begins to crush tissue. A No. 11 scalpel blade is preferable, because its long, straight cutting edge fosters slicing rather than chopping. As soon as it is clear that tissue is "dragging" under the blade, rather than cutting cleanly, the old blade should be discarded in favor of a new one. Fragments should be washed twice, in serum-free medium, to remove debris and endogenous serum proteins. Shaking them vigorously in a half-filled, 50-ml centrifuge tube, followed by removal of the wash medium, is a convenient way to accomplish this washing step.

C. *Disaggregation*

Place up to 1 gm of fragments in the disaggregation flask
and add 15 ml of the warmed (37°C) enzyme mixture. Place the
stirring assembly in the disaggregation flask, so as to seal
its mouth completely. Begin stirring in a 37°C incubator at
a speed sufficient to agitate fragments vigorously, but not so
fast as to cause frothing. Ensure that the suspended stirring
bar does not touch either the sides or bottom of the flask,
thereby avoiding mechanical crushing of the tissue. Continue
stirring for 20-30 min, after which time the supernatant medium, containing free cells, is removed by pipette. The harvested supernate is immediately added to 1.5 ml ice-cold fetal
bovine serum and the cells are removed by centrifugation.
Fresh enzyme mixture is added to the fragments for further
stirring. The entire process is repeated until the desired
number of cells has been obtained. Cell yields at each harvest may increase with time and can sometimes be accelerated
after 1-2 hr (when stromal attachments of cells have presumably been loosened) by the application of gentle, mechanical
force. The most effective means we have found is gentle aspiration into, and expulsion from, a plastic 10-ml pipette. We
enlarge the orifice of the pipette by reaming it out with a
sterile, No. 11 scalpel blade, thereby reducing shearing
forces to a minimum.

D. *Pooling of Harvested Cells*

After cells have been removed from the serum-neutralized
enzyme mixture, they are resuspended in ice-cold tissue culture medium containing 10% fetal bovine serum. While disaggregation progresses, the already harvested cells are held
in a polypropylene centrifuge tube, on ice, with occasional
gentle shaking to keep the cells from settling to the bottom.

E. *Preparation of Monolayers*

Of the cells in the resultant suspension, mononuclear
phagocytes are usually the first to adhere to glass or plastic
surfaces. Advantage can be taken of this fact to enrich the
mononuclear phagocyte population dramatically. If the number
of mononuclear phagocytes is low, or there are many cells of
other types that have the ability to adhere rapidly (e.g.,
some tumor cells or neutrophils), then an initial enrichment
step may be needed. We assume here that such a step is not
needed.

1. Preparation for Plating
Warm the tissue culture plate to 37°C. Warm the cell suspension, containing approximately 5×10^6 total cells/ml, to 37°C in a water bath. Minimize the time the cell suspension is held at 37°C, as after a short time mononuclear phagocytes will clump and begin to adhere, even to the walls of polypropylene or siliconized glass tubes.

2. Plating of Cell Suspension
Add 0.5 ml of the warmed cell suspension (2.5×10^6 cells) to each 16-mm diameter well. After all wells are seeded, replace the plate in the 37°C incubator. Shake it at right angles just before replacing the plate, as the motion generated by walking will have produced a slight vortex, tending to move cells to the center of the well. If the plate is not shaken, uneven distribution will result. After 5 min, remove the plate and vigorously shake it several times at right angles to resuspend weakly adherent and nonadherent cells. Replace the plate in the incubator for 5 min more. Repeat the shaking. Aspirate the medium containing nonadherent cells, add fresh medium, and shake again. Aspirate and wash again. Add the medium that is desired for culture.

3. Increasing the Population Density of the Monolayer
If too few cells have adhered, rather than wash after the first plating, add another 0.5 ml of the crude cell suspension per well and repeat the above process. Continue until the desired population density has been achieved. Then wash. This approach can also be used to produce a series of wells in the same plate of differing population densities, for example, one row of four platings, one of three, one of two, and one where a single exposure is used. When this course is taken, begin seeding with the row that will receive the most platings thereby eliminating cell losses that can be associated with excessive agitation of cell free medium on newly formed monolayers.

F. Quantification of Adherent Cells

1. Direct Counting
Using an inverted microscope and a calibrated, gridded ocular, the number of adherent cells can be estimated with a fair degree of accuracy. The accuracy of this approach decreases as the population density increases. Multiple counts should be made on the same well, after which the mean value is used. Knowing the area of the grid and the total area of the well bottom, the total number of cells in the well can be computed. Wells in which cells are not uniformly distributed should not be counted.

2. DNA Analysis
Using an assay for DNA, such as that described by Cookson
and Adams (8), the number of cells per well can be estimated
from a standard curve that is produced using known numbers of
cells of similar type.

3. Differential Analysis of Monolayers
It is essential that the percentage of macrophages in the
monolayers be determined. Other techniques described in this
volume can be used, but we have found morphologic examination
coupled with phagocytic uptake especially useful (see Taffet
and Russell, this volume). For microscopic examination of the
monolayers, well bottoms can be punched or cut out (using a
heated, No. 11 scalpel) after cells have been fixed (methanol)
and stained (Giemsa or Wright). For precise studies at high
power, immersion oil is placed on the fixed, stained monolayer,
after which a coverslip can be applied.

IV. CRITICAL COMMENTS

The pitfalls associated with the isolation of immune
effector cells from solid tumors have recently been reviewed
(9). To summarize, the principal considerations are (1) loss
of cells during disaggregation and possible introduction,
thereby, of selective bias; (2) the effects of enzymes on
isolated cells; and (3) contamination of the resultant effector cell population with cells of other types. In each of
these areas, there is no absolute way of solving the problems
that are inherent in isolating cells from tumors. Each investigator must, therefore, address these problems in the
specific tumor system he or she is using. For example, there
may be no need to use enzymes on a tumor that is friable and
subject, therefore, to gentle mechanical dispersion. Thus,
the method described here should be regarded as one that may
have to be modified in accordance with the needs of the individual investigator.

Acknowledgments

The author expresses his appreciation to Ms. Brenda Brown
for typing the manuscript.
Supported by United States Public Health Service Research
Grant CA 31199 and Research Career Development Award CA 00497.

REFERENCES

1. R. Evans. Macrophages in syngeneic animal tumors. *Transplantation 14:*468-473.

2. S. W. Russell, W. F. Doe, R. G. Hoskins, and C. G. Cochrane. Inflammatory cells in solid murine neoplasms. I. Tumor disaggregation and identification of constituent inflammatory cells. *Int. J. Cancer 18:*322-330, 1976.

3. S. W. Russell, G. Y. Gillespie, and A. T. McIntosh. Inflammatory cells in solid murine neoplasms. III. Cytotoxicity mediated *in vitro* by macrophages recovered from disaggregated regressing Moloney sarcomas. *J. Immunol. 118:*1574-1579, 1977.

4. S. W. Russell, and A. T. McIntosh. Macrophages isolated from regressing Moloney sarcomas are more cytotoxic than those recovered from progressing sarcomas. *Nature 268:* 69-71, 1977.

5. J. O. Shaw, S. W. Russell, M. P. Printz, and R. A. Skidgel. Macrophage-mediated tumor cell killing: Lack of dependence on the cyclooxygenase pathway of prostaglandin synthesis. *J. Immunol. 123:*50-54, 1979.

6. A. F. Esser, and S. W. Russell. Membrane perturbation of macrophages stimulated by bacterial lipopolysaccharide. *Biochem. Biophys. Res. Comm. 87:*532-540, 1979.

7. G. Y. Gillespie, and S. W. Russell. Level of activation determines whether inflammatory peritoneal and intratumoral macrophages will promote or suppress *in vitro* development of cytolytic T lymphocyte activity. *J. Reticuloendothel. Soc. 27:*535-545, 1980.

8. S. Cookson and D. O. Adams. A simple and sensitive assay for determining DNA in mononuclear phagocytes and other cells. *J. Immunol. Methods 23:*169-173, 1978.

9. S. W. Russell. A review of data, problems, and open questions pertaining to *in situ* tumor immunity. I. Problems (technical and interpretive) associated with the isolation of immune effector cells from tumors. *Comtemp. Topics Immunobiol. 10:*1-9, 1980.

13

OBTAINING MONONUCLEAR PHAGOCYTES FROM GRANULOMAS

Robert J. Bonney

I. INTRODUCTION

Granulomas are "focal chronic inflammatory reactions characterized by the accumulation and proliferation of leuko-cytes, principally of the mononuclear type" (1). Granuloma-tous inflammatory lesions can be divided into (a) nonimmuno-logical or foreign body responses and (b) immune-based re-sponses resulting from delayed hypersensitivity reactions. Although both types of granulomas contain macrophages as the predominant cell type, lymphocytes play a key role in the for-mation of the immune-based granuloma (2). The immune-based granulomas can be induced by slowly degradable antigens that normally elicit delayed hypersensitivity reactions in the host (3). Examples of such antigens are those of *Schistosoma mansoni* eggs (4), *Bacillus - Calmette Guerin* (5), *Bordetella pertussis* (6), spores of fungi such as Micropolyspora and *Thermoactinomyces* (7), and *Mycobacterium tuberculosis* (8). The granuloma lesion induced by *Schistosoma* eggs (4) or

METHODS FOR STUDYING
MONONUCLEAR PHAGOCYTES

111

Toxocara consists primarily of eosinophils initially, which
are recruited by the acute inflammatory infiltrate (9). The
eosinophils degranulate, and the resulting debris is taken up
by macrophages that become the predominant cell type. After
10 - 12 weeks the granulomas are fibrotic encapsulated epithelioid lesions (9). In contrast, nonimmunological granulomas are induced by relatively inert nondigestible or poorly
digestible particles, such as carrageenans (10), streptococcal
cell walls (11), cotton pellets (12), polyvinyl sponges (13),
and nylon and acrylic fibers (14). These lesions are composed
of neutrophils, macrophages, and fibroblasts and do not have a
prominent lymphoid cell component. Macrophages that comprise
these lesions are long-lived and usually contain the undigested
or partly digested inducing agent (10). For example, when carrageenan is injected subcutaneously into an air pouch in
rodents, an acute edematous reaction occurs in a few hours.
This is followed by accumulation of newly recruited bone
marrow-derived macrophages after a few days (15). Up to 100%
of the macrophages can be shown to contain carrageenan 2 - 3
weeks after the injection (10), and the lesion is slow to resolve, taking up to 3 months.

In order to study the functional capacity of the cells
that comprise these various lesions, it is advantageous to devise methods for their removal from the lesions and for their
purification and cultivation. Therefore, by utilizing techniques that have been used successfully to disperse parenchymal
cells from adult liver (16), synovial cells from human rheumatoid joints (17), and neoplastic cells (18), a method for preparing macrophages from granulomas has been devised (19). The
starting tissue is a 7-day granuloma induced in mice by one
subcutaneous injection of carrageenan that can be shown histo-
logically to be comprised predominantly of macrophages (19).
The principle underlying this method is a gentle enzymatic dispersion of the dissected granuloma followed by purification by
adherence and finally cultivation in serum-free medium (to
eliminate fibroblast proliferation). Thus, it is likely that
other foreign- body- as well as immune-based granulomas could
also be studied by these techniques.

II. REAGENTS

Carrageenan is a polysaccharide extracted from Irish moss
Chondrus crispus composed of a mixture of a α and β isomers of
sulfated D-polygalactose. Sodium carrageenan, Viscarin brand,
was used exclusively in this study and was a gift from Marine
Colloids, Inc., Springfield, New Jersey. Collagenase (CLS II),

175 U/mg, was from Worthington Biochemical Corporation, Free-hold, New Jersey. Dulbecco's modified Eagles medium, lactal-bumin hydrolysate, fetal calf serum, and penicillin/strepto-mycin were from Grand Island Biological Co., Grand Island, New York. The fetal calf serum was inactivated by heating to 56°C for 30 min (HIFCS). Nonclon tissue culture dishes were from Vangard International, Inc., Neptune, New Jersey.

Male SW-ICR mice were purchased from Hilltop Lab Animals, Inc., Scottdale, Pennsylvania and were fed a standard pellet diet and water *ad libitum.*

III. PROCEDURES

A. *Induction of Granulomas*

A solution of carrageenan (5 mg/ml) was prepared by slowly adding carrageenan to sterile distilled H_2O, which was being stirred with a magnetic bar. The solution was then warmed to 37°C and 0.5 ml injected subcutaneously into the abdominal area using a 1-ml syringe fitted with a 25-gauge needle. The mice weighed 20 - 25 gm and were 4 - 6 months old. After 7 days the lesion was comprised mainly of mature macrophages with small numbers of immature macrophages, fibroblasts, and few neutro-phils (19).

B. *Isolation of Granuloma Cells*

The 7-day-old granulomatous nodules from 30 mice were dis-sected with scissors under aseptic conditions from the subcu-taneous tissue underlying the skin and scraped with a scalpel into a bacterial petri dish containing sterile Dulbecco's phosphate-buffered saline (PBS) supplemented with 100 U/ml of penicillin and streptomycin. As outlined in Fig. 1, the tis-sue was sliced further into small pieces with scalpels and added to a 100-mm bacterial petri dish (Falcon) containing 20 ml of 0.2% collagenase in Dulbecco's modified Eagles medium (DMEM). The dish is placed on a stirrer inside a 37°C incu-bator equilibrated with 5% CO_2 in air and stirred slowly with a small magnetic stirrer for 45 - 60 min. The supernatant fluid containing released cells were removed into a sterile 50-ml conical centrifuge tube and chilled on ice. The diges-tion step is repeated for 1 hr with 20 ml of fresh digesting medium and the two supernatant fluids are combined. The cells are pelleted by centrifugation at 800 g for 10 min at 4°C and washed three times with ice-cold PBS. In three different ex-

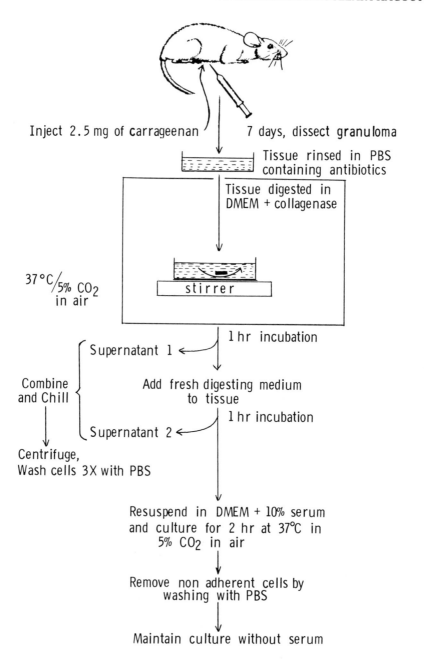

Fig. 1. *Schematic of procedures for isolating mononuclear phagocytes from carrageenan-induced granulomas in mice [reproduced from Bonney et al. (19)].*

periments, the yield was $4 \times 10^6 - 5 \times 10^6$ cells per granuloma
with 75 - 95% of cells excluding trypan blue. The cells were
resuspended in DMEM containing 10% HIFCS and added to 35 or
60 mm Nunclon tissue culture dishes or to 15-mm glass coverslips and incubated for 2 hr. The nonadherent cells were removed by washing the cell sheet four times with PBS, and the
adherent cells were incubated overnight in fresh DMEM containing 10% HIFCS. After 24 hr in the presence of serum, the cells
were washed again and maintained in DMEM + 0.2% lactalbumin
hydrolyzate.

IV. CHARACTERIZATION OF CULTURED CELLS

Cells isolated from carrageenan-induced granulomas in mice
by the procedures described above exhibit the characteristics
of mononuclear phagocytes (19). Table I summarizes several of
the activities exhibited by these cells in comparison with

TABLE I. *Activities Exhibited by Cultured Cells*

Characteristic	Granuloma	Macrophage	Fibroblast
Phagocytosis[a]	+	+	−
Lysozyme secretion[b]	+	+	−
Binding of ^{125}I-labeled IgG[c]	+	+	−
Secretion of LAF[d]	+	+	−
Trypsin detachment[e]	−	−	+
Elastase secretion[f]	+	+	−
High specific activities of lysosomal hydrolases	+	+	−

[a]Ingestion of several particles of 0.81 μm latex beads in
serum-free medium in 2 hr.
[b]Net increase in lysozyme activity in the culture medium
over 72 hr.
[c]Binding of ^{125}I-labeled IgG at 0°C and displacement by
unlabeled IgG.
[d]Secretion of lymphocyte-activating factor (LAF) induced
by lipopolysaccharide.
[e]Resistant to detachment by trypsin-EDTA for 24 hr; fibroblasts were completely removed in 10 min.
[f]Secreted an activity capable of hydrolyzing tritium-
labeled insoluble elastin.
[g]Specific activities of three lysosomal acid hydrolases
were four to eight times greater than that found in fibroblasts.

mouse peritoneal macrophages and a mouse fibroblast line (CC-1, NCTC clone 929). It has been recently reported that the activities of two membrane enzymes, 5'-nucleotidase (20) and leucine aminopeptidase (21) are vastly different in resident populations of macrophages compared to populations elicited by the injection into the peritoneal cavity of certain inflammatory stimuli. These enzymes were assayed in homogenates obtained from cultured macrophages isolated from the carrageenan granulomas, and it can be concluded that these cells resemble elicited population of macrophages (Table II).

The presence of 10% serum in the first 24 hr was essential for attachment and stability of the cells, perhaps due to residual proteolytic enzymes from the collagenase digestion medium. However, after 24 hr the cells can be maintained for up to 3 weeks without serum. Medium should be changed three times a week and should contain penicillin - streptomicin or gentamicin.

V. CRITICAL COMMENTS

In the past macrophages have been isolated from granulomatous lesions by mechanical treatment rather than by enzymatic dispersion (22). These workers dissected the granuloma induced by *Bordetella pertussis* and rubbed it against the ribbed internal surface of dissecting forceps in heparinized M199 medium. The resulting suspension was found to adhere to coverslips (22). Yields, viabilities, and contamination by

TABLE II. *Membrane Enzyme Activities of Granuloma Macrophages Compared to Resident and Elicited Mouse Peritoneal Macrophages[a]*

Macrophages	Enzyme-specific/Activity (U/mg protein)	
	5'-Nucleotidase	Aminopeptidase
Resident	13.28 ± 1.33	9.41 ± 4.50
Elicited	0.21 ± 0.15	41.67 ± 1.61
Granuloma	0.31 ± 0.12	36.67 ± 2.81

[a]*Cells were cultured for 24 hr, washed, and harvested in Triton-×100 (0.1%) and saline. The enzymes were assayed as described (19). The elicited cells were obtained from mice injected 4 days previously with thioglycollate broth. Reproduced from Bonney et al. (19).*

other cell types were not discussed. It is most likely that a more gentle dispersion such as that achieved by proteolytic action would yield a population of cells with higher viability that could be further purified by other techniques and subsequently cultivated. The methodology for enzymatic dispersion of granulomas described here is similar to that described by Russell *et al.* (18) for dispersing neoplasms and confirms the usefulness of their method.

The mononuclear phagocytes isolated from carrageenan-induced granulomas in mice by the technique described herein exhibit many of the characteristics of elicited populations of mouse peritoneal macrophages. The cultures are nearly homogeneous as determined by the percentage of cells capable of phagocytosing latex beads in serum-free medium (>95%). This method most likely would be applicable to granulomas induced by other agents (foreign body or hypersensitivity induced). Times of incubations with the proteolytic enzymes as well as the concentration of enzymes should be varied to obtain optimal conditions for each type of granuloma. In the case of carrageenan granulomas, it is most crucial to determine a nontoxic but effective dose of carrageenan to be injected into the mice. Macrophages isolated from lesions induced by 5 mg of carrageenan did not survive in culture, and an injection of less than 1 mg of carrageenan did not elicit a sizable lesion. This would be expected to vary with type of carrageenan and strain of mice.

REFERENCES

1. K. S. Warren. A functional classification of granulomatous inflammation. *Ann. NY Acad. Sci. 278*: 7-18, 1976.
2. W. G. Spector. Chronic inflammation. *In* "The Inflammatory Process" (B. Zweifach, L. Grant, and R. T. McCluskey, eds.), p. 277. Academic Press, New York, 1974.
3. D. L. Boros. Granulomatous inflammations. *Progr. Allergy 24*: k83-267, 1978.
4. D. L. Boros and K. S. Warren. Delayed hypersensitivity granuloma formation and dermal reaction induced by a soluble factor isolated from *Schistosoma mansoni* eggs. *J. Exp. Med. 132*: 488-507, 1970.
5. A. M. Danneberg, M. Ando, and K. Shima. Macrophage accumulation, division, maturation, and digestive and microbicidal capacities in tuberculous lesions. III. The turnover of macrophages and its relation to their activation and antimicrobial immunity in primary BCG lesions and those of reinfection. *J. Immunol. 109*: 1109-1121, 1972.

6. W. G. Spector and A. W. J. Lykke. The cellular evolution of inflammatory granulomata. *J. Pathol. Bacteriol.* 92: 163-177, 1966.

7. R. P. McCombs. Diseases due to immunological reactions in the lungs (two parts). *N. Engl. J. Med.* 286: 1186-1194 and 1245-1252, 1972.

8. M. B. Lurie. "Resistance to Tuberculosis: Experimental Studies in Native and Acquired Defensive Mechanisms," p. 6. Harvard University Press, Cambridge, Massachusetts, 1964.

9. S. G. Kayes and J. A. Oaks. Development of the granulomatous response in murine *Toxocariasis*. *Am. J. Pathol.* 93: 277-286, 1978.

10. W. G. Spector and G. B. Ryan. New evidence for the existence of long lived macrophages. *Nature 221*: 860, 1969.

11. I. Ginsburg. Mechanisms of cell and tissue injury induced by group A streptococci. Relation to post streptococcal sequence. *J. Infect. Dis.* 126: 294-340, 1972.

12. C. A. Winter, E. A. Risley, and G. W. Nuss. Antiinflammatory and antipyretic activities of indomethacin. *J. Pharmacol. Exp. Ther.* 141: 369-376, 1963.

13. E. Kulonen and M. Potila. Effect of administration of antirheumatic drugs and experimental granuloma in rat. *Biochem. Pharmacol.* 24: 219-225, 1975.

14. J. Cortez Pimentel. Sarcoid granulomas of the skin produced by acrylic and nylon fibers. *Br. J. Dermatol.* 96: 673-677, 1977.

15. B. Morris, T. Weinberg, and G. J. Spector. The carrageenan granuloma in the rat. A model for the study of the structure and function of macrophages. *Br. J. Exp. Pathol.* 49: 302-311, 1968.

16. R. J. Bonney, P. R. Walker, and V. R. Potter. Isoenzyme patterns in parenchymal and nonparenchymal cells from regenerating and regenerated liver. *Biochem. J. 136*: 947-954, 1973.

17. J. M. Dayer, S. M. Krane, R. G. G. Russel, and D. R. Robinson. Production of collagenase and prostaglandins by isolated adherent rheumatoid synovial ce-ls. *Proc. Nat. Acad. Sci. USA 73*: 945-949, 1976.

18. S. W. Russell, W. F. Doe, R. G. Hoskins, and C. G. Cochrane. Inflammatory cells in solid murine neoplasms. I. Tumor disaggregation and identification of constituent inflammatory cells. *Int. J. Cancer 18*: 322-330, 1976.

19. R. J. Bonney, I. Gery, T. Y. Lin, M. F. Meyenhofer, W. Acevedo, and P. Davies. Mononuclear phagocytes from carrageenan-induced granulomas: Isolation cultivation and characterization. *J. Exp. Med. 148*: 261-275, 1978.

20. P. J. Edelson and Z. A. Cohn. 5'-Nucleotidase activity of mouse peritoneal macrophages. I. Synthesis and degradation in resident and inflammatory populations. *J. Exp. Med. 144*: 1581–1595, 1976.
21. E. D. Wachsmuth. Aminopeptidase as a marker for macrophage differentiation. *Exp. Cell Res. 96*: 409–412, 1975.
22. G. B. Ryan and W. G. Spector. Natural selection of long-lived macrophages in experimental granulomata. *J. Pathol. 99*: 139–151, 1967.

14

TEFLON FILM AS A SUBSTRATE
FOR THE CULTURE OF MONONUCLEAR PHAGOCYTES

Jos W. M. van der Meer
Joke S. van de Gevel
Ralph van Furth

I. INTRODUCTION

Mononuclear phagocytes cultured *in vitro* on a glass or
plastic surface adhere and attach to the surface, and under
these conditions the morphology, cytochemistry, and functions
of the cells can be easily studied. It is, however, difficult
to recover the cells into suspension when required for certain
experiments. This chapter presents two methods in which a
hydrophobic Teflon membrane is used as the culture substrate.
Mononuclear phagocytes adhere poorly to Teflon membranes and
can easily be recovered intact for subculture or for experiments in which the cells must be in suspension (e.g., transfer
experiments, chemotactic studies, and assessment of intracellular killing of bacteria). These culture systems are suitable
for human and murine mononuclear phagocytes; those of other
species have not as yet been studied by us to any appreciable
extent.

121

II. MATERIALS

A. *Teflon Film*

     Disposable hydrophobic Teflon FEP film (fluorinated
ethylene propylene resin, DuPont de Nemours and Company; gauge
25 μm)* supplied by Janssens' M & L (St. Niklaas, Belgium) is
used as the culture substrate. This film is completely translucent and, since it is nontoxic, can be used without prior
cleaning procedures. It resists autoclaving without any change
in size, shape, or clarity. Since the film is permeable for
oxygen, carbon dioxide, and water vapor (1, 2), closed bags
(see below) can be used for culture of cells. The film is im-
permeable for water in the liquid phase, as well as for electrolytes and microorganisms.

B. *The Teflon Film Dish (TFD)*

     The TFD is a tissue culture chamber consisting of a re-
usable aluminum holder with a Teflon ring (inner diameter
40 mm) on which a piece of hydrophobic Teflon-FEP film is
mounted (3) (Fig. 1). The cover consists of a metal ring in
which a transparent glass disk is fixed. This tissue culture
chamber has also been used for slightly different purposes
(4 - 6) and can be obtained from Tecnomara AG, Zürich, CH
8059, Switzerland. The assembled chamber can be sterilized
by autoclaving.

C. *The Teflon Culture Bag (TCB)*

     Sheets of Teflon FEP film are sealed with a diathermic
sealing apparatus (Super Sealboy 235; 210 W, Audion Electron,
Amsterdam, The Netherlands) to form a triangular bag (2) (Figs.
2 and 3a and b). Usually bags measuring 4 × 15 × 15 cm are
made in our laboratory, but, of course, either larger or
smaller bags can be produced. A glass bead (diameter 4 mm)
is sealed in to allow easy introduction of the needle (19
gauge) through which the bag is filled with a cell suspension
(Fig. 3c). Before the cell suspensions are brought into the
bags, the bags are sterilized by autoclaving for 20 min at
120°C and 3 atm. After a bag has been filled with medium and

─────────────────────

     *Teflon FEP film, Type 100-gauge, from E. I. DuPont de
Nemours and Co., Wilmington, Delaware 19805, may be an acceptable substitute.

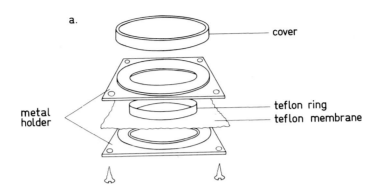

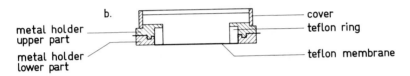

Fig. 1. Schematic drawing of the Teflon film dish.
(a) Dish in unassembled state. (b) Dish in cross section.
(Reproduced with permission of the J. Exp. Med. 147: 271-276,
1978.)

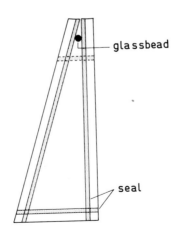

Fig. 2. The Teflon culture bag (TCB). (Reproduced with
permission of Cell. Immunol. 42: 208-212, 1979.)

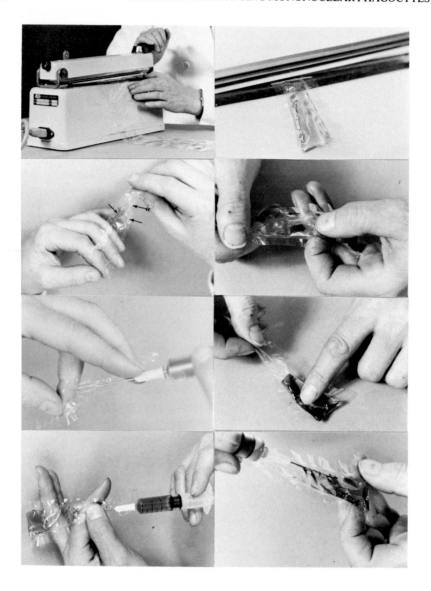

Fig. 3. (a) Teflon membranes are sealed with a diathermic sealing apparatus. (b) The seals (arrow) are made such that a triangular bag is formed, a glass bead (double-tailed arrow) is sealed in, to facilitate introduction of a needle. (c) and (d) Via the needle, the bag is filled with a cell suspension. (e) and (f) The opening in the bag is sealed diathermically (seal, arrow). (g) After incubation, the bags are gently rubbed and kneaded to detach loosely adherent cells. (h) A needle is introduced into the culture bag and the culture fluid is aspirated to harvest the cells.

cells (Fig. 3d), the opening is sealed diathermically (Fig. 3e and f). During incubation substances (e.g., drugs, nutrients, [^{3}H]-thymidine) or particles (latex spheres, opsonized bacteria, etc.) can be added or samples taken by perforating the Teflon film near this seal with the needle of the syringe and resealing the hole afterward.

III. PROCEDURE

A. Preparation of Cell Suspensions

Mononuclear phagocytes from various sources can be suspended in one of the currently available culture media supplemented with serum. The culture media and sera in use in our laboratory for the culture of mononuclear phagocytes of various kinds are given in Table I. The cells are usually seeded at a density of approximately $10^5 - 10^6$ cells/ml.

B. Incubation

The cultures are placed in an incubator with a humidified atmosphere at 37°C and 10% CO_2 added to the air.

C. Recovery of the Cells

Cells are recovered from the TFD by aspirating the culture fluid and by gently rinsing the Teflon surface with culture medium to remove loosely adhering cells as well. For recovery from a TCB, the bag is gently kneaded (Fig. 3g), a needle (19 gauge) attached to a syringe is introduced, and the culture fluid is aspirated (Fig. 3h), this fluid is gently reinjected and aspirated several times to remove all loosely adherent cells.

The cells recovered from a TFD, a TCB, or from glass or plastic are counted in a hemocytometer and viability is determined by (0.1%) trypan blue exclusion.

Light and Phase-Contrast Microscopy

During incubation, the cells in both the TFD and the TCB can be studied in an unfixed state with an inverted phase-contrast microscope. Cells recovered from the TFD or the TCB are studied light microscopically in cytocentrifuge prepara-

TABLE I. Media and Sera for Liquid Culture of Mononuclear Phagocytes

Kind of mononuclear phagocyte	Culture medium	Serum	Reference
Murine bone marrow cells	Dulbecco's MEM[a] + conditioned medium[b]	Horse serum[c] 20%	7, 8
Murine peritoneal macrophages	Medium 199[a]	Newborn calf serum[a,d] 20%	9
Murine pulmonary macrophages	Medium 199[a]	Newborn calf serum[a,d] 20%	10
Murine liver macrophages	Medium 199[a]	Newborn calf serum[a,d] 20%	11
Murine macrophage tumor cell lines	RPMI 1640[c]	Fetal calf serum[c] 10%	2, 3
Human bone marrow cells	Alpha MEM[c]	Horse serum[c,d] 35% + fetal calf serum[c,d] 15%	12
Human blood monocytes	Medium 199[a]	Newborn calf serum[a,d] 20%	13

[a]GIBCO, Grand Island, New York.
[b]Prepared from supernatants of cultures of embryonic mouse fibroblasts.
[c]Flow Laboratories, Irvine, Scotland.
[d]Inactivated by incubation at 56°C for 30 min.

tions (6) or in cultures of these cells on a flying glass coverslip in a Leighton tube. The cells on glass or plastic surfaces are rapidly air-dried and fixed (e.g., in methanol) and stained (e.g., with Giemsa stain).

E. Electron Microscopy

Electron microscopic studies can be done by fixing the cells in the TFD according to van Ewijk and Hösli (4). With this method, cells can be selected and marked under the inverted microscope; the cells are then fixed and dehydrated semiautomatically, while they are still *in situ* in the dish and without disturbance of their geographical relationship. Since the Teflon film does not stick to polymerized Epon, it can be easily peeled off. Ultrathin sections of the selected cells can be made according to any predetermined plan. Alternatively, the cells can be recovered from the TFD or TCB and the cell suspension processed for electron microscopy in the conventional way (14).

F. Replating of Cultures

After a certain incubation period, the cells can be harvested from the TFD or TCB to be subcultured. For this purpose the cells are centrifuged (110 *g* for 10 min), washed, resuspended in fresh medium, and incubated in a new TFD or TCB.

IV. CRITICAL COMMENTS

Methods are described for the culture of mononuclear phagocytes in suspension by incubation on a hydrophobic Teflon film to which the cells do not adhere. Such cells can be easily harvested from the culture without damage and used for further experiments or for subculture. Under these conditions more than 75% of the resident peritoneal macrophages can be harvested undamaged after 24 hr of culture.

Of the two methods, we now prefer the one using the Teflon culture bag because the bag is cheap, disposable, easily made in the laboratory, and its size can be varied; moreover the use of closed bags minimizes the risk of infection of the culture. However, the Teflon film dish with its flat bottom, despite its disadvantages (expensive aluminum holder, laborious cleaning and assembly of the device, greater likelihood of infection in the incubator), is more suitable for (time-lapse) photography and cinematography as well as for electron microscopic examination of individual cells (5, 6). Both systems are suitable for the culture of virtually all kinds of mononuclear phagocytes. We have shown that the characteristics of mononuclear phagocytes cultured on Teflon are similar to those seen after culture on a glass or plastic surface. Proliferation of murine bone marrow mononuclear phagocytes in the presence of colony-stimulating factor is the same on Teflon and on glass (2, 3, 8), and macrophage tumor cell lines also proliferate to the same degree on Teflon and on plastic (2, 3). Peroxidase activity, α-naphthyl butyrate esterase activity, Fc receptors, complement receptors, phagocytosis, and pinocytosis of both murine long-term resident peritoneal macrophages and of (long-term) proliferating bone marrow mononuclear phagocytes are the same on Teflon and on glass (3). Furthermore, peroxidatic activity patterns of mononuclear phagocytes, as studied under the electron microscope in these adherent and nonadherent cultures, are also the same (14). With replating at regular intervals, cultures of proliferating bone marrow mononuclear phagocytes have been maintained in our laboratory for more than 180 days. Several investigators, including the authors, have found the Teflon systems to be very convenient for short-term as well as long-term cultures of human blood monocytes (14, 15). Recently, we attempted to culture human marrow in the Teflon culture bag; the human monoblast could be recognized in these cultures, and cultures could be maintained for at least 3 - 4 weeks (12).

What are the disadvantages of these culture systems? First, they do not provide separation of mononuclear phagocytes from less adherent cells (lymphocytes and granulocytes). This poses no problem for the culture of mouse bone marrow mononuclear phagocytes, but in cultures of human blood monocytes and human bone marrow relatively large numbers of lymphocytes and granulocytes persist throughout the culture period. To obtain pure cultures of human monocytes, a separation step to eliminate lymphocytes must be included (15).

Second, since the cells do not adhere and spread as they do on a glass surface, the morphology is different. Consequently with cultures on glass or plastic, the stage of development (monoblast, promonocyte, monocyte, and macrophage) (7) cannot be determined at the light microscopic level.

Third, cells that adhere very strongly to glass, as thioglycollate-induced peritoneal macrophages, are also able to adhere to the Teflon membrane, but after 24 hr of culture the percentage of cells that can be harvested from the TCB equals that of resident peritoneal macrophages.

Last, the proliferation of thioglycollate-induced peritoneal macrophages in the presence of L cell conditioned medium is lower on Teflon than on glass (C. Stewart, personal communication). Fibroblasts (as well as mouse L cells) also tend to proliferate better on glass or plastic than on Teflon.

How do these Teflon culture systems compare with methods used to avoid adherence of mononuclear phagocytes or to detach these cells from a surface? Munder *et al.* (1) employed a hydrophilic Teflon membrane for cell support; however, mononuclear phagocytes adhere to these chemically etched membranes. Plastic petri dishes with a Teflon bottom (either hydrophilic Teflon for adherent cultures or hydrophobic for nonadherent cultures) are now commercially available (Petriperm, Heraeus, Hanau, West Germany). Our experience with these dishes is limited, but we have found that cells do adhere more firmly to the hydrophobic dish than to the Teflon film we use.

The Cuprophane sheet (a cellulose membrane for hemodialysis; Akzo, Wuppertal, West Germany) described by van Ginkel *et al.* (17) has the disadvantage of permeability for water and electrolytes. Mononuclear phagocytes are said to adhere poorly to polypropylene tubes (Corning Glass Works, Corning, New York). These tubes have the disadvantage of not being translucent, which prevents observation of cell cultures with the inverted microscope. Plastic petri dishes can be coated with Teflon from a spray (No. 6075, Crown Industrial Products Co., Hebron Illinois), but are then no longer translucent (18).

Methods to recover adherent cells from other surfaces, such as scraping with a rubber policeman at 4°C and treatment with trypsin, chelating agents, or cationic anesthetics (19), give either very incomplete recovery or damage the cells. Cultures in tumbler tubes or in siliconized glassware do not completely eliminate surface attachment of mononuclear phagocytes. The culture of mononuclear phagocytes on a surface coated with collagen or in a plasma clot and recovery of the cells by enzymatic digestion of the coating has several disadvantages, such as activation of the cells by material on the surface, ingestion of the coating substance by the cells, damage to the cell membrane by the enzymes used, and interference with direct microscopical observation of the attached cells during incubation. Furthermore, study of the morphology of fixed, cultured cells may be hampered by nontranslucent coating material. Even cells that normally do not attach easily to glass or plastic (e.g., lymphocytes) may attach to the coated surface.

REFERENCES

1. P. G. Munder, M. Modolell, and D. F. H. Wallach. Cell propagation on films of polymeric fluorocarbon as a means to regulate pericellular pH and pO_2 in cultured monolayers. *FEBS Letters 15*: 191-196, 1971.

2. J. W. M. van der Meer, J. S. van de Gevel, I. Elzenga-Claasen, and R. van Furth. Suspension cultures of mononuclear phagocytes in the Teflon culture bag. *Cell. Immunol. 42*: 208-212, 1979.

3. J. W. M. van der Meer, D. Bulterman, T. L. van Zwet, I. Elzenga-Claasen, and R. van Furth. Culture and mononuclear phagocytes on a Teflon surface to prevent adherence. *J. Exp. Med. 147*: 271-276, 1978.

4. P. Hösli. Microtechniques for rapid prenatal diagnosis in early pregnancy. *In* "Birth Defects." Proceedings of the Fourth International Conference, Vienna, Austria, 2-8 September 2973 (A. G. Motulsky and W. Lenz, eds.), p. 226. Excerpta Medica, Amsterdam, 1974.

5. W. van Ewijk and P. Hösli. A new method for comparative light and electron microscopic studies of individual cells, selected in the living state. *J. Microsc. 105, 1*: 19-31, 1975.

6. E. de Vries, J. P. van der Weij, A. C. van Buysen, and A. Cats. A Teflon culture and embedding device for the study of cells by light and electron microscopy. *J. Immunol. Methods 36*: 81-87, 1980.

7. Th. J. L. M. Goud, C. Schotte, and R. van Furth. Identification and characterization of the monoblast in mononuclear phagocyte colonies grown *in vitro*. *J. Exp. Med. 142*: 1180-1199, 1975.

8. J. W. M. van der Meer, J. S. van de Gevel, M. M. C. Diesselhoff-den Dulk, R. H. J. Beelen, and R. van Furth. Long-term cultures of murine bone marrow mononuclear phagocytes. *In* "Mononuclear Phagocytes - Functional Aspects" (R. van Furth, ed.), pp. 343-362. Martinus Nijhoff Publishers, The Hague, Boston, London, 1980.

9. R. van Furth and Z. A. Cohn. The origin and kinetics of mononuclear phagocytes. *J. Exp. Med. 128*: 415-435, 1968.

10. A. Blussé van Oud Alblas and R. van Furth. The origin, kinetics, and characteristics of pulmonary macrophages in the normal steady state. *J. Exp. Med. 149*: 1504-1518, 1979.

11. R. W. Crofton, M. M. C. Diesselhoff-den Dulk, and R. van Furth. The origin, kinetics, and characteristics of the Kupffer cells in the normal steady state. *J. Exp. Med. 148*: 1-17, 1978.

12. J. W. M. van der Meer, J. S. van de Gevel, R. H. J.

Beelen, D. Fluitsma, and R. van Furth. Culture of human bone marrow in the Teflon culture bag. Identification of the human monoblast. *In* "Proceedings International Workshop on Heterogeneity of Mononuclear Phagocytes." Baden, July 1980. In Press.

13. R. van Furth, J. A. Raeburn, and T. L. van Zwet. Characteristics of human mononuclear phagocytes. *Blood 54*, 2: 485-500, 1979.

14. R. H. J. Beelen, D. M. Fluitsma, J. W. M. van der Meer, and E. C. M. Hoefsmit. Development of different peroxidatic activity patterns in peritoneal macrophages *in vivo* and *in vitro*. *J. Reticuloendothel. Soc. 25*, 5: 513-523, 1979.

15. M. Glazenburg, M. de Boer, J. H. van Liebergen, P. H. Tegelaers, M. C. Brouwer, and D. Roos. Oxygen-dependent and -independent effector functions of human monocytes and macrophages. *In* "Proceedings International Workshop on Heterogeneity of Mononuclear Phagocytes." Baden, July 1980. In press.

16. W. P. Arend and C. G. Ragsdale. Neutral protease secretion and receptor expression in human monocytes: Effects of cell differentiation. *In* "Proceedings International Workshop on Heterogeneity of Mononuclear Phagocytes." Baden, July 1980. In Press.

17. C. J. W. Van Ginkel, W. G. van Aken, J. I. H. Oh, and J. Vreeken. Stimulation of monocyte procoagulant activity by adherence to different surfaces. *Br. J. Haematol. 37*: 35-45, 1977.

18. V. Klimetzek and H. Remold. The murine bone marrow macrophage. A sensitive indicator cell for murine migration inhibitory factor and a new method for their harvest. *Cell. Immunol. 53*: 257-266, 1980.

19. M. Rabinovitch and M. J. de Stefano. Use of the local anesthetic lidocaine for cell harvesting and subcultivation. *In vitro 11*: 379, 1975.

15

EFFECTS OF HUSBANDRY AND MOUSE STRAINS
ON MONONUCLEAR PHAGOCYTES

Monte S. Meltzer

Mouse peritoneal macrophages are widely used as a standard for study of mononuclear phagocyte function. To be useful as a standard, however, morphologic, functional, and biochemical properties of these cells should be reproducible: reproducible from day to day within one's own laboratory and between different laboratories. Two considerations that can profoundly affect reproducibility are the strains of mice selected for study and conditions under which the animals are bred and housed. Despite the importance of these factors, however, there have been very few systematic studies on macrophage function and the general health of laboratory mice. For example, male mice from certain strains housed 5 - 8 cage establish a pecking order by tail and ear biting. Once this pecking order is established, tail biting ceases. However, transfer of a new male mouse into that cage restarts the entire process. Macrophage function in these mice, animals with chronic superficial skin lesions, may be very different from "normal" mice.

For the most part, general information on the care and use of laboratory mice can be found in any of several standard textbooks and manuals and will not be discussed here (1 - 4). Animals with overt clinical signs of infection or abnormal development are usually recognized, and the causative event corrected or the animals excluded from study. More serious situations, however, arise from breakdown of proper laboratory animal management (housing, sanitation, and husbandry) and inapparent or subclinical infections. More often than not, these two problems are coincident.

Difficulties described for quantitation of macrophage-induced tumor cytotoxicity illustrate the complexity of this problem. There is general agreement that with normal mice, resident peritoneal macrophages or inflammatory macrophages induced in the peritoneal cavity by injection of sterile irritants are not cytopathic to tumor cells *in vitro*. Peritoneal macrophages, however, can develop tumoricidal activity after treatment *in vivo* or *in vitro* with any of a wide variety of activation agents. There have been instances when macrophages from apparently normal mice exerted tumoricidial activity. Boyle and Omerod (5) showed that macrophages from healthy mice housed in a conventional but "dirty" animal room were cytopathic to tumor cells *in vitro*; cells from matched mice kept isolated in a relatively "clean" animal room had no effect on tumor cell growth. Similar observations were made with nude mice: macrophages from nude mice housed in a clean conventional environment were tumoricidal; cells from germ-free nude mice had no cytotoxic activity (6). Both reports illustrate situations in which specific-pathogen-free animals were affected by their environment to develop alterations in macrophage function. In both cases, mice had no overt symptoms of infection.

It should be noted at this point that certain procedures intended to limit subclinical infections in an animal colony can also affect macrophage activity. The suppression of macrophage function in mice that receive hyperchlorinated (25 ppm) drinking water is an example of such procedures (7). Moreover, cells from germ-free animals are not comparable to cells from conventionally housed animals and, in fact, have been shown to have several functional defects (8).

Subclinical viral infections are a major cause of abnormal immune responses in apparently healthy mice. There are many rodent viruses which can be carried in an animal colony without overt symptoms of i-lness or even gross pathologic changes. Alterations in normal immune function have been reported for inapparent infections with murine leukemia virus (9), lymphocytic choriomeningitis virus (10), murine cytomegalovirus (11), reovirus 3 (12), ectromelia virus (13), murine hepatitis virus (14), minute virus of mice (15), lactic dehydrogenase-elevating virus (16), and Sendai virus (17). Many of these viruses are carried in transplantable tumors. One should, therefore, be especially vigilant in examination of macrophage function in tumor-bearing animals. Serodiagnostic services such as that offered by Microbiological Associates, Inc., Rockville, Maryland should be used to monitor periodically animals for a wide spectrum of murine viruses.

Genetic differences in macrophage function between strains of mice must also be considered in the study of mononuclear phagocytes. In attempts to establish a new assay, it is, of course, most prudent to use the strain of mice for which the particular assay of macrophage function was initially defined. This is not always possible. One should therefore be aware of possible genetic differences in macrophage response. Characterization of these genetic differences, however, is very incomplete. There are few systematic studies in the current literature which address this problem. One example of differences in macrophage function between mouse strains can be shown for development of nonspecific tumoricidal activity following *in vivo* or *in vitro* treatments (18) (Table I). It is likely that similar observations can be made with other mononuclear phagocyte functions.

TABLE I. *Genetic Variation in Development of Macrophage Tumoricidal Activity among Mouse Strains*

Responsive	Variable	Nonresponsive
C3H/HeN	BALB/cAnN	A/J
AKR/N	A/WySnJ	A/HeJ
CBA/CaHN	RII/AnN	A/HeN
CBA/N		AL/N
C57BL/6N		
C57BL/10J		C3H/HeJ
C57L/N		C57BL/10ScCR
DBA/1JN		C57BL/10ScN
DBA/2N		
NZW/N		P/J
NZB/N		P/JN
NIH Swiss (outbred)		
B10.A/SgSnJ		

aPeritoneal exudate macrophages from mice inoculated intraperitoneally 7 days previously with viable Mycobacterium bovis, strain BCG were adjusted to an equal macrophage concentration and cultured with prelabeled tumor target cells for 48 hr. Cytotoxicity was estimated by measurement of radiolabel release and confirmed by observation of cultures under phage microscopy.

REFERENCES

1. "Biology of the Laboratory Mouse" (E. L. Green, ed.),
    Second edition. Dover Publications, Inc., New York, 1975.
2. "Guide for the Care and Use of Laboratory Animals." U.S.
    Department of Health, Education and Welfare. Public Health
    Service, National Institutes of Health. DHEW Publication
    No. (NIH) 78-23, 1978.
3. "Long-Term Holding of Laboratory Rodents." ILAR News.
    Volume XIX, Number 4, 2076. (Institute of Laboratory Ani-
    mal Resources, Assembly of Life Sciences, National Research
    Counci..)
4. Laboratory animal management: Rodents. ILAR News, Vol.
    XX, Number 3, 1977.
5. M. D. P. Boyle and M. G. Ormerod. Destruction of alloge-
    neic tumor cells by peritoneal macrophages: Production of
    lytic effectors by immune mice. *Transplantation 21*: 242-
    246, 1976.
6. M. S. Meltzer. Tumoricidal responses *in vitro* of peri-
    toneal macrophages from conventionally housed and germ-free
    nude mice. *Cell. Immunol. 22*: 176-181, 1976.
7. Fidler, I. J. Depression of macrophages in mice by drink-
    ing hyperchlorinated water. *Nature 270*: 735-736, 1977.
8. T. T. MacDonald and P. B. Carter. Requirement for a bac-
    terial flora before mice generate cells capable of mediat-
    ing the delayed hypersensitivity reaction to sheep red
    blood cells. *J. Immunol. 122*: 2624-2629, 1979.
9. W. S. Ceglowski and H. Friedman. Immunosuppression by
    leukemia viruses. III. Adoptive transfer of antibody-
    forming cells to Friend disease virus-infected mice.
    J. Immunol. 103: 460-466, 1970.
10. C. A. Mims and S. Wainwright. The immunodepressive action
    of lymphocytic choriomeningitis virus in mice. *J. Immunol.*
    101: 7171-7172, 1968.
11. J. E. Osborn and J. Medearis. Studies of relationship
    between mouse cytomegalovirus and interferon. *Proc. Soc.*
    Exp. Biol. Med. 121: 819-824, 1966.
12. J. O. Klein, G. M. Green, J. K. C. Tilles, E. H. Kass, and
    M. Finland. Effect of intranasal reovirus infection on
    antibacterial activity of mouse lung. *J. Infect. Dis. 119*:
    43-50, 1969.
13. A. W. Gledhill, D. L. J. Bilbey, and J. S. F. Niven. Ef-
    fect of certain murine pathogens on pathocytic activity.
    Br. J. Exp. Pathol. 46: 433-442, 1965.
14. A. L. Notkins. Lactic dehydrogenase virus. *Bacteriol.*
    Rev. 29: 143-160, 1965.
15. G. D. Bonnard, E. K. Manders, D. A. Campbell, R. B. Herber-
    man, and M. J. Collins. Immunosuppressive activity of a

subline of the mouse EL-4 lymphoma. Evidence for minute virus of mice causing the inhibition. *J. Exp. Med. 143*: 187-199, 1976.

16. V. Riley. The LDH-virus: An interfering biological contaminant. *Science 200*: 124-126, 1978.

17. G. L. Jakak and G. M. Green. The effect of sendai virus infection on bacteriocidal and transport mechanisms of the mouse lung. *J. Clin. Invest. 51*: 1989-1998, 1972.

18. D. Boraschi and M. S. Meltzer. Macrophage activation for tumor cytotoxicity: Genetic variation in macrophage tumoricidal capacity among mouse strains. *Cell. Immunol. 45*: 188-194, 1979.

16

ENDOTOXIN CONTAMINATION AND *in vitro*
MONOCYTE-MACROPHAGE FUNCTION:
METHODS OF DETECTING, DETOXIFYING, AND ELIMINATING ENDOTOXIN

J. Brice Weinberg

I. INTRODUCTION

Bacterial endotoxin (ET) is a protein - lipopolysaccharide
complex that comes from the outer membrane of gram-negative
bacteria. Endotoxin has effects on various systems that indirectly or directly affect mononuclear phagocyte function.
Endotoxin can activate the classical and alternate pathways of
complement *in vivo* and *in vitro* (1, 2). Endotoxin also has
direct effects on different cell types including fibroblasts
(3), kidney cells (4), endothelial cells (5), ovary cells (6),
B lymphocytes (7), and monocyte-macrophages (8 - 11). In addition, through the induction of interleukin 1 [IL1, which is
probably the same as lymphocyte-activating factor and endogenous pyrogen (12)] released from monocyte-macrophage, ET
causes changes in T lymphocytes (13), brain cells (14), and
synovial cells (15). Although investigators in the past have
used ET in the microgram per milliliter range for *in vitro*
studies, recent experience has shown that ET in quantities of

picogram to nanogram per milliliter has potent effects on macrophage function including elaboration of IL1 (12) and tissue
factor (16), induction of macrophage-mediated tumor cytotoxicity (8 - 11), and modulation of macrophage neutral proteinase
secretion (17).

The realization that such low quantities of ET can so
dramatically influence macrophage function has made investigators more wary of ET contamination in media and various
reagents (10, 11, 18 - 23). Although the pharmaceutical indus-
try is aware of ET ("pyrogen") contamination and produces ET-
free products for clinical use, chemical companies do not
routinely monitor for the ET content in their products. I and
others have previously demonstrated that ET contamination of
tissue culture media, sera, and various reagents has dramatic
effects on *in vitro* assays of macrophage-mediated tumor cell
killing (9, 10). The purpose of this chapter is to describe
means of detecting, detoxifying, and eliminating ET.

II. REAGENTS

     (1) Glass tubes, 10 × 75 mm borosilicate (Scientific
Products, T1290-2)
     (2) Sterile plastic pipettes (Falcon Plastics)
     (3) Serum, adult bovine (Sterile Systems, Inc.)
     (4) Tissue culture medium: Dulbecco's modified Eagle
medium (DMEM) (GIBCO No. 430-1600) is made from powder using
ET-free water. The medium is sterilized by filtration through
0.22 µm diameter pore size Millipore filters. The final
medium also contains 20 mM HEPES buffer (Sigma Chemical Co.),
1.75 mgm/ml added dextrose (final concentration of dextrose
15 mM), 100 U/ml penicillin G potassium (Lilly and Co.), and
100 µg/ml streptomycin sulfate (Pfizer)
     (5) Water distilling apparatus: Water still AG-2 (Corning
Glass Works)
     (6) *Limulus* amebocyte lysate, PanMed, Inc., Three Oaks,
Michigan
     (7) Chromatography supplies: Sephadex G-200 gel and glass
columns (Pharmacia); sodium azide and Tris buffer (Sigma
Chemical Co.)
     (8) Polymyxin B sulfate, Burroughs Wellcome and Co.
     (9) ET-free saline, GIBCO/Invenex Division of Dexter Cor-
poration
     (10) Drying oven, Thelco Model 17, GCA/Precision Scien-
tific
     (11) Endotoxin, phenol-extracted *E. Coli* 0128:B12 (Sigma
Chemical Co.)
     (12) Human hemoglobin, type IV (Sigma Chemical Co.)

III. PROCEDURES

A. *Detection of ET* [*Limulus amebocyte lysate (LAL) assay*]

(1) The lyophilized LAL is dissolved into the prescribed amount of sterile, ET-free water or saline. Unused LAL is aliquotted into 0.2-ml portions and frozen at −20°C for later use. Sterile technique is used.

(2) LAL (0.03 ml) is placed into baked (see Section III. B. 1) 10 × 75 mm glass tubes, and then 0.03 ml of the substance in question is added to the tubes using separate pipettes for all additions. The pH of the sample should be between 6.8 − 7.6 (24), and is adjusted by addition of HCl or NaOH. The tubes are capped with aluminum foil (which has been previously baked 2 hr at 170°C) to avoid evaporation. The tubes are kept upright in a rack.

(3) After 60 min of undisturbed incubation in a 37°C water bath, each tube is observed individually for the formation of a clot by smoothly inverting the tube a full 180°.

(4) A positive test is one in which a solid clot is present and does not dislodge on inversion. Increased viscosity is considered negative.

(5) Controls should include a negative (commercially bought ET-free water or saline), a positive (commercially bought ET, usually 0.1, 1, 10, and 100 ng/ml), and tests for nonspecific inhibition (mixture of reagent in question with ET). When making serial dilutions of ET, it is important to use fresh pipettes between tubes to avoid carry-over inaccuracies. Table I shows an example of a typical LAL assay with appropriate controls.

(6) Semiquantitation of ET content can be done by serially diluting the positive sample and comparing to a standard curve prepared with ET.

(7) Serum and plasma contain lipoprotein inhibitors of ET, and unless special preparation of the sample is made, the ET content cannot be accurately assessed (24). Although chloroform extraction will remove the inhibitors, heat treatment is easier and yields comparable results (25). The serum is diluted 1 : 10 into ET-free saline, heated in a boiling water bath 7.5 min, cooled, centrifuged, and the supernatant is tested as described above (steps 1-6).

Of the various practical methods available to detect the presence of ET [e.g., pyrogenicity in rabbits, death in chicken embryos, and death in sensitized mice (26)], the LAL assay has proved the most useful. The technique described here requires no special equipment and detects ≥0.5 − 1.0 ng/ml of ET. Other LAL assays using nephelometry (27), determination of precipi-

TABLE I. *Typical LAL Assay*

	Reagent[a]	Result
1.	ET-free saline	−
2.	ET, 0.1 ng/ml	−
3.	ET, 0.5 ng/ml	+
4.	ET, 1.0 ng/ml	+
5.	ET, 10.0 ng/ml	+
6.	ET, 100.0 ng/ml	+
7.	Hb, 0.1 μg/ml	−
8.	Hb, 1.0 μg/ml	+
9.	Hb, 5.0 μg/ml	+
10.	Hb, 10.0 μg/ml	+
11.	Hb, 50.0 μg/ml	+
12.	Hb, 100.0 μg/ml	+
13.	$NaIO_4$, 5 mM	−
14.	$NaIO_4$, 10 mM	−
15.	$NaIO_4$, 20 mM	−
16.	$NaIO_4$ (5 mM) + ET (1 ng/ml)	+
17.	$NaIO_4$ (10 mM) + ET (1 ng/ml)	+
18.	$NaIO_4$ (20 mM) + ET (1 ng/ml)	+

[a]ET (endotoxin), Hb (hemoglobin), and $NaIO_4$ (sodium periodate) are dissolved into ET-free saline. Numbers 2 - 6 indicate that the LAL is sensitive to ≥ 0.5 ng/ml ET. Numbers
7 - 12 indicate that $\geq g$ μg/ml hemoglobin has the same clotting
activity as ≥ 0.5 ng/ml ET. Numbers 13 - 15 imply that 5 - 20
mM $NaIO_4$ has < 0.5 ng/ml ET, and numbers 16 - 18 indicates that
the negative result of $NaIO_4$ is not due to nonspecific inhibition by $NaIO_4$ of ET or the LAL reaction.

tated LAL protein (28), or determination of amidase activity
of LAL (29) may provide more sensitive quantitation of ET.
Difficulty with false positives (30) and false negatives has
been minimal in my hands. More precise and accurate quantitation of ET may be available by chemically determining the
presence of fatty acids unique to ET's (31), but the sensitivity is not as great as the LAL bioassay.

B. *Detoxification of ET*

1. *Destruction by Heat*

Endotoxin is resistant to boiling and autoclaving (121°C),
but dry heat at 170°C for 2 - 4 hr destroys the activity of
ET (26). Obviously this is useful only for nonvolatile, non-

combustible materials. All of the glassware used is prepared for tissue culture by washing with detergent, drying, and then baking at 170°C for 4 hr for sterilization and ET inactivation purposes.

2. Detoxification by Alkalai Treatment

Alkalai treatment cleaves the fatty acids from the lipid portion of ET and abolishes lipid A activity (32). In some instances when equipment will not tolerate 170°C (e.g., plastic ware), it can be treated with 1 N NaOH at 56°C for 90 min and then washed with ET-free water.

3. Detoxification by Polymyxin B

The amphipathic polypeptide antibiotic polymyxin B binds to lipid A and prevents its actions (33, 34) (Fig. 1). Inclusion of 1 - 10 µg/ml polymyxin B in *in vitro* experiments can counteract the lipid A effects of ET (10, 34 - 36).

4. Use of Lipid A-Resistant Mouse Strains

Some mouse strains including the C3H/HeJ strain are resistant to the effects of lipid A (37, 38). By using cells from C3H/HeJ mice, one can avoid lipid A effects. However, other components of ET such as the lipid A protein (LAP) affect C3H/HeJ cells as it does cells of lipid A responder mice (39, 40).

Heat at 170°C for 2 - 4 hr and alkali treatment are useful in destroying ET on glassware and other hardware, but they generally are too extreme for use with biological reagents. Although superficially it would appear that by using polymyxin B- and lipid A-unresponsive mice, one could avoid the problems of ET contamination, this is not so (41). ET with LAP does not bind polymyxin B, and ET with LAP effects lymphocytes and macrophages from C3H/HeJ mice (34, 39-41) (Fig. 1). Since the ET-contaminating reagents may be comparable to ET, which is extracted from bacteria by mild means (38, 41, 42), it would likely contain LAP. Therefore, naturally contaminating ET containing LAP would not be inhibited by polymyxin B, and cells of C3H/HeJ would respond to the ET.

C. Endotoxin-Free Tissue Culture Conditions

1. ET-Free Culture Ware

All of the glassware (flasks, beakers, pipettes, etc.) is baked 4 hr at 170°C in metal cannisters (pipettes) or with

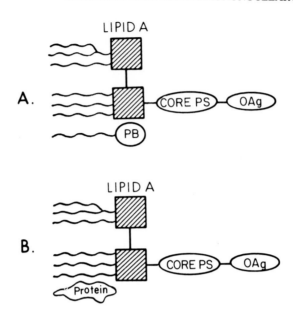

Fig. 1. Diagrammatic representation of endotoxin and lipid A associated protein (B) and endotoxin associating with polymyxin B (A) (45a, 33). The native endotoxin essentially exists as three parts: the polysaccharide (0 antigen), the core polysaccharide containing KDO, and the lipid portion (lipid A), which consists of a diglucosamine backbone with linked fatty acids with or without associated protein. The amount of the hydrophobic lipid A associated protein present in extracted endotoxins depends on the methods used to extract them from the bacteria (38). The endotoxins frequently exist as large polymers. Polymyxin B (PB) is an amphipathic antibiotic, which will bind to lipid A and prevent its biological effects (33, 34). Its binding, however, is apparently inversely proportional to the content of lipid A associated protein, so that endotoxins with a high content of lipid A associated protein are not affected by polymyxin B (40).

aluminum foil covering tops. To date, all sterile plastic ware (Falcon and Costar) I have tested for ET has been negative.

ET-free Water

All liquid tissue culture media that I have bought and tested has contained >1 ng/ml ET (10). Thus, powdered media are formulated with ET-free water and sterilized by filtration. Many water stills (including those produced by Corning, Bellco, and Barnstead) and a filtering-reverse osmosis device provided by Millipore will provide ET-free water. Special care must be taken in maintenance of sterile collection tubings and vessels. Low-volume usage encourages contamination. Some commercial suppliers sell ET-free liquid tissue culture media (e.g., Microbiological Associates).

3. ET-Free Sera

Serum from most commercial suppliers contains ET (10), apparently because of postbleeding contamination. Some serum companies will supply ET-free serum (e.g., Sterile Systems, Inc.). Although serum from portal blood of normal people may contain ET (43), serum from nonportal blood of normal animals is ET-free. Serum from patients with liver disease or sepsis may contain ET (43, 44).

D. Elimination of Contaminating ET

1. Removal by Column Chromatography

Endotoxin (as well as smaller biologically active subunits such as lipid A) exists in aqueous solutions as high molecular weight polymers ($>1 \times 10^6$ dalton) (20, 26, 45, 45a) (see Fig. 1). Thus, sieving chromatography has been used to remove ET from smaller molecular weight substances (10, 20). The difficulty here is to maintain sterile columns to avoid endogenous ET contamination during the procedure.

The column (2.5 × 60 cm glass) is cleaned with detergent, rinsed extensively with ET-free water, dried, assembled, and gas-sterilized with ethylene oxide. Sephadex G-200 gel is boiled, degassed, and poured into the column using sterile technique with the aid of sterile gloves. The column is equilibrated in 0.15 M NaCl, 0.02% sodium azide (as an antibacterial agent), and 5 mM Tris. All procedures are done at 4°C. The void volume (containing the ET) is discarded, and fractions containing the protein of interest are dialyzed against ET-free water, and lyophilized. Figure 2 illustrates the separation of ET from soybean trypsin inhibitor using Sephadex G-200 chromatography.

2. Removal by Ultracentrifugation

Because of the large polymeric nature of ET, it would be expected to sediment at high g forces leaving smaller proteins in suspension. Although others have been able to remove ET from protein solution using this technique (18, 46), I have not been able to.

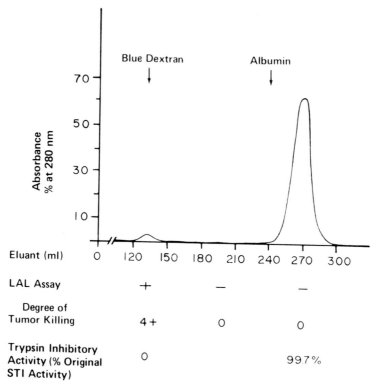

Fig. 2. *Separation of ET from ET-contaminated soybean trypsin inhibitor (STI) by G-200 gel chromatography in 5 mM Tris, 0.15 M NaCl, and 0.02% sodium azide buffer and relationship of separated LPS and STI to macrophage tumor cell killing. Twenty-five milligrams of commercially obtained STI were passed through the 2.5 × 60-cm column at 0.6 ml/min flow rate. Fractions of interest were lyophilized before testing. Nonfractionated STI was positive for ET in the LAL assay at ≥5 µg/ml, whereas fractionated STI (postalbumin fraction) was negative through 1000 µg/ml. The trypsin inhibitory activity of this fraction of STI (tested at 10, 100, and 1000 µg/ml) was unaltered as compared to the nonfractionated STI, whereas no inhibitory activity could be found in the void volume fraction (blue dextran marker). The LAL-negative fraction which contained the trypsin inhibitory activity had no influence on macrophage tumor cell-killing activity (neither enhancing nor inhibitory) when tested at 1 to 1000 g/ml, but the LAL positive void fraction, which contained no trypsin inhibitory activity, made nontumoricidal activated macrophages kill tumor cells in doses as low as 0.5 to 1.0 ng/ml. (From ref. 10, with permission.)*

3. Removal by Ultrafiltration

Variable success has resulted in attempts to remove ET from solutions by ultrafiltration (42, 49 - 52). Theoretically, the large ET aggregates should be retained behind filters with pore sizes of less than 100,000 dalton cutoff, but this is dependent on the solutions used (52). Preliminary studies in my laboratory using Amicon XM100 ultrafiltration membranes indicate the possibility of removing ET effectively by multiple passes through these membranes (Weinberg, Naramore, and Capel, manuscript in preparation).

Although gel chromatography separation of ET from reagents is possible, it is very difficult to maintain ET-free conditions in columns. Important steps are the inclusion of azide as an antibacterial agent, working at 4°C and essentially constant flow of the column buffer when not using the column. Other methods of ET removal have been tried with limited success. In using *Limulus* amebocyte lysate absorption (22, 47), one must cope with incomplete ET removal and inclusion of the LAL into the sample. Polymyxin B affinity columns (48) would not be expected to bind ET containing LAP (see Section III. B. 3). Since erythrocyte membranes bind ET (52a), one might be able to remove ET with erythrocyte absorptions. However, erythrocytes also bind other biological products [including migration inhibitory factor (52a) to type O cells] making accurate interpretations of some experiments difficult. Ultrafiltration may eventually be the most efficient means of removing ET.

IV. CONCLUDING REMARKS

Many reagents used in tissue culture studies of monocytes-macrophages are contaminated with enough ET to effect dramatically monocyte-macrophage function. Table II displays results of LAL testing of various agents. In general, protein reagents usually contain ET, and amino acids and salts are usually ET-free. Proteins purified by routine chromatography have always contained large amounts of ET; the "purer" the protein (the more steps in the purification scheme), the more ET that protein is likely to have.

Figure 2 demonstrates how ET contamination of a reagent can alter interpretation of studies of macrophage-mediated tumor cytotoxicity. Contaminating ET could not only give the false impression that a particular contaminated agent has an enhancing effect on macrophage function (e.g., macrophage-mediated tumor cell killing), but the ET could also mask the suppressive

TABLE II. *Results of LAL Assay on Various Reagents*[a]

Positive		Negative	
1.	Horseradish peroxidase (types II and VI)	16.	Fetal bovine serum (Flow)
2.	Catalase (Sigma)	17.	L-Histine-HCl
3.	Xanthine oxidase (grade IV)	18.	Dimedone
4.	Fetuin (types I and II)	19.	Reduced glutathione (grade IV)
5.	Bovine pancreatic inhibitor (type III)	20.	Sodium periodate
		21.	Imidazole (grade III)
6.	Ovomucoid (type II-O)	22.	Dipalmitoylphosphatidyl-choline
7.	Soybean trypsin inhibitor (type I-S)	23.	Catalase (Boehringer)
8.	Neuraminidase (type VIII)	24.	Phorbol myristate acetate
9.	Hemoglobin (type IV)	25.	Dextran sulfate
10.	Porphobilinogen	26.	Tissue culture media power (Gibco, Flow)
11.	Superoxide dismutase		
12.	α-1-Antitrypsin	27.	Fetal bovine serum (Sterile System)
13.	Bovine serum albumin		
14.	Concanavalin A	28.	Adult bovine serum (Sterile System)
15.	Fetal bovine serum (Gibco)		

[a]Reagents 1 - 10 and 17 - 22 were from Sigma; 11 from Truett Laboratories; 12 and 13 from Miles Laboratories; 14 from Calbiochem; 24 from P-L Biochemicals and Dr. Peter Borchert of Minneapolis, Minnesota; 25 from Pharmacia. 17 - 21 were tested at 5 mM; 26 was tested after formulation with ET-free water; sera were tested after chloroform extraction; all other agents were tested at 1 mg/ml. (Adopted from reference 10, with permission.)

effects of certain agents. In some experiments the effect of the covert ET could be manifested as an inhibition of a certain function (17). In experiments studying macrophage activation for tumor cytotoxicity, ET and lymphocyte-derived macrophage activating factor act synergistically to enhance macrophage tumoricidal activity (10, 53, 54). Amounts of ET that might be inconsequential in some *in vitro* assays could produce dramatic enhancing effects in the presence of macrophage activating factor. Thus, this synergistic activity makes it especially important to use ET-free preparations of lymphokines in studies of macrophage function (54).

   Useful tests to determine if the effects of a particular substance are due to ET include heat sensitivity and inhibita-

TABLE III. Effect of Heat and Polymyxin B (PB) on MAF-
and/or ET-Induced Tumor Cell Killing by BCG Macrophages from
C_3H/HeN Mice[a]

Pretreatment additive[c]	Degree of tumor cell killing[b]	
	0 PB	25 µg/ml PB[d]
Medium (DMEM)	0	0
Macrophage activating factor (MAF)	+++	+++
Heated MAF	0	0
ET	++++	0
Heated ET	++++	0
MAF + ET	++++	++++
Heated MAF + ET	++++	0

[a](3×10^5) peritoneal cells per chamber. From reference
10, with permission.
[b]Tumor cell killing quantitated by visual cell counting.
++++ tumor cell killing signifies 0 to 3 tumor cells/300×
microscopic field; +++, 4 to 14 cells/field; ++, 15 to 25 cells/
field; +, 26 to 36 cells/field; and 0, a multilayer of tumor
cells over the macrophage. For comparison, the initial tumor
cell density (time 0) was 33 to 37 tumor cells/300× field.
[c]Macrophages treated at 37°C for 2 hr with additives and
then additives removed and macrophages challenged with tumor
cells. MAF 5%, ET 100 ng/ml. Heating at 80°C for 10 min.
[d]Polymyxin B present in 2-hr pretreatment only.

bility by polymyxin B (10, 41). Table III shows how heat and
polymyxin B help distinguish between the effects of ET and
macrophage-activating factor in assays of macrophage-mediated
tumor cell killing. If heating an agent to temperature known
to denature or inactivate it does not change its effect on
macrophage function, the effect is probably due to contaminating
ET. If the effect of an agent can be blocked by polymyxin B,
that effect is most likely due to ET. However, the effects of
ET-contaminated agents that are not inhibitable by polymyxin B
could still be due to the contaminating ET with high LAP content, since ET with LAP is not inhibited by polymyxin B. For
practical purposes, meaningful evaluations of the effects of
agents on macrophage function can only be obtained when those
agents are free of ET as determined by the LAL assay.
    Although maintenance of ET-free culture conditions dra-
matically increases the work and complexity of operations, it
is necessary for the accurate interpretation of in vitro experiments investigating monocyte-macrophage function.

REFERENCES

1. D. C. Morrison and L. F. Kline. Activation of the classical and properdin pathways of complement by bacterial lipopolysaccharide (LPS). *J. Immunol. 118*: 362-368, 1977.

2. V. E. Gilbert and A. I. Braude. Reduction of serum complement in rabbits after injection of endotoxin. *J. Exp. Med. 116*: 477-490, 1962.

3. A. Vaheri, E. Ruoslahti, M. Sarvas, and M. Nurminen. Mitogenic effect by lipopolysaccharide and pokeweed lectin on density-inhibited chick embryo fibroblasts. *J. Exp. Med. 138*: 1356-1364, 1973.

4. A. McGivney and S. G. Bradley. Effects of bacterial endotoxin on lysosomal and mitochondrial enzyme activities of established cell cultures. *J. Reticuloendothel. Soc. 26*: 307-316, 1979.

5. H. S. Rubenstein, J. Fine, and A. H. Coons. Localization of endotoxin in the walls of the peripheral vascular system during lethol endotoxenus. *Proc. Soc. Exp. Biol. Med. 111*: 458-467, 1962.

6. K. W. Brunson and G. L. Nicolson. Lipopolysaccharide effects on sensitive and resistant variant chinese hamster ovary cell lines. *J. Supramolec. Structr. 9*: 231-242, 1978.

7. J. Andersson, F. Melchers, C. Galanos, and O. Luderity. The mitogenic effect of lipopolysaccharide on bone-marrow-derived mouse lymphocytes. Lipid A as the mitogenic part of the molecule. *J. Exp. Med. 137*: 943-953, 1973.

8. P. Alexander and R. Evans. Endotoxin and double-stranded RNA render macrophages cytotoxic. *Nature (New Biol.) 232*: 76-78, 1971.

9. J. B. Hibbs, Jr., R. R. Taintor, H. A. Chapman, Jr., and J. B. Weinberg. Macrophage tumor killing: Influence of the local environment. *Science 197*: 279-282, 1977.

10. J. B. Weinberg, H. A. Chapman, Jr., and J. B. Hibbs, Jr. Characterization of the effects of endotoxin on macrophage tumor cell killing. *J. Immunol. 121*: 72-80, 1978.

11. S. W. Russel, W. F. Doe, and A. T. McIntosh. Functional characterization of a stable, noncytolytic stage of macrophage activation in tumors. *J. Exp. Med. 146*: 1511-1520, 1977.

12. Anon. Revised nomenclature for antigen-nonspecific T cell proliferation and helper factors. *J. Immunol. 123*: 2928-2929, 1979.

13. I. Gery and B. H. Waksman. Potentiation of lymphocyte responses to mitogens. II. The cellular source of potentiating mediators. *J. Exp. Med. 136*: 143-155, 1972.

14. W. I. Cranston. Central mechanisms of fever. *Fed. Proc.* *38*: 49-51, 1979.

15. J. M. Dayer, J. H. Passwell, E. E. Schneeberger, and S. M. Krane. Interactions among rheumatoid synovial cells and monocyte-macrophages; production of collagenase-stimulating factor by human monocytes exposed to concanavalin A or immunoglobulin Fc fragments. *J. Immunol.* *124*: 1712-1720, 1980.

16. F. R. Rickles, J. Levin, J. A. Hardin, C. F. Barr, and M. E. Conrad, Jr. Tissue factor generation by human mononuclear cells: Effects of endotoxin and dissociation of tissue factor generation from mitogenic response. *J. Lab. Clin. Med.* 89: 792-803, 1977.

17. H. A. Chapman, Jr., Z. Vavrin, and J. B. Hibbs, Jr. Modulation of plasminogen activator secretion by activated macrophages: Influence of serum factors and correlation with tumoricidal potential. *Proc. Nat. Acad. Sci.* 76: 3899-3903, 1979.

18. H. F. Dvorak and R. C. Bast, Jr. Nature of the immunogen in crystalline serum albumins. *Immunochemistry* 7: 118-124, 1970.

19. K. W. Brunson and D. W. Watson. Concanavalin A preparations with activities related to bacterial lipopolysaccharide. *J. Immunol.* 115: 599-600, 1975.

20. M. Loos, S. Vadlamudi, M. Meltzer, S. Shifrin, T. Borsos, and A. Goldin. Detection of endotoxin in commercial L-aspariginase preparation by complement fixation and separation by chromatography. *Cancer Res.* 32: 2292-2296, 1972.

21. L. Z. Bito. Inflammatory effects of endotoxin-like contaminants in commonly used protein preparations. *Science* *196*: 83-85, 1977.

22. S. E. Graber, J. D. Bomboy, Jr., W. D. Salmon, Jr., and S. B. Krantz. Evidence that endotoxin is the cyclic 3':5'-GMP-promoting factor in erythroprotein preparations. *J. Lab. Clin. Med.* 93: 25-31, 1979.

23. D. Fumarola and E. Jirillo. Endotoxin contamination of some commercial preparations used in experimental research. *In* "Biomedical Applications of the Horseshoe Crab (Limulidae)" (E. Cohen, F. B. Bang, J. Levin, J. J. Marchalonis, T. G. Pistole, R. A. Prendergrast, C. Shuster, Jr., and S. W. Watson, eds.), pp. 379-385. Alan R. Liss, New York, 1979.

24. J. Levin, P. A. Tomasulo, and R. S. Oser. Detection of endotoxin in human blood and demonstration of an inhibitor. *J. Lab. Clin. Med.* 75: 903-911, 1970.

25. J. J. Corrigan, Jr., and J. F. Kiernat. Effect of polymyxin B sulfate on endotoxin activity in a gram-negative septicemia model. *Pediat. Res.* 13: 48-51, 1979.

26. K. C. Milner, J. A. Rudbach, and E. Ribi. Bacterial endotoxins. General characteristics. *In* "Microbial Toxins IV" (G. Weinbaum, S. Kadis, and S. I. Ajl, eds.), pp. 1-65. Academic Press, New York, 1971.

27. V. P. Hollander and W. C. Harding. A sensitive spectrophotometric method for measurement of plasma endotoxin. *Biochem. Med. 15*: 28-33, 1976.

28. R. Nandan and D. R. Brown. An improved *in vitro* pyrogen test: To detect picograms of endotoxin contamination in intravenous fluids using *Limulus* amebocyte lysate. *J. Lab. Clin. Med. 89*: 910-918, 1977.

29. T. Harada, T. Morita, S. Iwanga, S. Nakamura, and M. Neiva. A new chromogenic substrate method for assay of bacterial endotoxins using *Limulus* hemocyte lysate. *In* "Biomedical Applications of the Horseshoe Crab *(Limulidae)*" (E. Cohen, F. B. Bang, J. Levin, J. J. Marchalonis, T. G. Pistole, R. A. Prendergrast, C. Shuster, Jr., and S. W. Watson, eds.), pp. 209-220. Alan R. Liss, New York, 1979.

30. R. J. Elin and S. M. Wolff. Nonspecificity of the *Limulus* amebocyte lysate test: Positive reactions with polynucleotides and proteins. *J. Infect. Dis. 128*: 349-352, 1973.

31. S. K. Maitra, M. C. Schotz, T. T. Yoshikawa, and L. B. Guze. Determination of lipid A and endotoxin in serum by mass spectroscopy. *Proc. Nat. Acad. Sci. 75*: 3993-3997, 1978.

32. D. Tripodi and A. Nowotny. Relation of structure to function in bacterial O-antigens. V. Nature of active sites in endotoxic lipopolysaccharides of *Serratia marcescens*. *Ann. NY Acad. Sci. 133*: 604-621, 1966.

33. D. C. Morrison and D. M. Jacobs. Binding of polymyxin B to the lipid A portion of bacterial lipopolysaccharides. *Immunochemistry 13*: 813-818, 1976.

34. D. M. Jacobs and D. C. Morrison. Inhibition of the mitogenic response to lipopolysaccharide (LPS) in mouse spleen cells by polymyxin B. *J. Immunol. 118*: 21-27, 1977.

35. W. F. Doe, S. T. Yang, D. C. Morrison, S. J. Betz, and P. M. Henson. Macrophage stimulation by bacterial lipopolysaccharides. II. Evidence for independent differentiation signals delivered by lipid A and a protein rich fraction of LPS. *J. Exp. Med. 148*: 557-568, 1978.

36. L. P. Ruco and M. S. Meltzer. Macrophage activation for tumor cytotoxicity: Tumoricidal activity by macrophages from C3H/HeJ mice requires at least two activation stimuli. *Cell. Immunol. 41*: 35-51, 1978.

37. B. M. Sultzer. Genetic control of leucocyte responses to endotoxin. *Nature 219*: 1253-1254, 1968.

38. B. J. Skidmore, D. C. Morrison, J. M. Chiller, and W. O. Weigle. Immunologic properties of lipopolysaccharide

(LPS). II. The unresponsiveness of C3H/HeJ mouse spleen
cells to LPS-induced mitogenesis is dependent on the
method used to extract LPS. *J. Exp. Med. 142*: 1488-1508,
1975.

39. B. M. Sultzer and G. W. Goodman. Endotoxin protein: A
B-cell mitogen and polyclonal activator of C3H/HeJ lymphocytes. *J. Exp. Med. 144*: 821-827, 1976.

40. D. C. Morrison, S. J. Betz, and D. M. Jacobs. Isolation
of a lipid A bound polypeptide responsible for "LPS-
initiated" mitogenesis of C3H/HeJ spleen cells. *J. Exp.
Med. 144*: 840-846, 1976.

41. D. C. Morrison and B. J. Curry. The use of polymyxin B
and C3H/HeJ mouse spleen cells as criteria for endotoxin
contamination. *J. Immunol. Meth. 27*: 83-92, 1979.

42. D. C. Morrison and L. Leive. Isolation of lipopolysaccharides from bacteria. *Methods Enzymol. 28B*: 254-
262, 1972.

43. H. Ravin, D. Rowley, C. Jenkins, and J. Fine. On the
absorption of bacterial endotoxin from the gastrointes-
tinal tract of the normal and shocked animal. *J. Exp.
Med. 112*: 783-792, 1960.

44. J. Levin. The *Limulus* test: A status report. *In*
"Biomedical Applications of the Horseshoe Crab *(Limulidae)*"
(E. Cohen, F. B. Bang, J. Levin, J. J. Marchalonis, T. T.
Pistole, R. A. Prendergrast, C. Shuster, Jr., and S. W.
Watson, eds.), pp. 235-244. Alan R. Liss, New York, 1979.

45. J. A. Cameron. Bacterial lipopolysaccharide as a void
volume marker for agarose gel permeation chromatography.
J. Chromatogr. 37: 331-332, 1968.

45a. C. Galanos, O. Luderitz, E. T. Rietschel, and O. Westpal.
Newer aspects of the chemistry and biology of bacterial
lipopolysaccharides, with special reference to their
lipid A component. *Int. Rev. Biochem. 14*: 239-335, 1977.

46. R. K. Shadduck, A. Waheed, A. Porcellini, V. Rizzoli, and
J. Levin. A method for removal of endotoxin from purified
colony stimulating factor. *Proc. Soc. Exp. Biol. Med.
164*: 40-50, 1980.

47. S. E. Siegel, N. Shore, J. Ortega, and P. P. Dukes. Removal of endotoxin (pyrogen) from erythropoietin by
Limulus amebocyte lysate. *Fed. Proc. 33*: 608, 1974.

48. D. C. Morrison, J. F. Roser, C. G. Cochrane, and P. M.
Henson. The initiation of mast cell degranulation: Activation of the cell membrane. *J. Immunol. 114*: 966-970,
1975.

49. J. C. Craddock, L. A. Guder, D. L. Francis, and S. L.
Morgan. Reduction of pyrogens-application of molecular
filtration. *J. Pharm. Pharmacol. 30*: 198-199, 1978.

50. J. Hattingh, H. Laburn, and D. Mitchell. Fever induced
in rabbits by intravenous injection of bovine serum

albumin. *J. Physiol.* *290*: 69-77, 1979.

51. L. W. Henderson and E. Beans. Successful production of sterile pyrogen-free electrolyte solution by ultrafiltration. *Kidney Int.* *14*: 522-525, 1978.

52. K. J. Sweadner, M. Forte, and L. L. Nelson. Filtration removal of endotoxin (pyrogens) in solution in different states of aggregation. *Appl. Environ. Microbiol.* *34*: 382-385, 1977.

52a. G. F. Springer, J. C. Adye, A. Bezkorovainy, and B. Jirgensons. Properties and activity of the lipopolysaccharide-receptor from human erythrocytes. *Biochemistry* *13*: 1379, 1974.

52b. R. A. Fox, J. M. MacSween, and R. L. McGuire. Potentiation of the macrophage response to migration inhibition factor from fetal calf serum by blood group substances with human H activity. *Scand. J. Immunol.* *5*: 941, 1976.

17

CONTINUOUS CELL LINES WITH PROPERTIES OF MONONUCLEAR PHAGOCYTES

Peter Ralph

I. GENERAL INTRODUCTION

The creation of the murine IC-21 macrophage line 10 years ago, reviewed by Defendi (1), ushered in a new era in the study of mononuclear phagocytes. Many other lines have since been discovered including immature myeloblast lines, such as M1, in which some mature macrophage characteristics can be induced (2). This resource has now been introduced into most areas of re-search in the field. Many of the lines were derived from his-tiocytic tumors and maintain tumorigenicity. However, their popularity lies in their convenience as sources of pure popula-tions of macrophages and in the great range of macrophage-specific properties manifested.

The cell lines can be easily maintained by laboratory per-sonnel familiar with tissue culture methods. The lines differ in degree of maturity and functional properties, but almost all macrophage characteristics have been found in one or more of the lines. Most of the lines available are from the mouse, but

TABLE I. *Characterized monocyte - macrophage cell lines*

Name	Strain[a]	Etiology[b]	Biochemical properties[d,f,g]							RBC[e,f,h]		Ref.
			Lysozyme enzyme	Neutral proteases	Endogenous pyrogen	$\overline{O_2}$	PGE	CSF	LAF	Ingestion	Lysis	
Murine, immature												
M1	SL	S	+									2
R453	B	R-MuLV										9
RAW8	C	A-MuLV			+							8
Murine, mature												
IC-21	B	SV40[c]								+	+	1
M2	B/10	SV40[c]	+	+						+	+	12
WEHI-3	C	S	+	+	+	-		+		(+)	-	13
J774	C	Oil	+	+	+	+	+	+		+	(+)	13
P338D1	DBA/2	S?	+	+	+	+	+	+	+	+	+	14
FC-1	C	Fusion[c]	+	+				+		+	(+)	15
PU5-1.8	C	S?	+	+	+			+		+	(+)	13
RAW264	BAB/14	A-MuLV	+	+	+	+	+	+	+	+	+	13
SK2.2	CBA/J	S[c]					+	+		(+)	+	5
426C	DBA/2	OS virus[c]								+	(+)	5
427E	BDF₁	F-MuLV[c]								(+)	+	5
Human, immature												
U937		DHL	+	-	+	+	-	-		i	i	10

^{a} B, C57BL/6; C, BALB/c; B/10 = C57BL/10; D, DBA/2.

^{b}Tumors, except as noted. S, spontaneous; R-MuLV, Rauscher murine leukemia virus; A, Abelson; OS, osteogenic sarcoma; F, Friend; DHL, diffus histiocytic lymphoma.

^{c}Experimental infections or spontaneous outgrowth in culture.

^{d}Lysosomal enzymes (β-glucuronidase, arylsulfatase, acid phosphatase), neutral proteases, (plasminogen activator, collagenase, elastase), endogenous pyrogen; O_2^- superoxide anion; PGE, prostaglandin E; CSF, granulocyte/macrophage colony-stimulating factor; LAF, thymus lymphocyte-activating factor. Lines may require stimulation with LPS, phorbol myristate, etc., for measurable activity.

^{e}Antibody-dependent phagocytosis or lysis of chicken or sheep red blood cells (RBC). ^{i}, Requires activation by lymphokine for activity.

^{f}Blank, not tested. $-$, No activity under basal conditions or with some stimulating agents effective with other lines.

^{g}See, in addition, references 12, 16 - 28.

^{h}See, in addition, references 10, 13, 14, 15, 29, 30.

rabbit (3), hamster (4), and human (Table I) monocyte-related lines have also been described. Their potential goes far beyond being a convenient source of macrophages. The cell lines are unique for biochemical, immunological, development, and regulation studies in which the absence of other cell types is essential. The continuous growth of the cell lines allows selection of variants with altered macrophage properties for physiological studies during different stages of the cell cycle. Functions of macrophage cell lines have been recently reviewed (5, 5a).

II.   FUNCTIONAL TYPES OF MACROPHAGE CELL LINES

A.   *Constitutive Properties of Macrophage Cell Lines*

Extensively characterized cell lines are listed in Table I. Generally all lines express receptors for complement and for the Fc domain of IgG immunoglobulin (6), phagocytose latex beads and zymosan particles (7), and synthesize and secrete lysozyme (8). Lines designated immature usually express these functions only after incubation with colony-stimulating factor/ macrophage growth factor (CSF/MGF) or a variety of other agents presumably acting via induction of CSF/MGF (2, 9 - 11). Other macrophage-type characteristics found in most of the mature lines tested include several lysosomal enzymes and neutral proteases, endogenous pyrogen, nitroblue tetrazoleum reduction and O_2^- production. Prostaglandins, lymphocyte comitogen, and separate granulocyte and macrophage colony-stimulating factors (31) are also produced. Some of the cell lines (Table II) are positive for peroxidase, lipogenic enzymes, migration in response to chemotactic factors, spontaneous migration sensitive to MIF, and regulation by and receptors for corticosteroids and insulin. The lines have variable amounts of ectoenzymes and adenosine deaminase reported to be correlated with macrophage maturation or activation and display macrophage-specific antigen recognized by a hybridoma antibody and an antigen present only on activated macrophages. PU5-1.8 produces interferon in response to pI:C (41). Most of the mature lines mediate antibody-dependent phagocytosis and, by a different mechanism (42), exocytolysis of erythrocytes (Table I).

B.   *Tumor Cytotoxicity and Activation of Macrophage Cell Lines*

The activity of the mature lines appears to be intermediate between that of resident peritoneal cells and stimulated exudate

TABLE II. Specialized properties studied in macrophage cell lines[a]

Line	Peroxidase (9,18,32)	Lipogenic enzymes (33)	Chemotaxis (17)	MIF Sensitivity (34)	Corticosteroid regulation (13,20,21, 35,36)	insulin regulation (37,68)
R453	+					
M1		+			+	
IC-21						
WEHI-3	+				+	
J774			+	–	+	+
P388D1			–	–	+	+
FC-1				+		
PU5-1.8					+	
RAW264					+	
U937	+					

[a]Numbers in parenthesis are references
[b]Mφ, macrophage.

Ectoenzymes (38)
Adenosine deaminase (17)
Mφ[b] antigen (19,39)
Act. Mφ antigen (40)

macrophages, having a moderate basal level of secretion of lysosomal enzymes and neutral proteases. The expression of
these products and also of prostaglandin E, myeloid-CSF, mega-
karyocyte-CSF and - potentiation factors (19, 43), and LAF can
be greatly augmented by incubation with LPS, phorbol myristate,
and other stimulators. Production of myeloid CSF by the
PU5-1.8 line with LPS, and probably by several other lines with
a variety of stimulators (26), is a true induction since CSF is
normally undetectable, requires new protein and RNA synthesis,
and takes several days for full expression (44). Latex bead
phagocytosis and antibody-dependent lysis of RBC by line PU5-1.8
is stimulated twofold by LPS and tuberculin PPD (13, 45). J774
phagocytosis via C3 receptors is stimulated by LPS (46).

Cytotoxic activity against tumor targets is summarized in
Table III. Some lines, such as WEHI-3, show no activity for a
number of assays and targets tested. Spontaneous cytotoxicity
in apparent absence of activating agents is manifested by
several lines against some T and B lymphoid tumors, a myeloblast
leukemia, and transformed fibroblasts. Soluble factors released
by several lines are toxic to lymphoid RBL-5 and fibroblast 7943
targets (48, 49). Most tumor targets tested were not sensitive
to this spontaneous lytic mechanism, including the NK-sensitive
K562 line (19). Antibody-dependent killing occurs in several
macrophage lines against mouse and human lymphoid tumors
(Table III).

Lymphokine stimulation of cytotoxicity is expressed against
hemic and fibroblast targets, as well as killing induced or augmented by microbial, polysaccharide, and polynucleotide agents.
Generally, the same macrophage lines, particularly PU5-1.8 and
RAW264, are active in all systems. However, for certain pairs
of effector lines and tumor targets, an unexpected lack of cytotoxic effect suggests that macrophage lines have different
lytic mechanisms, depending on the tumor target and method of
activation (75). Among biochemical mechanisms proposed for
macrophage toxicity, O_2^- and H_2O_2 are unlikely to be responsible
for line J774 killing of tumor and RBC targets, since two variant
clones selected for undetectable extracellular production of
these oxygen metabolites (52) have full lytic activity (51).

C. Macrophage Cell Lines--Regulation of Lymphocyte Immune Responses

Several murine macrophage lines replace normal adherent
cells in induction of spleen cells to allogeneic T killers or
antibody to sheep RBC. Both of these effects are largely a
mercaptoethanol-replacing function. Soluble factors produced
by macrophage lines, for which mercaptoethanol will not substitute, induce spontaneous induction of T killers (53),

TABLE III. *Cytotoxic activity of macrophage cell lines toward tumor targets*

Line	Spontaneous	Antibody dependent	Lymphokine dependent[a]	Microbial/other stimulus[b]
IC21	+		+	− −
WEHI-3	−	− −	−	− +
J774	+ (+) (+)	− −	+ (+)	− (+)
P388D₁	(+) (+)	−	(+)	+ +
PU5-1.8	(+) + +	+ +	+ +	+ +
RAW264	(+) + +	+ +	+	+ − +
U837	−	i −	−	−
Target	M1 RBL-5 RBL-2 7943	CEM EL4 18-8 18-8	RBL-5 SV-3T3 CEM P815→ SL2	M1 RBL-5 CEM P815
type[c]	m,ℓ ℓ ℓ f	i[d] ℓ ℓ ℓ	ℓ f ℓ ℓ,m	m ℓ ℓ m
Ref.	75 47 48 49	10 13 50 75	5 51 47 35 48	75 13 47 48

[a] Con A or secondary antigen stimulation of spleen cells, or leukocyte-interferon preparation.
Blank = Not tested.
[b] LPS, PPD, Muramyl dipeptide, poly(I:C), zymosan, dextran sulfate, C. parvum or BCG stimulation in vitro.
[c] m, myeloid (tranulocyte/monocyte); ℓ, lymphocyte; f, fibroblast.
[d] i, activity induced by lymphokine, targets: TNP-modified HSB, EL4, RL ♂ 1, MOLT4.

replace T cells and macrophages in induction of antibody (54),
and stimulate human IgG production (55). In some cases the
cell lines themselves need to be incubated with inducing agents,
such as LPS or *Mycobacterium* BCG, to produce factors stimulating
the immune responses. No macrophage line has been found to display Ia surface antigens, which is the phenotype for accessory
cells that present antigen to B and T lymphocytes. Five lines
tested failed to present antigen for proliferation of primed T
cells (5, 56).

III. DERIVATION AND REPOSITORY OF CULTURE-ADAPTED MACROPHAGE
      LINES

A. *Adaptation of Murine Macrophage Tumors to Culture*

     Most of the lines listed in Table I arose as tumors in
mice. The first step for adaptation to growth in culture is
usually to obtain passage of the tumor as ascites cells upon
intraperitoneal (ip) injection. This is favorable to culture
growth for hemic tumor lines in general, simplifies handling,
and allows facile comparison with peritoneal macrophages (57).
Ascites cells collected sterilely are washed twice with a
balanced salt solution (BSS) and cultured at 1 - 2 × 10^6/ml in
a rich medium (see Section IV). Five to 10 vessels, e.g.,
petri dishes, are preferable to a single large one in case
some become contaminated. Large numbers of RBC in the ascites
can be removed by several low-speed centrifugations that leave
most of the RBC in the supernatant. Alternatively, the cell
pellet can be suspended in 1 - 2 ml H_2O and then 10 ml BSS
added after 30 sec. This lyses the RBC leaving the macrophage
cells viable and still functional, e.g., in antibody-dependent
lysis and phagocytosis of RBC. Up to 10 RBC per tumor cell can
be tolerated. Usually 90% of tumor cells will die during the
next few days in culture. Half the culture supernate should be
replaced with fresh medium twice a week, or more often if there
is extensive metabolism seen by change in the phenol red indicator to acid yellow. If considerable death occurs, cells
should be harvested, centrifuged, and recultured at higher cell
densities between 3 and 10 × 10^5/ml.
     If cells appear to be dying rapidly, or if a microbial con-
tamination occurs that cannot be eliminated with antibiotics,
the cells can be transplanted back into a mouse of original
strain. Priming mice with 1 ml mineral oil or pristane ip on,
or up to 1 month before, the day of tumor cell inoculation, appears to aid macrophage as well as myeloma and Abelson lymphoma
tumor growth (58). Several cycles of cell culture/*in vivo*

growth may be necessary before obtaining growth *in vitro*. As lines adapt to culture, viable cells will increase in number with population doubling times of 1 - 7 days. This will allow periodic splitting, making two cultures from one. Culturing on a sparse feeder layer of normal fibroblasts may be beneficial. Ascitic forms of cell lines already adapted to culture will begin rapid growth within several days of *in vitro* culture.

B. *Human Macrophagelike Cell Lines*

The human line U937 came from pleural effusion of a patient with diffuse histiocytic lymphoma. It was adapted to culture using special techniques, including feeder layers of normal human glial cells (32). Most tumors typed morphologically as histiocytic are actually of lymphoid origin, and no generalization can be made about the possibility of obtaining more human macrophage-related lines. Cell lines from histiocytic lymphoma (59), myeloid and monocytic leukemia (18, 60-64), and Hodgkin's disease (23, 65) have been obtained with some macrophagelike characteristics. However, each of these lines has characteristics either incompatible with the monocyte lineage or else more akin to granulocytes. The myeloblast line HL-60 can be induced for phagocytosis and macrophagelike enzyme activities (66), and may be a model for the common precursor of granulocytes and monocytes similar to the murine M1 line (2).

C. *In Vitro Derivation of Macrophage Cell Lines*

The first macrophage lines to be described were obtained by SV40 virus transformation *in vitro* (1). The key to this method is the use of a growth factor to induce cell division prior to viral infection (1, 12). In principle, macrophage lines could be obtained from any species using similar methods and suitable transforming viruses. Another murine line is FC-1 developed during an experimental fusion of a myeloma with spleen cells, which has many of the properties of macrophages (12, 15, 34). Long-term cultures of peritoneal or spleen cells have occasionally yielded permanent macrophage lines (30). The introduction of conditions for maintaining pluripotent bone marrow stem cell replication and differentiation into myeloid and monocyte lineages (67) has led to a number of macrophage lines as spontaneous outgrowths or during RNA viral infections (30).

D. *Repository of Murine Macrophage Lines*

Cell lines WEHI-3, J774, P388D1, PU5-1.8, and RAW264, covering a variety of macrophage properties, are maintained under a contract from the National Cancer Institute by Cell Distribution Center, The Salk Institute for Biological Studies, San Diego, California.

IV. CULTURE GROWTH CONDITIONS FOR MACROPHAGE CELL LINES

A. *Introduction*

Lines have been maintained in culture in a variety of ways depending on the preference of the investigator and beliefs about how to maintain strong expression of the macrophage property being studied. I will describe methods used in our laboratory that allow cell doubling times from 16 to 24 hr (20 - 30 hr for human U937), maximum cell numbers of $1 - 2 \times 10^6$/ml, and relatively constant expression of lysozyme, Fc, and C receptors, phagocytosis of latex beads and RBC, and tumor toxicity.

B. *Reagents*

1. *Fetal Calf Serum*

Fetal calf serum is available from Associated Biomedic Systems, Buffalo, New York; Flow Laboratories, Rockville, Maryland; GIBCO, Grand Island, New York; Microbiological Associates, Bethesda, Maryland; and Sterile Systems, Logan, Utah. All these sources have been suitable, but each serum lot has to be tested for good cell growth. Heat inactivation is unnecessary. Screening or irradiation for mycoplasma is prudent, but has not been necessary for mouse lines.

2. *Media*

Media used are MEM alpha (GIBCO, without nucleosides), RPMI 1640, or McCoy's 5A (available from several vendors, also as powdered formulations). The lines will grow in other media, such as Dulbecco's MEM, but seem to grow faster in a richer medium.

C. Procedure

Mature macrophage lines, in contrast to lymphoid cell lines, will remain viable for a week or more at saturating densities ($1 - 2 \times 10^6$/ml). However, for most studies cultures should be kept at lower concentrations, allowing logarithmic growth, or else fed three times a week. Lines can be subcultured by diluting the cells 1 : 10 or 1 : 100 into fresh media. Population doubling times should be 16 - 24 hr. At dilution to low cell concentrations, there may be a lag before initiation of rapid growth. The all-purpose medium is RPMI 1640, 10% fetal calf serum, with 20 mg L-glutamine per 100 ml added within 2 weeks of use. Penicillin (50 U/ml) and streptomycin (50 µg/ml) are useful in preventing microbial contaminations; 50 µg/ml Gentamicin (Schering Corp.) may be substituted as a more stable antibiotic with a broader spectrum of activity. In cases of fungal contamination, Fungizone (E. R. Squibb & Sons) at 2 - 5 µg/ml is suitable. Cells are grown in plastic petri dishes in volumes of 2 ml (e.g., Falcon Plastics No. 1008), 5 ml (No. 1007), 20 ml (No. 1005), or 100 ml (No. 1013). Petri dishes must be kept in a humidified 37°C incubator with 5 - 10% CO_2 - air. Closed flasks with cells maintained above 5×10^5/ml will generate enough CO_2 to maintain proper pH conditions without external CO_2. If cultured in glass or plastic tissue culture dishes (Falcon 3000 series), or flasks, cells of some lines will bind tightly to the substrate, spread out, grow slowly, and yield less than 30% of petri dish saturation densities. This may be an advantage for certain studies on macrophage physiology (68). Large volume spinner cultures have been used with macrophage cell lines (40).

D. Harvesting Macrophage Cell Lines

With plastic petri dishes, or flasks in most cases, the majority of cells can be harvested by vigorous pipetting. For complete single cell recovery without compromising viability or other functions, the petri dishes or flasks are scraped with a rubber policeman. Other methods of harvesting which may be necessary in special situations include the use of 0.125% trypsin (47) or 12 mM lidocaine (69).

E. Critical Comments

1. Mycoplasma Contamination

This contaminant may coexist with cell lines for years and be a scientific problem only in certain kinds of experiments.

However, since this represents an unknown variable, it is important to assay cultures for mycoplasma and replace contaminated cultures with axenic ones whenever possible. See (70) for further details.

2. *Stability of Cell Line Characteristics*

Long-term transplantable tumors and cell lines frequently drift away from a parental or normal phenotype over a period of years. Drift or selection of variants due to different culture conditions employed by each laboratory is a common problem and emphasizes the need to keep early freezings for reference and the desirability for frequent exchanges with other investigators. The occasional contamination of a cell line with another line that outgrows the first points out the need for caution, especially if a new morphology or other property appears in a culture. It cannot be assumed that a cell line obtained from laboratory A will be identical in all properties to that described in publications from laboratory B.

V.   UNIQUE USES OF MACROPHAGE CELL LINES

Macrophage cell lines offer several unique contributions to the science of mononuclear phagocytes. They are not contaminated by any other cell types. They are engaged in rapid cell division and can be cloned. Each line represents a subtype of normal macrophages ranging from very immature to well differentiated. Table IV lists results obtained using cell lines, which could not be derived from normal macrophage sources with the present technology. These studies include findings that macrophage subsets have separate, specific receptors for a number of immunostimulatory agents; they differ in sensitivity to the inhibitory effects of corticosteroids, and they differ in a number of other properties including antibody-dependent lysis and phagocytosis of targets. Heteroantiserum made against a cell line has been reported to be specific for tumoricidal, activated macrophages after suitable absorption with resident peritoneal cells or nontumoricidal, stimulated macrophages. Most of these experiments would be very difficult with normal sources of macrophages due to extensive heterogeneity in cell types.

Due to the fact that the lines are growing rapidly, it is possible to select for a loss or alteration in a physiological trait. Thus, variants for phagocytosis [and correction of the defect by cyclic AMP elevating agents (68)], for immunoglobulin receptors, and for NBT reduction have been described (Table IV).

TABLE IV. Special uses of macrophage cell lines

Property	Reference
Differential sensitivity to growth inhibition and CSA induction by LPS, PPD, zymosan, and dextran sulfate	26
Differences in immune effector functions	See Table III
Differences in expression and inducibility of neutral proteases	20, 21
Differences in sensitivity to corticosteroids	13, 20, 21
Separate receptors for immunoglobulin subclasses	69, 71, 72, 76
Variants defective in receptors for immunoglobulins	15, 73, 76
Phagocytosis and lysis of RBC directed by antibodies of all 4 mouse IgG classes	77
Variants defective in phagocytosis	15, 68
Variants defective in NBT reduction and O_2^- production	52
Cell cycle analysis of endocytosis	74

Variants lacking superoxide anion production can kill tumor targets as well as the parental cell line (51). There is also the possibility, due to their rapid growth, of selecting synchronized populations of cell lines for study of the effect of position in the cell cycle on macrophage functions.

REFERENCES

1. V. Defendi. Macrophage cell lines and their uses in immunobiology. *In* "Immunobiology of the Macrophage" (D. S. Nelson, ed.), pp. 275-290. Academic Press, New York, 1976.

2. L. Sachs. Control of normal cell differentiation and the phenotypic reversion of malignancy in the myeloid leukaemia. *Nature (London)* 274: 535-539, 1978.

3. M. Mangkornkanok, A. S. Maskowitz, and J. A. Esterly. Establishment of replicating long-term lines of rabbit macrophages and lymphocytes. *J. Immunol. Methods* 7: 327-336, 1975.

4. I. Miyoshi, S. Hiraki, I. Kubonishi, Y. Matsuda, R. Nakayama, H. Kishimoto, H. Masuji, and I. Kimura. Establishment and characterization of two hamster macrophage cell lines. *Cancer Lett.* 4: 253-257, 1978.

5. P. Ralph. Functions of macrophage cell lines. *In* "Mono-

nuclear Phagocytes - Functional Aspects" (R. van Furth, ed.) pp. 439-456. Martinius Nijhoff, The Hague, 1980.

5a. W. S. Walker. Phenotype of mouse macrophagelike cell lines. *J. Reticuloendothel. Soc. 27*: 228, 1980.

6. P. Ralph, I. Nakoinz, H. E. Broxmeyer, and S. Schrader. Immunological functions and *in vitro* activation of cultured macrophage tumor lines. *J. Natl. Cancer Inst. Monogr. 48*: 303-310, 1978.

7. P. Ralph and I. Nakoinz. Direct toxic effects of immuno-potentiators on monocytic, myelomonocytic, and histiocytic tumor cells in culture. *Cancer Res. 37*: 546-550, 1977.

8. P. Ralph, M. A. S. Moore, and K. Nilsson. Lysozyme synthesis by established human and murine histiocytic lymphoma cell lines. *J. Exp. Med. 143*: 1528-1533, 1976.

9. Y. Ichikawa, M. Maeda, and M. Horiuchi. *In vitro* differentiation of Rauscher virus-induced myeloid leukemia cells. *Int. J. Cancer 17*: 789-797, 1976.

10. H. S. Koren, S. J. Anderson, and J. W. Larrick. *In vitro* activation of a human macrophage-like cell line. *Nature (London) 279*: 328-331, 1979.

11. Y. Honma, T. Kasukabe, and M. Hozumi. Production of differentiation-stimulating factor in cultured mouse myeloid leukemia cells treated with glucocorticoids. *Exp. Cell Res. 111*: 261-267, 1978.

12. B. R. Bloom, B. Diamond, R. Muschel, N. Rosen, J. Schneck, G. Damiani, O. Rosen, and M. Scharff. Genetic approaches to the mechanisms of macrophage function. *Fed. Proc. 37*: 2765-2771, 1978.

13. P. Ralph, M. Ito, H. E. Broxmeyer, and I. Nakoinz. Corticosteroids block newly induced but not constitutive functions of macrophage cell lines: CSA production, latex phagocytosis, antibody-dependent lysis of RBC and tumor targets. *J. Immunol. 121*: 300-303, 1978.

14. H. S. Koren, B. S. Handwerger, and J. R. Wunderlich. Identification of macrophage-like characteristics in a cultured murine tumor line. *J. Immunol. 114*: 894-897, 1975.

15. B. Diamond, B. R. Bloom, and M. D. Scharff. The Fc receptors of primary and cultured phagocytic cells studied with homogeneous antibodies. *J. Immunol. 121*: 1329-1333, 1978.

16. B. Mørland and G. Kaplan. Properties of a murine monocytic tumor cell line J-774 *in vitro*. II. Enzyme activities. *Exp. Cell Res. 115*: 63-72, 1978.

17. R. M. Snyderman, M. C. Pike, D. G. Fischer, and H. S. Koren. Biologic and biochemical activities of continuous macrophage cell lines P388D1 and J774.1. *J. Immunol. 119*: 2060-2066, 1977.

18. J. S. Greenberger, P. C. Newberger, A. Karpas, and W. C. Moloney. Constitutive and inducible granulocyte-macrophage

functions in mouse, rat and human myeloid leukemia-derived continuous tissue culture lines. *Cancer Res. 38*: 3340-3348, 1978.

19. P. Ralph, I. Nakoinz, N. Williams, and H. Jackson. Unpublished results.

20. Z. Werb, R. Foley, and A. Munck. Glucocorticoid receptors and glucocorticoid-sensitive secretion of neutral proteinases in a macrophage cell line. *J. Immunol. 121:* 115-121, 1978.

21. J. A. Hamilton, P. Ralph, and M. A. S. Moore. A macrophage tumor cell line and plasminogen activator: A model system for macrophage regulation of enzyme production. *J. Exp. Med. 148*: 811-816, 1978.

22. P. Bodel. Spontaneous pyrogen production by mouse histiocytic and myelomonocytic tumor cell lines *in vitro*. *J. Exp. Med. 147*: 1503-1515, 1978.

23. P. Bodel, P. Ralph, K. Wenc, and J. C. Long. Endogenous pyrogen production by Hodgkin's disease and human histiocytic lymphoma cell lines *in vitro*. *J. Clin. Invest. 65*: 514-518, 1980.

24. R. B. Johnston, Jr., C. Godzik, and Z. Cohn. Increased superoxide anion production by immunologically activated and chemically elicited macrophages. *J. Exp. Med. 148*: 115-127, 1978.

25. J. I. Kurland, L. Pelus, P. Ralph, R. S. Bockman, and M. A. S. Moore. Synthesis of prostaglandin E by normal and neoplastic macrophages is dependent upon colony-stimulating factors (CSF). *Proc. Nat. Acad. Sci. USA 76*: 2326-2330, 1979.

26. P. Ralph, H. Broxmeyer, I. Nakoinz, and M. A. S. Moore. Induction of myeloid colony-stimulating activity (CSA) in murine monocyte tumor cell lines by macrophage activators, and in a T cell line by Con A. *Cancer Res. 38*: 1414-1419, 1978.

27. L. B. Lachman, M. P. Hacker, G. T. Blyden, and R. Handschumacher. Preparation of lymphocyte-activating factor from continuous murine macrophage cell lines. *Cell. Immunol. 34*: 416-419, 1977.

28. S. B. Mizel, D. L. Rosenstreich, and J. J. Oppenheim. Phorbol myristic acetate stimulates LAF production by the macrophage cell line P388D$_1$. *Cell. Immunol. 40*: 230-235, 1978.

29. W. S. Walker and A. Demus. Antibody-dependent cytolysis of chicken erythrocytes by an *in vitro*-established line of mouse peritoneal macrophages. *J. Immunol. 114*: 765-769, 1975.

30. P. Ralph, N. Williams, A. Sheridan, I. Nakoinz, H. Jackson, and M. Moore. Effector Cell Functions in Long-term Culture of Murine, Prosimian and Human Bone Marrow. *In* Mononuclear

Phagocytes - Functional Aspects" (R. van Furth, ed.), pp. 363-372. Martinius Nijhoff, The Hague, 1980.

31. N. Williams, R. R. Eger, M. A. S. Moore, and N. Mendelsohn. Differentiation of mouse bone marrow precursor cells into neutrophil granulocytes by an activity separation from WEHI-3 cell-conditioned medium. *Differentiation 11*: 59-63, 1978.

32. C. Sündstrom and K. Nilsson. Establishment and characterization of a human histiocytic lymphoma cell line (U/937). *Int. J. Cancer 17*: 565-577, 1976.

33. M. Okuma, Y. Ichikawa, S. Yamashito, K. Kitajima, and S. Numa. Studies on some lipogenic enzymes of cultured myeloid leukemic cells. *Blood 47*: 439-446, 1976.

34. W. Newman, B. Diamond, P. Flomenberg, M. D. Scharff, and B. R. Bloom. Response of a continuous macrophage-like cell line to MIF. *J. Immunol. 123*: 2292-2297, 1979.

35. H. vanLoveren, M. Snoek, and W. den Otter. Effects of silica on macrophages and lymphocytes. *J. Reticuloendothel. Soc. 22*: 523-531, 1977.

36. T. Jones and R. Byrne. The interaction between macrophages and intravacuolar microbes. *In* "Mononuclear Phagocytes - Functional Aspects" (R. van Furth, ed.), pp. 1116-1125. Martinius Nijhoff, The Hague, 1980.

37. R. S. Bar, C. R. Kahn, and H. S. Koren. Insulin inhibition of antibody-dependent cytotoxicity and insulin receptors in macrophages. *Nature 265:* 632-635, 1977.

38. P. J. Edelson. Plasma membrane ectoenzymes and their regulation. *In* "Mononuclear Phagocytes - Functional Aspects" (R. van Furth, ed.), pp. 665-681. Martinius Nijhoff, The Hague, 1980.

39. T. Springer, G. Galfré, D. S. Secher, and C. Milstein. Mac-1. Macrophage differentiation antigen identified by monoclonal antibody. *Eur. J. Immunol. 9*: 301-306, 1979.

40. A. M. Kaplan, H. D. Bear, L. Kirk, C. Cummins, and T. Mohanakumar. Relationship of expression of a cell-surface antigen on activated murine macrophages to tumor cell cytotoxicity. *J. Immunol. 120*: 2080-2085, 1978.

41. J. Y. Djeu, J. A. Heinbaugh, H. T. Holden, and R. B. Herberman. Role of macrophages in the augmentation of mouse natural killer cell activity by poly I:C and interferon. *J. Immunol. 122*: 182-188, 1979.

42. P. Ralph and I. Nakoinz. Environmental and chemical dissociation of antibody-dependent phagocytosis from lysis mediated by macrophages: Stimulation of lysis by sulfhydryl-blocking and esterase-inhibiting agents and depression by trypan blue and trypsin. *Cell. Immunol. 50*: 94-105, 1980.

43. N. Williams, H. Jackson, P. Ralph, and I. Nakoinz. Cell interactions influencing murine marrow megakaryocytes:

Nature of the potentiator cell in bone marrow. *Blood 57*: 157-163, 1981.

44. P. Ralph, H. Broxmeyer, and I. Nakoinz. Immunostimulators induce granulocyte/macrophage colony-stimulating activity and block proliferation in a monocyte tumor cell line. *J. Exp. Med. 146*: 611-616, 1977.

45. M. Ito, P. Ralph, and M. A. S. Moore. *In vitro* stimulation of phagocytosis in a macrophage cell line measured by a convenient radiolabeled latex bead assay. *Cell. Immunol. 46*: 48-56, 1979.

46. G. Kaplan and B. Mørland. Properties of a murine monocytic tumor cell line J-774 *in vitro*. I. Morphology and endocytosis. *Exp. Cell Res. 115*: 53-62, 1978.

47. T. Taniyama and H. T. Holden. Direct augmentation of cytolytic activity of tumor-derived macrophages and macrophage cell lines by muramyl dipeptide. *Cell Immunol. 48*: 369-374, 1979.

48. S. W. Russell, G. Y. Gillespie, and J. L. Pace. Comparison of responses made to activating agents by mouse peritoneal macrophages and cells of the macrophage line RAW264. *J. Reticuloendothel. Soc. 27*: 607-612, 1980.

49. R. R. Aksamit and K. J. Kim. Macrophage cell lines produce a cytotoxin. *J. Immunol. 122*: 1785-1790, 1979.

50. P. Ralph and I. Nakoinz. Antibody-dependent killing of erythrocyte and tumor targets by monocyte related cell lines: Enhancement by PPD and LPS. *J. Immunol. 119*: 950-954, 1977.

51. P. Ralph, I. Nakoinz, J. E. R. Potter, and M. A. S. Moore. Activity of macrophage cell lines in spontaneous and LPS, lymphokine or antibody-dependent killing of tumor targets. *In* Genetic Control of Natural Resistance to Infection and Malignancy" (E. Skamene, P. A. L. Kongshavn and M. Landy, eds.), pp. 519-529. Academic Press, New York, 1980.

52. G. Damiani, C. Kiyotaki, W. Soeller, M. Sasada, J. Peisach, and B. R. Bloom. Macrophage variants in oxygen metabolism. *J. Exp. Med. 152*: 808-822, 1980.

53. T. Igarashi, M. Okada, T. Kishimoto, and Y. Yamamura. *In vitro* induction of polyclonal killer T cells with 2-mercaptoethanol and the essential role of macrophages in this process. *J. Immunol. 118*: 1697-1703, 1977.

54. M. K. Hoffmann, S. Koenig, R. S. Mittler, H. F. Oettgen, P. Ralph, C. Galanos, and U. Hämmerling. Macrophage factor controlling differentiation of B cells. *J. Immunol. 122*: 497-502, 1979.

55. T. Kishimoto, T. Hirano, T. Kuritani, Y. Yamamura, P. Ralph, and R. A. Good. Induction of IgG production in human B lymphoblastoid cell lines with normal human T-cells. *Nature 271*: 756-758, 1978.

56. R. Schwartz. Unpublished.
57. P. Ralph, J. Prichard, and M. Cohn. Reticulum cell sarcoma: *In vitro* model for mediator of cellular immunity. *J. Immunol.* *114*: 898-905, 1975.
58. M. D. Sklar, E. M. Shevach, I. Green, and M. Potter. Transplantation and preliminary characteristics of lymphocyte surface markers of Abelson virus-induced lymphomas. *Nature 253*: 550-552, 1975.
59. A. L. Epstein, R. Levy, H. Kim, W. Henle, G. Henle, and H. S. Kaplan. Biology of the human malignant lymphomas. IV. Functional characterization of ten diffuse histiocytic lymphoma cell lines. *Cancer 42*: 2379-2392, 1978.
60. C. B. Lozzio and B. B. Lozzio. Human chronic myelogenous leukemia cell line with positive Philadelphia chromosome. *Blood 45*: 321-334.
61. A. Karpas, F. G. J. Hayhoe, J. S. Greenberger, C. R. Barker, J. C. Cawley, R. M. Lowenthal, and W. C. Moloney. The establishment and cytological, cytochemical, and immunological characterization of human haemic cell lines. *Leukemia Res. 1*: 35-49, 1977.
62. S. J. Collins, F. W. Ruscetti, R. E. Gallagher, and R. C. Gallo. Normal functional characteristics of cultured human promyelocytic leukemia cells (HL-60) after induction of differentiation by dimethyl sulfoxide. *J. Exp. Med. 149*: 969-975, 1979.
63. H. P. Koeffler and D. W. Golde. Acute myelogenous leukemia: A human cell line responsive to colony-stimulating activity. *Science 200*: 1153-1154, 1978.
64. J. F. DiPersio, J. K. Brennan, M. A. Lichtman, and B. L. Speiser. Human cell lines that elaborate colony-stimulating activity for the marrow cells of man and other species. *Blood 51*: 507-519, 1978.
65. J. C. Long, P. C. Zamenik, A. C. Aisenberg, and L. Atkins. Tissue culture studies in Hodgkin's disease. Morphologic, cytogenetic cell surface, and enzymatic properties of cultures derived from splenic tumors. *J. Exp. Med. 145*: 1484-1500, 1977.
66. G. Rovera, D. Santoli, and C. Damsky. Human promyelocytic leukemia cells in culture differentiate into macrophage-like cells when treated with a phorbol diester. *Proc. Nat. Acad. Sci. USA 76*: 2779-2783, 1979.
67. T. M. Dexter, T. D. Allen, and L. G. Lajtha. Conditions controlling the proliferation of haemopoietic stem cells *in vitro*. *J. Cell. Physiol. 91*: 335-341, 1977.
68. R. J. Muschel, N. Rosen, O. M. Rosen, and B. R. Bloom. Modulation of Fc-mediated phagocytosis by cyclic AMP and insulin in a macrophage-like cell line. *J. Immunol. 119*: 1813-1820, 1977.

69. J. C. Unkless. The presence of two Fc receptors on mouse macrophages: Evidence from a variant cell line and differential trypsin sensitivity. *J. Exp. Med. 145*: 931-947, 1977.

70. "Mycoplasma Infection of Cell Cultures" (G. J. McGarrity, D. G. Murphy, and W. W. Nichols, eds.). Plenum Press, New York, 1978.

71. W. S. Walker. Separate Fc-receptors for immunoglobulins IgG$_{2a}$ and IgG$_{2b}$ on an established cell line of mouse macrophages. *J. Immunol. 116*: 911-914, 1976.

72. C. L. Anderson and H. M. Grey. Physicochemical separation of two distinct Fc receptors on murine macrophage-like cell lines. *J. Immunol. 121*: 648-652, 1978.

73. J. C. Unkless. Characterization of a monoclonal antibody directed against mouse macrophage and lymphocyte Fc receptors. *J. Exp. Med. 150*: 580-596, 1979.

74. R. D. Berlin, J. M. Oliver, and R. J. Walter. Surface functions during mitosis: Phagocytosis, pinocytosis, and mobility of surface-bound Con A. *Cell 15*: 327-341, 1978.

75. P. Ralph and I. Nakoinz. Tumoricidal activity of macrophage cell lines: Differences in ADCC and activated killing. *Cancer Res. (in press)*, 1981.

76. B. Diamond and D. E. Yelton. A new Fc receptor on mouse macrophages binding IgG$_3$. *J. Exp. Med. 153*: 514-519, 1981.

18

SEPARATION OF MONONUCLEAR PHAGOCYTES FOR ENRICHMENT AND FOR DEPLETION: AN OVERVIEW

William S. Walker

Ideally, procedures for isolating any cell type should be simple and reproducible and should yield pure functionally competent populations of cells. Despite repeated attempts, there are still no completely reliable methods for separating mononuclear phagocytes (MP). However, these cells do have a number of physical and biological properties that allow for their enrichment or depletion from complex cell mixtures and for their separation into functionally enriched subpopulations of cells. More specifically, MP adhere tenaciously to certain surfaces where they resist removal by agents such as trypsin (1); they differ from other cell types in size and density (2 - 5); they can be maintained *in vitro* for long periods of time (6); they are phagocytic (7); they possess surface membrane receptors for a variety of ligands (8); and, a certain subpopulation of MP expresses Ia-antigens (9).

Most strategies for separating MP exploit the property of surface adherence. Yet this feature is not unique to MP and a procedure that relies solely on adherence, particularly for preparative purposes, will at best yield populations that are

enriched for the cell type of interest. The acceptable level
of contamination is therefore an important consideration in
selecting a separation method. The choice will depend on the
demands of the experiment and whether the goal of the separation is the functional depletion of a cell type (e.g., its reduction below a functionally detectable level) or its complete
elimination based on a combination of functional and morphologic criteria.

To achieve better enrichment, it is often advantageous to
use two or more methods sequentially, particularly when each
differs in its basis of separation. For instance, methods that
combine adherence followed by phagocytosis of magnetic carbonyl
iron particles will effectively remove MP from a suspension of
spleen cells (10). Unfortunately, both of these procedures
have shortcomings, including the appreciable loss of lymphocytes (11), which, depending on the experimental requirements,
may or may not be acceptable.

A combination of techniques can be used to obtain reasonably pure populations of MP. If a cell suspension containing
MP is cultured for 12 to 24 hrs, the contaminating polymorphonuclear leukocytes will not survive. The remaining adherent population of cells can then be vigorously washed to
remove the less adherent lymphocytes and any remaining T and B
lymphocytes are killed by the addition of specific antisera
and complement. Finally, if the MP are to be cultured for any
extended time, contaminating fibroblastic elements can be removed with trypsin. However, certain fractions of the macrophages may be lost over the 24-hr culture period.

The separation strategy just described draws attention to
yet another caveat - the effects of the procedures on cell
function and ultimately on the interpretation of data. An
awareness of this possibility is most important when working
with MP, as these cells undergo pronounced morphologic and
functional changes as a consequence of *in vitro* manipulation.

Separation procedures that rely on physical and functional
properties have definite limitations, either their lack of cell-
type selectivity or a tendency to alter cell function. A more
specific approach, but one that may also affect cell function,
makes use of the antigens and receptors displayed on the cell
surface - a strategy that has been successful with lymphoid
cells (12). Similar application of hybridoma technology (13)
to MP may also provide the means to identify and isolate
specifically these cells from complex mixtures (14). Moreover,
MP are functionally heterogeneous (15), a diversity that is
partly reflected by the array of antigens and receptors on the
cell surface (16).

The methods described in this section have all proved
valuable in defining the cellular requirements in homeostasis,

and in the induction and expression of immunity. The future should bring newer and more effective methods and hence refine our understanding of mononuclear phagocytes.

REFERENCES

1. V. Defendi. Macrophage cell lines and their use in immunobiology. *In* "Immunobiology of the Macrophage" (D. S. Nelson, ed.), pp. 275-290. Academic Press, New York, 1976.

2. K.-C. Lee, A. Wilkinson, and M. Wong. Antigen-specific murine T-cell proliferation: Role of macrophage surface Ia and factors. *Cell. Immunol. 48*: 79-84, 1979.

3. W. S. Walker. Functional heterogeneity of macrophages: Subclasses of peritoneal macrophages with different antigen-binding activities and immune complex receptors. *Immunology 26*: 1025-1037, 1974.

4. H. J. Cutts. "Cell Separation: Methods in Hematology." Academic Press, New York, 1970.

5. K. Shortman. Physical procedures for the separation of animal cells. *Ann. Rev. Biophys. Bioeng. 1*: 93-130, 1972.

6. Y. T. Chang. Long-term cultivation of mouse peritoneal macrophages. *J. Natl. Cancer Inst. 32*: 19-35, 1964.

7. S. C. Silverstein, R. M. Steinman and Z. A. Cohn. Endocytosis. *Ann. Rev. Biochem. 46*: 669-722, 1977.

8. S. H. Zuckerman and S. D. Douglas. Dynamics of the macrophage plasma membrane. *Ann. Rev. Microbiol. 33*: 267-307, 1979.

9. R. H. Schwartz, H. B. Dickler, D. H. Sachs, and B. D. Schwartz. Studies of Ia antigens on murine peritoneal macrophages. *Scand. J. Immunol. 5*: 731-743, 1976.

10. H. S. Koren and R. J. Hodes. Effect of tumor cells on the generation of cytotoxic T-lymphocytes *in vitro*. *Eur. J. Immunol. 7*: 394-400, 1977.

11. G. Lundgren, C. H. F. Zukoski, and G. Moller. Differential effects on human granulocytes and lymphocytes on human fibroblasts *in vitro*. *Clin. Exp. Immunol. 3*: 817-824, 1968.

12. J. A. Ledbetter and L. A. Herzenberg. Xenogeneic monoclonal antibodies to mouse lymphoid differentiation antigens. *Immunol. Rev. 47*: 63-90, 1979.

13. *Lymphocyte Hybridomas*. F. Melchers, M. Potter, and N. Warner, eds. Springer-Verlag, New York, 1978.

14. T. Springe, G. Galfré, D. S. Secher, and C. Milstein. MAC-1: A macrophage differentiation antigen identified

by monoclonal antibody. *Eur. J. Immunol. 9*: 301-306, 1979.

15. Walker, W. S. Functional heterogeneity of macrophages. *In* "Immunobiology of the Macrophage" (D. S. Nelson, ed.), pp. 91-111. Academic Press, New York, 1976.

16. W. S. Walker. Macrophage heterogeneity: Membrane markers and properties of macrophage subpopulations. *In* "Regulatory Role of Macrophages in Immunity (E. R. Unanue and A. S. Rosenthal, eds.), pp. 307-318. Academic Press, New York, 1980.

19

SEPARATION OF MURINE MACROPHAGES
BY ADHERENCE TO SOLID SUBSTRATES

Donald E. Mosier

I. INTRODUCTION

Physical separation of macrophage and lymphoid populations
has been essential in demonstrating principles of cell cooperation in immune responses. Evidence now exists that substrate
adherent macrophage populations either are required for most
forms of lymphocyte activation or significantly enhance lymphocyte transformation (1 - 12). This chapter deals with separation of macrophage populations on the basis of their ability
to adhere actively to a solid substrate such as plastic, glass,
or collagen. Such techniques are useful as a rapid and simple
method of macrophage purification (in the adherent fraction)
and depletion (in the nonadherent fraction), although more
rigorous macrophage depletion is best accomplished by a combination of these techniques with Sephadex G-10 column passage
[(13) and Chapter 25 this volume]. It is important to note
from the outset that the population of cells which adheres to

solid substrates is heterogenous and includes in addition to classic phagocytic mononuclear cells the Ia^+ antigen-presenting cells (14) and the dendritic cells described by Steinman *et al.* (15). Moreover, the fraction of adherent cells that function in specific antigen presentation to lymphocytes has been estimated by limiting dilution techniques to be as low as 1 per 10,000 (12). Any conclusions on the functional properties of adherence separated cell populations should take into account the possibility that a very small distinct subpopulation is entirely responsible for the observed results.

Separation of macrophages by adherence requires active cell metabolism, and attachment is temperature dependent (16, 17). The presence of serum is necessary for attachment, and it is likely that proteins such as fibronectin play an important role in substrate adherence. Cells that are in late G_2 or metaphase are less adherent to substrates and may detach during mitosis, as may cells that have "overindulged" in phagocytosis. The physiological basis for cell adhesiveness is not yet well understood, but these techniques should apply to all species.

II. REAGENTS AND MATERIALS

The hallmark of adherence techniques is their simplicity. Tissue culture grade plasticware or glass dishes or beads acid washed to tissue culture specifications [e.g. (18)] are required. There is some variation from lot to lot in 35- or 60-mm tissue culture dishes, and plasticware sterilized by gamma irradiation seems to be less variable than that sterilized with ethylene oxide. Most standard tissue culture media [e.g., modified MEM (1), RPMI 1640, M199] will support cell adherence. Medium designed for suspension culture has reduced Ca^{2+} and Mg^{2+} concentrations and is not suitable for adherence techniques. Serum is required for active adherence; 10% fetal calf serum is adequate, although higher serum concentrations promote cell spreading following initial adhesion (17).

The Shortman (18 - 21) glass bead column technique requires acid washed glass beads (about 450 μm in diameter, available from a variety of sources including 3-M, Minneapolis, Minnesota) and a 1.5 - 2.0 × 15 - 20 cm glass column. The glass beads should be siliconized before use (e.g., by treatment with Siliclad, available from Clay-Adams).

If recovery of adherent cells is a prime consideration, cells may be eluted from solid substrates by using tissue culture medium without serum and Ca^{2+} or Mg^{2+} salts and supplemented with 30 mM EDTA. Alternatively, cells may be adhered

to a collagen monolayer and eluted by collagenase treatment
(see below). Calf skin collagen (LS 0001660, Worthington)
and type-1 collagenase (LS 0004194, Worthington) are adequate
for this purpose. The merthiolate added as a preservative to
the collagen should be removed shortly before use by dialysis
against pH 4.4, 0.075 M sodium citrate.

III. PROCEDURES

A. *Adherence to Plastic Culture Dishes*

A single-cell suspension of murine spleen cells is prepared
by teasing the spleens with fine forceps in cold Hanks' balanced salt solution (HBSS). Large cell clumps are allowed to
settle 3 - 5 min, and the remaining cells in suspension are
transferred to a new tube and sedimented by centrifugation.
The cells are washed twice more in HBSS and then resuspended
in RPMI 1640 + 10% fetal calf serum. A viable cell count is
performed, and the cell density is adjusted to 10 - 20
$\times$ 10^6 ml^{-1}. One milliliter per 35-mm dish or 3 - 5 ml per
60-mm dish is dispensed, and the dishes are incubated in a 5%
CO_2 atmosphere at 37°C for 1 hr. Rocking the dishes on an os-
cillating platform as originally described (1) does not seem
to be required for active adherence of macrophages, although it
may diminish the number of lymphocytes that bind to macrophages (21). After 1 hr incubation, the dishes are gently
swirled to resuspend settled cells and the nonadherent population aspirated with a sterile Pasteur pipette. These cells
may be transferred to a new set of culture dishes after one
wash with HBSS and resuspension to one-half the original volume
to correct for the approximately 50% recovery of the starting
cell number. The cells remaining in the original culture dish
should be washed vigorously three times with cold HBSS. A
stream of HBSS should be directed at the entire surface of the
dish using a narrow bore Pasteur pipette. Macrophages are
firmly attached to the plastic by this point, and it is probably impossible to be too vigorous in this washing step, which
removes loosely adherent lymphocytes.

The population of cells originally nonadherent to plastic
may be cultured in additional dishes to improve depletion of
phagocytic cells. Alternatively, additional purification can
be achieved by passing plastic nonadherent cells over Sephadex
G-10 columns, a procedure we prefer for more vigorous depletion
of macrophages.

At each step, the percentage of macrophages should be monitored by assays of phagocytosis and/or nonspecific esterase

staining (see Chapter 28). Typically, one step of plastic
adherence leads to an 80 - 90% decrease in phagocytic cells
in the nonadherent population. The adherent population contains greater than 90% phagocytic, esterase-positive cells.

Recovery of the adherent population can be achieved by
replacing the complete medium with serum-free medium lacking
Ca^{2+} and Mg^{2+} and containing 30 mM EDTA. Adherent cells then
can be scraped free with a rubber policeman. Unfortunately,
this procedure leads to reduced viability and cell function
so we prefer to use adherent cells in the culture dish in
which they were originally prepared. They can be enumerated
in the culture dish using an inverted phase microscope. Between 1 and 5% of the initial cell number is recovered as
adherent macrophages depending upon the age and strain of
mouse used.

B. Adherence to Glass Bead Columns

Several versions of this technique are available, but the
one of Shortman *et al.* (18) seems to work the best for us, although there is considerable variability in the number of lymphocytes retained by the column. Acid-washed, siliconized
glass beads ($\sim$450 μm diameter) are added to a 2.4 × 14 cm
glass column that previously had been plugged with a small pad
of acid-washed glasswool and filled with sterile HBSS. The
beads are poured rapidly into the column and allowed to settle
by gravity. Prior to use, the column should be equilibrated
with serum-free medium, e.g., RPMI 1640, at 37°C. Maintenance
of pH at the appropriate range of 6.8 - 7.3 can be accomplished
by omitting $NaHCO_3$ from the medium and adding 25 mM HEPES buffer plus enough 1 N NaOH to achieve a pH of 7.2. This obviates
the need to run the column in a CO_2 incubator.

The column is loaded with cells suspended in RPMI 1640
+ 50% fetal calf serum (FCS). We have not found the use of
mouse serum to be essential to the technique. Just prior to
column loading, one column volume of RPMI 1640 + 60% FCS
should be added to the beads. From 2 to 10 × 10^8 spleen cells
(prepared as above) are then added in 4 - 5 ml with care taken
not to disturb the interface between 50 and 60% FCS. As the
cells enter the column, additional medium + 50% FCS should be
added and the upper portion of the column bed stirred with the
popette tip to dislodge nonspecifically trapped cells. The
cells should be allowed to enter the column quite rapidly
(e.g., 30 - 60 sec), and the column then loaded with one column
volume of RPMI 1640 + 25% FCS. The flow rate should be slowed
so that the cell band at the 50 - 60% FCS interface takes
about 10 min to traverse the column.

In contrast to elution of adherent cells from plastic dishes, the medium recommended by Shortman for elution of macrophages from glass bead columns contains 2% serum, in addition to 30 mM EDTA and no Ca^{2+} or Mg^{2+}. The procedure for eluting the cells from the column includes agitating the column while filled with the elution medium. This can be done by inverting the stoppered column or by stirring the beads with a sterile glass rod or pipette. Again, our experience has been that the function of eluted cells is impaired when compared to undisturbed adherent cells.

The relative yield of adherent and nonadherent cells from the Shortman column is somewhat variable. About a tenfold depletion in macrophages with a 40 – 70% recovery can be expected in the nonadherent fraction, while eluted cells are enriched 5 to 10-fold for macrophages. Again, recovered cells should be evaluated for purity by assays for phagocytosis, esterase activity, and function.

C. Adherence of Cells to Collagen Monolayers

The advantage of this technique is that adherent cells can be recovered with good viability and function. The disadvantage is that the purity of separation is not good, so that the main use of the technique is in recovering enriched populations of viable, functioning macrophages.

Soluble collagen at 1 – 2 mg/ml, pH 4.4, is adjusted to pH 7.0 with 0.5 M sodium carbonate and 1 ml immediately added to a prewarmed 60-mm plastic culture dish. The dish is incubated without agitating for 30 min at 37°C during which time the collagen gels. The dish is then washed gently with 37°C RPMI 1640 + 10% FCS twice, and allowed to incubate at 37°C for another 30 min with medium and FCS. At this point, the medium is gently decanted, and 3 ml of a spleen cell suspension containing 10 – 20 × 10^6 cells/ml is added slowly to prevent disruption of the collagen monolayer. The culture dishes are incubated at 37°C for 1 hr, and the nonadherent cells are decanted. The surface of the collagen is gently flushed with three washes of cold HBSS. The cells adherent to the collagen are recovered by adding 1 mg/ml type I collagenase in warm HBSS. Incubation is continued at 37°C for 1 – 2 hr with gentle swirling of the dish at frequent intervals. The cells are recovered by decanting and washed in RPMI 1640 + 10% FCS twice. The recovery is variable with this technique (10 – 20%), but one can achieve an enrichment for phagocytic cells of 3 to 5-fold. Lymphocytes still comprise the majority population, however. Activated macrophages secrete endogenous collagenase (22), which may mean they will not be recovered by these procedures.

IV. CALCULATION OF DATA

The calculation of percentage cell recovery, cell viability, phagocytic cells, etc., is straightforward provided one has performed cell counts at each step of the procedure.

V. CRITICAL COMMENTS

As emphasized above, none of these techniques yields absolutely pure cell populations, and the best strategy may be to combine two or more different procedures. The final criterion for purity of separation should be a functional assay, not morphological scanning. For example, the finding that adherent accessory cells are required for many, if not all, thymic-independent antibody responses *in vitro* was based upon improved methods for more rigorous depletion of adherent cells (7). An additional functional criterion of effective accessory cell depletion in *in vitro* systems is the inability of 2-mercapto-ethanol (2-ME) to replace macrophage function. In our laboratory, depletion of adherent cell function for primary *in vitro* antibody responses routinely is accomplished in medium supplemented with 2-ME.

All of these techniques show some variability that might be attributed to the biological status of the cell source or to variables in cell culture technique such as serum source or the type (or even age) of tissue culture vessels employed. Conversion of monocyte precursors (which might be expected to be non-adherent) to adherent macrophages does not occur with any detectable frequency in our experience, but it may occur in species other than the mouse or under different culture conditions. Such a differentiation process should be checked in other systems by assessing the number of macrophage-like cells appearing with time.

Finally, until more is known about the heterogeneity of macrophage subpopulations and their cell biology, these approaches remain empirical and should be subject to constant improvement.

REFERENCES

1. D. E. Mosier. A requirement for two cell types for antibody formation *In vitro*. *Science 158*: 1573-1575, 1967.
2. C. W. Pierce and B. Benacerraf. Immune response *in vitro*: Independence of "activated" lymphoid cells. *Science 166*: 1002-1004, 1969.
3. R. W. Dutton, M. M. McCarthy, R. I. Mishell, and D. J. Raidt. Cell components in the immune response. IV. Relationship and possible interactions. *Cell. Immunol. 1*: 196-206, 1970.
4. K. Shortman and J. Palmer. The requirement for macrophages in the *in vitro* immune response. *Cell. Immunol. 2*: 399-410, 1971.
5. M. Feldman and A. Basten. The relationship between antigenic structure and the requirement for thymus-derived cells in the immune response. *J. Exp. Med. 134*: 103-119, 1971.
6. E. Unanue and D. H. Katz. Immunogenicity of macrophage-bound antigens: The requirement for hapten and carrier determinants to be on the same molecule for T and B lymphocyte collaboration. *Eur. J. Immunol. 3*: 559-563, 1973.
7. T. M. Chused, S. S. Kassan, and D. E. Mosier. Macrophage requirement for the *in vitro* response to TNP Ficoll: A thymic-independent antigen. *J. Immunol. 116*: 1579-1581, 1976.
8. A. A. Nordin. The *in vitro* immune response to a T-independent antigen. I. The effect of macrophages and 2-mercaptoethanol. *Eur. J. Immunol. 8*: 776-781, 1978.
9. D. L. Rosenstreich and A. S. Rosenthal. Peritoneal exudate lymphocyte. II. *In vitro* lymphocyte proliferation induced by brief exposure to antigen. *J. Immunol. 110*: 934-942, 1973.
10. R. C. Seeger and J. J. Oppenheim. Synergistic interaction of macrophages and lymphocytes in antigen-induced transformation of lymphocytes. *J. Exp. Med. 132*: 44-65, 1970.
11. D. S. Nelson (ed.). "Immunobiology of the Macrophage." Academic Press, New York, 1976.
12. D. E. Mosier and L. W. Coppleson. A three-cell interaction required for the induction of the primary immune response *in vitro*. *Proc. Nat. Acad. Sci. USA 61*: 542-547, 1968.
13. I. Ly and R. I. Mishell. Separation of mouse spleen cells by passage through columns of Sephadex G-10. *J. Immunol. Methods 5*: 239-248, 1974.
14. C. Cowing, B. D. Schwartz, and H. B. Dickler. Macrophage Ia antigens. I. Macrophage populations differ in their expression of Ia antigens. *J. Immunol. 120*: 378-384, 1978.

15. R. M. Steinman and Z. A. Cohn. Identification of a novel
     cell type in peripheral lymphoid organs of mice. I.
     morphology, quantitation, tissue distribution. *J. Exp.*
     Med. *137*: 1142-1162, 1973.
16. S. Gordon and Z. A. Cohn. The macrophage. The macrophage
     as a tool in cell biology. *Int. Rev. Cytol.* *36*: 171-124,
     1973.
17. M. Rabinovitch and M. J. DeStefano. Macrophage spreading
     in vitro. I. Induces of spreading. *Exp. Cell. Res.* *77*:
     323-334, 1973.
18. K. Shortman, N. Williams, H. Jackson, P. Russell, P. Byrt
     and E. Diener. The separation of different cell classes
     from lymphoid organs. IV. The separation of lymphocytes
     from phagocytes on glass bead columns, and its effect on
     subpopulations of lymphocytes and antibody-forming cells.
     J. Cell Biol. *48*: 566-579, 1971.
19. K. Shortman. The separation of different cell classes
     from lymphoid organs. I. The use of glass bead columns to
     separate small lymphocytes, remove damaged cells, and
     fractionate cell suspensions. *J. Exp. Biol. Med. Sci.*
     44: 271-284, 1966.
20. Y. Rabinowitz. Separation of lymphocytes, polymorphonu-
     clear leukocytes, and monocytes on glass columns, includ-
     ing tissue culture observations. *Blood 23*: 811-828, 1964.
21. J. Ellner, P. E. Lipsky, and A. S. Rosenthal. Antigen
     handling by guinea pig macrophages: Further evidence for
     the sequestration of antigen relevant for activation of
     primed lymphocytes. *J. Immunol.* *118*: 2053-2057, 1977.
22. L. M. Wahl, S. M. Wahl, S. E. Mergenhagen, and G. M.
     Martin. Collagenase production by endotoxin-activated
     macrophages. *Proc. Nat. Acad. Sci. USA 71*: 3598-3601,
     1974.

20

SEPARATION OF HUMAN MONOCYTES AND GUINEA PIG MACROPHAGES
BY DENSITY GRADIENTS OF METRIZAMIDE

Barbara A. Sherry
*Mathew A. Vadas**
John R. David

I. INTRODUCTION

The use of slightly hypertonic discontinuous metrizamide gradients as an effective, reproducible method for the purification of normal human peripheral blood eosinophils and neutrophils was developed in our laboratory by Vadas *et al.* (1). High yields and purity were obtained without sacrificing the viability or functional integrity of the fractionated cells. This method employs density steps ranging between 1.10 gm/cm^3 and 1.13 gm/cm^3 [on a percentage basis steps are 18, 20, 22, 23, 24, and 25% (w/v) metrizamide]. In the course of experimentation, it was observed that a large percentage of human mononuclear cells did not enter the gradients at all, but rather formed a band above the 18% metrizamide step. It was

Present address: Walter and Eliza Hall Institute, Royal Melbourne Hospital, Parkville, 3050 VIC, Australia.

METHODS FOR STUDYING
MONONUCLEAR PHAGOCYTES

187

hypothesized that by modifying the method of Vadas *et al.* to incorporate a range of density steps between 1.088 and 1.108 gm/cm^3 [on a percentage basis steps would be 16, 17, 18, 19, 20, and 21% (w/v) metrizamide], a fraction enriched for human peripheral blood monocytes might be recovered.

Using these modified conditions, certain fractions were found to be considerably enriched in human monocytes. Ten experiments were performed using peripheral blood white cells from six separate donor individuals (see Table I). With a mean starting monocyte concentration in the buffy coat of 8.9% (individual values ranging between 4.0 and 15.4%), enriched fractions were recovered with a mean purity of 76.0% (values ranging between 61.0 and 88.2%). In these ten experiments, the mean percent recovery of total monocytes in the enriched fraction was 46.8% (values ranging between 19.0 and 85.7%). Cells from a single donor individual were fractionated on five separate occasions to test for reproducibility of the technique (see Table II). Starting monocyte concentrations in the buffy coat varied between 10.0 and 20.0% (mean 15.4%) depending upon the experiment. After purification of these cells on metrizamide gradients, enriched fractions were recovered that ranged between 83.0 and 93.0% monocytes (mean purity 88.2%). The percentage recovery of total monocytes in enriched fractions ranged between 21.0 and 51.0% (mean recovery 34.3%). Cells in experiments 1 - 3 were tested for viability by trypan blue exclusion both before and after fractionation. They were found in all cases to be greater than 94% viable. No cell damage was observed by morphologic criteria, and when cells were tested for function, as assessed by uptake of latex particles or phagocytosis of sensitized sheep red blood cells, they appeared to be functionally intact.

This modified method was expanded to the fractionation of guinea pig macrophages from casein-induced peritoneal exudate cells, and as is shown in Table III, purities ranging from 94.8 and 97.9% were achieved, with a percent recovery of macrophages in enriched fractions ranging between 13.2 and 93.8%. Data from all fractionation experiments can be reviewed in Tables I - III, along with results of functional assays and peroxidase staining.

II.   REAGENTS

MEM complete, minimal essential medium (Microbiological Associates, Inc., Bethesda, Maryland) supplemented with 10% heat-inactivated fetal calf serum, 100 U/ml penicillin G, 100 µg/ml streptomycin, 5 m*M* L-glutamine, 25 m*M* HEPES buffer

TABLE I. Purification of Human Monocytes

| | Experiment No. | | | | | | |
	$1-5^a$	6	7	8	9	10	Mean
Subject[b]	A	B	C	D	E	F	
Cells/gradient $(\times 10^6)$	52.0	58.6	55.1	76.2	73.3	61.0	62.7
Monocytes (%) in buffy coat	15.4	8.0	13.0	5.0	4.0	8.0	8.9
Monocytes (%) in purest fraction[c]	88.2	71.2	76.0	61.0	72.0	88.0	76.0
Monocyte (%) recovery in purest fraction[c]	34.3	60.1	35.7	46.0	85.7	19.0	46.8
EAC[c,d] (%)	e	–	–	–	68.0	–	
Latex incorporation[c,d] (%)	e	–	–	–	–	87.0	
Peroxidase[c,d] (%)	e	–	–	–	–	46.0	

[a]Values in column 1 refer to mean of five separate experiments utilizing peripheral blood from donor A. Remaining columns (donors B - F) reflect data obtained from single experiments utilizing peripheral blood from different individuals.
[b]Code letters specify individual blood donors.
[c]Purest fraction refers to the 16% metrizamide interface in experiments 1, 8, and 10, to a pool of the 16 and 17% interfaces in experiments 6 and 7, and to the 17% interface for experiment 9.
[d]Techniques used for functional tests are described in Section II.
[e]See Table II.

(all from Microbiological Associates, Inc., Bethesda, Maryland), and DNase, 30 mg/liter (Worthington Biochemical Corp., Freehold, New Jersey, 2045 U/mg), pH adjusted to 7.3.

Hank's balanced salt solution, HBSS (Microbiological Associates, Inc., Bethesda, Maryland).

5× Tyrode's stock solution, each liter containing 5 gm dextrose, 5 gm $NaHCO_3$, 1 gm KCl, 40 gm, NaCl, and 0.25 gm Na_2HPO_4 (anhydrous).

Tyrode's gel DNase, appropriate dilution of 5× Tyrode's stock solution supplemented with 0.1% gelatin and DNase 30 mg/liter (Worthington Biochemical Corp., Freehold, New Jersey), pH adjusted to 7.2.

Thirty percent working metrizamide solution. 30 gm metrizamide (centrifugation grade, Nyegaard and Co., A/S, Oslo) diluted to 100 ml with Tyrode's gel DNase, prepared fresh before each fractionation.

TABLE II. Purification of Human Monocytes

| | Experiment No.[a] | | | | | |
	1	2	3	4	5	Mean
Subject[b]	A	A	A	A	A	
Cells/gradient ($\times 10^6$)	38.2	53.8	55.6	61.8	50.4	52.0
Monocytes (%) in buffy coat	18.0	14.0	15.0	10.0	20.0	15.4
Monocytes (%) in purest fraction[c]	93.0	90.0	91.0	84.0	83.0	88.2
Monocyte (%) recovery in purest fraction[c]	33.3	51.0	38.4	27.9	21.0	34.3
EAC[c,d] (%)	-	-	85.0	-	77.0	
EA[c,d] (%)	-	-	-	-	80.0	
Latex incorporation[c,d] (%)	-	88.0	-	-	-	
Peroxidase[c,d] (%)	-	80.0	-	-	-	

[a]In experiments 1 - 3 cells from all fractions were found
to be 94% viable by trypan blue exclusion. Percent viability
not determined in experiments 4 and 5.
[b]Code letters specify individual blood donors. Same donor
in experiments 1 - 5 (A).
[c]Purest fraction refers to the 16% metrizamide interface in
experiments 1 - 4, and a pool of the 16 and 17% interfaces in
experiment 5.
[d]Techniques used for functional tests are described in
Section II.

Dextran (4.5%), 4.5 gm dextran T500 (Pharmacia Fine Chemicals, Inc., Piscataway, New Jersey, MW 500,000) diluted to
100 ml with PBS; Heparin (Sigma Chemical Co., St. Louis, Missouri) diluted to 1000 U/ml in saline.

III. PROCEDURES

A. Cell Isolation

    Collection of human peripheral blood white cells was ac-
complished by drawing 50 ml of blood from normal individuals
into a syringe containing 10 ml of 4.5% dextran and 0.5 ml
heparin [final dextran concentration equals 0.9% (w/v), final
heparin concentration equals 10 U/ml]. Blood was allowed to
sediment at 37°C for approximately 30 min with the syringe secured in a vertical position. When sedimentation was complete,

TABLE III. Purification of Guinea Pig Macrophages[a]

| | Experiment No.[a] | | | | |
	11	12	13	14	Mean
Cells/gradient (×10⁶)	61.8	50.0	25.0	55.9	48.2
Macrophages (%) in unfractionated PE cells	67.0	72.0	77.0	78.0	73.5
Macrophages (%) in purest fractions[b]	94.8	97.2	96.3	97.9	96.6
Recovery of macrophages in purest fractions[b] (%)	13.2	58.9	93.8	47.2	53.5

[a]Experiments 11 - 14 were done using guinea pig peritoneal exudate cells induced by injection of casein 4 days prior to harvest. Each experiment is based on the fractionation of cells from a single Hartley guinea pig.
[b]In all four experiments, relatively pure macrophages were found in two successive fractions. These fractions were pooled accordingly, and chart values reflect differentials and counts on pooled fractions. In experiment 11 17% and 18% metrizamide interfaces were pooled, in experiments 12 and 13 16% and 17% interfaces were pooled, and in experiment 14 15 and 16% interfaces were pooled.

the buffy coat material was expressed through an 18-gauge needle into a 50-ml conical centrifuge tube containing an equal volume of MEM complete. Cells were washed three times in MEM complete by centrifugation at 1000 rpm for 10 min. After the final wash, cells were counted and resuspended to between 38.0×10^6 and 72.0×10^6 cells/ml. One milliliter of resulting cell suspension was layered onto each metrizamide gradient.

Casein-induced peritoneal exudate cells were collected from normal Hartley guinea pigs according to the method of David and David (2). Cells were washed three times in HBSS by centrifugation at 1000 rpm for 5 min. After the final wash, cells were counted and resuspended to between 25.0×10^6 and 61.0×10^6 cells/ml. One milliliter of resulting cell suspension was layered onto each metrizamide gradient.

B. Purification of Cells on Metrizamide Gradients

Cells were fractionated on slightly hypertonic discontinuous metrizamide gradients. A 30% working metrizamide solution was freshly prepared, and dilutions, in Tyrode's gel DNase, of this stock solution were made on a percentage basis ranging between 16 and 21% metrizamide (densities ranging between 1.088 and 1.108 gm/cm^3). To prepare individual gradients, 2 ml volumes of decreasing metrizamide densities, 1% difference each, were layered into 15-ml conical centrifuge tubes (Falcon No. 2095), each tube ultimately containing six gradient steps. A 1-ml suspension of human buffy coat cells or guinea pig peritoneal exudate cells (optimal cell concentrations ranging between 40.0 × 10^6 and 60.0 × 10^6 cells/ml) was layered onto each gradient. Gradients were spun for 45 min at 1200 g in a centrifuge with a nonflexible shaft. Temperature was maintained at 20°C throughout centrifugation. Cells were collected from each interface using Pasteur pipettes, and washed three times in MEM complete by centrifugation at 1000 rpm for 10 min. Total cell yield per fraction was determined, and cytocentrifuge smear preparations of each fraction were made. Smears were fixed for 5 min in methanol, allowed to air dry, and stained for 5 min in an 8% giemsa solution. Differentials were read under 100× oil immersion. In certain experiments, cells were then taken from each fraction and tested for functional integrity.

Cytocentrifuge smears of each fraction were stained for peroxidase activity according to the method of Kaplow (3). The ability of the cells to ingest latex particles (4) and to phagocytose antibody-coated red cells (5) were also determined.

IV. CRITICAL COMMENTS

Although absolute purity cannot be achieved by this modified metrizamide gradient method, fractions were recovered in which monocyte purity was found to be enriched at least eightfold from the buffy coat values (as is shown in Table I). This enrichment is substantial in view of the fact that it is achieved by a routine, single-step fractionation technique that is independent of the adherent capacity of human monocytes. Because the ability to adhere to surfaces is not the determining factor in this purification method, the necessary and tedious process of recovering cells from monolayers with EDTA, rubber policemen, or lidocaine treatment, all of which could possibly have an adverse effect on cell viability as well as on functional integrity, is not required. Therefore, under certain conditions this density gradient technique might be preferable to plating techniques. In all cases tested, the percent phagocytosis of either latex particles or sensitized sheep red blood cells correlated directly with the percent monocytes in fraction being analyzed (experiment 10, 88% monocyte/87% phagocytosis; experiment 9, 72% monocyte/68% phagocytosis; experiment 2, 90% monocyte/88% phagocytosis; experiment 3, 91% monocyte/85% phagocytosis; experiment 5, 83% monocyte/77 and 80% phagocytosis). This is evidence that differential counts were accurate and that the monocytes present were viable and functionally competent. Purity of the monocyte-enriched fraction increases as percent monocytes in buffy coat increases. It must be noted, however, that percent recovery of total monocytes in the enriched fraction seems to decrease as purity of that fraction increases. The fact that this method also allows for a mean macrophage purity of 96.6% in the fractionation of guinea pig peritoneal exudate cells could be very useful in cases in which one requires pure guinea pig macrophages devoid of neutrophil contamination. A preliminary experiment showed that this method might also be useful in purifying mouse peritoneal exudate macrophages.

Acknowledgment

Supported by NIH grant No. AI 07685 and a grant from the Rockefeller Foundation.

REFERENCES

1. M. A. Vadas, J. R. David, A. Butterworth, N. T. Pisani, and T. A. Siongok. A new method for the purification of human eosinophils and neutrophils, and a comparison of the ability of these cells to damage schistosomula of *Schistosoma mansoni*. *J. Immunol. 122*: 1228, 1979.
2. J. R. David and R. A. David. *In* "In Vitro Methods in Cell Mediated Immunity" (B. R. Bloom and P. R. Glade, eds.), p. 249. Academic Press, New York, 1970.
3. L. S. Kaplow. Simplified myeloperoxidase stain using benzidine hydrochloride. *Blood 26*: 215, 1965.
4. J. Michl, D. J. Ohlbaum, and S. C. Silverstein. 2-Deoxyglucose selectivity inhibits Fc and complement receptor-mediated phagocytosis in mouse peritoneal macrophages. *J. Exp. Med. 144*: 1465, 1976.
5. D. T. Fearon, K. F. Austen, and S. Ruddy. Formation of a hemolytically active intermediate by the interaction between properdin factors B±D and the activated third component of complement. *J. Exp. Med. 138*: 1305, 1973.

21

SEPARATION OF MURINE MONONUCLEAR PHAGOCYTES
BY DENSITY GRADIENTS OF PERCOLL

Raymond B. Hester
William S. Walker

I. INTRODUCTION

The study of mononuclear phagocytes (MP) has been aided by
techniques that allow the phagocytes to be separated into
functionally enriched subpopulations of cells (1 - 7). In the
procedure to be described, resident peritoneal cells, rich in
MP, are separated into subpopulations based on differences in
cell density. It must be stressed, however, that this technique is based on a physical rather than a functional property
of MP, and as such will yield functionally enriched subpopulations only if the two properties are related.

The separation of cells by density gradients is governed
in part by Stoke's law (8), which states that the rate of cell
sedimentation in a centrifugal field is zero when the cell en-
counters a medium of identical density. In discontinuous
density gradients, cells migrate under the influence of the
centrifugal field until they reach the interface of a solution
with a density equal to or greater than their own; at that

point, they cease moving. Cells with different densities will
come to rest at different points along the gradient, where
they can be recovered with ease.

II.   REAGENTS

Percoll (Pharmacia, Piscataway, New Jersey is polyvinyl-
pyrrolidone-coated silica and is supplied as a sterile colloidal suspension (9). An osmotically balanced (approximately
300 mOsM) stock solution of Percoll is prepared by adding one
part of sterile 1.5 M NaCl (10$^\times$ saline) to nine parts of Percoll. Gradient solutions of 39, 45, 51, 57 and 63% Percoll
are then prepared by diluting the osmotically balanced stock
solution with sterile, physiological saline (0.15 M NaCl) and
adjusting the refractive index of each solution to 1.3410,
1.3420, 1.3430, 1.3440, and 1.3450, respectively (Abbe re-
fractometer at room temperature; the osmotically balanced
Percoll is considered to be 100% for the purpose of preparing
the various gradient solutions).

Phosphate-buffered saline (PBS): 0.385g KH_2PO_4, 1.249 g;
K_2HPO_4, 8.49g NaCl, and deionized water to 1000 mg; pH 7.2;
osmolarity, 290 to 310 mOsM.
Mice: Approximately 15, 6 to 8 weeks of age, are required
to ensure enough peritoneal cells for one gradient ($10-15 \times 10^6$).
Each mouse yields 1 to 2 x 10^6 resident peritoneal cells.
Gradient tubes: Round-bottomed centrifuge tubes (15 ml
volume, Corning No. 8441 or equivalent) that have been siliconized (Prosil 80, Curtin Matheson Scientific) serve well as
the gradient tubes.

III.   PROCEDURE

The separation procedure is presented in detail below.

(1). The gradient solutions, PBS (approximately 500 ml)
and gradient tubes are prechilled and maintained in an ice
bath.
(2). To harvest the peritoneal cells, kill a mouse by
cervical dislocation; pin the animal, ventral side up, on a
dissecting board and peel back the skin on the abdomen. Using
a 10-ml plastic, disposable syringe with an 18-gauge needle,
inject up to 10 ml of ice-cold PBS (depending on the size of
the mouse) into the peritoneal cavity. Without removing the
needle from the peritoneal cavity, draw the PBS into the
syringe and transfer the cell suspension to a polypropylene
tube (Falcon No. 2070). Harvest the peritoneal cells from

one mouse before killing the next.

(3). Centrifuge the tubes containing the peritoneal cells in a refrigerated centrifuge (IEC CRU-5000 or equivalent) at 4°C and 200 g for 5 min.

(4). Draw off the supernatant fluid and resuspend the cell pellet, using a siliconized Pasteur pipette, in a total of 1 to 2 ml of ice-cold PBS. Count the cells and set aside a small aliquot for a differential count.

(5). Place 10 to 15 x 10^6 cells in a polypropylene tube and centrifuge for 5 min at 4°C and 200 g.

(6). Remove the supernatant fluid and resuspend the cell pellet carefully and completely, again using a siliconized Pasteur pipette, in 3 ml of the most dense Percoll solution (63%, RI = 1.3450). Transfer this cell suspension to the siliconized gradient tube; take care to ensure that the cells do not run down the side of the tube.

(7). Using a separate 5-ml pipette for each solution, slowly overlay the 63% Percoll with 3 ml each of 57, 51, 45, and 39% Percoll, taking care to maintain the gradient inter-faces. This may require some practice to do properly.

(8). Centrifuge the gradient for 30 min at 4°C in a re-frigerated centrifuge with a swinging-bucket rotor, using adapters if necessary. The rotor should be accelerated slowly to a speed that yields 300 g at the bottom of the gradient tube. After centrifugation, allow the rotor to decelerate without using the brake.

(9). Carefully remove the gradient tube and note the distribution of the cells. Record any evidence of cell clumping or streaming.

(10). Using siliconized Pasteur pipettes, transfer the cells from each interface to an appropriately labeled poly-propylene tube (Falcon No. 2070) containing approximately 10 ml of PBS. Cap and invert the tubes several times to en-sure complete mixing of the cells and Percoll in the PBS. Centrifuge at 200 g for 10 min at 4°C.

(11). Wash the cells three times with 10 ml of PBS by centrifuging at 200 g for 5 min at 4°C. Insufficient washing can cause the cells to aggregate.

(12). After washing, resuspend each pellet in 1 ml of PBS and count.

IV. CALCULATION OF DATA

When using density gradients to separate MP into subpopu-lations of cells, you must know the percentage of cells re-covered from the gradient, the distribution of the cells in the gradient, and the percentage of MP in each subpopulation.

(1). To determine the percent recovery, count the cells in each gradient fraction and divide this total (times 100) by the number of cells applied to the gradient.

(2). To determine the distribution of the cells in the different subpopulations, divide the number of cells in each fraction by the total number of cells *recovered* from the gradient.

(3). Any of a number of cell markers may be used to determine the percentage of MP in each fraction (see chapter by Russell and Bianco, this volume).

(4). Summarized in Table I are the results from a series of experiments testing the ability of subpopulations of resident peritoneal cells to render murine thymocytes functionally mature as measured by their acquisition of Con A responsiveness.

V. CRITICAL COMMENTS

The efficiency of cell recovery from a gradient will depend on whether the purity of a subpopulation takes precedent over the recovery of the maximum number of cells. Experience to date indicates that recoveries between 50 and 75% of the cells applied to the gradient can be expected with little chance for the contamination of the subpopulations. Furthermore, the proper attention to detail will usually result in reproducible numerical and functional distributions of the type shown in Table 1. The major source of variation is usually the use of unhealthy animals as cell donors and to the failure to prepare the gradient media properly.

The gradients are readily modified to accommodate MP from other sources, including established cell lines of macrophages (2). However, separation of peritoneal exudate cells (e.g., thioglycollate-elicited cells) by density gradient procedures can be more difficult because of the tendency of these cells to aggregate during isolation and separation.

Finally, we would like to reiterate that the use of density gradients to enrich for functionally distinct subpopulations of cells depends on (a) whether the activity of interest is restricted to a subpopulation, and (b) the relevant cells having buoyant densities sufficiently different to allow for their separation from the other cells. If these conditions can be met, then Percoll is a convenient and inexpensive medium to use in constructing gradients and will yield functionally enriched subpopulations of MP.

TABLE 1. *Functional Heterogeneity of Mouse Resident Peritoneal Cells in the Induction of Thymic Lymphocyte Maturation*

Percoll interface	Percentage of recovered cells	Percentage macrophages[a]	Percentage Ia+ cells[b]	Thymic lymphocyte maturation[c]
39/45	10	50	50	2+
45/51	25	50	50	4+
51/57	55	60	35	+-
57/63	10	15	70	-

[a]Determined by light microscopy and the uptake of latex particles.
[b]The percent of cells killed by an A.TH anti-A.TL antiserum and complement as determined by trypan blue dye exclusion.
[c]The response to concanavalin A by CBA mouse thymocytes following coculture with cells recovered from the indicated Percoll interfaces. The data are summarized based on a scale of 1+ to 4+ for increasing activity.

REFERENCES

    1. W. S. Walker. Functional heterogeneity of macrophages.
In "Immunobiology of the Macrophage" (D. S. Nelson, ed.),
pp. 91-111. Academic Press, New York, 1976.
    2. C. S. Serio, D. M. Gandour, and W. S. Walker.
Macrophage functional heterogeneity: Evidence for different
antibody-dependent effector cell activities and expression of
Fc receptors among macrophage subpopulations. *J. Reticuloendothel. Soc. 25*:197-206, 1979.
    3. K.-C. Lee, A. Wilkinson, and M. Wong. Antigen-
specific murine T-cell proliferation: Role of macrophage
surface Ia and factors. *Cell. Immunol. 48*:79-90, 1979.
    4. W. S. Walker. Functional heterogeneity of macrophages:
Subclasses of peritoneal macrophages with different antigen-
binding activities and immune complex receptors. *Immunology
26*:1025-1037, 1974.
    5. H. V. Raff, K. C. Cochrum, and J. D. Stobo.
Macrophage - T cell interactions in the Con A induction of
human suppressive T cells. *J. Immunol. 121*:2311-2315, 1978.
    6. K.-C. Lee and D. Berry. Functional heterogeneity in
macrophages activated by *Corynebacterium parvuum:* Characterization of subpopulations with different activities in promoting
immune responses and suppressing tumor cell growth. *J. Immunol.
118*:1530-1540, 1977.
    7. D. S. Weinberg, M. Fishman, and B. C. Veit. Functional
heterogeneity among peritoneal macrophages. I. Effector cell
activity of macrophages against syngeneic and xenogeneic tumor
cells. *Cell. Immunol. 38*:94-104, 1978.
    8. K. Shortman. Physical procedures for the separation
of animal cells. *Ann. Rev. Biophys. Bioeng. 1*:93-130, 1972.
    9. H. Pertoff, and T. C. Laurent. Isopycnic separation
of cells and organelles by centrifugation in modified silica
gradients. *In* "Methods of Cell Separation" (N. Catsimpoolas,
ed.), pp. 25-61. Plenum, New York, 1977.

22

SEPARATION OF MONOCYTES BY DENSITY GRADIENTS OF PERCOLL

R. Seljelid

H. Pertoft

The ideal method for the isolation of monocytes should be
applicable to blood from all species, be simple and require
only standard laboratory equipment, produce pure cells at
maximum yield, and not influence the biological and chemical
properties of the monocytes. Such a method does not exist.
By far the most widely used method for isolation of monocytes
from human blood is centrifugation on Ficoll-Isopaque (1).
The method is simple and reproducible, but has a few disadvantages, e.g., careful washing of the cells is necessary for
most purposes. Washing is potentially harmful to the cells
and also causes considerable cell loss (2). The method produces a mixture of monocytes and lymphocytes and a varying
number of granulocytes. Recently, a novel gradient medium,
Percoll, has been employed for the separation of blood monocytes (3). Percoll appears to be nontoxic, has a low
viscosity, and little osmotic effect, and these last two
properties permit the preparation of blood-isotonic solutions
through a wide density range (4,5). This chapter describes

a one-step procedure for obtaining a high yield suspension of
monocytes of about 20% purity, and a two-step procedure for
obtaining better than 90% monocytes at a lower yield. Both
methods are described here with human blood as starting
material; the methods may be used with rat and mouse blood
with minor modifications of the densities of the gradient
medium.

I. THE ONE-STEP PROCEDURE (HIGH YIELD)

A. *Introduction*

    This procedure is similar to the widely used Isopaque-
Ficoll separation and should be preferred when an admixture
of nonadherent lymphocytes does not constitute a problem,
e.g., for routine work *in vitro*.

B. *Reagents*

    Stock isotonic Percoll (SIP). Nine volumes of commercial
Percoll (Pharmacia Fine Chemicals AB, Uppsala, Sweden) are
diluted with one volume of 15 M NaCl to make a density of
1.124 gm/ml, pH 8.2, isosmotic to blood plasma. The commercial Percoll varies in density from batch to batch (1.130-
1.135 gm/ml), so that each new solution of SIP must be checked
and adjusted to 1.124 gm/ml before use. Densities may be
accurately measured at 22°C by use of organic density columns,
refractive index (4) or density-marker beads (Pharmacia Fine
Chemicals, AB, Uppsala, Sweden).

C. *Procedures*

    (1). Blood is collected into evacuated glass tubes con-
taining polystyrene beads (Becton Dickinson-France S.A.,
Grenoble, France), and defibrinated by rotation (5 rpm) for
15 min. The blood may also be defibrinated by use of a glass
rod or glass beads.
    (2). Seven milliliters of defibrinated blood is layered
on top of 4 ml of a 60% (v/v) SIP in 0.15 M NaCl, density
1.076 gm/ml, in a 12-ml conical polystyrene tube.
    (3). The tube is centrifuged at 800 $g$av for 30 min at
room temperature in any standard laboratory centrifuge
equipped with a swing-out rotor. A clear supernatant of pure

serum (which can be used in cell culture) is produced, with a
clearly discernible band (volume 1.5-2 ml) consisting of mononuclear cells located in the interface below the middle of the
tube and a pellet at the bottom consisting mainly of lymphocytes, granulocytes, and erythrocytes.

   (4). The serum and the interface band may be collected by
use of a Pasteur pipette. If the cells in the interface are
not to be used immediately in an *in vitro* experiment, they
should be kept in a cooled test tube to prevent adherence of
monocytes to the tube wall and subsequent loss of cells. In
some cases small aggregates of cells may be formed during the
centrifugation, but usually these can easily be dispersed by
use of a pipette.

D. *Identification of Cells and Calculation of Data*

   It is important to perform a May-Grünewald-Giemsa staining
on a smear of the original blood as well as the mononuclear
cell fraction. A May-Grüwald-Giemsa stained preparation provides a survey of the morphology and permits detection of
contaminating granulocytes. Esterase staining with α-naphthyl
acetate as substrate can be used to differentiate between
monocytes (strongly esterase positive) and lymphocytes (6-8).
Although a definitive identification of mononuclear phagocytes
requires determination of the cells' ability to phagocytose
by way of the Fc receptor, one is usually well served by the
esterase staining for routine use.

E. *Critical Comments*

   One can usually obtain around 20% purity of monocytes
(16-32%) (3). The yield is more difficult to assess since
the original number of monocytes in whole blood is controversial. Assuming that 5% of the white blood cells in whole
blood are monocytes (2), the yield is practically 100%.

   Probably the most important potential pitfall in the procedure is the defibrination of the blood. Monocytes adhere
strongly to small, perhaps microscopic blood clots. Also the
viability of the cells is decreased substantially after contact with blood clots.

   If the monocytes are to be used *in vitro* for short- or
long-term cultures, they may be transferred directly from the
centrifuge tube to the tissue culture without washing. Autologous serum is provided by the same centrifugation. It is
well to remember that the presence of Percoll in the cell suspension will increase the density of the tissue culture medium

and thus slow down the sedimentation of the cells. Monocytes are best cultivated at high serum concentration (around 50%) in any conventional tissue culture medium and may be kept this way without change of medium for weeks. The reproducibility of the procedure can be improved somewhat by adjustment of the Percoll density before centrifugation according to the hematocrit value, so that the Percoll density after centrifugation is kept constant. This is not necessary for routine use with blood of normal hematocrit values, for details, see (3).

II.   THE TWO-STEP PROCEDURE

A.   *Introduction*

In some cases one would like to have a high purity suspension of monocytes for immediate biochemical studies of the cells as they appear in the blood without adaptation to *in vitro* conditions, etc. The following method was developed to meet this need.

B.   *Reagents*

The same SIP is used as described in Section I.B.

C.   *Procedure*

The mononuclear bands from two tubes contrifuged according to the one-step procedure are collected and diluted to 7 ml with 0.15 M NaCl and layered on top of 3 ml of a 50% (v/v) solution of SIP in 0.15 ml M NaCl (density 1.064 gm/ml). Centrifugation for 60 min at 800 $g$av at 4°C produces an interface band (in some experiments two closely situated bands are formed), which contains monocytes, and a pellet that contains lymphocytes, erythrocytes, and, in some experiments, a few granulocytes.

D.   *Calculation of Data*

Data calculated as described in Section I.D.

E. Critical Comments

With the two-step procedure, one can routinely obtain monocytes at purity better than 90%. The yield is more controversial as commented upon in Section I.D. It is essential to have a single cell suspension before starting centrifugation No. 2. If there is a little aggregation after the first centrifugation, the cells should be gently dispersed with a pipette. For the same reason, the second step should be performed at 4°C (3).

REFERENCES

1. A. Bøyum. Isolation of mononuclear cells and granulocytes from human blood. Isolation of mononuclear cells by one centrifugation and of granulocytes by combining centrifugation and sedimentation at 1 g. *Scand. J. Clin. Lab. Invest. 21:* Suppl 97: 77-89, 1968.
2. W. D. Johnson, B. Mei, and Z. A. Cohn. The separation, long-term cultivation, and maturation of the human monocyte. *J. Exp. Med. 146:* 1613-1626, 1977.
3. H. Pertoft, A. Johnsson, B. Wärmegård, and R. Seljelid. Separation of human monocytes on density gradients of Percoll. *J. Immunol. Methods.* In press, 1980.
4. H. Pertoft, and T. C. Laurent. Isopycnic separation of cells and cell organelles by centrifugation in modified colloidal silica gradients. *In* "Methods of Cell Separation" (N. Catsimpoolas, ed.), pp. 25-65. Plenum, New York, 1977.
5. H. Pertoft, T. C. Laurent, T. Låås, and L. Kågedal. Density gradients prepared from colloidal silica particles coated by polyvinylpyrrolidone (Percoll). *Anal. Biochem. 88:* 271-282, 1978.
6. T. Barka and P. J. Anderson. "Histochemistry. Theory, Practice, and Bibliography." Hoeber Medical Division, Harper & Row, New York, Evanston, and London, 1963.
7. T. H. Tötterman, A. Ranki, and P. Häyry. Expression of the acid α-naphthyl acetate esterase marker by activated and secondary T-lymphocytes in man. *Scand. J. Immunol. 6:* 305-310, 1977.
8. P. G. Gill, C. A. Waller, and I. C. M. Maclennan. Relationships between different functional properties of human monocytes. *Immunology 33:* 873-880, 1977.

23

SEPARATION OF MURINE MONONUCLEAR PHAGOCYTES
BY VELOCITY SEDIMENTATION AT UNIT GRAVITY

Louis M. Pelus
Malcolm A. S. Moore

I. INTRODUCTION

The study of many problems in cell biology are often complicated by the fact that starting cell populations are complex, consisting of a variety of functionally different cells.
Physical separation into cell subpopulations retaining functional integrity would clearly provide a more specific means
of pursuing cellular investigations. The fact that cell function can often be associated with changes in cell size has led
to the development and refinement of cell separation by velocity sedimentation (1).

The principle of velocity sedimentation separation at unit
gravity is based primarily upon the fact that, in a shallow
gradient of low density, variations in terminal velocity result
from differences in cell size. Using a continuous step gradient
of 0.3 - 2.0% bovine serum albumin (BSA), in isotonic buffered
saline, a gradient having an average density of 1.010 (1.0074 -
1.0113) gm/cm^3 is formed (2). Since most mammalian cells have

a cell diameter of 5.0 to 20.0 μm and densities in the range
of 1.05 to 1.10 gm/cm^3, it becomes apparent that cell size will
be the determining factor effecting terminal velocity and thus
the separation. [A complete discussion of the theory involved
in unit gravity velocity sedimentation can be found in (2).]

The technique of velocity sedimentation has been widely applied in the field of hematology and more recently immunology.
It has been successfully used to separate and enrich for various hematopoietic stem cell populations (3-6) and to separate
bone marrow monocytoid cells that stimulate myeloid colony formation from marrow myeloid colony-forming cells (6, 7). More
recently, velocity sedimentation has been used to separate populations of elicited murine peritoneal cells differing in their
cytotoxic capacity and ability to promote the *in vitro* antibody-
forming response (8), and to separate resident mouse peritoneal
mononuclear cells differing in their production of granulocyte-
macrophage colony-stimulating factors (GM-CSF) (9, 10) and responding to modulation by lactoferrin (10).

II. REAGENTS

Velocity sedimentation at unit gravity is performed using
the Sta-Put cell separator, available from O. H. John's Scientific, Toronto, Canada. The apparatus has three main parts, a
sedimentation chamber [available in three sizes (11, 17, and
25 cm) to suit individual needs for small- to large-scale
separation], an intermediate loading vessel, and a gradient
maker. The procedure detailed herein will describe cell separation using the 25-cm sedimentation chamber having a fluid
column capacity of 1200 ml and capable of separating a maximum
of 300 × 10^6 cells. [The major limitation to cell separation
by velocity sedimentation is the phenomenon of streaming.
Beyond a critical cell concentration no separation can be obtained. The phenomenon of streaming and "streaming limit" is
discussed elsewhere (2).]

Cell separation can be satisfactorily performed in gradients of fetal calf serum (FCS), BSA, Ficoll, or Percoll. We
routinely use BSA as the gradient material (Cohn fraction V).
In order not to create an appreciable tonicity gradient, lyophilized BSA is prepared in isotonic phosphate-buffered saline
(PBS) (∿320 mOsm for murine cells and ∿280 mOsm for human
cells). A stock solution of 10% BSA (w/v) in PBS is prepared,
membrane sterilized, and stored either at 4°C or frozen until
used.

Nonspecific cell sticking to glass, particularly the sedimentation chamber cone and intermediate vessel, can result in

cell loss and random contamination of cell fractions. In order
to minimize cell sticking, especially when the separation involves mononuclear phagocytes, the sedimentation chamber and
intermediate vessel are siliconized. Siliconization is performed by immersion in a 1% solution of Prosil-28 (PCR Research
Chemicals, Inc., Gainesville, Florida), followed by thorough
rinsing in distilled water. In addition, all chamber inter-
connections should be made with silicone tubing (Silastic, Dow
Corning).

Albumin solutions of 1% (600 ml), 2% (600 ml), 0.2% (50 ml),
and 0.3% (50 ml) should be prepared in isotonic PBS by dilution
from the 10% stock BSA solution. All solutions should be stored
at 4°C until used.

Isolation of resident murine peritoneal cells are obtained
by peritoneal lavage with cold McCoy's modified 5A medium containing antibiotics, 2% FCS, and 2 U/ml preservative-free heparin. Other methods for mononuclear phagocyte cell isolation
can be found elsewhere in this volume.

III. PROCEDURES

The separation procedure is presented in detail below.

(1) Locate and level the Sta-Put apparatus within a 4°C
cold room (to reduce the metabolic activity of the cells) in
an area free from mechanical vibration and jarring.

(2) Prior to use, the sedimentation chamber, intermediate
vessel, and gradient makers should be washed, the appropriate
parts siliconized as described, and completely connected. The
assembled apparatus consists of the sedimentation chamber with
steel baffle, connected by means of a three-way valve and tubing to the intermediate vessel (with spin-bar), which in turn
is connected to the two large gradient chambers [left column A
(with spin-bar) and right chamber B]. Tubing clamps are located between the three-way valve and intermediate vessel, intermediate vessel and gradient chamber A, and on either side of
chamber B. The assembled apparatus is then appropriately
wrapped, steam or gas sterilized (if necessary), and placed onto
the Sta-Put cabinet. For sterilization, the sedimentation
chamber is disconnected and sterilized apart from the rest of
the apparatus.

(3) It is imperative, that the stainless steel flow baffle
be carefully centered inside the cone of the sedimentation
chamber. This baffle is used to deflect incoming fluid during
loading, and is necessary to avoid gradient mixing. With practice, the baffle can be easily positioned using a sterile pipette or glass rod.

(4) Load 50 ml of PBS into the sedimentation chamber through the intermediate vessel, making sure that all tubing on the sedimentation chamber side of the intermediate vessel is filled with PBS and free of air bubbles. Reclamp tubing before the loading vessel empties. This fluid layer functions to prevent disturbance of the cell band by air currents and the rising fluid column.

(5) Clamp the lines between the loading vessel and the gradient chambers. Load 600 ml of 1.0% BSA in the left chamber and 600 ml of 2.0% BSA in the right chamber. Unclamp the lines slightly in order to fill the connecting tubing, making sure no air bubbles remain in the lines, and reclamp. At this point, the velocity sedimentation chamber is ready for the introduction of the cell population. As stated earlier, this chamber can accommodate a maximum of 300×10^6 total cells. However, depending upon the number of cells required for functional analysis, the starting cell population can often be manipulated to enrich for particular cells, before loading into the chamber, provided that those cells so removed have no accessory function. When separating resident or elicited murine peritoneal cells, we have found it advantageous to remove contaminating red blood cells. This is performed by pelleting the cells and resuspending in 5.0 ml of $0.174 \, M \, NH_4Cl$ on ice for 5 min. A layer of 5.0 ml of fetal calf serum is then introduced under the suspension, and viable nucleated cells are recovered by centrifugation through the serum cushion. For human peripheral blood or bone marrow cell separation, neutral density centrifugation through BSA at $1.070 \, gm/cm^3$ or Ficoll, $1.077 \, gm/cm^3$, has proved useful for mononuclear cell enrichment provided that granulocytes are not required. Cell suspensions are adjusted to a concentration of 300×10^6 cells in 40 ml of isotonic PBS. An appropriate number of cells should be set aside at this point to serve as an unseparated control.

(6) Load the cells through the intermediate vessel and reclamp the line as soon as the chamber is near empty. A flow rate of 10 ml/min is adequate. Passage of the cell suspension through a 22-gauge spinal needle under slight positive pressure during loading will break up small cell aggregates and cell doublets and will ensure a uniform single cell suspension.

(7) Rinse the intermediate vessel twice with 25 ml of 0.2% BSA in PBS (50 ml total) using a syringe and spinal needle. Make certain that no air bubbles are introduced. Adjust the flow rate to approximately 2 - 3 ml/min.

(8) Fill the intermediate vessel with 0.3% BSA in PBS to the height of the fluid column in the gradient chambers and start the magnetic stirrers (avoid foaming). The time elapsed between introducing the cells and starting the gradient should be less than 10 min.

(9) Remove all clamps and record the time (t_1). Once the

cells have been lifted off the bottom of the sedimentation
cone, the flow rate can be continuously increased. Loading
should be as rapid as possible (30 min) without disturbing
the cell band.

(10) Record the time the fluid column reaches the top of
the sedimentation cone (t_2). From this point on, the gradient
can be left to load itself.

(11) After an appropriate sedimentation time (usually 3.5
to 4 hr), the chamber is unloaded through the three-way valve,
at a flow rate of 35 to 40 ml/min. Record time (t_3) when un-
loading is started. The first 250 ml is the cone volume and
is discarded.

(12) Collect the remainder of the gradient in equal 35-ml
fractions. We have found that conical graduated Falcon centrifuge tubes (No. 2070, Falcon Plastics, Division of Becton Dickinson and Co., Oxnard, California) particularly useful for both
quantitation of fraction volume and estimation of flow rate.
Record the time the collection of the first fraction is started
(t_4) and the last fraction is finished (t_5), as well as the
number (N_f) and volume (v_f) of the final fraction.

(13) All individual cell fractions should be kept on ice
to prevent cell aggregation. Wash each fraction three times
in cold media containing 2% FCS and finally resuspend in 5 ml
of complete media containing 15% FCS.

(14) Determine the cell concentration and viability in each
fraction. We routinely use vital dye exclusion and counting by
hemacytometer; however, electronic cell counting can be used.
In our hands, cell recoveries of 85 - 95% and with greater than
95% viability are routinely obtained.

(15) Adjust all fractions to uniform cell concentration depending upon the individual assay procedure to be employed. We
have found a cell density of 10^6/ml to be a suitable starting
concentration for most procedures. However, to obtain this
concentration, it is often necessary to pool fractions, particularly in the most rapid and slow sedimentation cell fractions.
In pooling fractions, no more than three consecutive fractions,
corresponding to approximately a 1 mm/hr sedimentation rate difference (see Section IV), should be combined.

IV. CALCULATION OF DATA

A. *Calculation of Sedimentation Velocity*

Populations of separated cells can be best characterized by
their sedimentation velocity (s) in millimeters per hour, related to a standard set of conditions, which for this procedure

have been adopted as 4°C and a gradient with an average density
of approximately 1.010 gm/cm^3. Under these conditions, absolute
s values are accurate within 5% (2).

The calculation of sedimentation velocity is performed using
a mathematical equation, determined by Miller and Phillips (2),
which describes the distance the cells have fallen through the
gradient. The sedimentation velocity in millimeters per hour
for fraction N is given by

$$s(N) = \frac{(N_f - N - \frac{1}{2})v - (V_0 + \frac{1}{2}V_{cb} - v_f)}{\alpha[(t_4 - t_1) - 0.4(t_4 + t_2 - t_3 - t_1) + N(t_5 - t_4)/N_f]}$$

where the times (t_1 through t_5 in hours) are the times at which
loading was started (t_1), the cells reached the top of the sedimentation chamber cone (t_2), draining was started (t_3), the
first fraction was collected (t_4), and completion of the un-
loading procedure (t_5). The chamber constant (α) or milliliters
per millimeter of length in the cylindrical portion of the chamber is given as α = 22.5 for the 25-cm chamber, N is the fraction number you are calculating an s value for, v the volume of
fraction N, and N_f and v_f describe the final fraction number and
volume, respectively. The volume of fluid above the cell band
is given by V_0 (50 ml of PBS) and the volume of the cell band
by V_{cb} (40 ml).

B. Expression of Data

The biophysical properties of the given cell populations
are adequately expressed as their sedimentations velocities.
However, this expression is only meaningful when used in combination with a description of the functions and/or properties of
a given cell population. This leads us to consider how one expresses the functional data concerning each cell fraction in a
manner that best describes cellular enrichment, functional activity, and relation to control cells, as well as in a form that
allows individual assays to be compared.

Individual cell fractions contain widely varying cell numbers, expecially when starting with a mixed cell population (see
Fig. 1). Therefore, one must express data as a function of
cells. For those cell populations in which one cannot directly
identify each cell possessing the measurable property, this can
be quantitated in either of two ways. Data can be expressed as
a function of a standard number of cells from each fraction.
Thus when plotted, all data will be expressed as activity per
unit number of cells with a particular sedimentation velocity.
This method of data expression is best used for generating an
enrichment profile, or detecting maximal activity in circumstances in which even after cell separation, the active cells
represent a minor component of the total fraction cell number.

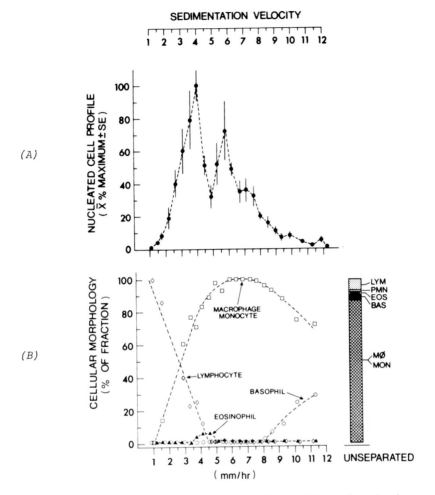

Fig. 1.   (A) Total nucleated cell profile of velocity
sedimentation separated BDF₁, resident nucleated peritoneal
cells. Data are normalized to the maximal cell containing
fraction and expressed as $\overline{X} \pm S.E.M.$ for four experiments.
(B) Total nucleated cell profile and morphological evaluation
of separated cells in a representative experiment. Morphology
was determined by oil microscopy (×960) on a minimum of 300
cells from each of duplicate Wright stained cytocentrifuge
slide preparations.

The second method of data expression compares individual fractions of cells. In this method, functional activity again is
based upon assay of a standard number of cells, however, it is
corrected to represent total cells within the fraction. Critical to this method, is the necessity of measuring cellular ac-

tivity on the linear portion of the dose - response curve. After correction, the data can be normalized by assigning an activity of 100% to that cell fraction having maximal activity, and expressing each fraction as a percent of maximum. This normalization is performed by dividing the activity of each fraction by the maximum activity. When plotted, the resulting profile allows one at a glance to determine where maximal activity lies and to assess the relative contribution of all cell fractions. The major advantage of this method lies in the ability to compare directly individual assays.

In reporting data on morphology, phagocytosis, or any cell function where one can directly quantitate the number of cells which possess a particular property, the results should be expressed as the percentage of cells positive for the given characteristic as a function of sedimentation velocity.

V. CRITICAL COMMENTS

Velocity sedimentation is not a preparative cell isolation procedure, but rather is analytical in nature, designed to compare and contrast populations of cells differing in size. We have found this technique to be highly reproducible when applied to the study of the mononuclear phagocytic cell lineage and to resolve effectively monocytoid cell populations with differential characteristics and functions.

In four separate experiments, two major populations of nucleated cells could be separated (Fig. 1A). The maximal recoverable cell population characteristically sedimented with a modal velocity of 4.0 mm/hr and consisted primarily of small monocytes and less differentiated monocytoid cells, with some lymphocyte contamination (Fig. 1B). Relatively pure populations of lymphoid cells were found in the sedimentation range of 1.0 - 3.0 mm/hr with 30 - 45% of these cells sensitive to monoclonal anti-Thy 1.2 antibody plus complement treatment.

The second major population of cells sedimented with a modal velocity of 5.8 mm/hr and corresponded to relatively pure populations of monocytes and macrophages sedimenting in the range of 5.0 - 8.0 mm/hr. Cell fractions with a sedimentation velocity greater than 9.0 mm/hr contained less than 3% of the total recoverable cells and were comprised of large well-differentiated macrophages with increasing numbers of basophils and mast cells.

Biophysical cell separation does not "*a priori*" guarantee a separation of cell function. It is up to the investigator carefully to define and compare isolated cell fractions using a variety of assays characteristic of or specific for the range of cell populations that might be present. Only in this way can subpopulations of cells or cells at different stages of differentiation be identified.

TABLE I. *Characterization of Mononuclear Cell Populations*

Sedimentation velocity	Recovered cells (range, 4 Expts) (%)	Phagocytosis (% positive per fraction)	Fc receptor (% positive per fraction)	Nonspecific esterase (% positive per fraction)
11.0 - 12.0	0.1 - 0.5	67	89	69
10.0 - 11.0	0.1 - 0.6	73	87	77
9.0 - 10.0	0.8 - 2	74	81	82
8.0 - 9.0	3 - 7	84	72	95
7.0 - 8.0	6 - 9	93	58	98
6.0 - 7.0	10 - 19	88	59	99
5.0 - 6.0	17 - 23	68	73	96
4.0 - 5.0	10 - 24	25	82	87
3.0 - 4.0	18 - 31	6	61	67
2.0 - 3.0	8 - 10	2	32	28
1.0 - 2.0	0.2 - 1.5	0	10	18
Unseparated	—	51	71	80

Adherence (% per fraction)	Lysozyme (ng/ml/10^5 cells)	N-Acetyl-β-D-glucosa-minidase (nM/hr/10^6 cells)	Ectoenzyme 5'-nucleo-tidase (nM/min/10^6 cells)	Neutral pro-tease activity (% fibrinolysis/ 2.5 × 10^5 cells)
96	47	1522	167	1
96	10	1637	193	2
97	34	1368	200	2
94	51	328	227	2
94	37	568	234	2
87	53	673	223	2
77	30	321	113	3
54	<10	200	30	13
17	<10	96	15	20
0	<10	72	31	3
0	<10	107	47	0
58	12	900	127	3

TABLE II.   *Cytotoxic Activity of Mononuclear Cell Populations[a]*

Sedimentation velocity	Natural cytotoxicity (NC)	Natural killer (NK)	ADCC	Spontaneous killing
11.0 - 12.0	-	-	++	++
10.0 - 11.0	-	-	++	++
9.0 - 10.0	-	-	++	++
8.0 - 9.0	-	-	++	+
7.0 - 8.0	-	-	+	++
6.0 - 7.0	-	-	++	+
5.0 - 6.0	-	-	++	++
4.0 - 5.0	-	++	-	+
3.0 - 4.0	++	++	-	-
2.0 - 3.0	++	+	-	-
1.0 - 2.0	++	-	-	-

[a] ++, Enrichment, significantly greater than unseparated cells; +, equivalent to unseparated cells; -, 0, or significantly lower than unseparated cells。

Separated resident murine peritoneal cells have been evaluated using a number of functional assays characteristic for the monocytoid cell lineage (Tables I and II). Although the sedimentation range for maximal activity varied with the particular function assayed, expression of properties characteristic of monocytoid cells were found in cells in a broad sedimentation range of 4.0 - 12.0 mm/hr, with elevated functional monocytoid expression observed with increasing cell size. Thus, cells in the sedimentation range of 6.0 - 12.0 mm/hr were highly adherent, phagocytic, Fc receptor positive cells, which stained intensely for cytoplasmic nonspecific esterase activity and negative for peroxidase (not shown). Moreover, high lysozyme, acid hydrolase, and membrane ectoenzyme activity and low neutral proteolytic capacity was observed (Table I). Antibody-dependent cellular cytotoxicity (ADCC) and nonspecific spontaneous tumor target cytotoxicity could be demonstrated throughout this range (Table II). In all cases, significant enrichment of activity in comparison to unseparated cells was evident.

In the 4.0 - 6.0 mm/hr sedimentation range, more variability or heterogeneity in functional activity was observed. Most cells in this range possessed Fc receptors and stained positively but diffusely for nonspecific esterases, however they were less adherent, and with reduced phagocytic capacity, low lysozyme and acid hydrolase activity, and lower overall ADCC and spontaneous cytotoxicity in comparison to the more rapidly sedimenting fractions. Morphologically, the major proportion of these cells appeared to be early members of the monocytoid cell lineage, having a high nuclear-to-cytoplasmic ration, highly lobulated nucleus, and lacy chromatin pattern. Furthermore, these cells were non-T, non-B by appropriate antibody plus complement treatment. The high neutral proteolytic and low ectoenzyme activities of these cells further support a monocytoid origin at an early stage of differentiation. Moreover, both populations of cells have the capacity to produce constitutively granulocyte-macrophage colony-stimulating factor (GM-CSF) required for myeloid stem cell proliferation; however only GM-CSF production by those cells in the 5.0 - 8.0 mm/hr sedimentation range can be regulated by lactoferrin, a PMN-derived inhibitor of macrophage GM-CSF production (10). The ability of lactoferrin to inhibit GM-CSF is dependent on specific cell surface receptors that are not expressed on the more slowly sedimenting GM-CSF producing cells and perhaps become expressed with differentiations. It appears that like the bone marrow myeloid stem cell (CFU-GM), which acquires the responsiveness to growth promotion by GM-CSF before becoming sensitive to growth inhibitions (11), so too, the monocytoid cell acquires the ability to produce GM-CSF before entering a stage of responsiveness to regulation.

A central and yet unresolved question concerning the monocytoid cell lineage is that of heterogeneous cell populations. The unitarian concept would argue that the cells pass through different stages of differentiation and that each function becomes more or less prominent at each stage. An alternate view recognizes functionally distinct and specialized macrophage subsets, not necessarily related in a differentiation sequence. Although the concept of discrete subpopulations of monocytoid cells cannot be excluded by the data presented, the observed characteristics, at least for resident murine peritoneal monocytoid cells separated by velocity sedimentation, indicate an apparent continuum of monocytoid differentiation associated with increasing cell size. A definitive resolution to macrophage heterogeneity will require a combination of cell separatory procedures such as velocity sedimentation plus continuous or discontinuous density gradient centrifugation, as well as the comparative study of monocytoid cells inhabiting discrete anatomical locations, and the study of committed bone marrow stem cells.

Acknowledgments

Supported by Grants CA 28512 and CA 19052 from the National Cancer Institute, DHEW, and the Gar Reichman Foundation. The authors wish to thank Drs. J. Hamilton and P. Ralph of this de-

partment for analysis of neutral proteolytic activity and lysozyme, respectively, and Dr. Bonney of the Merck Institute
for Therapeutic Research, Rahway, New Jersey for measuring
acid hydrolase activity.

LMP is a Special Fellow of the Leukemia Society of
America, Inc.

REFERENCES

1. R. G. Miller and R. A. Phillips. Separation of cells by
   velocity sedimentation. *J. Cell Physiol*. *73*: 191-198,
   1969.
2. R. G. Miller. Separation of cells by velocity sedimentation. *In* "New Techniques in Biophysics and Cell Biology"
   (R. H. Pain and B. J. Smith, eds.), pp. 87-112. Wiley,
   London, 1973.
3. D. J. A. Sutherland, J. E. Till, and E. A. McCulloch.
   Short term cultures of mouse marrow cells separated by
   velocity sedimentation. *Cell Tissue Kinet*. *4*: 479-490,
   1971.
4. R. G. Worton, E. A. McCulloch, and J. E. Till. Physical
   separation of hematopoietic stem cells from cells forming
   colonies in culture. *J. Cell Physiol*. *74*: 171-182, 1969.
5. N. Jacobsen, H. E. Broxmeyer, E. Crossbard, and M. A. S.
   Moore. Colony-forming units in diffusion chambers
   (CFU-D) and colony-forming units in agar culture (CFU-C)
   obtained from normal human bone marrow: A possible
   parent-progeny relationship. *Cell Tissue Kinet*. *12*:
   213-226, 1979.
6. N. Williams and R. R. Eger. Purification and characterization of granulocyte-macrophage precursor cell populations. *In* "Hematopoietic Cell Differentiation" (D. W.
   Golden, M. Cline, D. Metcalf, and C. F. Fox, eds.), pp.
   385-398. Academic Press, New York, 1978.
7. N. Williams and M. A. S. Moore. Sedimentation velocity
   characterization of the cell cycle of granulocyte progenitor cells in monkey hemopoietic tissue. *J. Cell Physiol*.
   82: 81-92, 1973.
8. K. C. Lee and D. Berry. Functional heterogeneity in
   macrophages activated by *Corynebacterium parvum*: Characterization of subpopulations with different activities in
   promoting immune responses and suppressing tumor cell
   growth. *J. Immunol*. *118*: 1530-1540, 1977.
9. J. I. Kurland, L. M. Pelus, P. Ralph, R. S. Bockman, and
   M. A. S. Moore. Induction of prostaglandin E synthesis
   in normal and neoplastic macrophages: Role for colony-

stimulating factor(s) distinct from effects on myeloid progenitor cell proliferation. *Proc. Nat. Acad. Sci. USA 76*: 2326-2330, 1979.

10. L. M. Pelus, H. E. Broxmeyer, M. deSousa, and M. A. S. Moore. Heterogeneity among resident murine peritoned macrophages: Separation and functional characterization of monocytoid cells producing granulocyte-macrophage colony stimulating factor (GM-CSF), and responding to regulation by lactoferrin. *J. Immunol. 126*: 1016-1021, 1981.

11. L. M. Pelus, H. E. Broxmeyer, and M. A. S. Moore. Regulation of human myelopoiesis by prostanglandin E and lactoferrin. *Cell Tissue Kinet.*, in press.

24

USE OF LIDOCAINE FOR DETACHMENT
OF ADHERENT MONONUCLEAR PHAGOCYTES

Carl F. Nathan

I. INTRODUCTION

It is frequently desirable to obtain in suspension mononuclear phagocytes that have adhered to glass or plastic surfaces. Trypsinization is usually ineffective; at the same
time, it alters phagocytic receptors and other surface structures. Scraping with a rubber policeman in divalent cation-
deficient media at low temperatures often gives low yields
and poor viability when used with mouse peritoneal macrophages, although it may be more successful with human blood
monocytes. In 1975, Rabinovitch and DeStefano introduced the
use of the local anesthetic, lidocaine, for the detachment of
adherent cells (1). Lidocaine causes macrophages to round up
and often permits them to be dislodged with mechanical
measures that would otherwise be ineffective.

The lidocaine method gives nearly quantitative recoveries
only under carefully defined conditions, which must be worked
out for each experimental situation. The best results have

been obtained with resident mouse peritoneal macrophages, human blood monocytes, and murine macrophagelike cell lines. Results have frequently been unsatisfactory using elicited or activated peritoneal macrophages of the mouse and guinea pig. In addition, after phagocytosis, macrophages tend to become refractory to detachment by lidocaine. Nonphagocytic adherent cells may still be recovered almost quantitatively (2), but the macrophages themselves are damaged.

II. REAGENTS

Preservative-free lidocaine hydrochloride is obtained from Astra Pharmaceuticals, Worcester, Massachusetts. A stock solution of 360 mM is prepared in normal saline and carefully titrated to pH 6.55 with NaOH. At more alkaline pH, the drug precipitates. The stock solution may be sterilized by autoclaving or by filtration. It is stable for many months at 4° or -20°C.

III. PROCEDURE

The following procedure applies to resident mouse peritoneal macrophages. The cells are adherent in 35- or 60-mm plastic dishes in tissue culture medium containing 20% fetal bovine serum at 37°C. Sufficient lidocaine is added to make the medium 4 to 12 mM, and the cells are incubated at 37°C for 5.0 min. The medium is then recovered, and the monolayer jetted with 8 ml of normal saline (37°C) expressed from a syringe with a No. 20 needle. After directing the jet of saline over the entire surface of the monolayer, the saline is collected and pooled with the original medium; the saline rinse is repeated twice more. Alternatively, a rubber policeman may be used with adherent macrophage cell lines. The collected fluid is centrifuged at 4°C, and the pellet is washed. The cells are counted in a hemocytometer with trypan blue.

IV. CALCULATION OF RECOVERY

It is important to monitor recoveries quantitatively, since slight variation of the conditions may result in complete lysis of a proportion of the mononuclear phagocytes, such that they do not appear as trypan blue-positive cells. One method is to compare the protein content of well-rinsed, adherent monolayers with the recovered protein in the cell pellet, the latter having been washed to remove serum proteins. In addition, the number of adherent cells can be determined by difference from the number plated and the number that were nonadherent. The number of adherent cells can then be compared to the number of viable cells recovered after the lidocaine procedure.

V. CRITICAL COMMENTS

Resident mouse peritoneal macrophages are recovered in high yield and subsequently show 80 - 100% of normal capacity to readhere, phagocytize ^{14}C-acetylated starch granules, and consume glucose. The macrophages are easier to dislodge after overnight incubation than they are after only several hours of adherence. With macrophages from BCG-treated mice, however, viability of macrophages recovered in suspension with lidocaine was only 71%, and H_2O_2 release in response to phorbol myristate acetate was reduced by 65% (3). Departures from the above conditions, in terms of lidocaine concentration, temperature, medium composition, and incubation times, resulted in poorer results. Thus, the method must be adapted carefully to each intended use and can be expected to give satisfactory results only in selected situations.

ACKNOWLEDGMENTS

C. N. is a Scholar of the Leukemia Society of America and a Research Career Awardee of the Irma T. Hirschl Trust.

REFERENCES

1. M. Rabinovitch and M. J. DeStefano. Use of the local
    anesthetic lidocaine for cell harvesting and subcultiva-
    tion. *In Vitro 11*: 379-381, 1975.
2. C. F. Nathan, R. Asofsky, and W. D. Terry. Characteriza-
    tion of the nonphagocytic adherent cell from the peritoneal
    cavity of normal and BCG-treated mice. *J. Immunol. 118*:
    1612-1621, 1977.
3. C. F. Nathan and R. K. Root. Hydrogen peroxide release
    from mouse peritoneal macrophages: Dependence on sequen-
    tial activation and triggering. *J. Exp. Med. 146*: 1648-
    1662, 1977.

25

USE OF SEPHADEX COLUMNS TO DEPLETE
MONONUCLEAR PHAGOTCYES

Robert I. Mishell

Barbara B. Mishell

I. INTRODUCTION

Mononuclear phagocytes can be removed from murine and
human lymphoid cell suspensions by passage over columns of
Sephadex G-10 (1). This procedure is particularly useful for
rapid and gentle processing of large numbers of cells under
sterile conditions. Recoveries typically range from 30 to 40%
with murine spleen and lymph node cells (1 - 4). Somewhat
higher recoveries have been reported with human peripheral
blood leukocytes, which were initially purified on Ficoll -
Hypaque (5,6). Depletion of macrophages as judged histolog-
ically and by phagocytosis of latex particles ranges from
90 to 99% (5 - 9). Analysis with surface markers and by
functional criteria (1,6,7,9,10) indicate that approximately
normal proportions of T and B lymphocytes are recovered in the
effluent population.

In addition to macrophages, G-10 passage removes most
antibody-forming cells from spleens of immune mice (1); and

225

it has been reported that macrophage granulocyte progenitors
(3), some of the cells which mediate antibody-dependent cytolysis (2), and recently activated suppressor T cell blasts (11)
are also removed.

The procedure has been employed primarily to evaluate the
functions of macrophages in the induction of *in vitro* immune
responses. These include proliferative responses to plant
mitogens (9,12,13) and alloantigens (5,9), primary humoral
immunity to heterologous red cells (1), T-dependent synthetic
polymers (7) and T-independent antigens (4), and primary cell-
mediated immunity to major and minor histocompatibility antigens (10). G-10 passage has also been used to study the
contributions of macrophages in mediating the immunoregulatory
effects of lipopolysaccharide (8,14) and for evaluating and
removing suppressor cells from both immune and normal popul-
lations (15 - 17).

II. REAGENTS

A. *Preparation of Sephadex G-10*

    Saline, 0.85% NaCl (w/v)
    Sephadex G-10 (Pharmacia Fine Chemicals, Piscataway, NJ
    Flask, 6 liters
    Centrifuge tubes, 50 ml, autoclavable

B. *Preparation of Glass Beads*

    Nitric acid, concentrated
    Sulfuric acid, concentrated
    Sodium bicarbonate, 1% (w/v) in double-distilled water
    Hydrochloric acid (concentrated acid diluted 1:100
in double-distilled water)
    Glass beads (Microbeads subdivision of Cataphote Division,
Ferro Corp., Ferro Corporation, Jackson, Mississippi)
      250 - 350 μm, Class IV-A No. 456 Unisphere beads
      500 - 710 μm, Class IV-A No. 235.5 Unisphere beads
    Glass test tubes, 11 × 75mm, with stainless steel closures
(No. 2005-00013, Bellco Glass Co., Inc., Vineland, New Jersey)
    Drying oven

C. *Cell Separation*

    Balanced salt solution (BSS) (18), with penicillin
(50 U/ml), streptomycin (50 μg/ml) and 5 - 10% heat-inactivated
fetal calf serum (56°C, 30 min). Approximately 250 ml/column
    Sephadex G-10
    Glass beads, 1 tube (approximately 5 gm) of each size
    Syringe, disposable, 50 ml

Beaker, 150 ml
Tissue culture dish, 60 mm
Three-way stopcock (No. K-75, Pharmaseal Laboratories
Division, American Hospital Supply Corp., Gendale, California)
Pasteur pipettes with rubber bulbs
Pipettes: 10 ml, 5 ml, 1 ml
Centrifuge tube, graduated, for collection of effluent
Clamp and ring stand
Cell suspension, 1.5×10^8 cells/ml in BSS ($4 - 6 \times 10^8$
cells/column)

III. PROCEDURES

A. *Preparation of Sephadex G-10*

(1) Place approximately 2 liters of saline in a 6-liter
flask and add approximately 250 gm of Sephadex G-10.

(2) Stir the mixture gently, cover the flask, and allow
the Sephadex to swell overnight at 4°C.

(3) Remove the saline from the settled Sephadex with suction and gently resuspend the Sephadex in a volume of saline
that is approximately four times the estimated bed volume.

(4) Allow most of the Sephadex to settle; remove the saline
and the unsettled fine particles of Sephadex with suction.
Repeat this step three or four times or until the fine particles of Sephadex have been removed.

(5) Add a volume of saline equal to 30 - 50% of the estimated bed volume. Adjust the ratio of Sephadex to saline such
that 40 - 45 ml of slurry contain 30 - 35 ml of packed Sephadex.
Centrifuge a sample at low speed (just enough to lightly pack
the gel) to check the ratio and accordingly add or remove saline.

(6) Distribute the slurry in 40 - 45 ml volumes to 50 ml
tubes. Loosely cap the tubes. Autoclave at 110°C for 40 min
with slow exhaust. It is best to place the rack of tubes in
a large pan in the autoclave to protect it against occasional
spillage. When the tubes have cooled sufficiently, tighten
the caps and store the sterile Sephadex at room temperature
indefinitely.

B. *Preparation of Glass Beads*

(1) Prepare separately each bead size. In a fume hood,
soak the beads in equal volumes of concentrated sulfuric acid
and nitric acid for 24 hr. Rinse them under gently running
tap water for 8 hrs.

(2) Soak the beads in a large volume of 1% sodium bicarbonate for 24 hr, followed by k0 rinses in double-distilled
water.

(3) Soak the beads in diluted hydrochloric acid for 24 hr.
Rinse them in double-distilled water until the pH of the rinse

water is above 6 and dry them in a drying oven.

(4) Aliquot approximately 5 gm of beads per tube, top the tubes with stainless steel closures and autoclave them at 121°C for 20 min (fast exhaust).

C. Cell Separation

(1) Clamp the 50-ml syringe to the ring stand. Discard the plunger and cover the top of the syringe column with the sterile lid of a 60-mm culture dish. To the tip of the syringe, attach the stopcock in closed position.

(2) First pour the larger glass beads and then the smaller ones into the syringe. It may be necessary to first loosen the beads. This can be done with a sterile 1-ml plastic pipette or glass stirring rod. Rinse the beads from the sides of the syringe by adding approximately 10 ml of BSS that contains fetal calf serum and antibodies (BSS-FCS).

(3) Gently pipette the Sephadex on top of the glass beads (one tube containing 40 - 45 ml of slurry per 50-ml syringe). After the Sephadex has settled, place a beaker under the column and open the stopcock.

(4) Wash the column with a total of 100 - 150 ml BSS-FCS. When the last of the BSS-FCS has been added to the column, stir the top of the Sephadex with a pipette to level the top of the column.

(5) When all the fluid has penetrated the column, quickly load the cells onto the Sephadex with a Pasteur pipette, taking care not to disturb the top of the column. Once the cells have penetrated the column, continually add small amounts of BSS-FCS until the band of cells is midway down the column. At this point, gently add 15 - 20 ml of BSS-FCS. Begin collecting the effluent cells into a graduated centrifuge tube when the cells reach the glass bead layer. Collect only the first 10 - 15 ml for best depletions.

(6) Allow any contaminating Sephadex to settle for 2 - 3 min, transfer the cells to another tube and centrifuge at 200 g for 10 min.

IV. CRITICAL COMMENTS

When judged by functional criteria, the degree of depletion is variable. This can be demonstrated by using 2-mercapto-ethanol as a culture medium supplement that enables partially depleted populations to generate primary humoral immune responses *in vitro*. With more adequate depletion, 2-mercapto-ethanol does not restore immune competence (1, 10). The causes of variability are not understood. We have found that spleen cells from mice maintained under conditions that mini-mize bacterial exposure are more difficult to deplete than those from mice maintained under conventional conditions. Thus cells that have not been stimulated may more easily pass through the columns. The likelihood that depleted cells still contain some functional mononuclear phagocytic cells or their precursors should be considered in using the G-10 procedure and in evaluating data obtained with it.

Other investigators have sequentially passed cells through two columns (7) and have conducted depletions at 42°C (11, 15) in order to improve depletion. In our experience, similar modifications have not significantly affected the degree of contamination when judged by the aforementioned criteria. Other approaches for dealing with the problem of residual contamination are to choose cell sources, such as lymph nodes, which may be easier to deplete (3), to dilute out the effects of the contaminating cells by conducting the assay at low cell concentrations, or to use antigens of limited complexity for immune induction since these apparently require more macrophages (7).

Because G-10 passage is generally used to evaluate mononuclear phagocytic cells, the resulting biological effects, for example, inability of filtered cells to respond to concanavalin A, are usually attributed to the loss of these cells. However, since G-10 passage may remove other biologically important adherent accessory cells, interpretations should take this possibility into account.

We have had little experience in trying to recover the adherent population. A method for this purpose is described by Schwartz et al. (6).

REFERENCES

1. I. A. Ly and R. I. Mishell. Separation of mouse spleen cells by passage through columns of Sephadex G-10. *J. Immunol. Methods* 5: 239-247, 1974.
2. S. B. Pollack, K. Nelson, and J. O. Grausz. Separation of effector cells mediating antibody-dependent cellular cytotoxicity (ADC) to erythrocyte targets from those mediating ADC to tumor targets. *J. Immunol.* 116: 944-946, 1976.
3. J. I. Kurland, P. W. Kincade, and M. A. S. Moore. Regulation of B-lymphocyte clonal proliferation by stimulatory and inhibitory macrophage-derived factors. *J. Exp. Med.* 146: 1420-1435, 1977.
4. T. M. Chused, S. S. Kassan, and D. E. Mosier. Macrophage requirement for the *in vitro* responses to TNP-Ficoll: A thymic independent antigen. *J. Immunol.* 116: 1579-1581, 1976.
5. N. T. Berlinger, C. Lopez, and R. A. Good. Facilitation or attenuation of mixed leukocyte culture responsiveness by adherent cells. *Nature* 260: 145-146, 1976.
6. R. H. Schwartz, A. R. Bianco, B. S. Handwerger, and C. R. Kahn. Demonstration that monocytes rather than lymphocytes are the insulin-binding cells in preparations of

human peripheral blood mononuclear leukocytes: Implications for studies of insulin-resisdant states in man. *Proc. Nat. Acad. Sci. USA 79:* 474-478, 1975.

7. A. Singer, C. Cowing, K. S. Hathcock, H. B. Dicler, and R. J. Hodes. Cellular and genetic control of antibody responses *in vitro.* III. Immune response gene regulation of accessory cell function. *J. Exp. Med. 147:* 1611-1620, 1978.

8. D. L. Rosenstreich, S. N. Vogel, A. R. Jacques, L. M. Wahl, and J. J. Oppenheim. Macrophage sensitivity to endotoxin: Genetic control by a single codominant gene. *J. Immunol. 121:* 1644-1670, 1978.

9. C. Martinez Alonso, R. R. Beruabé, E. Moreno, and F. Diaz de Espada. Depletion of monocytes from human peripheral blood leukocytes by passage through Sephadex G-10 columns. *J. Immuno. Methods 22:* 361-368, 1976.

10. C. L. Miller and R. I. Mishell. Differential regulatory effects of accessory cells on the generation of cell-mediated immune reactions. *J. Immunol. 114:* 692-695, 1975.

11. K. Pickel and M. K. Hoffman. Suppressor T cells arising in mice undergoing graft versus host response. *J. Immunol. 118:* 653-656, 1977.

12. G. B. Ahmann, D. H. Sachs, and R. J. Hodes. Requirement for an Ia-bearing accessory cell in concanavalin A-induced T cell proliferation. *J. Immunol. 121:* 1981-1989, 1978.

13. L. Harwell, J. W. Kappler, and P. Marrack. Antigen specific and nonspecific mediators of T cell/B cell cooperation. III. Characterization of the nonspecific meadiator(s) from different sources. *J. Immunol. 116:* 1379-1384, 1976.

14. M. K. Hoffmann, C. Galanos, S. Koenig, and H. F. Oettgen. B-cell activation by lipopolysaccharide. Distinct pathways for induction of mitosis and antibody production. *J. Exp. Med. 146:* 1640-1647, 1977.

15. J. P. Kolb, S. Arrian, and S. Zolla-Pazner. Suppression of the humoral immune response by plasmacytomas: Mediation by adherent mononuclear cells. *J. Immunol. 118:* 707-709, 1977.

16. Y. P. Yung and G. Cudkowicz. Suppression of cytotoxic T lymphocytes by carrageenan-activated macrophage-like cells. *J. Immunol. 121:* 1990-1997, 1978.

17. N. T. Berlinger, C. Lopez, M. Lipkin, J. E. Vogel, and R. A. Good. Defective recognitive immunity in family aggregates of colon carcinoma. *J. Clin. Invest. 59:* 761-769, 1977.

18. B. B. Mishell and S. M. Shiigi (eds.). "Selected Methods in Cellular Immunology," pp. 447-448. W. H. Freeman, San Francisco, California, 1980.

26

DEPLETION OF MONONUCLEAR PHAGOCYTES:
PITFALLS IN THE USE OF CARBONYL IRON, CARRAGEENAN,
SILICA, TRYPAN BLUE, OR ANTIMONONUCLEAR PHAGOCYTE SERUM

Paul A. LeBlanc
Stephen W. Russell

I. INTRODUCTION

Selective depletion has been used to characterize the
biologic functions of a number of different cell types, most
notably lymphocytes. The approach has proved to be especially
instructive when the function of a depleted population has
then been reconstituted by adding back cells of the enriched
subpopulation that is under investigation.

Selective depletion, by definition, works best when a
unique characteristic of the cell of interest can be exploited.
This approach has recently become relatively straightforward
for lymphocytes, because these cells are now known either to
follow distinct differentiation pathways that can be inter-
rupted or to express specific antigens that can be targeted,
resulting in the destruction of a single subpopulation. Information that would suggest different pathways of differentiation or antigenic markers for individual subsets has yet to
be obtained for mononuclear phagocytes. The means used to

231

deplete mononuclear phagocytes have, therefore, been plagued by a common difficulty, namely, lack of specificity. The brief descriptions that follow consider the most commonly used approaches.

II. CARBONYL IRON

A. Introduction

Removal of mononuclear phagocytes with carbonyl iron theoretically depends on phagocytic uptake of the iron, after which iron-containing cells are removed in a magnetic field. The method was first described by Rous and Beard (1) for the isolation of Kupffer cells from perfusate of rabbit liver. The carbonyl iron approach has not proved useful for depletion of mononuclear phagocytes *in vivo*.

B. Reagents

Carbonyl iron in powder form (General Aniline and Film Co., New York, New York) is used.

C. Method

Cells (10^6/ml) are incubated with carbonyl iron (4 mg/ml) for 1 hr at 37°C with gentle agitation every 15 min. At the end of the incubation period a magnet is applied to the side of the tube for 1 min. The cells in suspension are gently withdrawn with a pipette to a new tube and the magnet reapplied. This cycle is repeated five times.

D. Critical Comments

Carbonyl iron has been found to remove up to 98% of the macrophages from thioglycollate-elicited peritoneal cells (2). However, the overall recovery of cells in these studies was low. Such low recoveries are a major problem with the technique, as iron particles often are entrapped in clumps of cells or adhere to the surfaces of nonphagocytic cells. Thus, nonphagocytic, as well as phagocytic, cells may be nonspecifically lost. In addition, phagocytic cells other than mononuclear phagocytes, e.g., neutrophils (3, 4), will be removed. Finally, immature mononuclear phagocytes may not be avidly phagocytic and may not, therefore, be subject to removal by this technique.

III. CARRAGEENAN

A. *Introduction*

Carrageenan was first described as a mononuclear phagocyte toxin by Allison *et al.* (5). The toxic effect of carrageenan was ascribed by these authors to destabilization of the membranes of secondary lysosomes, resulting in release of hydrolytic enzymes into the cytoplasm of treated cells.

B. *Reagent*

Carrageenan (Marine Colloids, Inc., Rockland, Maine) is used. The lambda form of carrageenan appears in several reports to be the most potent macrophage toxin, compared to other forms of this material (6, 7). The reagent is dissolved (1 - 2 mg/ml) in phosphate-buffered saline by heating to boiling. The final preparation may be sterilized by autoclaving.

C. *Method*

1. *Use in Vivo (6)*

The usual routes of administration are intravenous or intraperitoneal. The intravenous dose is 0.5 ml of a 1 mg/ml solution of carrageenan. For intraperitoneal use, the recommended dose is generally higher, i.e., 3 to 5 mg/mouse. The choice of route is based largely on whether a systemic or local, e.g., intraperitoneal, effect is desired. Substantial effects are seen during the first 48 hr after carrageenan is administered.

2. *Use in Vitro (5)*

Effective doses have varied from 25 µg/ml to 1 mg/ml; however, the most used concentration has been 100 µg/ml, in conjunction with 24-hr preincubation.

D. *Critical Comments*

Carrageenan has a broad spectrum of effects apart from its suppression of mononuclear phagocytes. For example, it can have either a depressive or adjuvant effect on antibody production to either cellular or soluble antigens (6, 8, 9). The dif-

ferent forms of carrageenan have suppressive effects on cytotoxic T cells that have been reported to vary independently of
their antimacrophage effects (7). Carrageenan initiates the
cleavage of Hageman factor and triggers the complement sequence
by the alternative pathway (10). Carrageenan also binds to
Cla, C2, and C4 (11). Its effects *in vivo* are so diverse that,
rather than deplete macrophages, some investigators have used
this agent successfully to induce inflammatory reactions that
are rich in mononuclear phagocytes, i.e., so-called carrageenan granulomas (12). In light of these facts, carrageenan must
be viewed as one of the least specific of macrophage inhibitors.

IV. SILICA

A. *Introduction*

The antimacrophage effects of silica were also first described by Allison *et al.* (5), as part of an investigation of
the fibrogenic properties of this particulate compound. Toxicity for phagocytic cells was thought to stem from the induction of membrane destabilization and rupture of secondary lysosomes.

B. *Reagent*

Silica, quartz form, with a particle size of 1 - 5 μm
(Whittaker, Clarke, and Daniels, Inc., White Plains, New York)
is used. Surface contamination with iron oxide is removed by
repeated boiling in 1 N hydrochloric acid until no further
color change (green) is detectable. The cleansed particulate
material is washed extensively (no further chloride reaction)
in distilled water and then dry-heat sterilized for storage.
For use, the agent is suspended in tissue culture medium, after
which clumps are dispersed by sonication. Suspensions should
be made freshly for each use.

C. *Method*

1. *Use in Vivo (13, 14)*

The silica suspension should be sonicated immediately before use to prevent possible embolism due to intravenously injected clumps. The dose of silica will vary batch to batch;
however, a useful starting range for mice has been from 1 to
40 mg. Both single and divided doses have proved effective.

2. *Use in Vitro (15)*

Silica for use *in vitro* should be suspended in serum-containing medium. This maneuver tends to reduce the direct toxicity of silica for cells. The dose used in culture is usually 50 - 100 µg/ml with cells at a population density of 10^6/ml. Effects are seen after overnight incubation at $37°C$.

D. *Critical Comments*

There are two major difficulties with silica. First, many of the same criticisms previously lodged against carrageenan apply equally to silica. For example, adverse effects on other cell types, most notably lymphocytes (16, 17), have been reported. Second, in many experiments conducted *in vivo*, efficacious levels of silica have proved lethal to a portion of the animals injected. Results obtained from survivors of such a treatment would have to be treated with reservations. Finally, different batches of silica may have varying levels of anti-mononuclear phagocyte activity, even to the extent of lacking activity altogether (15).

V. TRYPAN BLUE DYE

A. *Introduction*

Trypan blue has been reported to interfere with the rejection of allogeneic skin (18) and tumors (19), as well as the elimination of antigenic, syngeneic neoplasms (20). Treatment of animals with the dye has also resulted in reduced resistance to *Trypanosoma musculi* (21). Because of these, and other findings, it has been suggested that trypan blue may be a selective inhibitor of macrophage function (18). While there is little doubt that this agent affects macrophages, as will be seen from the comments in Section V.D, it has a wide spectrum of effects and should not, therefore, be viewed as selectively affecting macrophages.

B. *Reagent*

Trypan blue can be obtained either as a solution from a variety of vendors of tissue culture supplies or as a powder (Sigma, St. Louis, Missouri). All preparations should be dialyzed exhaustively against distilled water to remove impurities (19). The dye is then lyophilized to dryness. For use, the powdered dye can be resolubilized in an appropriate buffer and sterilized by autoclaving.

C. Methods

1. Use In Vivo

Short-term suppression of macrophage function has been reported using a single injection of 1 mg/mouse (22). Sustained effects have been produced by Hibbs (19), using a loading dose of 4 mg/mouse and a biweekly maintenance dose of 1 mg/mouse, thereafter. The route of injection for the loading dose is intraperitoneal, while the maintenance dose is given subcutaneously.

2. Use In Vitro

A concentration of 1 mg/ml, using a 2- to 4-hr period of pretreatment, has proved effective (22).

D. Critical Comments

The mechanism by which trypan blue exerts its effects is not known. It is an inhibitor of certain hydrolytic lysosomal enzymes (23). In addition, however, it inhibits fibrinolysis (24) and the activation of plasminogen (24), and interferes with the functions of a number of other proteins, such as antibody and most of the components of the complement system (25). This broad spectrum of activities has led one group of investigators to suggest that trypan blue mediates many of its biologic effects through a general affinity for proteins (25). Clearly, the activity or activities of this dye should not be considered specific for macrophages or macrophage-related proteins.

VI. ANTIMONONUCLEAR PHAGOCYTE SERUM

A. Introduction

Of all of the methods that are currently available for effecting the depletion of mononuclear phagocytes, conventional antiserum or monoclonal antibody raised against this cell type offers the greatest potential for achieving true specificity. Even here, however, there are serious problems that center on cross-reactivity or sharing of antigens with other cell types.

B. Reagent

Either conventional antisera or monoclonal antibodies can be raised against mononuclear phagocytes.

1. Conventional Antiserum

Antimononuclear phagocyte serum can be produced in any convenient laboratory animal species. Xenogeneic antiserum is used as there are no allotypic markers yet defined for mononuclear phagocytes. Every effort should be made to enrich the immunizing cell population for mononuclear phagocytes. Extensive washing of an adherent population is the most commonly used approach to enrichment. The protocol for immunization has varied from investigator to investigator. For use *in vivo* in mice, we have found "early" IgG produced in rabbits to be most effective at depleting mononuclear phagocytes. Immunization is started with a single, intramuscular injection of cells emulsified in Freund's complete adjuvant. This injection is followed by two intravenous administrations of cells suspended in saline, given at weekly intervals. Serum is harvested 1 week later and fractionated to yield the IgG fraction. Extensive absorption of the antiserum is then required to render it specific.

2. Monoclonal Antibody

The standard hybridization technique (26) can be used to produce the clones. If antibody against mouse mononuclear phagocytes is desired, rats can be immunized. The rat spleen cells are then fused to mouse myeloma cells. The fusion efficiency and stability of the resulting interspecies hybrids have been good; however, the need for a HAT sensitive rat myeloma line suitable for rat-rat fusions is clear. At this writing there is the expectation that such a line will be available soon. If antibodies against the mononuclear phagocytes of other species are desired, mice can be immunized, allowing mouse - mouse hybrids to be used for the production of antibody. When an antibody of interest has been identified, it can be concentrated from tissue culture supernate or produced in quantity in ascites fluid (27).

C. Methods

1. Use In Vivo

An appropriate amount (0.1 - 0.5 ml) of the antiserum is injected. If recruitment of mononuclear phagocytes into a lesion is to be interdicted, the route of administration should probably be intravenous. If local depletion is the aim, it may be preferrable to inject locally, for example, intraperitoneally. Repeated administration will be necessary to sustain *in vivo* depletion.

2. Use In Vitro

For eliminating mononuclear phagocytes *in vitro*, the standard approach to producing antibody/complement-mediated cytotoxicity is followed.

D. Critical Comments

Achieving true specificity for mononuclear phagocytes with conventionally raised antisera is extremely difficult. The difficulty is caused by the fact that mononuclear phagocytes share antigens or bear antigens that cross-react with those of other cell types, e.g., neutrophils (28) and lymphocytes (27). Claims for specificity attained after few or no absorptions are quite simply the result either of not looking at enough other cell types or not using an assay sensitive enough to detect cross-reactivity. In this latter regard, we have found assays such as antibody/complement-mediated cytotoxicity or immunofluorescence to be relatively insensitive. Assays that measure interference with the functions of cell types other than mononuclear phagocytes have proved to be much more sensitive indicators of nonspecific effects. As an example of how extensive the process of absorption must be, rabbit antiserum produced against murine bone marrow mononuclear phagocytes in our laboratory has routinely required 15 separate absorptions with packed mouse erythrocytes and absorption with an additional 10^{10} cultured mouse tumor cells before antispecies activity has been completely removed.

Many of the problems of nonspecificity might be overcome with the use of monoclonal antibodies, providing screening is adequate to eliminate those that bind to cell types other than mononuclear phagocytes. Monoclonal antibodies of interest are now being developed in several laboratories. When working with a single species of antibody that is directed against a single antigenic determinant, new problems may arise. Chief among these is that the conditions of cell - antibody interaction may simply not be adequate to effect depletion, either *in vivo* or *in vitro*. In such cases it might be necessary to use a "cocktail" consisting of several different monoclonal antibodies. There is also the potential problem of the antibody that will not fix complement. This may present no real difficulty *in vivo* because it is not clear that depletion *in vivo*

is effected by this means. If the density of antigenic determinants bound by a complement-fixing antibody is too low to
permit cytolysis, or the antibody is not of the complement-
fixing type, then the addition of a "second layer" of complement-fixing antibody to the system might serve to eliminate
mononuclear phagocytes *in vitro*.

In either case, there is the problem of sustaining depletion *in vivo*. Because xenogeneic antibodies are employed, the
recipient will respond with antibodies of its own that will be
directed against the foreign protein(s). Immune elimination
of the injected antibody could result. It may be possible to
blunt or to circumvent completely the recipient's response if
antibody is first deaggregated before it is injected. This approach has been used successfully in the therapeutic application
of antilymphocyte globulin (29), and is used routinely as a
means of inducing tolerance in experimental animals (30). If
such steps are not taken, the recipient's antibody response
might neutralize the antimononuclear phagocyte globulin allowing
the bone marrow to replenish the depleted population.

VII. CONCLUDING REMARKS

The state of the art is such that we simply cannot yet make
the claim that an easy approach is available to the depletion
of mononuclear phagocytes *in vivo*. Of the methods considered
here, certainly antibody (especially monoclonal antibody) holds
the greatest promise for the future. We are hopeful, given the
current amount of interest in the field, that within the next
few years a monoclonal antibody preparation that is suitable for
depletion studies and that has absolute specificity for mononuclear phagocytes will become available. Perhaps, then it will
be possible to answer definitively those questions that stand
unanswered today because of the problems of nonspecificity.

Acknowledgment

The authors would like to thank Ms. Brenda Brown for typing
the manuscript. Supported by NIH Research Grant CA-31199 and
NRSA CA-06088 and Contract CB-84271. S.W.R. is the recipient
of Research Career Development Award CA 00497.

REFERENCES

1. P. Rous and J. W. Beard. Selection with the magnet and cultivation of reticuloendothelial cells (Kupffer's cells). *J. Exp. Med. 59*: 557–591, 1934.

2. P. Goldstein and H. Blomgren. Further evidence for autonomy of T cells mediating specific *in vitro* cytotoxicity: Efficiency of very small amounts of highly purified T cells. *Cell. Immunol. 9*: 127–141, 1973.

3. G. Lundgren, CH. F. Zukoski, and G. Möller. Differential effects of human granulocytes and lymphocytes on human fibroblasts *in vitro*. *Clin. Exp. Immunol. 3*: 817–836, 1968.

4. R. E. Falk, L. Collste, and G. Möller. *In vitro* detection of transplantation immunity: The inhibition of migration of immune spleen cells and peripheral blood leukocytes by specific antigen. *J. Immunol. 104*: 1287–1292, 1970.

5. A. C. Allison, J. S. Harington, and M. Birbeck. An examination of the cytotoxic effects of silica on macrophages. *J. Exp. Med. 124*: 141–153, 1966.

6. L. J. Becker and J. A. Rudbach. Altered antibody responses in mice treated with toxins for macrophages. *J. Reticuloendothelial Soc. 25*: 443–454, 1979.

7. Y. P. Yung and G. Cudkowicz. Depressive effects of carrageenans on cell-mediated lympholysis induced *in vitro*: Antimacrophage and antilymphocyte activities. *J. Reticuloendothel. Soc. 24*: 461–475, 1978.

8. E. V. Turner and R. D. Higginbotham. Carrageenan-induced alterations of antigen distribution and immune responses in mice. *J. Reticuloendothel. Soc. 22*: 545–554, 1977.

9. L. Aschheim and S. Raffel. The immunodepressant effect of carrageenan. *J. Reticuloendothel. Soc. 11*: 253–262, 1972.

10. H. J. Schwartz and R. W. Kellermeyer. Carrageenan and delayed hypersensitivity. II. Activation of Hageman factor by carrageenan and its possible significance. *Proc. Soc. Exp. Biol. Med. 132*: 1021–1024, 1969.

11. T. Borsos, J. H. Rapp, and C. Crisler. The interaction between carrageenan and the first component of complement. *J. Immunol. 94*: 662–665, 1965.

12. R. J. Bonney, I. Gery, T. Lin, M. F. Meyenhofer, W. Acevedo, and P. Davies. Mononuclear phagocytes from carrageenan-induced granulomas. *J. Exp. Med. 148*: 261–275, 1978.

13. N. N. Pearsall and R. S. Weiser. The macrophage in allograft immunity. I. Effect of silica as a specific macrophage toxin. *J. Reticuloendothelial Soc. 5*: 107–120, 1968.

14. R. Keller. Abrogation of antitumor effects of *Coryne-
     bacterium parvum* and BCG by antimacrophage agents. *J.
     Nat. Cancer Inst. 59*: 1751-1753, 1977.

15. A. C. Allison. Fluorescence microscopy of lymphocytes
     and mononuclear phagocytes and the use of silica to elimi-
     nate the latter. *In "In Vitro* Methods in Cell-Mediated
     and Tumor Immunity" (B. R. Bloom and J. R. David, eds.),
     pp. 395-404. Academic Press, New York, 1976.

16. H. VanLoveren, M. Snoek, and W. Den Otter. Effects of
     silica on macrophages and lymphocytes. *J. Reticuloendo-
     thelial Soc. 22*: 523-531, 1977.

17. S. D. Miller and A. Zarkower. Alteration of murine im-
     munologic responses after silica dust inhalation. *J.
     Immunol. 113*: 1533-1543, 1974.

18. M. L. Kripke, K. C. Norbury, E. Gruys, and J. B. Hibbs,
     Jr. Effects of trypan blue treatment on the immune re-
     sponses of mice. *Infect. Immun. 17*: 121-129, 1977.

19. J. B. Hibbs, Jr. Activated macrophages as cytotoxic ef-
     fector cells. I. Inhibition of specific and nonspecific
     tumor resistance by trypan blue. *Transplantation 19*:
     77-81, 1975.

20. J. W. Kreider, G. L. Bartlett, and E. DeFreilas. Abroga-
     tion of tumor rejection by trypan blue. *Cancer Res. 38*:
     1036-1040, 1978.

21. B. O. Brooks and N. D. Reed. The effect of trypan blue
     on the early control of *Trypansoma musculi* parasitemia in
     mice. *J. Reticuloendothelial Soc. 25*: 325-328, 1979.

22. R. P. Strauss, N. Patel, and C. Patel. Suppression of the
     immune response in BALB/c mice by trypan blue. *J. Reticu-
     loendothelial Soc. 22*: 533-543, 1977.

23. F. Beck, J. B. Lloyd, and A. Griffiths. Lysosomal enzyme
     inhibition by trypan blue: A theory of teratogenesis.
     Science 157: 1180-1182, 1967.

24. K. Dano and E. Reich. Inhibitors of plasminogen activa-
     tion. *In* "Proteases and Biological Control" (E. Reich,
     D. B. Rifkin, and E. Shaw, eds.), pp. 357-366. Cold Spring
     Harbor Laboratory, 1975.

25. J. C. Scornik, P. Ruiz, and E. M. Hoffman. Suppression of
     cell-mediated tumor cell lysis and complement-induced cyto-
     toxicity by trypan blue. *J. Immunol. 123*: 1278-1284, 1979.

26. R. H. Kennett, K. A. Denis, A. S. Tung, and N. R. Klinman.
     Hybrid plasmacytoma production: Fusions with adult spleen
     cells, monoclonal spleen fragments, neonatal spleen cells
     and human spleen cells. *Curr. Top. Microbiol. Immunol. 81*:
     77-91, 1978.

27. J. C. Unkeless. Characterization of a monoclonal antibody
     directed against mouse macrophage and lymphocyte Fc recep-
     tors. *J. Exp. Med. 150*: 580-596, 1976.

28. T. Springer, G. Galfre, D. S. Secher, and C. Milstein.

Mac-1: A macrophage differentiation antigen identified by monoclonal antibody. *Eur. J. Immunol. 9*: 301-306, 1979.

29. J. Ring, J. Seifert, F. Seiler, and W. Brendel. Improved compatibility of ALG therapy by application of aggregate free therapy. *Int. Arch. Allergy Appl. Immunol. 52*: 227-234, 1976.

30. D. W. Dresser. Specific inhibition of antibody production II. Paralysis induced in adult mice by small quantities of protein antigen. *Immunology 5*: 378-388, 1962.

27

IDENTIFICATION OF MONONUCLEAR PHAGOCYTES:
OVERVIEW AND DEFINITIONS

R. van Furth

For the study of the physiological functions of mononuclear phagocytes as well as their role in pathophysiology,
adequate characterization of the cells under study is necessary. Until recently, use was often made of suspensions of
mononuclear cells, in which both monocytes (or macrophages)
and (T/B) lymphocytes occur. Although these cells seem to
resemble each other, the use of techniques more advanced than
routine histological staining (e.g., cytochemical and immunochemical staining of cellular enzymes) and the demonstration
of cell receptors makes it possible to distinguish relatively
easily cells of the mononuclear phagocyte cell-line from lymphoid cells.

To appreciate the importance of such optimal characterization, it is necessary to know something about the origin
and kinetics of cells that seem to be morphologically similar.
Mononuclear phagocytes form a cell line that originates from
the pluripotent stem cell in the bone marrow (Fig. 1) (1).
The most immature cell of this line is the monoblast. *In vivo,*

Copyright © 1981 by Academic Press, Inc.
All rights of reproduction in any form reserved.
ISBN 0-12-044220-5

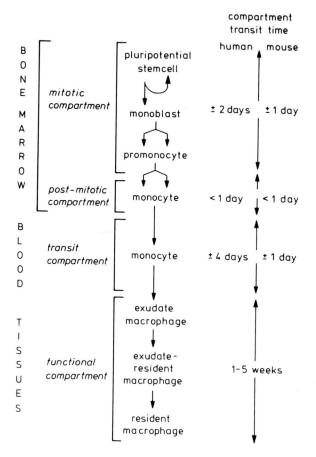

Fig. 1. Schematic representation of the origin and kinetics of mononuclear phagocytes and some kinetic parameters.

the two daughter cells produced by division of a monoblast are promonocytes, which in turn divide and give rise to two monocytes. Thus, from monoblast to monocytes, a fourfold amplification occurs. Monocytes reside in the bone marrow for a relatively short time (Fig. 1), and are then transported via the circulation to the functional compartment of the mononuclear phagocytes, i.e., the tissues, and there they are called macrophages. Monocytes leave the circulation by a random process and first become exudate macrophages (i.e., cells with characteristics similar to those of monocytes), after which they undergo characteristic changes (e.g., decrease of the number of peroxidase-positive granules, reappearance of peroxidatic activity in the rough endoplasmic reticulum and nu-

clear envelope) and are then called exudate-resident macrophages (Fig. 2) (2); ultimately, they acquire all of the
characteristics of resident macrophages.

The proliferative cells of the mononuclear phagocyte
cell-line (i.e., monoblasts and promonocytes) reside in the
bone marrow (Fig. 1), and under normal conditions the monocytes and macrophages do not divide again. However, a small
proportion (less than 5%) of the mononuclear phagocytes in
tissues can incorporate [^{3}H] thymidine (1). These cells have
recently left the bone marrow and divide once after arriving
in the tissues. In the normal steady state, the renewal of
macrophages in the tissues occurs mainly via the influx of
monocytes, but a small contribution is made by the division
of immature mononuclear phagocytes in the tissues. The turnover time of macrophages in tissues was formerly thought to
be of the order of 1 to 2 months, but newer approaches have
shown it to be 1-5 weeks (Fig. 1). In an inflammatory exudate,
the number of dividing immature mononuclear phagocytes recruited from the bone marrow may be increased, but the main
source of macrophages is still the influx of nondividing monocytes.

It is understandable that on the basis of morphological
criteria alone, monocytes are often confused with (circulating)
lymphocytes, and macrophages with such cells as reticulum cells,
dendritic cells, fibroblasts, which occur in connective tissues
and lymphatic organs. However, cells belonging to this last
category do not originate from the haemopoietic stem cell, but
renew themselves by division in the tissues (Fig. 3). As already mentioned, this is not the way in which macrophages renew
themselves.

Properties that can be used for the identification of
mononuclear phagocytes are summarized in Table I. Because
neither the specificity of the available markers nor the sensitivity of the techniques used is optimal yet, classification

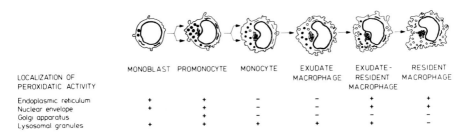

LOCALIZATION OF PEROXIDATIC ACTIVITY	MONOBLAST	PROMONOCYTE	MONOCYTE	EXUDATE MACROPHAGE	EXUDATE-RESIDENT MACROPHAGE	RESIDENT MACROPHAGE
Endoplasmic reticulum	+	+	−	−	+	+
Nuclear envelope	+	+	−	−	+	+
Golgi apparatus		+	−	−	−	−
Lysosomal granules	+	+	+	+	+	−

Fig. 2. Peroxidase activity patterns and sequence of
development of monocytes and macrophages.

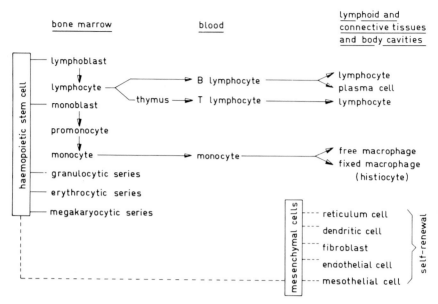

Fig. 3. Schematic representation of the origin and localization of cells in lymphoid and connective tissues and serous cavities. The macrophages and lymphoid cells are steadily replaced by bone marrow-derived precursors from the circulation, whereas reticulum cells, dendritic cells, fibroblasts, and endothelial and mesothelial cells do not have precursors in the bone marrow but renew themselves by division in the tissues (1).

must be based on more than one property. The most frequently used methods for the determination of the morphological, cytochemical, and functional characteristics are discussed in detail in Section V on the morphology of mononuclear phagocytes of this volume. The demonstration of ectoenzymes by cytochemical and biochemical methods is described in the same section and elsewhere (3). So far, the use of antisera to demonstrate cell-specific antigens has contributed little to the characterization of mononuclear phagocytes, because it is still difficult to produce antisera specific for mononuclear phagocytes. Many of these polyclonal antisera contain antibodies that cross-react with other kinds of cell. Monospecific monoclonal antibodies with hybridomas should greatly facilitate the identification of mononuclear phagocytes in tissue and the determination of their developmental stage. The proliferation of a cell population can be assessed by the counting of cells in culture. At the cellular level, the distinction between cells that divide and cells that merely survive can be made on the

TABLE I. *Outline for the Identification of Mononuclear Phagocytes*

Structure	Features in light, phase-contrast, and electron microscopy
Cytoplasmic and lysosomal enzymes	Nonspecific esterase lysozyme peroxidase
Ectoenzymes	5'-Nucleotidase Leucine aminopeptidase Alkaline phosphodiesterase I
Membrane characteristics	Fc and C receptors Specific antigens
Function	Immune phagocytosis Pinocytosis
Cell proliferation	[^{3}H]-Thymidine incorporation DNA content of nucleus Survival or multiplication in culture

basis of the incorporation of a DNA precursor (e.g. [3H]-thymidine) (ref. 1 and Section XI on the kinetics of mononuclear phagocytes of this volume) or by the determination of the DNA content of the nucleus.

On the basis of experience with the characterization of cells, it is possible to define the minimum requirements to be satisfied before a cell can be called a mononuclear phagocyte (4). These requirements are, in the first place, morphological characteristics, but also the presence in the cytoplasm of non-specific esterases (demonstrated with α-naphthyl butyrate or α-naphthyl acetate as substrate), peroxidase-positive granules and/or peroxidatic activity in the rough-endoplasmic reticulum, nuclear envelope, and Golgi region (2), the presence of lyso-zyme, and the presence of Fc (IgG) and C3 receptors in the cell membrane, and in addition the phagocytosis of IgG-coated red cells or opsonized bacteria, the absence of phagocytosis of C-coated red cells (only in nonactivated mononuclear phago-cytes), and the occurrence of avid pinocytosis. The question as to whether all cells in a homogenous population must be positive for one of these criteria has not been definitely an-swered yet, but it is generally accepted that positivity of 90% or more of the cells is sufficient. In many cases cells are not positive for all of the criteria mentioned here, or not all characteristics are investigated. However, *at least three characteristics must be positive.*

The mononuclear phagocytes participating in an inflammatory reaction (whether spontaneous or induced) are often not care-fully defined. The characteristics of these cells in an exu-date depend on the inducing agent, the method of isolation, the developmental stage, and the functional state of the cells. This means that the cells in an inflammatory exudate can be rather heterogeneous, and should therefore be cautiously char-acterized.

The terminology applied to the cells in an inflammatory exudate is generally unclear. For example, terms such as stimulated, activated, elicited, induced, and angry are inter-changeably used. Often, too, a distinction is not made between the developmental stage of the mononuclear phagocyte and the functional state. To deal with these problems, the following definitions have been proposed (4):

Resident macrophage: Macrophage present at any given site in the absence of an exogenous or endogenous inflammatory stimulus. These cells are sometimes called normal macrophages; they can also occur in an inflammatory exudate as a small sub-population already present before the stimulus was applied. Their pattern of peroxidatic activity differs from those of exudate and exudate-resident macrophages.

Exudate macrophage: Macrophage occurring in an exudate and identified by a specific marker, i.e., peroxidatic activity, and by cell-kinetic analysis. Exudate macrophages derive from monocytes and have almost the same characteristics as the latter. This term should be reserved for this developmental stage of the macrophage, and not applied to the functional state.

Exudate-resident macrophage: Transitional form between the resident and the exudate macrophage, which can only be characterized electron-microscopically after staining for peroxidatic activity.

Activated macrophage: Macrophage with increased functional activity induced by a given stimulus. Activation thus implies a new functional activity or an increase in one or more of the functional activities of a cell. Before activation this cell may have been a resident or an exudate macrophage. The term can be applied to mononuclear phagocytes stimulated *in vivo* and *in vitro,* but explicit mention should be made of how this was accomplished as well as how activation was measured.

Elicited macrophage: Macrophage attracted to a given site by a given substance. This term refers only to mononuclear phagocytes accumulating at a particular site and does not indicate the developmental stage of the cells or their functional state. An elicited population of cells is usually heterogenous in these respects. Since elicited and *evoked* have the same meaning, use of the latter term is acceptable.

The term *stimulated* macrophage is imprecise, because stimulation means the application of a stimulus that may result in the elicitation and/or activation of cells. The term *induced* macrophages is also inexact, since it can imply either elicited or activated. Therefore, neither of these adjectives should be used. The term *angry* macrophage is sometimes used instead of activated macrophage, but this practice cannot be recommended. The term *mononuclear cells* should be discarded because it covers cells of different cell lines (i.e., monocytes/macrophages and T/B lymphocytes) with entirely different functions.

The terms *accumulation* and *proliferation* of cells are often erroneously used. Proliferation should be reserved for cases in which the increase in the number of cells is known to be due to division of cells already present at or recruited to a site, and the term accumulation for increases caused by migration of (nondividing) cells from other sites.

A distinction should also be made between *differentiation* and *specialization.* Differentiation refers to a change in the morphological development in the direction of another morphological stage, whereas specialization means a change in the functional state of a cell in the direction of a special function.

The cells included at present in the mononuclear phagocyte system (MPS) are listed in Fig. 4; the grounds for inclusion of cells in or exclusion from the MPS have been discussed in detail elsewhere (4,5).

In experimental animals it is often relatively easy to obtain mononuclear phagocytes from various sites, and therefore

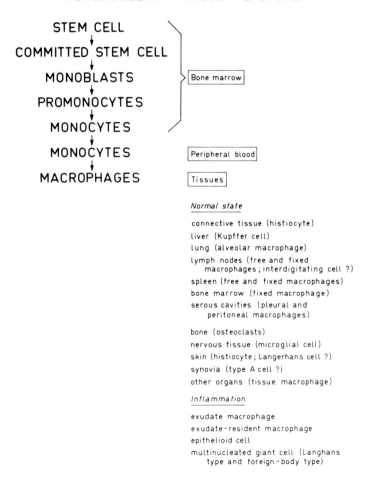

Fig. 4. Cells belonging to the mononuclear phagocyte system and occurring in normal and inflamed tissues (1).

much information is available about these cells. In man, to
the contrary, macrophages are difficult to obtain (6). However, on the basis of the concept of the MPS, monocytes can be
considered and used as representative of the cells of this
system, at least if it is kept in mind that monocytes are not
macrophages, and that morphological changes occur together with
the functional changes taking place during the transition from
monocyte into macrophage in the tissues. Such changes probably
occur very rapidly, even within a few hours.

REFERENCES

1. R. van Furth. Mononuclear phagocytes in inflammation.
    In "Handbook of Experimental Pharmacology" (J. R. Vane
    and S. H. Fereira, eds.), Chapter 3, pp. 68-108. Springer
    Verlag, Berlin, Heidelberg, New York, 1978.
2. R. H. J. Beelen, D. M. Fluitsma, J. W. M. van der Meer,
    and E. C. M. Hoefsmit. Development of exudate-resident
    macrophages, on the basis of the pattern of peroxidatic
    activity *in vivo* and *in vitro*. *In* "Mononuclear Phago-
    cytes-Functional Aspects" (R. van Furth, ed.), pp. 87-
    112. Martinus Nijhoff, The Hague, Boston, London, 1980.
3. J. W. M. van der Meer. Characteristics of mononuclear
    phagocytes in culture. *In* "The Reticuloendothelial Sys-
    tem." Comprehensive Treatise, No. 1. Morphology (I.
    Carr and W. Th. Daems, eds.), pp. 735-771. Plenum Press,
    New York, London, 1980.
4. R. van Furth. Cells of the mononuclear phagocyte system.
    Nomenclature in terms of sites and conditions,
    In "Mononuclear Phagocytes-Functional Aspects" (R. van
    Furth, ed.), pp. 1-30. Martinus Nijhoff Publishers.
    The Hague, Boston, London, 1980.
5. R. van Furth, Z. A. Cohn, J. G. Hirsch, J. H. Humphrey,
    W. G. Spector, and H. L. Langevoort. The mononuclear
    phagocyte system. A new classification of macrophages,
    monocytes and their precursor cells. *Bull. WHO 46:*845-
    852, 1972.
6. R. van Furth, J. A. Raeburn, and Th. L. van Zwet.
    Characteristics of human mononuclear phagocytes.
    *Blood 54:*485-500, 1979.

28

CHARACTERISTICS OF MONONUCLEAR PHAGOCYTES
FROM DIFFERENT TISSUES

M. M. C. Diesselhoff-den Dulk
R. van Furth

I. INTRODUCTION

To be classified as a mononuclear phagocyte, a cell must
have a number of characteristics (see Chapter 27). The morphological picture is not sufficient, because the group of
mononuclear phagocytes includes many different forms. For
example, comparison of the structure of monoblasts, promonocytes, monocytes, and macrophages (including the alveolar,
pleural, and peritoneal macrophages; Kupffer cells; type A
synovial cells; Langerhans cells; microglia cells; osteoclasts;
epithelioid cells; and multinucleated giant cells) will not
easily lead to the conclusion that these cells all belong to
the same cell line. Therefore, additional properties must be
taken into account, such as the presence of enzymes in the cytoplasm and of receptors on the surface and also various cell
functions. During the last decade such properties have been
studied in more detail in human and murine mononuclear phagocytes and, less intensively, in a number of other species.

METHODS FOR STUDYING
MONONUCLEAR PHAGOCYTES

253

This chapter includes a detailed description of the methods employed in this work and the results obtained in mononuclear phagocytes isolated from various organs.

II. MATERIALS AND PROCEDURES

A. *Cell Isolation*

1. *Bone Marrow*

(a) *Mouse*. After removal of a hindlimb and thorough cleaning of the femur, both ends of the bone are cut off and a needle (26 gauge) on a 2-ml syringe is inserted to flush the shaft with 2 ml of culture medium. The bone marrow cells are collected in a Falcon tube (Falcon Plastics, California) and dispersed by repeated aspiration in a pipette. One femur yields approximately 1.5×10^7 nucleated cells. The cell number is adjusted to 1×10^7 cells/ml culture medium (1).

(b) *Guinea Pig*. The marrow is obtained with the same procedure as in the mouse except that 10 ml of culture medium is used to flush the femur shaft, which requires a 19-gauge needle on a 10-ml syringe. One guinea pig femur yields approximately 2×10^8 nucleated cells, and the number is adjusted to 1×10^7 cells/ml culture medium (2).

(c) *Human*. Fragments of spongiosa bone (approximately 125 mm^3) collected in saline containing 40 U/ml heparin are transferred to a petri dish containing medium 199 (Microbiological Associates, Walkersville, Maryland), and marrow is removed from the bone by teasing with sterile scalpels. This material is stirred and then kept in an upright test tube for at least 1 min to allow the bone fragments and fibrous debris to sediment. The supernatant is then removed and spun at 110 g for 10 min, after which the cells are washed once with phosphate-buffered saline (pH 7.2) and brought into medium containing serum. After dispersal of the cells by repeated up and down movement in a 1-ml glass pipette for at least 1 min, the suspension is diluted to a cell concentration of $6.0 - 8.0 \times 10^6$/ml.

Sternal marrow aspirates collected in saline containing 40 U/ml heparin are placed in a petri dish containing medium 199 and 0.5 U/ml heparin, after which the bone marrow flocks are aspirated with a capillary pipette and brought into a plastic tube. Medium 199 is then added, the flocks spun at 110 g for 10 min and the supernatant discarded; the flocks are washed once more with medium 199 containing 0.5 U/ml heparin, dispersed very thoroughly in culture medium, and diluted as described above (3).

2. Peripheral Blood

(a) *Mouse.* Blood obtained by cardiac puncture from chloro-form-anesthetized mice is collected in heparin (20 U/ml blood). Leukocyte suspensions are made by preparing a buffy coat. For the latter purpose, 5-ml aliquots of heparinized blood are cen-trifuged three times for 3 min at 180 g, and after each run the supernatant plasma is collected. The collected plasma is pooled, centrifuged for 7 min at 180 g, and washed with medium, after which the leukocytes are resuspended in culture medium to a concentration of 2 × 10^6 cells/ml.

(b) *Guinea Pig.* Blood obtained by cardiac puncture of ether-anesthetized animals is collected in heparin (20 U/ml blood). A leukocyte-rich suspension is prepared by density centrifugation in a Ficoll – Hypaque suspension consisting of 12 parts Ficoll 400 (Pharmacia, Uppsala, Sweden) and 5 parts sodium metrizoate Isopaque (Nyegaard & Co., Oslo, Norway) (4). Next, 3.5 ml blood diluted 1 : 1 in phosphate-buffered saline is layered on 4 ml Ficoll – Hypaque and centrifuged for 20 min at 420 g. The leukocyte-rich cell layer is collected in sili-conized tubes, centrifuged for 10 min at 250 g, and washed four times with phosphate-buffered saline containing 0.5 U hepa-rin/ml. The washed cells are then resuspended in culture me-dium and counted. Approximately 2 × 10^7 nucleated cells are obtained from each animal, and the number is adjusted to 2 × 10^6/ml culture medium (2).

(c) *Human.* Monocytes are obtained from venous blood samples containing 20 U heparin/ml blood. A monocyte – lym-phocyte-rich suspension is prepared by density centrifugation on a Ficoll – Hypaque gradient as described above, except that 5 ml undiluted blood is layered on 4 ml of Ficoll – Hypaque. The cell number is adjusted to 2 × 10^6/ml culture medium (3).

3. Peritoneal Cavity

(a) *Mouse.* The animals are killed with chloroform. The skin over the abdomen is reflected and 2 ml of phosphate-buffered saline containing 50 U/ml heparin is injected into the peritoneal cavity. After gentle massage of the abdomen, the cell suspension is collected in a Falcon tube, centrifuged for 8 min at 150 g, and resuspended in culture medium at a con-centration of 1 × 10^6 cells/ml (1).

(b) *Guinea Pig, Rat, and Hamster.* The same procedure is followed, except that for the guinea pig 50 ml of phosphate-buffered saline with heparin is used to wash out the peritoneal cavity; for the rat and hamster 40 ml is used. The cell num-ber is adjusted to 1 × 10^6 cells/ml culture medium.

(c) *Human.* The fluid present in the peritoneal cavity of woman undergoing laparoscopy is aspirated by suction and placed in a Falcon tube. The cells are sedimented by centrifugation for 10 min at 110 g and resuspended in culture medium in a concentration of 1×10^6 cells/ml. The total number of nucleated cells is about 10^7, comprising 58.2% macrophages, 13.8% granulocytes, and 28% lymphocytes (3).

4. Liver

Cell isolation from the liver was only done in mice. The animals are anesthetized with 6 mg phenobarbital natrium (S.A. Abbot N.V., Amsterdam) given intraperitoneally. The abdomen is opened and the intestines reflected to expose the superior mesenteric vein. This vein is cannulated with a 27-gauge needle on a syringe and the liver perfused with 0.2% (w/v) pronase E (E. Merck, Darmstadt, W. Germany) in Hanks' solution (Oxoid Ltd., England) at a flow rate of 1 - 2 ml/min and a temperature of 37°C. Once perfusion is established, the inferior vena cava is cut, after which the liver becomes pale. Perfusion is continued for 3 - 4 min until the animal is completely exsanguinated. The liver is then removed and weighed after excision of nonhepatic tissue. Any segments that have not been perfused are removed and the liver is weighed again before being chopped into small pieces, which are washed three times in Hanks' solution.

The fragments are digested for 1 hr under constant stirring in 0.2% (w/v) pronase (10 ml/g liver) at pH 7.4 and 37°C. The pH is monitored continuously and adjusted when necessary with 0.1 N sodium hydroxide. At 20 and 40 min after the start of the incubation, 0.5 mg DNase (E. Merck) in 1 ml Hanks' solution is added to digest cellular debris. Sterilized and siliconized glassware is used throughout.

After incubation, the cell suspension is filtered through two layers of gauze, centrifuged for 4 min at 360 g, and washed three times in Hanks' solution, after which the nonparenchymal cells in the final suspension are counted in a Bürker hemocytometer. The viability of the cells is determined by incubating the cells with 0.1% trypan blue in saline for 30 sec at room temperature and counting the cells that exclude the dye. This suspension is used to make cytocentrifuge preparations and for cultures made with a suspension of $1 - 1.5 \times 10^6$ cells to study the glass-adherent cells (5, 6).

5. Lung

Cell isolation from the lung was only done in mice. The animals are anesthetized with 5 mg phenobarbital (Abbott N.V.) given intraperitoneally. The abdomen is opened and the diaphragm exposed and pierced. After collapse of the lungs, a triangular section of the thoracic cage is cut out, and the ex-

posed aorta, esophagus, and inferior caval vein are cut. The
right ventricle is then punctured with a 21-gauge needle on a
syringe containing 5 ml of a solution of 0.6 mM EDTA in
phosphate-buffered saline (PBS), and the contents are slowly
injected into the beating heart. The major blood vessels in
the neck and shoulders are cut to diminish backflow to the
heart. During the perfusion, the pink color of the lungs
changes to pale white. If part of the lung remains pink, which
indicates incomplete perfusion, the animal is discarded.

Next, the trachea is exposed and cannulated with a 20-gauge
Teflon catheter (Abbocath-T. Abbott N.V.) connected to a three-
way stopcock on which a syringe containing 15 ml of lavage
fluid at 37°C and an empty syringe for collection of fluid from
the lungs are mounted. The lavage fluid is composed of 0.6 mM
EDTA in PBS. Portions of 1 ml of lavage fluid at a time are introduced and recovered. The cells in the pooled lavage fluid
from one mouse are counted immediately in a Bürker hemocytometer in duplicate and then washed once in PBS. Viability is
determined by trypan blue exclusion. Cytocentrifuge preparations are made for characterization of the cells. For culture,
the cells are suspended in culture medium at a concentration of
about 5×10^5 viable cells/ml (7).

B. Morphology

1. Cytocentrifuge Preparations

Preparations of all cell suspensions are made by spinning
down the cells onto a glass coverslip. For this purpose, a
round coverslip with a diameter of 12 mm is placed in a flat-
bottomed centrifuge tube (diameter 15 mm, height 5.5 cm), and
then 3 ml of phosphate-buffered saline containing 5% newborn
calf serum is pipetted into the tube. Approximately 1 - 2
$\times 10^5$ cells are then added, and the tube is gently shaken and
centrifuged for 10 min at 180 g. The supernatant is discarded,
the coverslip carefully removed and quickly dried in an air
stream, after which the coverslip is attached with Depex to a
microscope slide with the cell-bearing side exposed for further
fixation and staining.

2. Cultures on Glass

To study adherent cells, cell suspensions in the required
concentration are incubated in Leighton tubes with a flying
coverslip (10 × 35 mm). The tubes are either incubated in a
CO_2 incubator or gassed with 5% CO_2 in air and tightly stoppered with nontoxic stoppers. For murine and human cells, the
culture medium is composed of medium 199 (Microbiological

Associates) with 20% heat-inactivated newborn calf serum
(GIBCO Europe, Glasgow, Scotland). For guinea pig cells, use
is made of Dulbecco's medium (GIBCO Europe, Glasgow, Scotland)
containing 20% heat-inactivated newborn calf serum (2).
Penicillin 1000 U/ml and streptomycin 50 µg/ml are added to
the culture medium. When enzyme digestion is used, as for
liver and lung tissue, the streptomycin is replaced by 20 µg/ml
gentamycin. After incubation, the coverslips are washed with
serum-free medium, removed from the tube, quickly air-dried,
and mounted cell side up on slides for staining.

3. Staining

The morphology is studied in preparations stained with
Giemsa stain (1 drop of Giemsa on 1 ml water). After fixation
in methyl alcohol for 15 min, blood smears are stained for
20 min and monolayers on coverslips or cytocentrifuge preparations for 7 min. For cells showing pinocytosis of dextran
sulfate, the preparations are stained with either Giemsa stain
for 5 min or toluidine blue (1% toluidine blue in 30% methyl
alcohol) for 15 min.

C. Cytochemistry

1. Esterase

Esterase activity of mononuclear phagocytes is investigated
according to Ornstein (3, 8, 9). The reagent is prepared by
mixing 0.8 ml of a pararosaniline hydrochloride solution with
0.8 ml of a sodium nitrite solution (Table I). After 30 sec,
4.5 ml 0.40 M sodium cacodylate is added and the pH checked
and, if necessary, brought to 6.0 with sodium cacodylate. The
volume is then adjusted to 15 ml with distilled water and
0.15 ml 10% Tween 20 is added. This solution is added to a
mixture of 2 ml 0.52% (w/v) α-naphthyl butyrate in dioxane and
3 ml methanol; next, distilled water is added to give a final
volume of 40 ml. This reagent remains stable for up to 6 hr.
The air-dried preparations are fixed in formalin vapor for
60 sec, washed in water, dried, and covered with the reagent
at room temperature for 25 min. The slides are then rinsed,
dried, and counterstained with Giemsa stain for 6 - 10 min.
Blood smears are counterstained with Giemsa for 15 min.

2. Peroxidase

Peroxidase is determined according to Kaplow (10). Air-
dried preparations are fixed in 10% formalin in absolute alcohol for 1 min, rinsed in tap water, and dried. Kaplow's

TABLE I. Reagents for Esterase and Peroxidase Staining

Esterase staining:[a]

Stock solutions
1. α-Naphthyl butyrate (0.26 gm) (Sigma Chemical Co.,
   St. Louis, Missouri) in 50 ml dioxane
2. Pararosaniline hydrochloride (1.0 gm) (Sigma) in 30 ml
   2 N HCl
3. NaNO₂ (1.0 gm) in 30 ml water (make fresh weekly)
4. Sodium cacodylate, 0.40 M
5. 10% Tween 20

Peroxidase staining:[b]

Incubation mixture
  30% Ethyl alcohol, 100 ml
  Benzidine dihydrochloride (Fluka AG, Buchs, Switzerland),
    0.3 gm
  0.132 M (3.8% w/v)ZnSO₄·7H₂O, 1.0 ml
  Sodium acetate (NaC₂H₃O₂·3H₂O), 1.0 gm
  3% Hydrogen peroxide, 0.7 ml
  1.0 N Sodium hydroxide, 1.5 ml
  Safranine 0, 0.2 gm

   The reagents should be added in the order listed and
mixed well with each addition. The benzidine salt may contain
a small amount of inert residue that will not dissolve. A
precipitate forms upon addition of the zinc sulfate, but dissolves after addition of the remaining reagents. If a nuclear
counterstain is not required, the safranine can be omitted.
The final pH is 6.00 ± 0.05. The solution should be filtered
and stored in a Coplin jar or bottle at room temperature. The
same solution can be used for as long as 6 months. Heparin,
oxalate, and EDTA are not inhibitory.
   [a]According to Ornstein (8, 9). The solution should be
prepared as described in the text.
   [b]According to Kaplow (10).

reagent, composed of 0.3% (w/v) benzidine dihydrochloride and
0.02% (v/v) hydrogen peroxide (pH 6.0), is poured over the
slides and washed off with tap water after 30 sec. The preparations are then dried, counterstained for 6 min with Giemsa
stain, washed, and dried. Blood smears are counterstained
with Giemsa for 20 min. If staining for peroxidase cannot be
performed immediately, the preparations should be kept in the
dark.

3. Lysozyme

The presence of lysozyme is demonstrated by the immunoperoxidase method (11). Antirat lysozyme serum was produced
in rabbits by repeated intramuscular immunization with rat
lysozyme (kindly supplied by E. F. Ossermann, Columbia College
of Physicians and Surgeons, New York) together with Freunds'
complete adjuvant (Difco Laboratories, Detroit, Michigan).
This antiserum has been used for studies in rat and mouse
cells. For human cells, rabbit immunoglobulins to human muramidase (Dako Copenhagen, Denmark), diluted 1 : 40, is used as
antiserum. Air-dried preparations are fixed in methanol for
15 min and then in methanol containing 0.03% hydrogen peroxide
for 10 min, washed in phosphate-buffered saline, and incubated
for 10 min with goat serum (diluted 1 : 8). After incubation
with rabbit antilysozyme serum (dilution 1 : 15) for 30 min at
room temperature, the preparations are thoroughly washed with
PBS and incubated with peroxidase-conjugated goat antirabbit
IgG (Miles Yeda Ltd., Israel) (dilution 1:100) for 30 min at
room temperature, washed in PBS, and stained for 6 min with
6 mg 3,3'-diaminobenzidine tetrahydrochloride (Fluka A. G.,
Buchs, Switzerland) in 10 ml 0.05 M tris buffer (pH 7.6) with
hydrogen peroxide added to a final concentration of 0.015%.
This reagent should be made just before use. The antiserum is
checked by substituting normal rabbit serum, the substrate by
substituting PBS for the antiserum, and the peroxidase reaction by determination of endogen peroxidase in cells.

4. Fc and C3 Receptors

The presence of Fc receptors can be detected with IgG-
coated sheep erythrocytes. Washed sheep erythrocytes are made
up into a 5% (about 2×10^9 erythrocytes/ml) solution in buffered saline, 0.2 ml is added to 0.04 ml heat-inactivated
mouse antisheep erythrocyte serum (prepared by repeated intravenous immunization of mice with sheep erythrocytes, hemagglutination titer of the antiserum 1:1500), and the volume is
made up to 1 ml with medium 199. This suspension is incubated
for 30 min at 37°C, after which the erythrocytes are washed
twice in buffered saline and resuspended in medium 199 to a
final concentration of 0.2%. Each culture receives 1 ml of
this suspension and is incubated for 1 hr at 37°C to allow
phagocytosis. The culture is then thoroughly washed with
medium 199, dried, fixed, and stained with Giemsa (5).

The presence of complement (C3) receptors can be detected
by using sheep erythrocytes coated with IgM and C (5). The
erythrocytes are first coated with IgM by incubating 0.2 ml of
a 5% sheep erythrocytes suspension with an equal volume of an
IgM fraction of rabbit antisheep erythrocyte serum for 15 min

at 37°C and then washed twice with buffered saline. A mixture of equal volumes of 2.5% IgM-coated erythrocytes in medium 199 and fresh mouse serum as a source of complement is incubated for 10 min at 37°C, washed twice with saline, and resuspended in medium 199 to a final concentration of 0.2%. Complement receptors are identified by using the procedure described for Fc receptors.

Rabbit IgM antisheep erythrocytes antibodies are prepared from rabbit serum obtained 3 days after a single intravenous injection of sheep erythrocytes by passing the latter twice through a Sephadex G-200 column. After concentration of the appropriate fractions by freeze-drying, possible IgG contamination was assessed by immunodiffusion using antirabbit IgG antiserum (Dako) and by assaying the ingestion of sheep erythrocytes coated with IgM (EIgM) or with IgM and complement (EIgMC) in 24-hr cultures of peritoneal macrophages. IgM is used in a dilution such that when EIgM are prepared, no rosetting or ingestion of coated erythrocytes by peritoneal macrophages is found and when used for the preparation of EIgMC shows rosettes on 100% of the macrophages and no more than 5% ingestion.

To detect C receptors in guinea pig cells, IgM-coated sheep erythrocytes were first incubated with guinea pig C1, C4, and C2 followed by a final incubation of the EIgMC1,4,2 with purified guinea pig C3 (2, 12).

D. Function Tests

1. Phagocytosis

Bacteria from an overnight culture in nutrient broth No. 2 (Oxoid Ltd., London) are washed twice with phosphate-buffered saline, and a suspension is made in medium 199 containing 10% noninactivated newborn calf serum. For human cells 10% AB serum is used. The bacteria-to-cell ratio is 100 : 1 for *Staphylococcus aureus* and 10 : 1 for *Staphylococcus epidermidis*. Monolayers are incubated for 1 hr at 37°C. When *S. epidermidis* is used, the monolayers are thoroughly washed, quickly air-dried, fixed, and stained. For *S. aureus,* the cultures are washed once and incubated with 10 U lysostaphin (Sigma Chemical Co., St. Louis, Missouri) in 1 ml medium for 5 min at 37°C to lyse the extracellular bacteria (13, 14). The cultures are then washed twice, air-dried, fixed, and stained. To investigate phagocytosis of IgG-coated sheep erythrocytes, cultures treated as described earlier under detection of Fc receptors are incubated with 0.83% NH_4Cl for 20 - 30 sec at room temperature to lyse extracellular erythrocytes, after which they are washed twice, air-dried, fixed, and stained.

2. Pinocytosis

The glass-adherent cells on coverslips are incubated in
1 ml culture medium with 25, 50, or 100 µg dextran sulfate
(MW 500,000, Pharmacia Fine Chemicals, Inc., Uppsala, Sweden)
for 24 hr at 37°C, washed, air-dried, fixed, and stained for
15 min in 1% toluidine blue.

III. RESULTS

A. Morphology

In Giemsa-stained direct preparations of bone marrow, blood,
and peritoneal fluid, the mononuclear phagocytes of the different species show great similarity, but their behavior on a glass
surface differs in some respects. Mouse peritoneal macrophages
have proved to be the best stretchers; after 24 hr these cells
are well spread and elongated on the glass surface. Mononuclear
phagocytes from bone marrow and blood spread somewhat more slowly, but after 48 hr in culture they are also well spread and
elongated and look very much like peritoneal cells after the
same culture period. In the guinea pig, mononuclear phagocytes
from bone marrow and peritoneal fluid have been studied in 96-hr
cultures on glass and those from blood in 48-hr cultures (2).
Although there are some well-spread cells after this period, the
majority of the mononuclear phagocytes are round or oval. The
same holds for rat peritoneal cells cultured for 24 and 48 hr
on glass. Some of the cells are well spread, but the majority
of the macrophages are round or oval. Hamster peritoneal macrophages cultured for 24 hr are well spread and closely resemble mouse peritoneal macrophages.
The morphology and other characteristics of the mononuclear
phagocytes of human bone marrow are best studied in 6-hr cultures. In Giemsa-stained preparations, the promonocytes show a
large round or indented nucleus and dark-blue cytoplasm containing a few dense granules. Bone marrow monocytes are slightly
smaller than the promonocytes and have an indented nucleus and
more cytoplasm, which is slightly paler and contains more
granules than that of the promonocytes. After an incubation
period of 48 hr, the promonocytes and monocytes show little
stretching (3). Peripheral blood monocytes after culture *in
vitro* for more than 6 hr show a certain amount of stretching of
the cytoplasm and the formation of pseudopods, but much less
than is seen in murine macrophages (3).
Human peritoneal macrophages in cytocentrifuge preparations
are round and show some variation in size. During incubation

in vitro for up to 48 hr, the peritoneal macrophages spread and put out pseudopods (3).

B. Cytochemical Characteristics

1. Esterase

Esterase activity is found in all cultured glass adherent cells (Tables II and III). The different species show differences in the intensity of staining. In mice, cytocentrifuge preparations of bone marrow and peritoneal fluid show very weak esterase staining, and no positive staining could be detected in blood smears, but the intensity of the esterase activity and the number of positive cells increases with the duration of incubation *in vitro* (Table III). Exceptions are freshly isolated Kupffer cells and alveolar macrophages, which are strongly positive from the start, which permits the use of shorter staining periods, i.e., 5 – 15 min (5, 7). In the guinea pig cells esterase activity is very strong, especially in the cultures of bone marrow and peritoneal macrophages. An incubation time of 15 min suffices for positive staining (2). In rat peritoneal cells, the staining is clearly positive in direct preparations and remains constant during culturing. These cells are more strongly positive than guinea pig and hamster cells. In the latter, the peritoneal macrophages are also strongly positive (Table II).

Human mononuclear phagocytes from bone marrow, blood, and peritoneal cavity are strongly esterase-positive (Tables II and III). Peripheral blood monocytes cultured for 48 hr on glass show a slightly lower degree of positivity, but the percentage of positive cells remains constant (3).

2. Peroxidase

In mice there is a high percentage of peroxidase-positive mononuclear phagocytes in the bone marrow and peripheral blood, but not in those from the peritoneal cavity, liver, and lung (Tables II and III). The peroxidase activity in blood decreases during incubation *in vitro* from 87% after 2 hr to 59.8% after 24 hr (15). Exudate macrophages collected 12 hr after an intraperitoneal injection of newborn calf serum show about 88% peroxidase-positive cells. However, this value declines to about 6% 72 hr after the serum injection. Since an intraperitoneal injection of newborn calf serum evokes a short-lasting influx of mainly mononuclear phagocytes from the peripheral blood into the peritoneal cavity, the high percentage of positive cells 12 hr after the injection of newborn calf serum indicates that the peroxidase-positive macrophages in the inflam-

TABLE II. Cytochemical Characteristics

	Mouse				Guinea Pig		Rat	Hamster	Human	
	Blood mono-cytes[a] (%)	Peri-toneal macro-phages[a] (%)	Kupffer cells[a] (%)	Alveolar macro-phages[a] (%)	Blood mono-cytes[b] (%)	Peri-toneal macro-phages[c] (%)	Peri-toneal macro-phages[a] (%)	Peri-toneal macro-phages[a] (%)	Blood mono-cytes[d] (%)	Peri-toneal macro-phages[d] (%)
Esterase	95.0	99.3	99.0	100.0	99.5	100.0	96.2	100.0	97.0	99.0
Peroxidase	59.8	0.4	0.0	0.9	10.0	2.5	3.0	n.d.	94.3	70.0
Lysozyme	96.5	100.0	n.d.[e]	n.d.	+[f]	+[f]	100.0	+[f]	92.2	n.d.

[a]Determined in 24-hr cultures.
[b]Determined in 48-hr cultures.
[c]Determined in 96-hr cultures.
[d]Determined in 6-hr cultures.
[e]n.d., not done.
[f]+, no specific antiserum available.

TABLE III. *Functional and Cytochemical Characteristics of Murine and Human Bone Marrow Mononuclear Phagocytes*

	Murine				Human	
	Promonocytes		Monocytes		Promonocytes	Monocytes
	6 hr (%)	24 hr (%)	6 hr (%)	24 hr (%)	6 hr (%)	6 hr (%)
Esterase	30.0	91.2	40.0	97.4	89.8	93.2
Peroxidase	96.3	93.6	90.9	87.0	98.1	97.9
Lysozyme[a]	n.d.[c]	99.7	n.d.	99.7	95.6	95.6
Fc receptor	56.4	93.0	56.1	93.0	97.6	90.3
C receptor	31.6	79.5	42.6	79.5	98.1	89.5
Phagocytosis opsonized bacteria	69.0	77.0	72.0	74.0	92.7	95.8
IgG-coated red cells[b]	39.3	93.0	36.9	93.0	97.6	88.0
Pinocytosis	79.0	91.0	87.0	91.0	72.8	72.4

[a]*Determined in 24-hr cultures in which a distinction cannot be made between promonocytes and monocytes.*
[b]*Sheep red cells coated with mouse IgG antibodies.*
[c]*n.d., not done.*

matory exudate are recent emigrees from the blood (15).

In the guinea pig the peroxidase activity of bone marrow and blood mononuclear phagocytes is lower than that in mice and also shows a decrease after incubation *in vitro.* The percentage of positive bone marrow cells fell from 40% at 48 hr to 19% at 96 hr of culture. In peripheral blood smears 52% of the monocytes are positive, but in 48-hr cultures of blood monocytes only 10% are positive. Peritoneal macrophages show only a very low percentage of positive cells (Table II) (2). Rat peritoneal macrophages also show a low percentage of peroxidase-positive cells (Table II).

In human bone marrow almost all of the promonocytes and monocytes are peroxidase-positive (Table III). Peroxidase positivity is similar in blood monocytes and bone marrow monocytes (Tables II and III). After culture on glass for up to 4 days, the percentage of positive cells significantly decreases (3). The decrease of peroxidase positivity after longer culture periods is probably explained by degranulation during fusion of lysosomes with pinocytic vesicles and subsequent degratation of the enzyme.

3. Lysozyme

This enzyme is found in high percentages in mononuclear phagocytes from mouse, rat, and man (Tables II and III). The guinea pig and hamster are not investigated with respect to lysozyme because no specific antiserum is available.

C. Functional Characteristics

1. Receptors

In the mouse almost all mononuclear phagocytes from the bone marrow, and peritoneal cavity show Fc and C receptors (Tables III and IV). In the bone marrow, the number of positive cells and the density of rosettes increase with increasing duration of culture on glass. In the liver, the percentage of Fc and C receptors increases during incubation *in vitro* but remains lower than in peritoneal macrophages (Table IV). This might be due to membrane damage caused by pronase digestion (5). The enzyme-treated pulmonary macrophages also show an increase of receptor-bearing cells during incubation *in vitro*. In the lung, the percentage of cells with C receptors is low (Table IV), and a difference is seen between cells obtained by lavage of the lung and those from enzyme-treated lung tissue (7).

Peritoneal macrophages of the rat also show high percentages of cells positive for both receptors (Table IV).

In the guinea pig, Fc receptors are detected on almost 100% of the mononuclear phagocytes from the bone marrow, peripheral blood, and peritoneal cavity (Table IV). After 24 hr of culture on glass, cells from bone marrow, blood, and peritoneal cavity show high percentages of C-receptor-bearing cells (Table IV) (2).

In human bone marrow, blood, and peritoneal cavity, 90 – 98% of the mononuclear phagocytes have Fc receptors, as shown with sheep red cells coated with mouse IgG antibodies (Tables III and IV). With the use of sheep red cells coated with IgM and mouse complement, C receptors are found on 98% of the promonocytes of the bone marrow and on almost 90% of the monocytes from bone marrow and blood (Tables III and IV). Almost 100% of the peritoneal macrophages show receptors on their surface (Table IV) (3).

2. Phagocytosis

In the mouse, IgG-coated sheep erythrocytes are readily ingested by mononuclear phagocytes from various sources (Tables III and IV). Sheep erythrocytes coated with IgM and C are only ingested in small percentages. The attached red cells appar-

TABLE IV. Functional Characteristics

	Mouse				Guinea Pig		Rat	Human	
	Blood mono-cytes[a] (%)	Peri-toneal macro-phages[a] (%)	Kupffer cells[a] (%)	Alveolar macro-phages[a] (%)	Blood mono-cytes[b] (%)	Peri-toneal macro-phages[c] (%)	Peri-toneal macro-phages[a] (%)	Blood mono-cytes[d] (%)	Peri-toneal macro-phages[d] (%)
Fc receptor	99.0	100.0	84.3	72.4	98.5	100.0	99.7	92.3	97.3
C receptor	96.3	100.0	37.5	2.2	84.5[a]	99.5[a]	88.2	88.1	92.8
Phagocytosis opsonized bacteria	90.0	98.0	81.5	94.2	>83.3	96.5	94.0	91.3	83.8
IgG-coated red cells	99.0	90.6	56.9	61.5	97.0	99.0	60.2	91.0	60.7
Pinocytosis	98.0	99.0	90.4	89.7	91.0	95.5	96.9	68.0	85.2

[a]Determined in 24-hr cultures.
[b]Determined in 48-hr cultures.
[c]Determined in 96-hr cultures.
[d]Determined in 6-hr cultures.

ently do not trigger ingestion in nonstimulated mononuclear phagocytes (16). However, thioglycollate-induced peritoneal macrophages do ingest complement-coated erythrocytes (17). Phagocytosis of opsonized bacteria increases with maturation of the cells, i.e., from about 75% in the bone marrow to 98% for the peritoneal macrophages (Tables III and IV). Nonopsonized *S. aureus* are also phagocytized by peritoneal macrophages, but the number of bacteria per cell is low. Latex beads, whether opsonized or nonopsonized, are phagocytized by peritoneal macrophages at a level of almost 100% (14).

In the guinea pig, IgG-coated erythrocytes and opsonized bacteria are phagocytized by almost 100% of the mononuclear phagocytes from the bone marrow, blood, and peritoneal cavity (Table IV) (2).

Rat peritoneal macrophages phagocytize opsonized bacteria at a level of more than 90%, but phagocytosis of IgG-coated erythrocytes is lower (Table IV).

Human mononuclear phagocytes from the bone marrow, blood, and the peritoneal cavity phagocytize high percentages of opsonized bacteria and IgG-coated sheep erythrocytes (Tables III and IV). Phagocytosis of sheep erythrocytes coated with IgM and mouse complement occurs only in about 10% of the bone marrow cells and 16% of the peripheral blood monocytes. Human peritoneal macrophages show in 74% ingestion of complement-coated erythrocytes, probably due to the activated state of the macrophages (3).

3. Pinocytosis

In the mouse pinocytosis of dextran sulfate amounts to more than 90% for mononuclear phagocytes from the bone marrow, blood, and peritoneal cavity (Tables III and IV). In the guinea pig and rat, too, pinocytosis is observed for the majority of the cells (Table IV).

For human bone marrow promonocytes and monocytes and peripheral blood monocytes, about 70% of the cells pinocytose dextran sulfate (Tables III and IV). After prolonged incubation with 100 µg dextran sulfate, the percentage of pinocytosing monocytes rises until, after 24 and 48 hr of incubation, the percentages of positive cells are 92 and 95%, respectively. Of the peritoneal macrophages, 85% show pinocytic activity (Table IV).

D. Comparison of Mononuclear Phagocytes with Lymphocytes and Fibroblasts

Aside from the study of morphological differences, investigation of cytochemical and functional aspects of cells and their behavior on a glass surface greatly facilitates differentiation between mononuclear phagocytes and other mononuclear cells, such as lymphocytes and fibroblasts. Lymphocytes do not adhere avidly to glass, except in the absence of serum, and they can be easily washed off a surface after adherence of the mononuclear phagocytes. T lymphocytes do have esterase activity, but only as a few distinct spots in the cytoplasm, whereas the mononuclear phagocytes show diffuse cytoplasmic esterase staining. Peroxidase and lysozyme staining is not positive in lymphocytes. Although lymphocytes have Fc receptors and can form rosettes with IgG-coated erythrocytes, they do not phagocytize opsonized erythrocytes or bacteria. Pinocytosis of dextran sulfate is also absent.

Fibroblasts are mononuclear cells, and differentiation from mononuclear phagocytes is often difficult. In cytocentrifuge preparations the former are round cells and have a large round nucleus with distinct nucleoli. After culture on a glass surface they are stretched but with a sheathlike shape differing from the stretching of macrophages. Esterase staining is not a very good marker for the differentiation from mononuclear phagocytes because fibroblasts also show the reaction, although not very strongly. Peroxidase staining is not a good marker either, fibroblasts are peroxidase negative, but so are tissue macrophages. Of the functional characteristics, pinocytosis of dextran sulfate cannot be used because it occurs in both fibroblasts and macrophages, although the former pinocytose less actively. The presence of receptors and immune phagocytosis are very good markers for distinguishing fibroblasts from macrophages, because fibroblasts have no Fc and C receptors, do not phagocytize opsonized erythrocytes, and only phagocytose opsonized *S. aureus* at a very low level (about 3%), which differs distinctly from the data found for macrophages (Table IV).

IV. DISCUSSION

Comparison of mononuclear phagocytes from different organs of various species clearly shows the divergence in their morphological appearance, but a detailed discussion on the morphological characteristics of these cells would take us beyond the scope of this chapter. From the morphological pattern it is not apparent that these cells all belong to one cell line, the mononuclear phagocyte system (MPS) (18), but many extensive studies done with, for instance, cell markers in radiation chimeras and parabiotic animals and on cell kinetics with various kinds of label, have proved that the monoblasts, promonocytes, monocytes, and macrophages occurring in tissues and serous cavities belong to the MPS (19).

Although immature dividing mononuclear phagocytes (monoblasts and promonocytes) occur mainly in the bone marrow, they
can also occur in the tissues in very small numbers, especially
in pathological conditions, recruited from the bone marrow. It
is of interest to know which features represent developmental
stages of the mononuclear phagocytes. A useful characteristic
is the presence of C receptors, which occur less frequently on
immature than on mature mononuclear phagocytes, but a much better characteristic for determination of the developmental stage
is the synthesis of DNA, which can be studied on the basis of
either [^{3}H]-thymidine incorporation into the nucleus or the
amount of DNA of the nucleus: The majority of the immature mononuclear phagocytes (monoblasts and promonocytes) synthesize
DNA, whereas monocytes and macrophages do not (20). However,
more studies are needed to find other characteristics making it
possible to distinguish mononuclear phagocytes from other cells
and to determine the degree of differentiation of the mononuclear phagocyte.

When we consider the more mature nondividing mononuclear
phagocytes (monocytes, macrophages), the question arises as to
whether there are characteristics that can be used to differentiate between mononuclear phagocytes, on the one hand, and
cells which resemble them morphologically, on the other hand
(e.g., lymphoid cells, fibroblasts, reticulum cells, dendritic
cells). Examples of characteristics permitting distinction between monocytes, macrophages, lymphocytes, and fibroblasts
(for instance, staining for esterase, peroxidase, or lysozyme;
the presence of Fc and C receptors; immune phagocytosis; and
pinocytosis) have been discussed in the preceding paragraphs.

In this chapter mention is made of only a limited number
of such characteristics. Promising features requiring further
investigation include other enzymes present in mononuclear phagocytes, i.e., aminopeptidase, 5'-nucleotidase, leucine aminopeptidase, α_1-antitrypsin, alkaline phosphodiesterase I, and
such properties as Ia antigens, and cell line- and cell type-
specific antigens determined with monoclonal antibodies.

An important question to be considered is how high the percentage of marker-bearing cells in a population must be before
that population can be called a mononuclear phagocyte population. Since almost none of the currently used markers give 100%
positivity, 90% seems to be acceptable for the present. In
this connection the developmental stage of the cells and their
state of activation must also be taken into account, because in
immature cells certain characteristics may be only poorly developed or not yet present. For some characteristics, furthermore, there is divergence between normal and activated cells in
the sense that in the latter, properties may have just appeared,
become more pronounced, or have disappeared after stimulation.

REFERENCES

1. R. van Furth and Z. A. Cohn. The origin and kinetics of mononuclear phagocytes. *J. Exp. Med. 128*: 415, 1968.
2. V. Brade, M. M. C. Diesselhoff-den Dulk, and R. van Furth. Isolation and characterization of mononuclear phagocytes from the bone marrow, blood, and peritoneal cavity of the guinea pig. *J. Pathology* (in press).
3. R. van Furth, J. A. Raeburn, and T. L. van Zwet. Characteristics of human mononuclear phagocytes. *Blood 54*: 485, 1979.
4. A. Bøyum. Separation of leucocytes from blood and bone marrow. *Scand. J. Clin. Lab. Invest. 27* (suppl.): 29, 1968.
5. R. W. Crofton, M. M. C. Diesselhoff-den Dulk, and R. van Furth. The origin, kinetics, and characteristics of the Kupffer cells in the normal steady state. *J. Exp. Med. 148*: 1, 1978.
6. J. J. Emeis and B. Planqué. Heterogeneity of cells isolated from rat liver by pronase digestion: Ultrastructure, cytochemistry, and cell culture. *J. Reticuloendothel. Soc. 20*: 11, 1976.
7. A. Blussé van Oud Alblas and R. van Furth. Origin, kinetics, and characteristics of pulmonary macrophages in the normal steady state. *J. Exp. Med. 149*: 1504, 1979.
8. H. Ansley and L. Ornstein. Enzymohistochemistry and differential white cell counts on the Technicon Hemalog D. *Adv. Automated Anal. 1*: 5, 1970.
9. L. Ornstein, H. Ansley, and A. Saunders. Improving manual differential white cell counts with cytochemistry. *Blood Cells 2*: 557, 1976.
10. L. S. Kaplow. Simplified myeloperoxidase stain using benzidine dihydrochloride. *Blood 26*: 215, 1965.
11. P. K. Nakane and G. B. Pierce. Enzyme-labeled antibodies: Preparation and application for the localization of antigens. *J. Histochem. Cytochem. 14*: 929, 1966.
12. V. Brade, C. Bentley, D. Bitter-Suermann, and U. Hadding. Interaction of zymosan and of activated properdin with factor D-depleted guinea pig serum: Implications for the mechanism of initial C3 cleavage via the alternative complement pathway. *Z. Immun. Forsch. 152*: 402, 1977.
13. J. S. Tan, C. Watanakunakorn, and J. P. Phair. A modified assay of neutrophil function: Use of lysostaphin to differentiate defective phagocytosis from impaired intracellular killing. *J. Lab. Clin. Med. 78*: 316, 1971.
14. R. van Furth and M. M. C. Diesselhoff-den Dulk. Methods to prove ingestion of particles by macrophages with light microscopy. *Scand. J. Immunol. 12*: 265, 1980.

15. R. van Furth, J. G. Hirsch, and M. E. Fedorko. Morphology
    and peroxidase cytochemistry of mouse promonocytes, mono-
    cytes, and macrophages. *J. Exp. Med. 132*: 794, 1970.
16. F. M. Griffin, C. Bianco, and S. C. Silverstein. Charac-
    terization of the macrophage receptor for complement and
    demonstration of its functional independence from the re-
    ceptor for the Fc portion of immunoglobulin G. *J. Exp.
    Med. 141*: 1269, 1975.
17. C. Bianco, F. M. Griffin, and S. C. Silverstein. Studies
    of the macrophage complement receptor. Alteration of re-
    ceptor functions upon macrophage activation. *J. Exp. Med.
    141*: 1278, 1975.
18. R. van Furth, Z. A. Cohn, J. G. Hirsch, J. H. Humphrey,
    W. G. Spector, and H. L. Langevoort. The mononuclear
    phagocyte system: A new classification of macrophages,
    monocytes, and their precursor cells. *Bull. WHO 46*: 845,
    1972.
19. R. van Furth. Cells of the mononuclear phagocyte system.
    Nomenclature in terms of sites and conditions. *In*
    "Mononuclear Phagocytes - Functional Aspects" (R. van
    Furth, ed.), p. 1. Martinus Nijhoff Publishers, The
    Hague, Boston, London, 1980.
20. R. van Furth. Mononuclear phagocytes in inflammation.
    In "Handbook of Experimental Pharmacology" (J. R. Vane
    and S. H. Ferreira, eds.). Springer Verlag, Berlin,
    1978, *50*: 1.

29

Fc AND C3 RECEPTORS

Celso Bianco
Bronislaw Pytowski

I. BACKGROUND

The hallmark of mononuclear phagocyte function is phagocytosis (reviewed in 1,2). However, it should be emphasized
here that phagocytosis is a general phenomenon in the biological world, and that many cells other than mononuclear
phagocytes are able to ingest particles. For instance, among
mammalian species, several cell types ingest latex beads, including peripheral blood lymphocytes and fibroblasts. The
only endocytic event that seems to be peculiar to mononuclear
phagocytes and polymorphonuclear leukocytes is the ingestion
via plasma membrane receptors for the Fc fragment of the IgG
molecule. At certain stages of differentiation, C3b fragments
of the C3 component of complement can also mediate phagocytic
uptake. These observations are discussed in detail in several
publications and reviews (3-5,6).

The procedures described below utilize erythrocytes as
indicator particles. They allow easy visual examination and

METHODS FOR STUDYING
MONONUCLEAR PHAGOCYTES

273

quantitation. Furthermore, under usual circumstances, the uncoated particles are not recognized by monocytes and macrophages, and precise analysis of the ligand-mediated ingestion can be performed.

The following are a series of statements that the authors consider important regarding phagocytic assays. They are not intended as a review of the subject. Further references can be obtained from the original articles and reviews.

(a) The phagocytic process can be divided in two stages: attachment (recognition) and ingestion (interiorization) (1). Many ligands mediate attachment without inducing ingestion. For instance, mouse resident macrophages do not ingest particles via their C3 receptor in the absence of IgG (6). The fibronectin receptor of human monocytes does not mediate ingestion (7).

(b) C3 by itself does not usually mediate ingestion by monocytes, resident macrophages, and neutrophils. However, activated macrophages are able to ingest particles via their C3 receptors (6).

(c) C3b-mediated attachment enhances IgG-mediated uptake (8). This synergistic effect may be important in the uptake of immune complexes. However, it appears that large amounts of C3 interfere with the availability of Fc fragments on the target particle for interaction with Fc receptors (9).

(d) Depending on the species studied, several subclasses of IgG seem to mediate phagocytosis. In the mouse, both the "aggregate" and the "monomeric" Fc receptors of macrophages described by Unkeless (10) seem to mediate phagocytosis (11).

(e) No single procedure can be used for the identification of mononuclear phagocytes with absolute reliability. However, in many cases, a mononuclear cell able to ingest a particle via the Fc receptor of IgG can be considered a mononuclear phagocyte. The Fc receptor can be detected at any stage of differentiation of this cell series.

II. MATERIALS

A. *Reagents*

(1) Phosphate-buffered saline (PBS) (Grand Island Biological Co., New York).

(2) Hanks' balanced salt solution with divalent cations (Hanks') (Grand Island Biological Co., New York).

(3) Dulbecco's Modified Eagle's Minimum Essential Medium (Dulbecco's) (Grand Island Biological Co., New York).

(4) Alsever's: glucose, 24:6 gm; sodium citrate (dihydrate), 9.6 gm; NaCl, 5.04 gm; add 1.2 liter double distilled H_2O and adjust to pH 6.1 with saturated citric acid. Sterilize by filtration.

(5) Veronal-buffered saline with Ca^{2+}, Mg^{2+}, and glucose (VBG): This solution should be prepared from stock solutions shortly before the preparation of indicator erythrocytes (see below).

Stock veronal: NaCl, 83 gm; Na-5,5-diethyl barbiturate, 10.19 gm; double distilled H_2O, 1.5 liter. Adjust pH to 7.35 and volume to 2 liter.

Stock Ca^{2+} and Mg^{2+}: 1 M $MgCl_2$ and 0.15 M $CaCl_2$ in double-distilled H_2O; add 10 ml of veronal stock to 25 ml of 10% glucose and 100 μl of Ca^{2+}, Mg^{2+} stock. Add 0.1 gm of gelatin dissolved in 1 ml of hot H_2O. Adjust volume to 100 ml with double-distilled H_2O. Keep on ice.

(6) Fetal calf serum (FCS) (Grand Island Biological Co., New York). Heat inactivate for 1 hr at 56°C.

(7) Brewer's Thioglycollate Medium (Difco Laboratories, Detroit, Michigan): 4% (w/v) solution in double-distilled H_2O. Boil briefly and sterilize by autoclaving. Keep at room temperature in the dark.

(8) Glutaraldehyde, 1.25%: Dilute 25% stock (Fisher Scientific Co., Fair Lawn, New Jersey) in PBS.

(9) Hypaque-Ficoll mixture: Lymphocyte separation medium (Bionetics, Bethesda, Maryland).

(10) EDTA (Disodium ethylenediamine tetraacetate). Prepare 0.1 M stock in double-distilled H_2O. Addition of NaOH will facilitate dissolving. Adjust pH to 7.35 with NaOH and sterilize by filtration. This solution is isotonic.

(11) Sodium suramin (FBA Pharmaceuticals, New York, New York). Inhibits serum C3b inactivator enzyme.

(12) Pansorbin: 10% suspension of *Staphylococcus aureus* cells (Calbiochem-Behring Corp., La Jolla, California). Used for removal of trace IgG from IgM preparations.

(13) ^{51}Cr, Isotonic solution of sodium chromate, 10 mCi/ml, half-life = 27.9 days (Amersham-Searle Co., Arlington Heights, Illinois).

B. Cells

1. Murine Macrophages

Murine peritoneal macrophages are prepared by washing the peritoneal cavity twice with 5 ml PBS. The cells are washed twice with PBS and once with Dulbecco's. For plating on coverslips, the macrophages are resuspended in Dulbecco's with 5% heat-inactivated FCS to a concentration of 1×10^6/ml. Round (12 mm) glass coverslips are prepared by washing with

70% ethanol and flaming; 100 µl of cell suspension is then placed on each coverslip. After 1 hr at 37°C, the coverslips are picked up with forceps and washed by vigorous immersion in Dulbecco's to remove nonadherent cells. The coverslips are placed, cell side up, in Linbro wells each containing 1 ml Dulbecco's medium.

Activated macrophages are obtained, in the same manner, 4 days following an intraperitoneal injection of 1 ml Brewer's Thioglycollate medium (4% w/v) and plated in the identical manner.

2. Human Monocytes and Lymphocytes

Typically, 20 ml of human blood is drawn into a syringe containing 400 µl of 0.5 M EDTA and diluted with equal volume of Hanks'. The blood is then carefully layered on top of 20 ml of Hypaque-Ficoll and centrifuged at 12°C for 40 min at 400 g (as measured at interphase). Erythrocytes and granulocytes form a pellet. The monocytes and lymphocytes form a band at the interphase. The cells are collected into a large volume of Hanks' to dilute the high-density Hypaque-Ficoll mixture and washed 3 times with Hanks'. Plating on coverslips is the same as for macrophages (sect. 2.2.1) except that human serum should be used instead of FCS. This will prevent the lymphocytes from adhering to glass resulting in a monolayer constituted predominantly of monocytes.

3. Erythrocytes (E)

Sheep blood diluted 1:1 in Alsever's should be used between 3 and 14 days of collection. Blood (3 ml) in Alsever's is diluted in a large volume of Hanks' and the erythrocytes washed 3 times in Hanks'. The pellet is resuspended in Hanks' to a 5% packed cell volume. This suspension contains approximately 10^9 cells/ml and should be prepared on the day of the experiment.

If human lymphocytes are present in the preparation, the 5% erythrocytes should be treated with 1 mg/ml of trypsin at 37°C for 1 hr. This should be followed with a wash in Hanks' containing 1 mg/ml of soybean trypsin inhibitor. These erythrocytes will not bind to human T cells.

In certain situations, ox erythrocytes are more convenient particles to use in the described assays. Because of charge characteristics of their surface, they do not agglutinate even when rather high concentrations of antibodies to ox erythrocytes are used. This allows the preparation of indicator particles with high concentrations of IgG for Fc receptor assays. The procedures used are identical. Commercial preparations of antisera to ox erythrocytes are available from many sources.

Latex beads are commonly used in phagocytic assays. However, they are normally ingested by mononuclear phagocytes and by many other cell types including fibroblasts and lymphocytes in the absence of humoral factors. This lack of specificity limits their use to only certain experiments. Latex ingestion is not a reliable marker of cells of the mononuclear phagocytic series.

C. Antisera and Complement Components

1. Antibodies to Sheep Erythrocytes
The IgM and IgG fractions of rabbit antiserum to sheep erythrocytes (E) can be obtained from Cordis Corporation, Miami, Florida. Alternatively, antibody fractions may be purified by chromatography of whole antiserum on DEAE-cellulose followed by a passage through G-200 Sephadex. Removal of trace IgG from the IgM fraction is described in Section III.A. Both antiserum fractions should be tested by hemagglutination against 0.25% E. The lowest nonagglutinating dilution is multiplied by 20 because the methods described below require 5% E suspension.

2. Partially Purified Complement Components
C1, C4, C2, and C3 components of human and guinea pig complement may be obtained from Cordis Laboratories, Miami, Florida. These should be stored at -70°C and reconstituted for use with 5 ml/vial of cold, sterile, double-distilled H_2O; volumes given in subsequent section refer to these preparations.

3. Mouse Complement
Since mouse complement is in general poorly lytic at the required concentrations, pooled sera from most inbred and outbred strains may be used. However, the optimal sources are inbred strains such as AKR/J and A/J, which are genetically deficient in C5. The blood is collected from ether-anesthetized mice either by heart puncture or by sectioning the axillary veins. The blood is kept for 15 min at room temperature, left on ice for 1 hr, and then centrifuged at 8700 g for 2 min in a Microfuge (Beckman Instruments). The serum may be used immediately or stored up to 60 days at -70°C. Freezing and thawing should be avoided.

4. C3b Inactivator for the Preparation of E (IgM) C3d
Human blood that has been allowed to clot at 37°C for 1 hr is spun at 1000 g for 15 min. The serum is heat-inactivated for 30 min at 56°C and EDTA added to the final concentration of 10 mM. The serum is then absorbed in the cold with 1/5 volume of packed E. Partially purified preparation of C3b inactivator can be obtained from Cordis Laboratories, Miami, Florida.

III.   METHODS

A. *Purification of IgM*

Trace amounts of IgG in E(IgM)C preparation described below, will lead to the binding and ingestion of the erythrocytes by human monocytes and mouse resident macrophages. We
find it essential to remove trace IgG from commercial and
laboratory preparations of IgM by absorption with protein A.
Pansorbin stock (0.6 ml of 10%) is washed 3 times with sterile
PBS by spinning at 8700 g for 2 min. Pansorbin is resuspended
in 0.2 ml PBS, 0.6 ml of IgM added, and the mixture resuspended in a vortex mixer. During the 20 min incubation at room
temperature, the tube is placed in the vortex 3 or 4 times.
The Pansorbin is spun in a Microfuge. Unused IgM should be
stored at -20°C.

B. *Preparation of Indicator Erythrocytes*

1. *E(IgG)*
One ml of 5% E in Hanks' is combined with an equal volume
of a dilution of IgG anti-E as determined by hemagglutination
and incubated for 15 min at 37°C. E(IgG) is washed 3 times
by centrifugation in Hanks' and resuspended to 10 ml with Dulbecco's. This constitutes the 0.5% E(IgG).
2. *E(IgM)*
Two ml of 5% E in Hanks' are added to an equal volume of a
dilution of IgM anti-E as determined by hemagglutination and
incubated for 15 min at 37°C. E(IgM) is washed once by centrifugation and resuspended to 2 ml in VBG. One ml is washed 3
times in Hanks' and resuspended to 10 ml with Dulbecco's.
This constitutes the 0.5% E(IgM). The remaining 1 ml of E(IgM)
is used for the preparation of E(IgM)C.
3. *E(IgM)C (Prepared with Mouse Complement)*
One ml of E(IgM) in VBG is added to 1 ml of mouse serum
diluted 1:5 in VBG and incubated 10 min at 37°C. Cold VBG is
immediately added. E(IgM)C is washed 3 times in the cold and
resuspended in 10 ml Dulbecco's. This is 0.5% E(IgM)C, containing predominantly C3b. Note: During the 10 min incubation,
some C3b will be converted to C3d. This can be prevented by
supplementing the serum dilution with 2 mg/ml Suramin.
4. *E(IgM)C3d*
Where the preparation of E(IgM)C3d is desired, the incubation period is extended to 30 min and no Suramin is added.
The resulting preparation should be further incubated in mouse
serum diluted 1:1 with saline containing 10 mM EDTA.

5. E(IgM)Cl4 (Prepared with Partially Purified Human and Guinea Pig Complement Components)

One ml of E(IgM) 5% in VBG is added to 1 ml of Cl. The mixture is incubated for 45 min in an ice bath followed by 5 min at 37°C. The cells are spun down in the cold and the supernatant discarded. Cold VBG (0.5 ml) is added followed by 1 ml of cold C4 and the mixture is incubated for 30 min at 0°C. The preparation is then washed 3 times in the cold and resuspended with Dulbecco's to the final volume of 10 ml (0.5%).

6. E(IgM)Cl423b

One ml of C2 is added to 1 ml of E(IgM)Cl4 (5%) followed by 1 ml of C3. The mixture is incubated for 45 min at 30°C, washed twice in the cold, and resuspended in 10 ml of Dulbecco's.

7. E(IgM)Cl423d

One ml of heat-inactivated (56°C, 30 min) human or guinea pig serum is preabsorbed with 1/5 packed volume of E for 10 min on ice. The serum is diluted 1:1 in saline and added to 1 ml of 5% E(IgM)Cl423b. The mixture is incubated at 37°C for 45 min, washed twice, and the cells resuspended in 10 ml of Dulbecco's. Partially purified C3b inactivator (Cordis Laboratories, Miami, Florida) can be used effectively in this step.

8. Chromium Labeling of Indicator Erythrocytes

Opsonized erythrocytes are spun down (300 g, 10 min) to a packed cell volume of 50 µl. The pellet is resuspended in 50 µl of Hanks' and 100 µCi of ^{51}Cr. The mixture is incubated for 40 min at 37°C with shaking. One ml of Dulbecco's is added at the end of the incubation and the mixture is layered carefully on top of 5 ml of Hypaque-Ficoll. Following centrifugation at 500 g for 15 min, the supernatant is discarded and the labeled erythrocytes washed once in Dulbecco's. The preparation is then incubated for 30 min on ice, washed 3 times and resuspended with 10 ml (0.5% final concentration) of Dulbecco's.

C. Assays

1. Monocyte and Macrophage Monolayers

The coverslips with cell monolayers are placed in culture plates and washed once with Dulbecco's. The medium is replaced with 0.5 ml of erythrocyte suspension (0.5%). After 1 hr incubation at 37°C, the coverslips are washed repeatedly with Dulbecco's and one set of duplicates fixed with 1.25% gluteraldehyde. Prior to fixation, the second set of duplicates is washed for 15 sec in Hanks' diluted 1:4 with water. This lyses all uningested erythrocytes. Following fixation, the coverslips should be washed with water and stored in cold water with 0.01% NaN_3 to prevent contamination. If the erythrocytes used in the assay were labeled with ^{51}Cr, the coverslips are placed directly in a gamma counter. For microscopic examination, the coverslips are placed cells down on a wet slide and viewed under phase contrast illumination. Giemsa staining of monolayers facilitates observation.

2. *Cell Suspensions*

Suspensions are adjusted to a concentration of 2×10^6/ml and 0.5 ml of the suspension is placed in a 5-ml plastic tube. The erythrocyte complex (0.5 ml of 0.5%) is added and the mixture spun at 40 g for 5 min. Pelleted cells are incubated for 15 min at 37°C without disturbing. After incubation, the pellet is gently disrupted by shaking and the cells examined under phase.

IV.   QUANTITATION OF RESULTS

A.   *Rosetting*

The degree of binding of opsonized erythrocytes to phagocytic cells is most conveniently expressed as a percentage of cells forming rosettes. A rosette is defined as a cell that has bound three or more target erythrocytes. A more useful number is expressed as the number of erythrocytes bound per 100 cells. Large numbers of assays can be performed by using ^{51}Cr label to estimate the number of erythrocytes bound per coverslip. This is then divided by the number of cells attached per coverslip obtained by visual examination and the resulting ratio multiplied by 100.

B.   *Ingestion*

The best method of expressing the degree of ingestion in a phagocytic event is to calculate the index of ingestion. This is defined as the number of erythrocytes ingested divided by the number of phagocytic cells counted times 100. To minimize the errors in counting the ingested erythrocytes, the bound uningested erythrocytes must be lysed by a hypotonic wash (Section III. C.1). For accurate results, 200 cells should be counted. When ^{51}Cr-labeled erythrocytes are used, the uningested erythrocytes are lysed and the index calculated as described for the binding assay (Section IV. A).

V. QUALITY OF THE REAGENTS

A. *Erythrocytes*

Mouse macrophages bind and ingest nonopsonized old erythrocytes. Thus, the sheep blood should be used 1-2 weeks after collection.

B. *Purity of IgM*

As mentioned previously, IgM preparations should be absolutely free of IgG. If no routine absorption with *S. aureus* is performed, the degree of IgG contamination should be assessed by passive hemagglutination of E(IgM) with a high-titer, heavy-chain specific antiserum to rabbit IgG.

C. *Complement*

If the complement is stored frozen, each batch should be pretested for activity prior to use in the above assays. Storage for more than two months or at a temperature higher than -70°C is not recommended.

VI. USE OF ^{51}Cr-LABELED ERYTHROCYTES

It is suggested that the binding and ingestion assays be standardized by visual quantitation prior to the use of the ^{51}Cr label. This method is very useful when a large number of assays is involved. When the number of erythrocytes to be counted is small, the accuracy of this method is markedly decreased. In addition, erythrocytes may bind nonspecifically to the coverslips. This may be overcome by pretreatment of the coverslips with serum and by the use of control coverslips containing no cells.

REFERENCES

1. M. Rabinovitch. Phagocytic recognition. *In* "Mononuclear Phagocytes" (R. van Furth, ed.), p. 299. Blackwell Scientific, Oxford, England, 1970.
2. S. C. Silverstein, R. S. Steinman, and Z. A. Cohn. Endocytosis. *Annu. Rev. Biochem.* *46:*699 1977.

3. C. Bianco. Plasma membrane receptors for complement. *In* "Biological Amplification Systems in Immunology" (N. K. Day and R. A. Good, eds.)m p. 69. Plenum Medical Book Company, New York, 1977

4. C. Bianco. Methods for the study of macrophage Fc and C3 receptors. *In* "*In Vitro* Methods for the study of Cell mediated and Tumor Immunity" (B. R. Bloom and J. R. David, eds.). Academic Press, New York, 1976.

5. C. Bianco and P. J. Edelson. Plasma membrane expression of macrophage differentiation. *In* "Molecular Basis of Cell-Cell Interaction" (R. H. Lerner, ed.), p. 119. Alan Liss, New York, 1978.

6. C. Bianco, F. M. Griffin, Jr., and S. C. Silverstein. Studies on the macrophage complement receptor. Alteration of receptor function upon macrophage activation. *J. Exp. Med.* *141:*1278, 1975.

7. M. P. Bevilacqua, D. Amrani, M. W. Mosesson, and C. Bianco. Receptors for cold-insoluble globulin (Plasma Fibronectin) on human monocytes. *J. Exp. Med.* *153:*42, 1981.

8. B. Mantovani, M. Rabinovitch, and V. Nussenzweig. Phagocytosis of immune complexes by macrophages. *J. Exp. Med.* *135:*780, 1972.

9. J. Michl, M. M. Pieczonka, J. C. Unkeless, and S. C. Silverstein. Effects of immobilized immune complexes on Fc- and complement-receptor function in resident and thioglycollate-elicited mouse peritoneal macrophages. *J. Exp. Med.* *150:*607, 1979.

10. J. C. Unkeless. The presence of two Fc receptors on mouse macrophages: Evidence from a variant cell line and differential trypsin sensitivity. *J. Exp. Med.* *146:*931, 1978.

11. B. D. Diamond, B. R. Bloom, and M. D. Scharff. A comparison of the Fc receptors of primary and cultured phagocytic lines examined with homogenous antibodies. *J. Immunol.* *121:*1329, 1978.

30

IDENTIFICATION OF MONONUCLEAR PHAGOCYTES BY INGESTION OF PARTICULATE MATERIALS, SUCH AS ERYTHROCYTES, CARBON, ZYMOSAN, OR LATEX

Steven M. Taffet
Stephen W. Russell

I. GENERAL INTRODUCTION

Mononuclear phagocytes and neutrophils are "professional" phagocytes. This colorful description was first applied by Rabinovitch (1) to distinguish these cell types from others that can ingest particles, but that are far less efficient at doing so. The description is useful to us here because it calls attention to two points: (i) there is another inflammatory cell type that is avidly phagocytic, namely, the neutrophil; and (ii) given the right conditions, still other cell types can engulf particulate material. Thus, phagocytosis is by no means a specific marker for mononuclear phagocytes. Rather, it must be considered as but one of several, or more, criteria that need to be applied to identify a cell positively as a mononuclear phagocyte. As long as this caveat is remembered, phagocytic capacity can be a useful, stable marker that is of help in identifying mature mononuclear phagocytes.

METHODS FOR STUDYING
MONONUCLEAR PHAGOCYTES

283

II. PREPARATION AND PROCESSING OF MACROPHAGE MONOLAYERS

A. *Introduction*

Mononuclear phagocytes are generally less avidly phagocytic when in suspension, especially if particles do not bind
strongly to their surfaces. In addition to increasing the efficiency with which uptake occurs, by forming a monolayer, one
enriches for mononuclear phagocytes and other adherent cells,
eliminates loss of adherent cells from suspensions during incubation steps, and facilitates the removal of uningested particles after incubation has been completed. Whenever possible,
we recommend use of monolayers in this assay rather than suspensions. Monolayers can be established on either glass
coverslips or the bottoms of plastic wells. Of the two, coverslips are easier to handle and, hence, the approach of choice.
If it is necessary to use plastic wells, the bottoms can be
punched out or excised with a heated scalpel after the adherent cells have been fixed and stained.

B. *Reagents*

(1) Medium: Modified Eagle's medium supplemented with
15 mM HEPES, 100 U/ml penicillin, 100 µg/ml streptomycin, and
10% fetal bovine serum (FBS). The FBS should be free of detectable endotoxin (Sterile Systems, Logan, Utah).
(2) Tissue culture plate containing twenty-four 16 mm-
diameter wells (e.g., Costar, Catalog No. 3524, Cambridge,
Massachusetts).
(3) Coverslips (Bellco, Vineland, New Jersey), 12 mm-
diameter. These are washed by boiling repeatedly in distilled
water and sterilized by autoclaving. Sticking of the coverslips together during autoclaving can be prevented by layering
them on gauze in a Petri dish.
(4) Diff-Quik stain set (Harleco, Gibbstown, New Jersey)
(5) A small, curved, fine-tipped forceps
(6) Glass microscope slides
(7) Mounting medium (e.g., Permount, Fisher Scientific,
Fair Lawn, New Jersey)

C. *Procedure*

(1) Place one coverslip in each assay well.
(2) After performing a differential count, seed the cells,
based on how many mononuclear phagocytes are present in the
suspension. While the number needed will vary depending on the

source of the cells and how they have been treated, 10^5 mononuclear phagocytes per well is appropriate for many preparations. The object is to plate fewer adherent cells than the
number that will yield a confluent monolayer. As confluency
is approached, it becomes more difficult to distinguish clearly
between what is inside and what is adherent to the outside of
individual cells.

(3) After allowing the cells to settle and adhere for
0.5 - 2 hr (the time needed varies with the population), nonadherent cells are washed away. Repeated, gentle jetting of
medium from a Pasteur pipette usually will suffice. Care must
be taken at this step not to wash away significant numbers of
mononuclear phagocytes, should they be lightly adherent. Two
coverslips, one for exposure to the particulate material and
one to be carried in parallel for differential analysis, should
be processed for each sample.

(4) When the phagocytosis assay has been completed, the
monolayers are washed to remove free particulate material.
Generally at this point it is well to continue the incubation
for 30 - 60 min, so that uningested material that is adherent
to the surfaces of cells can be engulfed. This step is unnecessary when erythrocytes are used, because they can be removed by
hypotonic lysis.

(5) The coverslip is removed from the well with the fine-
tipped forceps, fixed and stained, according to the instructions provided with the Diff-Quik stain set.

(6) After the two stained coverslips for each sample have
been air dried, they are mounted, using a medium such as Permount (or, in the case of plastic, immersion oil), so that the
cells can be examined microscopically. The coverslip that was
exposed to the particulate material is used to enumerate phagocytic cells, while the coverslip that was carried in parallel
through the washings and incubations but never exposed to particles is used to determine the percentage of neutrophils in
the monolayer. From these data, the number of phagocytic cells
that are mononuclear phagocytes can be estimated (see below).

(7) The person who is counting cells in monolayers will
find the job easier and the data more reproducible if a gridded
ocular is used in the microscope. This will be especially true
if many cells are present in each field, or counting is done at
a relatively low power. Counting at a higher power has the
added advantage of facilitating differentiation between particles that are inside or outside of cells.

D. *Critical Comments*

Two major pitfalls associated with forming monolayers center
around cell loss caused by excessively vigorous washings and

overcrowding. How each of these problems is to be avoided will vary with the population of cells being used. These considerations must, therefore, be addressed and worked out empirically in pilot experiments before a phagocytic assay is undertaken. If serum is excluded from the medium during the adherence step, nonspecific adherence of lymphocytes will dramatically increase.

III. Fc-MEDIATED PHAGOCYTOSIS OF SHEEP ERYTHROCYTES

A. *Introduction*

The professional phagocytes bear Fc receptors and are capable, therefore, of efficiently phagocytosing antibody-coated particles. Use of this approach, especially with large particles (usually erythrocytes), virtually excludes uptake by cell types that lack the Fc receptor.

B. *Reagents*

Tissue culture medium, e.g., modified Eagle's medium supplemented with 15 mM HEPES and heat-inactivated fetal bovine serum (final concentration, 10%).

Sheep erythrocytes (sRBC) (available from many supply houses). These should be as fresh as possible (<2 weeks) to reduce nonspecific uptake. Wash them several times in medium and resuspend the packed sRBC in medium (5%, v/v).

Rabbit antibody (IgG fraction) against sRBC is obtainable from Cordis Laboratories (Miami, Florida). The antibody should be diluted to the extent that it just fails to agglutinate the sRBC.

C. *Procedure*

(1) Macrophage monolayers are prepared as above. Each well should contain 0.5 ml of medium.

(2) Antibody-coated sRBC (EA) are prepared by incubating 1 ml of sRBC suspension with 1 ml of appropriately diluted antibody (30 min, 37°C). EA are washed 3 times and resuspended in 5 ml of medium.

(3) 0.05 ml of the EA suspension is added to each well, after which monolayers are incubated for 1 hr (37°C).

(4) The monolayers are then washed gently 3 times to remove unattached EA.

(5) Coverslips are removed from the wells using fine

pointed, small curved forceps and dipped in distilled water to lyse attached EA that have not been ingested.

(6) Monolayers can be fixed and stained for examination, as described in Section II, or examined by phase microscopy as a wet mount. The percentage of cells that contain erythrocytes is determined. In technically good preparations, the number of EA that each cell has engulfed can be counted.

D. Critical Comments

While the assay for Fc-mediated phagocytosis is relatively simple to perform, there are pitfalls. Chief among these is reduced uptake due either to insufficient antibody or to the wrong antibody used to sensitize the indicator erythrocyte. With regard to antibody density, it is essential to be at a level that is just below that which will cause agglutination. Certain bovine erythrocytes can be loaded with extraordinary amounts of IgG without agglutinating (2) and may, therefore be better indicator cells than sRBC. Preparation of such an indicator cell would include finding an animal whose RBC have poor agglutinating properties and preparing a rabbit antiserum against that animal's erythrocytes. Antibody type is also critical. For example, rabbit IgM will not bind to the Fc receptors of mouse mononuclear phagocytes (3).

A final comment regards the use of Fc receptor-mediated phagocytosis as a means of identifying mononuclear phagocytes. Not all mononuclear phagocytes are avidly phagocytic within the duration of the assay described here. This fact serves to reemphasize the need to use more than a single identifying criterion.

IV. CARBON PARTICLES (CHINA INK)

A. Introduction

China ink, a suspension of carbon particles, is a useful marker for phagocytic cells (4). Phagocytes are seen, when the technique works properly, as black due to their content of carbon compared to nonphagocytic cells that stain normally. The major advantage of this technique is the ease and rapidity with which it can be performed.

B. Reagents

(1) Tissue culture medium (Section II.B.(1)
(2) China Ink - Pellikan 50 special black (Gunther Wagner, Germany).
This product is available at most art supply stores. The china ink is dialyzed against two changes of phosphate-buffered saline.

C. Procedure

(1) Monolayers are prepared as in Section II.
(2) To each well containing 0.5 ml of medium, add 0.1 ml of the dialyzed ink. Incubate monolayers with the carbon particles for 30 min at 37°C.
(3) Wash the monolayers 4 times to remove unabsorbed carbon particles. Incubate the washed cells for an additional 30 - 60 min in fresh medium at 37°C to allow engulfment of particles that are still attached to cell surfaces.
(4) Remove the coverslips and prepare them for examination, as described in Section II.

D. Critical Comments

The principal problem with carbon particles centers on their tendency to obscure the cells with which they are associated. Neutrophils engulf this material and, when engorged with it, can be indistinguishable from mononuclear phagocytes that are similarly filled. If neutrophils contaminate the monolayer, it is essential that the result with carbon be interpreted as indicative of the total number of phagocytic cells in the monolayer. This figure can be corrected, if the percentage of neutrophils is obtained by differential analysis of a second, parallel monolayer that has not been exposed to carbon. The identity of a cell can also be obscured if carbon particles are adherent to its surface. Thus, it may not be possible to distinguish between a phagocyte and a nonphagocytic cell type if particles remain on cell surfaces.

V. ZYMOSAN

A. *Introduction*

Zymosan particles are yeast cell walls. They are large, easily seen, and are rapidly taken up by phagocytic cells. As with carbon, uptake of zymosan offers a rapid, relatively simple assay of phagocytic activity.

B. *Reagents*

(1) Tissue culture medium (see above)
(2) Zymosan (ICN Pharmaceuticals, Cleveland, Ohio). This reagent is prepared by suspending the particles in phosphate-buffered saline (PBS) at a concentration of 20 mg/ml. The covered container is then placed in a boiling water bath for 1 hr, with shaking every 5-10 min. Particles are centrifuged out of suspension and washed 5 times by centrifugation through PBS. The washed zymosan is resuspended in PBS (50 mg/ml), stored in aliquots, and frozen ($-20°C$).

C. *Procedure*

(1) The amount of zymosan to be used in each well should be empirically determined. The amount should be the least that will allow uptake of the particles by all cells that will do so, but not so much that later differentiation of the cells becomes a problem due to residual zymosan. We routinely use 10 - 50 µl of the stock solution per well.
(2) Incubate monolayers with the zymosan for 30 min at 37°C. Wash to remove nonadherent particles.
(3) Continue the incubation in fresh medium for 30 - 60 min to allow for particles that are adherent to cell surfaces to be ingested.
(4) Process the monolayers for microscopic examination, as described above.
(5) The zymosan associated with monolayers will not stain by the Diff-Quik procedure. The particles within stained cells will appear transparent to opalescent blue, giving the appearance of a vacuole in many instances.

D. *Critical Comments*

The principal problem is that cells in the monolayer may be obscured by uningested particles. To avoid this difficulty, the addition of excess zymosan must be avoided, and time must be allowed after washing for particles to be ingested that are still adherent to cell surfaces. The nuclei of phagocytic cells may be pressed eccentrically against their plasma membranes after ingestion has occurred, making it difficult to distinguish neutrophils from mononuclear phagocytes. It is important, therefore, to examine a second, untreated monolayer carried in parallel with the treated monolayer to determine the degree of neutrophilic contamination (5).

VI. LATEX PARTICLES

A. Introduction

Latex or polystyrene particles have become a popular probe for phagocytosis, principally because of the ease with which they can be used.

B. Reagents

(1) Tissue culture medium (see above)
(2) Latex particles, 1.1 μm in diameter (Dow Chemical Company, Indianapolis, Indiana).

C. Procedure

(1) Macrophage monolayers are prepared as above.
(2) Wash the latex particles 3 times by centrifugation (1200 g, 30 min). Resuspend them (5×10^8 particles/ml) in medium.
(3) 0.1 ml of the suspension of latex particles is added to each well.
(4) After 1 hr at 37°C, the monolayers are washed and the medium is changed.
(5) Continue the incubation in fresh medium (30 - 60 min) to allow time for ingestion of residual particles.
(6) Prepare the monolayers for microscopic examination, as described above. The latex particles will appear as vacuoles or refractile bodies in the stained cells. Latex preparations can also be examined as wet mounts, using phase microscopy.

D. *Critical Comments*

Latex particles can be ingested by nonprofessional phagocytes because of their small size. For example, latex has
been used extensively to investigate endocytosis by L cells
(6). Thus, the difference between the professional and nonprofessional phagocyte is the extent of uptake, rather than
the presence or absence of this property. Care must be taken,
therefore, when examining monolayers with this technique to
ensure that mononuclear cells containing but a few particles
are really mononuclear phagocytes.

VII. CALCULATION OF DATA

If neutrophil contamination is not a problem, the percentage of mononuclear phagocytes can be estimated as

$$\frac{\text{number of cells containing particles}}{\text{total cells counted}} \times 100 \ .$$

As stated above, however, a major problem in some preparations will be contamination of the monolayer with a significant
number of neutrophils. These must be differentiated from mononuclear phagocytes, and this is often difficult to do with certainty if only cells engorged with particles are examined. If
neutrophil contamination is found to be a problem, a reasonably
accurate estimation of the percentage of total phagocytic cells
that is mononuclear phagocytes can be obtained.

(1) Examine a coverslip that has been carried through the
washing and incubation steps, but that has not been exposed to
particles. From this coverslip, determine the percentage of
neutrophils in the monolayer.

(2) Next, examine the coverslip that has been exposed to
particles. Determine the total percentage of phagocytic cells.
Also, determine the percentage of neutrophils (PMN) that failed
to ingest particles (the larger the particle, the higher this
value will be).

(3) Estimate the percentage of mononuclear phagocytes:

$$\begin{array}{l}\text{\% mononuclear} \\ \text{phagocytes}\end{array} = \begin{array}{l}\text{\% total} \\ \text{phagocytes}\end{array} - \left(\begin{array}{l}\text{total} \\ \text{\% PMN}\end{array} - \begin{array}{l}\text{\% PMN empty} \\ \text{of particles}\end{array}\right),$$

where the total percentage of PMN was obtained from the
particle-free coverslip.

VIII. CONCLUDING REMARKS

We would like to reemphasize the major technical and interpretive pitfalls of phagocytic assays: (1) monolayers may be overcrowded, causing difficulty in distinguishing between particles that are inside or outside of cells; (2) particles may remain adherent to the surfaces of cells, obscuring the interiors of the cells and thereby limiting one's ability to identify them and to determine whether or not they have ingested particles; (3) cells other than mononuclear phagocytes are capable of engulfing particulate material and must be distinguished from mononuclear phagocytes; and (4) not all mononuclear phagocytes in a population may ingest the indicator particle, especially if a high percentage of the mononuclear phagocytes is relatively immature. The last two points again bring us to the most important point that can be made regarding phagocytic assays: The criterion of phagocytosis cannot be regarded as a specific assay for mononuclear phagocytes, but is an excellent tool if used in conjunction with other, confirmatory assays.

Acknowledgment

Supported in part by United States Public Health Service research grant CA 31199 and training grant CA 09057. S.W.R. is the recipient of Research Career Development Award CA 00497.

REFERENCES

1. M. Rabinovitch. Phagocytosis, the engulfment stage. *Sem. Hematol.* *5*: 134-155, 1968.
2. G. Uhlenbruck, G. V. F. Seaman, and R. R. A. Coombs. Factors influencing the agglutinability of red cells. III. Physicochemical studies on ox red cells of different classes of agglutinability. *Vox Sanguinis.* *12*: 420-428, 1967.
3. W. H. Lay and V. Nussenzweig. Ca^{2+}-dependent binding of antigen-19S antibody complexes to macrophages. *J. Immunol.* *102*: 1172-1178, 1969.
4. F. DeHalleux, H. S. Taper, and C. Deckers. A simple procedure for identification of macrophages in peritoneal exudeates. *Br. J. Exp. Pathol.* *54*: 352-358, 1973.
5. S. W. Russell, W. F. Doe, R. G. Hoskins, and C. G. Cochrane. Inflammatory cells in solid murine neoplasms. I. Tumor disaggregation and identification of constituent inflammatory

cells. *Int. J. Cancer 18*: 322-330, 1976.

6.   M. Rabinovitch. Phagocytosis of modified erythrocytes by macrophages and L2 cells. *Exp. Cell. Res. 56*: 326-332, 1969.

31

HETEROANTISERA RAISED AGAINST MONONUCLEAR PHAGOCYTES

Alan M. Kaplan
T. Mohanakumar

I. INTRODUCTION

The use of highly specific alloantisera has provided a powerful tool to dissect both the differentiation pathways and heterogeneity of thymus and bone marrow-derived lymphocytes. Antisera of appropriate macrophage specificity would be of value in specific *in vivo* depletion of macrophages, in analyzing the relationship of various macrophage functions to cellular heterogeneity, and in determining the membrane events and biochemical requirements for macrophage differentiation and activation. Unfortunately, the production of alloantisera to macrophage differentiation antigens has been generally unsuccessful with only a single mouse alloantigen, Mph-1, having been described by Archer and Davies (1). More recently, Springer *et al*. (2) have described a purported macrophage differentiation antigen (Mac-1) identified by a monoclonal rat-mouse hybridoma. However the antigen was also present on neutrophils and 44% of bone marrow cells, suggesting a broad specificity range. Other

monoclonal antibodies against mononuclear phagocytes are being
developed in other laboratories (2a).

While, unquestionably, the future development of specific
antimacrophage antibodies rests within hybridoma technology,
several xenoantisera have been described that identify both
serologically and biochemically macrophage-specific antigens.
Stinnertt *et al.* (3, 4) described a mouse macrophage antigen,
detected by an extensively absorbed rabbit antimouse macrophage
serum. This antigen (MSMA) was shown to have a molecular weight
of 83,000 in ^{125}I-radiolabeled mouse peritoneal macrophage membrane extracts and was present on normal, elicited, and "activated" peritoneal macrophages, a mouse macrophage cell line
(P388D$_1$), and exhibited some cross-reactivity with peritoneal
macrophages from closely related species (rats and hamsters).
More recently, Kaplan *et al.* (5, 6) have described a cell surface antigen (AMØCSA) associated with "activated" macrophages
that could be induced *in vivo* on murine peritoneal macrophages
by pyran copolymer or *Corynebacterium parvum* but not by glycogen or thioglycollate. The induction of AMØCSA by a series of
C. parvum vaccines correlated with the ability of the vaccines
to induce (1) regression of a methylcholanthrene fibrosarcoma
when inoculated intralesionally; (2) splenomegaly; and (3) peritoneal macrophages cytotoxic to tumor cells *in vitro*, suggesting
a relationship between AMØCSA induction and the functional activation of macrophages. These observations suggest that xenoantisera directed against specific macrophage membrane antigens
may be useful in elucidating structure - function relationships
with regard to a number of macrophage activities. While it is
generally easy to prepare xenoantisera with antimacrophage activity, extensive absorptions are required to render such sera
macrophage specific and it is difficult to produce large quantities of absorbed material.

II. MATERIALS

A. *Antiserum Production*

   Adult rabbits 3 - 4 kg weight
   Mice
   Mouse peritoneal macrophages or appropriate cell lines with
macrophage characteristics
   Hanks' balanced salt solution (HBSS) and RPMI-1640 media
   Syringes, 5 and 10 ml, and needles, 20- and 25-gauge
   Centrifuge tubes
   Petri dishes, 100 × 15 mm (Falcon)
   Ammonium sulfate or sodium sulfate

Glycogen (type II from oyster, Sigma G-8751, Sigma
Chemical Co., St. Louis, Missouri)

Thioglycollate (Brewer's thioglycollate, Difco Laboratories,
Detroit, Michigan)

Fetal calf serum

Pyran copolymer (lot XA124-177, Hercules, Inc., Wilmington,
Delaware)

Corynebacterium parvum (Burroughs-Wellcome, Research
Triangle, North Carolina)

B. *Antiserum Assay*

Terasaki plates (microtest plate, Falcon No. 3034, Falcon
Plastics, Bio Quest, Oxnard, California)

Rabbit complement (Low Tox-H, pretested, No. ACL3331,
Accurate Chemical and Scientific Corp., Hicksville, New York)
(Note: Absorption of even the Low Tox complement with pooled
spleen cells and agarose is frequently helpful in reducing the
background.)

Trypan Blue

Barbital buffer with 2% EDTA, pH 7.0 - 7.4 (Barbitone
C.F.T. Diluent, K-C Biologicals, Lenexa, Kansas)

Paraffin Oil (S894, J. T. Baker Chemical Co., Phillipsburg,
New Jersey)

Lidocaine hydrochloride (Xylocaine, Astra Pharmaceutical
Co., Worcester, Massachusetts)

Sodium azide

Seakem Agarose (Pacific Biomarine, Venice, California)

Fluorescein isothiocyanate-conjugated goat antirabbit IgG
$[F(ab)_2$ fragments$]$

Fluorescent microscope

Pooled cells for absorption (mouse erythrocytes, thymus
cells, and P388 leukemia cells)

III. PROCEDURES

A. *Preparation of Cells for Inoculation*

Peritoneal exudate cells (PEC) are obtained from mice 4 - 5
days after ip inoculation of glycogen (0.5 ml/mouse of a 2.5%
solution) or thioglycollate (1 ml/mouse of a 10% solution) and
7 days after ip inoculation of pyran copolymer (25 mg/kg in
0.2 ml) or *C. parvum* (17.5 mg/kg in 0.2 ml) by washing the
peritoneal cavity twice with 4 ml of RPMI-1640 or HBSS. (We
do not routinely use heparin in the wash fluid but 10 U of

preservative free heparin frequently reduces clotting.) The
PEC are pooled in 50 cc plastic centrifuge tubes and collected
by centrifugation at 200 g for 10 min, washed twice with HBSS,
and resuspended in RPMI-1640 with 20% FCS. Recent reports (7)
and our own experience suggest that lower concentrations of
FCS (1%) may be more effective for the initial adherence step.
To obtain peritoneal macrophages (PEM), 4×10^7 PEC are incubated in plastic petri plates (100 × 15 mm) for 2 hr at 37°C in
5% CO_2. Nonadherent cells are washed off exhaustively with
RPMI-1640 and adherent PEM removed from the plates by gently
scraping with a rubber policeman. The cells are centrifuged
at 500 g for 10 min, washed twice with HBSS, and resuspended
in HBSS for inoculation. Generally, greater than 95% of the
adherent cells phagocytosize latex particles and are esterase
positive (8). Alternatively the peritoneal macrophages may be
cultured *in vitro* for varying lengths of time to allow differentiation to occur and to allow weakly adherent cells to become dislodged. The macrophage cell line, $P388D_1$, is maintained
in spinner flasks in either Eagle's minimum essential medium or
RPMI-1640 supplemented with 20% FCS, 2 mM glutamine, and containing 100 U of penicillin and 100 μg streptomycin at 37°C in
5% CO_2. The cells are centrifuged at 200 g and washed three
times with HBSS before use for inoculation.

B. *Preparation of Antiserum*

Xenogeneic rabbit antimacrophage serum is prepared by inoculating rabbits iv into an ear vein with varying concentrations (usually between 2×10^7 and 10^8 cells in 1 ml) of PEM
or $P388D_1$ cells at varying intervals over a one-year period.
In some immunizations the primary inoculation is given multi-
site subcutaneously in an equal volume of complete Freund's
adjuvant. Rabbits are bled from the ear artery for 30 to 50 ml
of blood 7 to 10 days after inoculation of cells, generally
starting after the second inoculation. Antisera are tested for
their cytotoxic activity against PEM or $P388D_1$ targets and those
sera with high cytotoxic titers subjected to absorption and
further analysis as outlined below. In general, there is a
great deal of variation among rabbits both with respect to the
final cytotoxic titer of an antiserum and the kinetics of the
development of antibody.
The blood is allowed to clot at room temperature for one
hour and kept at 4°C overnight. After centrifugation, the immune serum is collected and heat inactivated at 56°C for 30 to
45 min. γ-Globulin is precipitated from the serum with either
14% Na_2SO_4 or 33% $(NH_4)_2SO_4$. Crystalline Na_2SO_4 (14 gm/100 ml)
is added slowly (over 20 min) to the serum at room temperature
with gentle stirring with a magnetic stirring bar. When the

Na_2SO_4 is dissolved, the precipitated γ-globulin is recovered by centrifugation at 5000 g for 30 min at room temperature and the precipitate dissolved in a volume of deionized H_2O equal to approximately 20% of the initial volume. The precipitation is repeated with 14% Na_2SO_4 (w/v) and the final precipitate dialyzed for 24 to 48 hr at 4°C against a minimum of four changes of 0.15 M, pH 7.2 phosphate buffered saline. The procedure with $(NH_4)_2SO_4$ is carried out in a similar fashion except that a saturated solution of $(NH_4)_2SO_4$ is added to the serum to achieve a final concentration of 33% (v/v).

C. Absorptions

Unabsorbed antisera generally have binding and cytotoxic activity against PEC, thymocytes, spleen cell suspensions, bone marrow cells, and most mouse cells tested. Regardless of which cell population is used for immunization, (PEM or $P388D_1$), absorption of cytotoxic antibody directed to either thymus cells or nonadherent peritoneal exudate cells appears to be most effectively removed with thymocytes. After a series of absorptions, the sera are tested for cytotoxic antibody against the $P388D_1$, thymus cells, and PEC. All screening of the serum for cytotoxic activity during the absorption process is done by the Amos two-stage technique to conserve serum (9). The absorptions are carried out until the sera are negative by cytotoxicity for thymus cells, nonadherent PEC, and/or spleen cells.

Absorptions are carried out by incubating approximately 1/3 ml of packed, washed mouse erythrocytes with 1 ml of dialyzed γ-globulin for 30 to 45 min at 4°C. The absorbing cells are removed by centrifugation at 300 g for 10 min at 4°C. Erythrocyte absorption is generally carried out until all hemagglutinating activity is removed. (Note: the buffy coat should be carefully removed from the packed erythrocytes before being used for absorption.) After completion of erythrocyte absorption, the serum is absorbed with packed, washed thymus cells using the same procedure as described for erythrocytes. In preparation of the thymus cells, care must be taken not to include parathymic lymph nodes. In our hands, rabbit antimouse macrophage sera prepared against any of the cells outlined above have required between 20 and 40 absorptions with thymus cells before they are macrophage specific. This has also been true of sera from rabbits immunized with the $P388D_1$ macrophage cell line where there are no contaminating lymphocytes.

To make an antiserum to the macrophage-specific activation antigen, rabbits should be inoculated with either $P388D_1$ cells or pyran or C. parvum-activated PEM. Absorption to achieve a macrophage-specific antiserum is carried out as described above. Generally, two absorptions with 10^8 normal PEC are suf-

ficient to remove the antimacrophage activity from 1 ml of
macrophage-specific γ-globulin, however this will vary with the
titer of the antiserum. These absorptions are carried out at
4°C for 30 to 45 min as described above. (Note: care should
be taken to ensure that the source of normal PEC is from non-
infected mice so that their PEM are not already activated.)

D. *Assay of Antimacrophage and Antiactivated Macrophage*
    Antiserum

     Target cells for analysis by either cytotoxicity or immuno-
fluorescence are prepared as described above except that the
washed cells are resuspended in HBSS with 5% FCS previously ab-
sorved with mouse spleen cells (AFCS). Target cells have included thymus cells, nonadherent spleen cells, nonadherent PEC,
total PEC, adherent PEC, and various macrophagelike cell lines.
While it is usually sufficient to scrape off gently adherent
macrophages for inoculation into rabbits, this procedure provides cells of poor viability that are not optimal for use in
cytotoxicity assays. Therefore, when purified PEM are required
for analysis, they are removed from plates after adherence purification by treatment with 12 mM lidocaine (10). Medium is aspirated from the adherent macrophage culture and replaced with
a sufficient volume of RPMI-1640 with 10% FCS and 12 mM lidocaine to cover the plate. The plates are allowed to incubate
at room temperature for 5 to 10 min after which the cells are
dislodged by several jets of medium from a syringe. The cells
are washed twice and resuspended in HBSS with 5% AFCS. Viability is determined by trypan blue dye exclusion and is generally
greater than 90%. When unseparated PEC rather than adherence-
purified PEM are used for immunofluorescence or cytotoxic assays, the plateau level of percentage positive fluorescent cells
or percentage cytotoxicity reflects the content of macrophages
in the PEC and may vary from 40 to 80%, depending on whether or
not the PEC are from normal mice or from mice induced with
agents like thioglycollate, pyran, etc.
     Cytotoxicity testing is performed by a standard Amos two-
stage technique in order to conserve reagents (9). Briefly,
1 µl of target cells (10^6/ml) is added to 1 µl of antiserum in
microtest plates and incubated at room temperature for 30 min.
The wells were washed with medium and 5 µl of appropriately absorbed (see below) rabbit complement are added. Incubation is
continued for an additional 60 min, then 0.3% trypan blue in
1% EDTA-barbital buffer is added to stop the reaction. After
10 min, the trays are flicked and wells filled with barbital
buffer (pH 7.4). Percent cytotoxicity is determined under an
inverted phase contrast microscope.
     Alternatively, cytotoxicity is measured in 10 × 75 mm tubes

using 0.1 ml of target cells at 10^7 cells/ml, and varying dilutions of 0.1 ml of antiserum. Incubation is carried out at room temperature for 30 min after which the cells are centrifuged at 500 g for 10 min, washed once with HBSS, and resuspended in a final volume of 0.3 ml prescreened, low-toxicity rabbit complement absorbed with mouse spleen and/or thymus cells and 80 mg agarose per ml of complement (11). (Note: agarose-absorbed complement cannot be refrozen without loss of activity.) The cells are then incubated at 37°C for 45 min and percent cytotoxicity determined with trypan blue at a final concentration of 0.2%.

Indirect immunofluorescence is performed using fluorescein isothiocyanate-conjugated antirabbit IgG F(ab)$_2$ fragments absorbed with P388D$_1$ cells or mouse spleen cells. The assay is carried out at 4°C in HBSS with 5% AFCS and 0.1% sodium azide.

IV. CALCULATION AND INTERPRETATION OF DATA

The production of antimacrophage sera by this technique is laborious, expensive, and time-consuming; however, if adequate absorptions are carried out, a useful, specific reagent can be derived. The minimum number of absorptions with thymus cells that we have found sufficient to render a xenogeneic rabbit antimouse macrophage serum specific for macrophages is 20 and frequently over 40 absorptions are required. Sera produced by this procedure frequently have 50% cytotoxic titers in the range of 1 : 80 to 1 : 320. The specificity of antimacrophage sera have been verified both serologically and biochemically with NP-40 extracts of ^{125}I-labeled macrophage membranes in an SDS-polyacrylamide gel electrophoresis system (3). The specificity of antiactivated macrophage membrane antigen antiserum has been verified serologically and indirectly by correlation with the functional properties of macrophages. Numerous attempts to precipitate membrane antigens specific to activated macrophages from cells labeled with ^{125}I or cells cultured with labeled amino acids have been unsuccessful. Problems frequently arise in the cytotoxicity and indirect immunofluorescence assays when reagents are not adequately absorbed or when target cell viability is less than 90%. Also, sera should be stored in small aliquots and not thawed and refrozen unless absolutely necessary. Absorptions work more effectively when carried out in small volumes (less than 1 ml).

V. CRITICAL COMMENTS

It is not unrealistic to expect to be able to obtain limited quantities of macrophage specific antiserum by these methods. Using these techniques, we have recently produced two rabbit antihuman macrophage antisera that can differentiate between human monocytes and splenic and/or peritoneal macrophages (11a,b). The antisera must be assessed rigorously and quantitative absorptions are valuable in differentiating between varying antigen density on cell types as opposed to the absence of an antigen.

Several alternative approaches for producing specific antimacrophage serum are currently under investigation. The use of rats to produce antimouse macrophage serum may provide sera with greater specificity and requiring less absorption due to the phylogenetic relationship of mice and rats. Preliminary attempts by Archer and Davies (1) at producing macrophage-specific alloantisera were promising and, based on analogy to lymphocyte alloantigens, this would seem to be a potentially productive avenue, particularly with the use of macrophagelike cell lines as immunogens. Lastly, the use of rat lymphocyte-mouse myeloma hybrids would appear to provide the most promising method for producing monoclonal-specific antiserum to the antigens associated with various subclasses and/or maturation states of the monocyte macrophage series. This approach has recently been used by Unkeless (12) to produce a monoclonal antibody to the trypsin-resistant macrophage Fc receptor that is specific for immune aggregates of mouse IgG_1 and IgG_{2b}.

Acknowledgment

Supported in part by grants Nos. 1M-183 and 1M-190 from the American Cancer Society and NIH grant CA 28308.

REFERENCES

1. J. R. Archer and D. A. L. Davies. Demonstration of an alloantigen on the peritoneal exudate cells of inbred strains of mice and its association with chromosome 7 (Linkage group 1). *J. Immunogenetics 1*: 113-123, 1974.
2. T. Springer, G. Galfré, D. S. Secher, and C. Milstein. Mac-1:A macrophage differentiation antigen identified by monoclonal antibody. *Eur. J. Immunol. 9*: 301-306, 1979.
2a. O. Forster (Ed.). "Heterogeneity of Mononuclear Phago-

cytes." Academic Press, New York, 1980.

3. J. W. Stinnett, A. M. Kaplan, and P. S. Morahan. Identification of a macrophage-specific cell surface antigen. *J. Immunol.* *116*: 273-278, 1976.

4. J. W. Stinnett, P. S. Morahan, and A. M. Kaplan. A macrophage cell surface antigen. *In* "The Reticuloendothelial System in Health and Disease: Functions and Characteristics" (S. M. Richard, M. R. Escobar, and H. Friedman, eds.), pp. 69-68. Plenum, New York, 1976.

5. A. M. Kaplan and T. Mohanakumar. Expression of a new cell surface antigen on activated murine macrophages. *J. Exp. Med.* *146*: 1461-1466, 1977.

6. A. M. Kaplan, H. D. Bear, L. Kirk, C. Cummins, and T. Mohanakumar. Relationship of expression of a cell-surface antigen on activated murine macrophages to tumor cell cytotoxicity. *J. Immunol.* *120*: 2080-2085, 1978.

7. R. A. Musson and P. M. Henson. Humoral and formed elements of blood modulate the response of peripheral blood monocytes. I. Plasma and serum inhibit and platelets enhance monocyte adherence. *J. Immunol.* *122*: 2026-2031, 1979.

8. C. Y. Li, K. W. Lam, and L. T. Yam. Esterases in human leukocytes. *J. Histochem. Cytochem.* *21*: 1-12, 1973.

9. B. D. Amos, H. Bosher, W. Boyle, M. Macqueen, and A. Tiilikamen. A simple microcytotoxicity test. *Transplantation 1*: 220-223, 1969.

10. M. Rabinovitch and M. J. DeStefano. The use of the local anesthetic lidocaine for cell harvesting and subcultivation. *In Vitro 11*: 379-381, 1975.

11. A. Cohen and M. Schleisinger. Absorption of guinea pig serum with agar. A method for elimination of its cytotoxicity for murine thymus cells. *Transplantation 10*: 130-132, 1970.

11a. J. C. Waldrep, A. M. Kaplan, and T. Mohanakumar. Human mononuclear phagocyte-associated antigens. I. Identification and characterization. *Cell. Immunol.* *50*: 399.

11b. J. C. Waldrep, T. Mohanakumar, and A. M. Kaplan. Human mononuclear phagocyte-associated antigens. II. Lymphokine inducible antigens on the macrophage cell line, U937. *Cell. Immunol.* In Press.

12. J. Unkeless. Characterization of a monoclonal antibody directed against mouse and lymphocyte Fe receptors. *J. Exp. Med.* *150*: 580-596, 1979.

32

MONOCLONAL ANTIBODIES AS TOOLS FOR THE
STUDY OF MONONUCLEAR PHAGOCYTES

Timothy A. Springer

The myeloma X immune spleen cell hybrid technique of Köhler and Milstein (1, reviewed in 2) has given great impetus to the analysis of complex biological systems. For example, macrophages of one species such as the mouse may be injected into another species such as the rat. The resultant multispecific response to a large array of different macrophage surface molecules may then be resolved by cloning into a set of hybrid lines, each secreting a monoclonal antibody (MAb) recognizing a single antigenic determinant on a single cell surface molecule. Recently, a substantial number of antimacrophage MAb have been obtained that are already proving to be invaluable reagents of extraordinary specificity for the study of macrophage differentiation, function, and surface antigen structure.

The properties of monoclonal antibodies defining murine and human macrophage differentiation antigens are summarized in Tables I and II, respectively. Most antibodies have been characterized for expression on different leukocytes and cell lines, but not on nonhematopoietic tissues or on mononuclear phagocytes other than macrophages. None of these monoclonals binds to lym-

METHODS FOR STUDYING
MONONUCLEAR PHAGOCYTES

305

TABLE I. Rat Monoclonal Antibodies Defining Murine Monocytic Differentiation Antigens

Monoclonal antibody	Antigen designation	Antibody Chains	Antibody Subclass	Lysis	Antigen Polypeptide chains
M1/70	Mac-1	HL^a	IgG_{2b}	weak	105,000 190,000
1.21J	Mac-1	NR^b	NR^b	NR^b	{ 94,000 180,000
M3/38 M3/31	Mac-2	HLK,HL^a HLK^a	IgG_{2a} IgM	NR^b	32,000
M3/84	Mac-3	HL^a	IgG_1	NR^b	110,000
54-2	Mac-4	NR^b	IgG_{2a}	NR^b	NR^d
M3/37	Mac-4	NR^b	NR^b	NR^b	180,000
F480					160,000
2.4G2	Fc receptor II		IgG		47,000– 70,000[e]

[a] H and L, specific heavy and light chains; K, myeloma Kappa chain.
[b] NR: Not reported.
[c] Thioglycollate-induced.
[d] 54-2 and M3/37 precipitate polypeptides which coelectrophorese (M. Ho, unpublished).
[e] Depending upon the cell population.
[f] M. K. Ho and T. Springer. Mac-2, a novel 32,000 M_r macrophage subpopulation-specific antigen defined by monoclonal antibody, manuscript in preparation.

Tissue distribution

Positive	*Negative*	*Reference*
Exudate and resident peritoneal macrophages, 50% bone marrow cells, $P388D_1$, J774	Thymocytes, lymph node cells, 90-95% spleen cells, P815, B and T lymphoid lines	11, 14, footnote 1
J774 macrophagelike line		3
TG^C macrophages	Resident peritoneal macrophages, bone marrow cells, lymph node and spleen cells, thymocytes	2, 14, 15, f
TG^C macrophages	Bone marrow cells, lymph node and spleen cells, thymocytes	2, 14
Cultured bone marrow macrophages, TG^C macrophages, mast cells	Spleen, lymph node, thymus, bone marrow cells, neutrophils, resident peritoneal and alveolar macrophages, blood monocytes	16, 17
TG^C macrophages	Bone marrow cells, lymph node and spleen cells, thymocytes	15
Blood monocytes, resident and induced macrophages, J774, P815	Lymphocytes	19
Macrophages, B lymphocytes	T lymphocytes	5, 18

TABLE II. Monoclonal antibodies defining human monocytic differentiation antigens

Monoclonal antibody	Antigen designation	Subclass	Lysis	Antigen polypeptide chain
OKM1[a]	OKM1	IgG_{2b}	+	NR[b]
M1/70[d]	Mac-1	IgG_{2b}	NR[b]	NR[b]
anti-Mol[a]	Mol	IgM	+	NR[b]
anti-Mo2[a]	Mo2	IgM	+	NR[b]
Mac-120[a]	Mac-120	NR[b]	+	$120,000\ M_r$
63D3[a]		IgG_1	NR[b]	$200,000\ M_r$

NR[b]

[a]*Mouse antibody.*
[b]*NR: Not reported.*
[c]*L: Leukemia*

[d]*Rat antimouse antibody, cross-reactive with human cells.*
[e]*ADCC: Antibody-dependent cellular cytotoxicity.*

| Tissue distribution | | Functional | |
Positive	Negative	studies	Reference
Blood monocytes, granulocytes, null cells, acute myelomono-cytic L[c]	B and T lines, T, B-ALL, T, B-CLL, K562, HL-60	Proliferation to antigen	20
Blood monocytes, granulocytes, NK, ADCC ef-fectors		Natural killing, ADCC[e]	6
Blood monocytes, granulocytes, null cells, monocytic L, 21% bone marrow	K562, HL-60, U937		21
Blood monocytes, 11% bone marrow, monocytic L, U937 weak	Granulocytes, B and T lympho-cytes, B and T lines, K562, HL-60		21
30% Blood mono-cytes	B and T lympho-cytes, neutro-phils, HL-60, T and B lines	Proliferation to Con A and an-tigen, lympho-kine produc-tion	10
Blood monocytes, granulocytes weak	B lymphocytes? T lymphocytes, endothelial cells, lympho-blastoid lines, HL-60, U937		22
Spreading mono-cyte fibrils, neuronal cell processes	Blood monocytes		23

phocytes except 2.4G2, directed to the Fc receptor II, which
is expressed on B but not on T lymphocytes. The anti-Mac-1
MAb (M1/70) cross-reacts with both mouse and human macrophages.
Mac-1 in the mouse and human and OKM1 and Mo1 in the human show
highly similar expression on macrophages, granulocytes, and
null cells, suggesting they may define homologous antigens.
Several MAb define macrophage subpopulations, including M3/38
and 54-2 in the mouse and Mac-120 in the human. The Mac-4
antigen defined by 54-2 is expressed on both macrophage subpopulations and on mast cells. As is illustrated also by the
pattern of expression of the Fc receptor II (Table I) and of
'jumping' or heterohistophile antigens such as Thy-1 (2), the
sharing of a single antigen by two different cell types does
not necessarily connote close ontogenetic relationship. Other
MAb to murine macrophages that immunoprecipitate polypeptides
of 82,000, 42,000, or 20,000 have been described in relation
to their use for the study of the composition of pinocytic
vesicles (3).

The ability to obtain large quantities of monospecific
antibodies after growth *in vivo* or *in vitro* is a great advantage of hybridoma lines. The M1/70 line is currently available
from the Cell Distribution Center, Salk Institute, P.O. Box
1809, San Diego, California 92112, and other lines should be
available in the future. Since some lines can undergo chromosome losses leading to loss of antibody secretion (4), it is
good practice to freeze aliquots of a line soon after receipt
and to check specific antibody secretion after more than 6
months of growth in culture. Mouse - mouse or mouse - rat
hybrids can be grown in syngeneic or irradiated hosts (5),
respectively, to obtain ascites antibody, or *in vitro* to obtain 20 - 200 µg antibody/ml (2, 4). Methods for purifying
MAb (6, 7) have been described.

Differences in the use of MAb and classical sera relate to
the homogeneity of MAb in both affinity and subclass. Some
MAb have low affinity such that in the concentration ranges
normally used ($\sim 10^{-9}$ - 10^{-6} M), the IgG or F(ab')$_2$ fragments
will bind to cell surfaces (bivalent interaction), but Fab'
fragments will not bind to cell surfaces nor will IgG immunoprecipitate monovalent antigen (monovalent interaction).
M1/70 is an example of an MAb which can bind monovalently to
the homologous mouse antigen but only bivalently to the cross-
reacting human antigen (6).

MAb vary from excellent to poor in complement-mediated
lysis (Tables I and II), depending on subclass. Lytic efficiency of the different rat MAb subclasses has been reported elsewhere (2, 8). Synergy for complement-mediated lysis between
2 MAb binding to different sites on the same surface molecule
has been reported (9). Second-layer anti-Ig reagents have been
used with the Mac-120 MAb to increase lytic efficiency (10).

Most studies with mouse MAb have relied more heavily on immunofluorescence than on complement-mediated lysis. Immunofluorescent labeling with MAb is far cleaner than with conventional sera, and has allowed the full resolving power of the fluorescence activated cell sorter to be realized (2). For rat anti-mouse MAb, both FITC-labeled SJL mouse anti-rat IgG (8) and mouse IgG-absorbed rabbit anti-rat IgG (11) have been used as second reagents. Immunofluorescent staining of thin sections with M1/70 MAb has recently been used to study the distribution of macrophages in spleen.[1]

Another difference between classical and MAb is that many hybrid lines secrete a mixture of hybrid molecules containing myeloma and specific chains. For example, an HLK line, i.e., secreting specific heavy (H) and light (L) and myeloma kappa (K) chains, would theoretically make only 25% of bivalently active H_2L_2 antibodies. In actuality, L and K chain secretion is often imbalanced (4) and thus the percentage of H_2L_2 molecules may considerably vary.

Purified MAb directly labeled with ^{125}I exhibit extraordinary specificity in binding assays (6, 12), particularly when antibody secreted by H_2L_2 variant clones (4) is used. Indirect binding assays with anti-Ig (2, 12) or *S. aureus* protein A (13) are also useful. In the case of *S. aureus* protein A, mouse IgG subclasses 1, 2a, and 2b (7), but only rat IgG 1 and 2c subclasses are reactive (2, 8).

Acknowledgment

This work was supported by USPHS Grant CA-27547 and Council for Tobacco Research Grant 1307.

REFERENCES

1. G. Köhler and C. Milstein. Derivation of specific antibody-producing tissue culture and tumor lines by cell fusion. *Eur. J. Immunol.* 6: 511-519, 1976.
2. T. A. Springer. Cell-surface differentiation in the mouse. Characterization of "jumping" and "lineage" anti-

[1]*M. K. Ho and T. A. Springer. Rat anti-mouse macrophage monoclonal antibodies and their use in immunofluorescent studies of macrophages in tissue sections. In "Monoclonal Antibodies and T Cell Hybridomas: (U. Hammerling, G. Hammerling, and J. Kearney, eds.). Elsevier, New York, 1981.*

gens using xenogeneic rat monoclonal antibodies. *In* "Monoclonal Antibodies: (R. H. Kennett, T. J. McKearn, and K. B. Bechtol, eds.), pp. 185-217. Plenum, New York, 1980.

3. I. S. Mellman, R. M. Steinman, J. C. Unkeless, and Z. A. Cohn. Selective iodination and polypeptide composition of pinocytic vesicles. *J. Cell. Biol. 86*: 712-722, 1980.

4. T. A. Springer. Quantitation of light chain synthesis in myeloma x spleen cell hybrids and identification of myeloma chain loss variants using radioimmunoassay. *J. Immunol. Methods 37*: 139-152, 1980.

5. J. Unkeless. Characterization of a monoclonal antibody directed against mouse macrophage and lymphocyte Fc receptors. *J. Exp. Med. 150*: 580-596, 1979.

6. K. A. Ault and T. A. Springer. Cross-reaction of a rat-antimouse phagocyte-specific monoclonal antibody (anti-Mac-1) with human monocytes and natural killer cells. *J. Immunol. 126*: 359-364, 1980.

7. P. L. Ey, S. J. Prowse, and C. R. Jenkin. Isolation of pure IgG$_1$, IgG$_{2a}$, and IgG$_{2b}$ immunoglobulins from mouse serum using protein A-sepharose. *Immunochemistry 15*: 429-436, 1978.

8. J. A. Ledbetter and L. A. Herzenberg. Xenogeneic monoclonal antibodies to mouse lymphoid differentiation antigens. *Immunol. Rev. 47*: 63-89, 1979.

9. J. C. Howard, G. W. Butcher, G. Galfre, C. Milstein, and C. P. Milstein. Monoclonal antibodies as tools to analyse the serological and genetic complexities of major transplantation antigens. *Immunol. Rev. 47*: 139-174, 1979.

10. H. V. Raff, L. J. Picker, and J. D. Stobo. Macrophage heterogeneity in man. A subpopulation of HLA-DR bearing macrophages required for antigen-induced T cell activation also contains stimulators for autologous-reactive T cells. *J. Exp. Med. 152*: 581-593, 1980.

11. T. Springer, G. Galfre, D. S. Secher, and C. Milstein. Mac-1: A macrophage differentiation antigen identified by monoclonal antibody. *Eur. J. Immunol. 9*: 301-306, 1979.

12. D. W. Mason and A. F. Williams. The kinetics of antibody binding to membrane antigens in solution and at the cell surface. *Biochem. J. 187*: 1-20, 1980.

13. G. Dorval, K. I. Welsh, and H. Wigzell. A radioimmunoassay of cellular surface antigens on living cells using iodinated soluble protein A from staphylococcus aureus. *J. Immunol. Methods 7*: 237-250, 1974.

14. T. A. Springer. Mac-1,2,3, and 4: Murine macrophage differentiation antigens identified by monoclonal antibodies. *In* "Heterogeneity of Mononuclear Phagocytes" (O. Förster, ed.). Academic Press, New York 1981 in press.

15. T. Springer. Monoclonal antibody analysis of complex bio-
     logical systems: Combination of cell hybridization and
     immunoadsorbents in a novel cascade procedure and its ap-
     plication to the macrophage cell surface. *J. Biol. Chem.*
     256: 3833-3839, 1981.

16. P. A. Leblanc, H. R. Katz, and S. W. Russell. A discrete
     population of mononuclear phagocytes detected by monoclonal
     antibody. *Infect. Immun. 8*: 520-525, 1980.

17. H. R. Katz, P. A. LeBlanc, and S. W. Russell. Antigenic
     determinant on mouse peritoneal mast cells. *J. Reticulo-
     endothel. Soc.*, in press, 1981.

18. I. S. Mellman and J. C. Unkeless. Purification of a
     functional mouse Fc receptor through the use of monoclonal
     antibody. *J. Exp. Med. 152*: 1048-1069, 1980.

19. J. Austyn and S. Gordon. F4/80 - A specific rat monoclonal
     antimouse macrophage antibody. *In* "Heterogeneity of Mono-
     nuclear Phagocytes" (O. Forster, ed.). Academic Press,
     New York, 1981, in press.

20. J. Breard, E. L. Reinherz, P. C. Kung, G. Goldstein, and
     S. F. Schlossman. A monoclonal antibody reactive with hu-
     man peripheral blood monocytes. *J. Immunol. 124*: 1943-
     1948, 1980.

21. R. F. Todd, III, L. M. Nadler, and S. F. Schlossman.
     Antigens on human monocytes identified by monoclonal anti-
     bodies. *J. Immunol. 126*: 1435-1442, 1981.

22. V. Ugolini, G. Nunez, R. G. Smith, P. Stastny, and J. D.
     Capra. Initial characterization of monoclonal antibodies
     against human monocytes. *Proc. Nat. Acad. Sci. USA 77*:
     6764-6768, 1980.

23. N. Hogg and M. Slusarenko. Monoclonal antibodies to sub-
     sets of human blood monocytes. *Fourth Intl. Cong. Immunol.*
     Abst. 11.1.08, 1980.

33

ANTISERA AGAINST Ia ANTIGENS

Carol Cowing

I. GENERAL INTRODUCTION

The *I* region of the murine major histocompatibility complex (MHC) codes for polymorphic cell surface molecules, the
*I*a antigens, which play an important role in cell collaboration in the immune response and in recognition of allogeneic
cells. The *I* region has been subdivided into five subregions:
I-A, I-B, I-J, I-E, and *I-C*. An extensive series of MHC con-
genic and recombinant mice bred on the C57BL/10 background
have allowed for the production of alloantisera specific for
Ia antigens and which react with gene products of *I-A, I-J,*
and *I-E* from various haplotypes (1). Ia antigens are expressed on only a limited number of cell types, including a
portion of the mononuclear phagocytes. This chapter will describe two procedures for the detection of Ia antigens on
murine mononuclear phagocytes: Indirect immunofluorescence
amd microcytotoxicity using anti-Ia alloantisera. Similar

315

Copyright © 1981 by Academic Press, Inc.
ISBN 0-12-044220-5

methods have been used for the detection of analogous MHC gene
products in other species (man, guinea pigs, rats) and on other
cell types.

II. ENRICHING MONONUCLEAR PHAGOCYTES FROM MOUSE SPLEEN

A. *Introduction*

The most readily obtained mononuclear phagocytes, normal
and induced peritoneal cells, are a poor source of cells for
the detection of Ia antigens because only a small percentage
(8-15%) are Ia$^+$ (2). However, mononuclear phagocytes in the
spleen (3) and liver (4) are about 50% Ia$^+$, which makes the
detection of Ia antigens a great deal easier even though it
necessitates an enrichment step. The simplest enrichment
procedure we have found is to incubate spleen cell suspensions
on glass petri dishes for 3-4 hr with several washes to remove
nonadherent cells; adherent cells are then resuspended with
EDTA and the phagocytes are tagged by ingestion of latex particles (3). One mouse spleen will yield about 1×10^6 adherent cells of which 40-60% will be mononuclear phagocytes and
about 50% of these express Ia antigens.

B. *Reagents*

EDTA: ethylene diaminetetraacetic acid (1:5000 Versene,
Grand Island Biological Company).
Latex particles: 10% suspension of 1.1 µm diameter poly-
strene beads (Dow Chemical Company).

C. *Procedures*

(1). Spleen cell suspensions should be free of RBC and
adjusted to 2×10^7 cells/ml in any complete medium containing
antibiotics, 20 mM HEPES buffer and 5-10% heterologous serum
(medium).
(2). The cells are then plated on 100 mm sterile glass
petri dishes. The dishes should be free of both detergent and
lipid; the easiest way to check this is to put 5 ml of medium
first in each dish: The medium should not cover the bottom
until the dish is swirled and then should completely cover it.
Then add 3 ml of cell suspension to the medium in each dish
and swirl to distribute the cells (6×10^7 cells in 8 ml/dish.
Incubate the dishes in a moist incubator at 37°C for 1.5 hr
in 5% CO_2 and air.

(3). Swirl the petri dishes to dislodge nonadherent cells and aspirate off the medium. Wash the dishes twice with 8 ml of warm (37°) medium, swirling each time. Finally add 8 ml of medium and reincubate the dishes for a second 1.5 hr. After the second incubation, repeat the washes and drain off any remaining medium.

(4). Place 5 ml of EDTA in each dish and swirl to cover the bottom. Incubate at 37°C for 15 min, then shake the dishes vigorously to detach the adherent cells and transfer them to an iced tube containing 5 ml of medium per dish (i.e., volume is equal to the EDTA). Centrifuge at 1500 rpm in the cold for 10 min. Resuspend the pellet in medium at 1×10^6 cells/ml and add latex particles (6 µl of a 10% suspension/ml cells). Place the tubes on a roller drum (Belco Glass, Inc.) overnight at 0.5-1.0 rpm and 37°C.

(5). The next day wash the cells three times by centrifuging the suspension through an underlayer (1-2 ml) of undiluted serum; this will remove free latex particles. Finally, resuspend the cells at 2×10^7/ml in PBA (see Section III. B.) for immunofluorescence or at 5×10^6 cells/ml in medium for microcytotoxicity.

D. Critical Comments

The purity of the phagocytic cell population obtained by this method is dependent on two factors: The duration of adherence and the extent of the washes. As you increase each, the percentage of mononuclear phagocytes will increase, but the final yield will diminish. For the detection of Ia antigens by the two methods described below, a pure population of phagocytes is unnecessary because only cells ingesting latex will be scored. The percentage of mononuclear phagocytes expressing membrane Ia antigens does not alter between fresh, nonadherent spleen cell suspensions and those adherent at 24 hr; but beyond 24 hr the percentage of Ia^+ phagocytes in the adherent population diminishes (3).

The concentration of latex particles and the duration of incubation of the cells with latex are greater than those normally used. However, the benefit of the conditions described in Section II. C. (4) is that all of the mononuclear phagocytes will be filled with particles and can be unequivocally distinguished from nonphagocytic cells. That all of the cells ingesting latex under these conditions are mononuclear phagocytes can be verified by their ability to bind antigen-antibody complexes (5).

III.   METHOD FOR DETECTION OF Ia ANTIGENS BY INDIRECT
       IMMUNOFLUORESCENCE

A. *Introduction*

     Indirect immunofluorescence involves incubation sequen-
tially of cells with two antisera. The first antiserum is
unlabeled antibody directed against the antigen you wish to
detect; the second antiserum is fluorescein isothiocyanate-
conjugated (FL-) antibody specific for the Fc portion of the
first antibody. It is essential that the second antiserum
does not react with the cells in the absence of the first
antiserum; this can occur by virtue of an unexpected cross-
reactivity with cell surface antigens. The problem can be
overcome by preabsorbing the second antibody with the cells
or by the use of an affinity-purified second antibody. When
the first antiserum is an alloantiserum, there is the additional potential for the second antibody to react with Fc-
bound immunoglobulin (Ig) on Fc receptor-bearing cells. To
an extent, the failure of an antiserum specific for the Fc
portion of the alloantibody to react with Fc-bound Ig is pure-
ly fortuitous; therefore the choice of the second antibody may
involve titrating several different reagents.

B. *Reagents*

     (1). PBA: Phosphate-buffered (0.05 M) saline, pH 7.2,
containing 2% w/v bovine serum albumin and 0.02% w/v sodium
azide. This is the diluent to be used throughout the procedures; it should be passed through a millipore filler,
stored frozen, and maintained on ice during use.
     (2). Anti-H-2 alloantisera: These may be prepared in
your own laboratory (6,7) or obtained from the NIAID Serum
Bank (Dr. John G. Ray, Jr., Program Officer, Immunobiology
and Immunochemistry Br., IAIDP, NIAID, NIH, Westwood Bldg.,
Room 754, Bethesda, Maryland 20205). You will need anti-Ia
antisera of the appropriate specificity to react with your
cells, anti-/H-2 K or D reagents as a positive control and
anti-Ia of a specificity that should not react with your cells
as a negative control. These reagents should be stored frozen
and used undiluted in most cases. Monoclonal anti-H-2 alloantibodies can be obtained from the Salk Institute (Project
Manager, Cell Distribution Center, The Salk Institute, PO Box
1809, San Diego, California 92112) and must be titrated because
some monoclonals show pronounced prozones.
     (3). Fluorescein-conjugated antimouse IgG. As most anti-
MHC alloantibodies are IgG, this reagent should be specific

for the Fc portion of IgG heavy chains. A fluorescein-conjugated goat antibody of this specificity can be obtained from
Cappel Laboratories, Inc., Cochranville, Pennsylvania or from
Tago Inc., Burlingame, California. Alternatively, a fluorescein isothiocyanate-conjugated rabbit (Fab')$_2$ anti-mouse IgG1
and rabbit F(ab')$_2$ anti-mouse IgG2 can be prepared in the
following manner: Inject rabbits with 1 mg of chromatographi-
cally purified MOPC 21 (IgG1,K) or MOPC 141 (IgG2b,K) in complete Freunds adjuvant three times at 2 week intervals and
bleed the animals 2 weeks after the third injection. Isolate
IgG fractions of the sera by DEAE chromatography and absorb
with myelomas insolubilized by covalent coupling to agarose
via the cyanogen bromide procedure (8). Anti-MOPC 21 can be
absorbed with RPC5 (IgG2a, K) and anti-MOPC 141 with MOPC 21
to yield anti-IgG1 and anti-IgG2, respectively. F(ab')$_2$ fragments can be prepared by pepsin digestion (9) and conjugated
to fluorescein (10). Plasmacytomas can be obtained from
Litton Bionetics (Kensington, Maryland). These reagents
should be stored frozen. The appropriate concentrations for
use of these reagents must be individually determined by titration on your cells with and without prior incubation with
anti-MHC alloantisera. All dilutions should be made immediately prior to use in PBA.

C. *Procedure*

(1). All reagents and cell suspensions (see Section II.C.
(5)), appropriately diluted in PBA, must be maintained on ice
throughout the procedures. Cell washes should be done in a
cold centrifuge at 1500 rpm for 10 min.

(2). Anti-MHC alloantisera and Fl- anti-mouse IgG must be
ultracentrifuged to remove material >10 S immediately prior
to use, unless the reagent is an F(ab')$_2$. Since only very
small volumes of reagents will be used, an airfuge (Beckman)
is ideal for this purpose (175 µl per tube, top speed setting,
27 min, use top 100 µl from tube).

(3). Incubations should be done on ice in 10 × 75 mm
glass tubes. First, put 25 µl of cell suspension in each
tube, then add 100 µl of anti-MHC alloantisera or PBA to the
cells and vortex well. Tubes should include: anti-H-2K or -D
of appropriate specificity, an inappropriate anti-Ia (as a specificity control for the anti-MHC reagents), and PBA (as a control for binding of the FL- anti-mouse IgG). Incubate the tubes
for 30 min on ice, vortexing every 10 min.

(4). Wash the cells three times in 1.0 ml iced PBA per tube,
vortexing the pellet each time you resuspend. After the final
wash, pour off the PBA and drain the pellet well.

(5). Add 25 µl of FL- anti-mouse IgG to each tube and vortex well. Incubate on ice 30 min, vortexing every 10 min. We have found that a combination of affinity-purified FL-anti-mouse IgG' and anti-mouse IgG2 at approximately 100 µg/ml each is the optimal concentration for maximum detection of Ia and minimum background (cells + FL-antigen-IgG alone) staining. However, this concentration will vary for each FL-anti-IgG reagent and must be independently determined. A good fluorescent reagent used alone should not stain more than 1-2% of the cells; whereas, when used after incubation with an anti-H-2K or -D alloantiserum, it should stain virtually 100% of the cells.

(6). Repeat step (4).

(7). Vortex each pellet very well just prior to putting 9 µl of cells on a microscope slide. Place a 22 × 22 mm cover glass on top of the cells and immediately seal the edges with nail polish.

(8). Examine the cells by phase and fluorescence microscopy for viability, latex ingestion, and surface fluorescence; a minimun of 200 viable cells should be counted.

D. Calculation of Data

Data are simply reported as number of cells with surface fluorescence per 100 latex-ingesting cells.

E. Critical Comments

As mentioned in Section III, C. (5), FL-anti-IgG should not stain more than 1-2% of mononuclear phagocytes, while anti-H-2K or anti-H-2D followed by FL-anti-IgG should stain virtually 100% of the cells. The percentage of cells stained by an anti-Ia antiserum will vary with the source of the cells and the specificity of the antibody (2-4). Of the three subregions that can be serologically detected, only products of *I-A* and *I-E* have been observed on mononuclear phagocytes by indirect immunofluorescence. The expression of *I-J* subregion products on these cells has been reported (11), but detection of *I-J* on the membrane has been problematic and may depend upon the particular antiserum used.

The success of this procedure depends on several factors. First of all, it is only as good as the specificity of the reagents used. It is important that the cells be stained in suspension rather than while adherent because the FL-anti-IgG background tends to be quite elevated on adherent mononuclear phagocytes. Prior incubation of the cells with latex is valuable not only because it allows assay of impure populations, but also because it diminishes ingestion of Ia-anti-Ia complexes by the phagocytes during the staining process. Strict maintenance of temperature at 4°C also reduces this. Cytoplasmic autofluorescence of mononuclear phagocytes may be distracting in the assessment of surface fluorescence; if this is a problem, the autofluorescence can be reduced by using medium lacking phenol red for preparation of the cells. Fluorescence microscopy has the advantage of enabling one to detect infrequent positive cells, but it has the disadvantage of subjectivity; this can only be overcome by doing repeated observations on coded samples using consistent criteria.

The procedure described above, applied to highly purified populations of mononuclear phagocytes, can also be used for flow microfluorometric analysis of Ia antigens on mononuclear phagocytes; in this case it is essential to reduce autofluorescence to a minimum.

IV. METHOD FOR DETECTION OF Ia ANTIGENS BY MICROCYTOTOXICITY

A. Introduction

Anti-Ia and C killing of mononuclear phagocytes will yield results parallel to those of the indirect immunofluorescence method (3). This method is easier in that only one antibody is required, but it is less sensitive because C alone gives a higher background than FL-anti-Ig.

B. Reagents

Medium: Described in Section II, C. (1).

Complement: This is a critical reagent as it must not be toxic to the cells by itself but must be effective in allo-antibody-mediated cell lysis. Individual C sources may be screened for low toxicity (< 10% lysis when used alone) and high C activity (> 90% lysis when used after anti-H-2K or anti-H-2D). We have found the best source to be serum from rabbits 3-4 weeks old. It is essential to screen C sources on the target cells to be used, as a good C for lymphocytes may not be good for mononuclear phagocytes, and we have even found it to vary with the tissue source of the phagocytes. In general, it is easier to screen several sera and choose one good one, than to do absorptions of sera whose toxicity is unacceptably high.

Anti-H-2 alloantisera: see Section III. B. (2).

C. Procedures

(1). This is a standard two-stage cytotoxicity procedure performed in round bottom microtiter plates (12). Serial two-fold dilutions of anti-H-2 alloantisera are made in medium (Section II. C. (1)) in a total volume of 25 µl. Two series of dilutions of each antiserum should be made and two wells should contain medium alone. The plates should be kept on a bed of ice.

(2). Add 25 µl of cell suspension from Section II. C. (5) (5×10^6 cells/ml in medium) to every well and mix on a micromixer (Cooke Engineering) for 10 sec at speed 3. Add cover to microtiter plate and leave on ice for 30 min.

(3). Add 150 µl of iced medium to all wells and centrifuge plates at 1000 rpm for 5 min in the cold, using microtiter plate holders.

(4). Remove supernatant by quickly flicking plates into a sink, then place plates on ice again.

(5). Add 25 µl of C source appropriately diluted in iced medium (see Section IV. B) to one of every two rows of alloantisera dilutions and to one of the two wells receiving medium alone. Add 25 µl of iced medium to all remaining wells. Cover plates and mix for 30 sec at full speed on a micromixer, then incubate at 37°C for 30 min.

(6). Centrifuge plates at 1500 rpm for 5 min in the cold, then replace on bed of ice.

(7). Counting can be done in a hemocytometer, but is more rapidly done on an F500 white slide (Roboz Surgical) using round (12 mm diam) No. 1 cover glasses (Kimble). Remove supernatant from 5 wells. Add 10 µl of trypan blue (0.2% in saline, freshly diluted) to each well, mix, remove 5 µl from each well, and place on slide, immediately adding cover glass. Count 200 cells containing latex particles and score for percent dead cells.

D. Calculation of Data

Data are reported as percentage lysis of latex-ingesting cells versus reciprocal antiserum dilution. The percent lysis with C alone and percent lysis with an inappropriate anti-MHC alloantiserum should be included in the results.

E. Critical Comments

In order for the cytotoxicity data to be meaningful, cell viability in medium alone, C alone, and alloantiserum alone must remain high (approx. 90%) throughout the assay; these

controls should be counted regularly during cytotoxicity
counting, as the percentage dead cells can increase with time.
It is not uncommon for high concentrations of alloantisera to
give unexpectedly low percentage lysis. This can occur for
two reasons: The serum can be anticomplementary at high concentrations, or cell lysis can be so extensive that many of
the dead cells are blown up and lost leaving a field with few
cells, lots of free latex particles, and an artificially low
dead cell count. Also, if a large number of contaminating
lymphocytes have been killed by an antiserum, there is a tendency for the mononuclear phagocytes to be found in clumps
with dead lymphocytes and it may be difficult to tell if these
cells are dead or alive. Generally these problems only occur
at very high antibody concentrations; more reliable cell
counts are obtained at lower antibody concentrations when the
percentage lysis is still on a plateau.

V. CONCLUDING REMARKS

Immunofluorescence and microcytotoxicity are the two
simplest methods for detection of Ia antigens on mononuclear
phagocytes. A more sensitive and precise analysis of Ia expression on these cells can be obtained using a fluorescence-
activated cell sorter. Finally, biochemical analyses of Ia
antigens synthesized by mononuclear phagocytes can be done on
immunoprecipitated molecules purified from cells grown with
radiolabeled amino acids (3).

REFERENCES

1. J. Klein, L. Flaherty, J. L. VandeBerg, and D. C.
    Shreffler. *H2* haplotypes, genes, regions, and antigens:
    First Listing. *Immunogenetics* 6:489, 1978.
2. R. H. Schwartz, H. B. Dickler, D. H. Sachs, and B. D.
    Schwartz. Studies of Ia antigens on murine peritoneal
    macrophages. *Scand. J. Immunol.* 5:731, 1976.
3. C. Cowing, B. D. Schwartz, and H. B. Dickler. Macrophage
    Ia antigens. 1. Macrophage populations differ in their
    expression of Ia antigens. *J. Immunol.* 120:378, 1978.
4. L. K. Richman, J. Klingenstein, J. A. Richman, W. Strober,
    and J. A. Berzofsky. The murine Kupffer cell. 1. Char-
    acterization of the cell serving accessory cell function
    in antigen-specific T cell proliferation. *J. Immunol.*
    123:2602, 1979.

5. R. D. Arbeit, P. A. Henkart, and H. B. Dickler.
    Lymphocyte binding of heat-aggregated and antigen-com-
    plexed immunoglobulin. *In "In Vitro* Methods in Cell-
    Mediated Immunity," Vol 11. (B. Bloom and J. David, eds.).
    Academic Press, New York, 1976.

6. D. H. Sachs and J. L. Cone. A mouse B cell alloantigen
    determined by gene(s) linked to the major histocompati-
    bility complex. *J. Exp. Med. 138:*1289, 1973.

7. C. S. David, D. C. Shreffler, and J. A. Frelinger.
    New lymphocyte antigen system controlled by the *Ir*
    region of the mouse H-2 complex. *Proc. Natl. Acad. Sci.
    USA 70:*2509, 1973.

8. P. Cuatrecasas, M. Wilchek, and C. B. Anfinsen.
    Selective enzyme purification by affinity chromatography.
    *Proc. Natl. Acad. Sci. USA 61:*636, 1968.

9. A. Nisonoff, F. C. Wissler, and L. N. Lipman. Properties
    of the major component of a peptic digest of rabbit anti-
    body. *Science 132:*1770, 1960.

10. J. H. Peters and A. H. Coons. Fluorescent antibody as
    specific cytochemical reagents. *In* "Methods in Immunol-
    ogy and Immunochemistry," Vol. V. (C. A. Williams and
    M. W. Chase, eds.), Academic Press, New York, 1976.

11. J. E. Niederhuber, P. Allen, and L. Mayo. The expression
    of *Ia* antigenic determinants on macrophages required for
    the *in vitro* antibody response. *J. Immunol. 122:*1342,
    1979.

12. D. H. Sachs, H. J. Winn, and P. S. Russell. The immuno-
    logic response to xenografts. *J. Immunol. 107:*481,
    1971.

34

QUANTITATION OF ADHERENT MONONUCLEAR PHAGOCYTES
BY INVERTED PHASE MICROSCOPY

D. O. Adams

I. PRINCIPLE

Establishing the number of *adherent* mononuclear phagocytes in a given culture vessel is often necessary for determining the specific activity of intracellular and secreted
macrophage constituents and for comparing on a per cell basis
various functional assays--such as target cytolysis, endocytosis, secretion or binding of ligands. Determining the DNA
or protein content of adherent mononuclear phagocytes is an
accurate but time-consuming technique and does not provide
immediate results. Counting the number of adherent macrophages
in a given culture by inverted phase microscopy offers a simple,
rapid, and reasonably accurate method for estimating the number of mononuclear phagocytes in a given culture (1,2).
The number of cells present within the confines of an ocular micrometer is determined for several randomly selected,
well-dispersed fields in the culture. This number, when multi-

plied by a calibrating factor, establishes the number of adherent macrophages per square centimeter in the culture vessel (Table I).

The principal pitfall in this method is nonhomogeneous
distribution of macrophages in the monolayers. The monolayers
must be completely even throughout the culture plate for the
randomly sampled fields to be representative. A principal
cause of unevenly distributed macrophages is vortex currents
around the edge of the culture vessel that are set up during
the transfer of culture plate from tissue culture hood to incubator. The result of such currents is peripheral accumulation and central sparseness of mononuclear phagocytes. The
problem is particularly prevalent in round culture vessels.
This problem can be avoided by stopping immediately in front
of the incubator and shaking each plate vigorously 2-3 times
from side to side and then from front to back. Immediately
and gently place the plate into the incubator. Use of this
technique and avoiding cell clumps in the suspension should
lead to even monolayers.

II. MATERIALS

     Culture plates. The method is applicable to various types
of macrophages or other cells cultured in 6 or 16 mm wells, in
petri dishes of various sizes or in T flasks.
     Fixative. 2.0% Glutaraldehyde in cacodylate buffer at
pH 7.4 is employed.
     Inverted phase microscope. The inverted phase microscope
should be equipped with 10×, 20×, and 40× objectives or their
approximate equivalents.

Table I. Surface Area of Some Commonly Employed Culture
          Vessels for Mononuclear Phagocytes

Vessel	Area (cm^2)
6-mm well (cluster plate)	0.28
16-mm well (cluster plate)	2.0
35-mm petri dish	8.0
35-mm well (cluster plate)	9.6
60-mm petri dish	21
60-mm well (cluster dish)	28.2
100-mm petri dish	55

An ocular micrometer. An ocular micrometer is inserted into one eyepiece of the inverted microscope. The Howard micrometer (Catalog No.6585-H20, Arthur H. Thomas Co.) is suitable for this purpose, though a larger grid is often more useful (Catalog No.422, Fisher Scientific).

Cell counter

Stage micrometer. A stage micrometer graduated in milli-meters will be needed once for calibration of the ocular micro-meter and, thus, can be borrowed.

III. CALIBRATION OF EYEPIECE MICROMETER

The eyepiece micrometer is inserted into one eyepiece. The stage micrometer is placed on the microscope. The area (in square millimeter) contained within the large square of the ocular micrometer at the level of the stage is determined for the 10×, 20×, and 40× objectives. To do so, focus the microscope on the stage micrometer. Using the scale on the stage micrometer, measure the width of the ocular micrometer square five times. The width squared equals the area observed through the ocular micrometer for that magnification. The calibration factor, which represents the number of micrometer squares contained within 1 cm^2, is calculated for each objec-tive.

Calibration factor for each objective =

$$\frac{100}{\text{Area in } mm^2 \text{ of the ocular micrometer at the level of the stage for that objective}}$$

IV. PROCEDURE

(1). The plates of macrophages may be counted immediately so that they can be subsequently used for various functional assays or they may be fixed in glutaraldehyde for later count-ing.

(2). Scan carefully at 10× the culture plates to be count-ed. Make sure that the cells are evenly distributed throughout the wells to be counted as well as throughout the other wells. If the cells are not evenly distributed, the method cannot be applied.

(3). Using the 20× objective, select a field at random. Count the number of cells contained within the large square of the micrometer. In the case of cells overlying the edges

of the square, count those cells overlapping the top and left
edges of the square but do not count cells overlapping the
right and bottom edges of the square. Repeat this for at
least three other fields. Count a minimum of 400 cells.

V. CALCULATION OF DATA

Determine the average number of cells per large square.
Multiply this by the calibration factor for the 20× objective.
The result is equal to the number of adherent cells per square
centimeter.

VI. COMMENT

The assay provides a good estimate of the number of macrophages present (Fig. 1). The data obtained in this assay correlate well with the content of DNA in the culture vessel
(Fig. 2). The accuracy of the assay depends primarily upon
the accuracy of the calibration. The reproducibility of the
assay depends on the accuracy of the cell counts, the unifor-
mity of the monolayer, and the error of the Poisson distribution. By counting 400 cells, the error due the Poisson distribution can be reduced to ± 5% of the total. The assay is
readily applicable to counts of other adherent cell types such
as tumor cells.

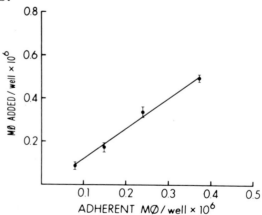

*Fig. 1. Various numbers of BCG-elicited macrophages
were added to 16 mm culture wells. After 4 hr, the nonadherent leukocytes were washed off. The number of adherent
macrophages/well was determined by counting the adherent cells
with an inverted microscope.*

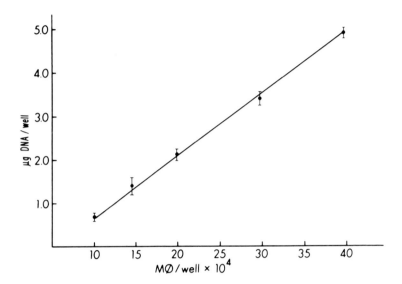

Fig. 2. Various numbers of BCG-activated macrophages were added to 16 mm wells. After 4 hr, the nonadherent cells were removed and the content of DNA in the wells determined (3) after counts of adherent cells had been performed by inverted microscopy.

Acknowledgment

Supported in part by USPHS Grant 16784.

REFERENCES

1. D. O. Adams. Macrophages. *In* "Methods in Enzymology," Vol. LVIII, Cell Culture (W. Jakoby and I. Pastan, eds.), pp. 494–505. Academic Press, New York, 1979.
2. D. O. Adams. Effector mechanisms of cytolytically activated macrophages. I. Secretion of neutral proteases and effect of protease inhibitors. *J. Immunol. 124:*286, 1980.
3. S. L. Cookson and D. O. Adams. A simple, sensitive assay for determining DNA in mononuclear phagocytes and other leukocytes. *J. Immunol. Methods 23:*169–173, 1978.

35

QUANTITATION OF DNA IN MONONUCLEAR PHAGOCYTES

D. O. Adams

I. PRINCIPLE

The specific activity of a given constituent within macrophages can be expressed in relation either to content of protein or to cell number. Determination of cell number is often advantageous, because cultivated macrophages may either produce large amounts of protein in culture, or lose protein after lysosomal discharge (1, 2). Thus, the specific activity of a given constituent may rise or fall in the face of a falling or rising total amount of a particular enzyme. Determining cell number by hemacytometer count is often inaccurate in this circumstance, because a large but variable number of macrophages may be lysed while removing them from the culture vessel (3). Determination of DNA content provides an accurate, reliable, and sensitive method for quantifying cell number (6). On the other hand, determination of specific activity in regard to cellular protein does take into account variations in the size of different macrophages.

The present assay, devised specifically for quantifying
DNA in mononuclear phagocytes, offers the advantages of simplicity and sensitivity (4). The DNA of macrophages lysed in
detergent is precipitated by cold PCA, extracted in hot PCA,
and quantified by spectrophotometry after reaction with diphenylamine (5). The assay can be applied to macrophages in
suspension or adherent to culture vessels such as petri dishes
or 16 mm wells. As few as 1×10^5 macrophages can be quantified by this procedure, and the assay is linear over the range
1 - 50 µg of DNA/sample.

II. REAGENTS

PCA. 7 M Perchloric Acid (PCA) and 1 M PCA
Diphenylamine: 3 gm % Diphenylamine (Eastman Kodak,
Rochester, New York). Under a fume hood, dissolve 3 mg/100 ml
glacial acetic acid. Store under a fume hood in an amber
bottle at room temperature. This reagent is generally good for
2 - 3 months.
Acetaldehyde: 1.6 gm % Acetaldehyde (Eastman Kodak). On
ice under a fume hood, add 0.5 ml of acetaldehyde stock to
24.5 ml of distilled water. Store in an amber bottle with a
screw top at 4°C. This is usually good to 2 - 3 months but
often deteriorates to acetic acid. If the assay begins to
give erratic results, check the acetaldehyde first.
DNA Standard. Dissolve 8 mg of DNA (Sigma No. D-1501;
Type 1, Na salt) in 20 ml of 5 mM NaOH. When thoroughly dissolved, make a 1 : 5 dilution in 5 mM NaOH. Determine A_{260nm}
and A_{280nm}. The DNA content of the dilution in microgram per
milliliter is then calculated using the nomogram of Warburg
and Christian (Fig. 1) (6). Store the stock at 4°C, where it
is good for about 6 months.

III. PROCEDURE

A. Cell Preparation

(1) It is important to keep the cells at 4°C at all times.
(2) Method 1: Wash cultured cells in wells or plates and
then freeze at -70°C in an appropriate volume of PBS (i.e.,
0.5 ml PBS/16 mm well). Thaw on ice. To each well, add
0.5 ml of freshly prepared 0.4% Triton X-100. Incubate on ice

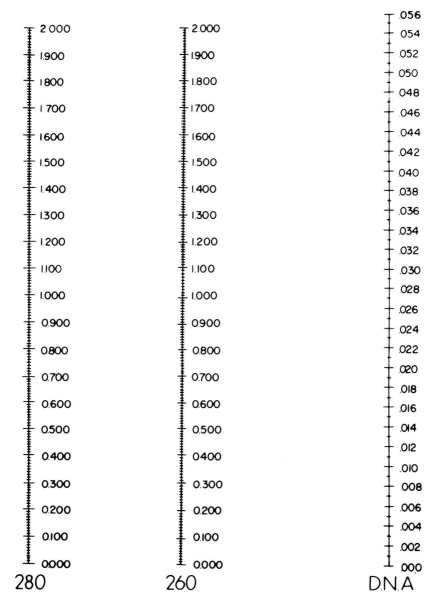

Fig. 1. Determination of DNA by A_{260} and A_{280} (6). Using a cuvette with a 1-cm light path, determine A_{260nm} and A_{280nm}. From these, the concentration of DNA (milligram per liter) can be determined. Based on a nomogram prepared by E. Adams from Calbiochem Corp. for biochemical research. (With permission of Calbiochem Corp.)

for 30 min. Scrape up cells with a rubber policeman. Transfer samples completely to test tubes on ice.

(3) Method 2: To cells at 4°C in a culture dish, add 0.4% Triton X-100 to a final concentration of 0.2%. Incubate 30 min at 4°C. Remove by scraping. Freeze in a Dry Ice - acetone slurry. Transfer samples completely to and store in polypropylene tubes at -70°C. Thaw on ice.

B. *Determination of DNA*

(1) Samples and standards are assayed in triplicate.

(2) Standards are made from DNA stock in 5 mM NaOH; 14, 7, 3.5, 1.75, and 0.87 µg of DNA/ml provide a useful range. Place 1.0 ml of each standard in 10 × 75 disposable culture tubes. Prepare blanks of 1.0 ml of NaOH and PBS. Add 20 µℓ of 10% Triton X-100 to each standard and incubate on ice 30 min. Add 30 µℓ of 7 M PCA to each standard. Mix thoroughly.

(3) To 10 × 75 mm disposable tubes on ice containing 30 µℓ 7 M PCA, add 1.0 ml of each lysate sample. Mix thoroughly on a vortex mixer.

(4) The DNA should now be stable. However, keep samples on ice. From this point on, all standards and unknown are identically treated.

(5) Incubate PCA-treated samples on ice for 30 min. Spin samples at 10,000 g for 15 min at 4°C. The DNA is now pelleted.

(6) Gently aspirate the supernatant with a Pasteur pipette while continuously observing the residual pellet. Discard supernatant carefully.

(7) Add 0.5 ml of hot PCA (70°C) and incubate 30 min at 70°C after covering the tubes with parafilm to hydrolyze the residual DNA.

(8) Remove the hydrolysate containing the DNA completely from each tube and place it in a clean 10 × 75 mm glass tube.

(9) Prepare the colorimetric reagent just before use: 10 ml of 3% diphenylamine, 0.2 ml of conc. H_2SO_4, 0.1 ml of 1.6% acetaldehyde.

(10) Add 0.5 ml of the above reagent to each sample, blank or standard. Seal tubes with parafilm. Incubate 16-24 hr at 37°C. The time can be varied as long as all samples are similarly treated.

(11) Spin at 10,000 g for 10 min at 4°C.

(12) Determine A_{600nm} against a water blank.

IV.   CALCULATION OF DATA

Plot net A_{600nm} of standards (versus NaOH blank) against the concentration of DNA in microgram per milliliter.   Calculate extinction coefficient (slope of regression line:

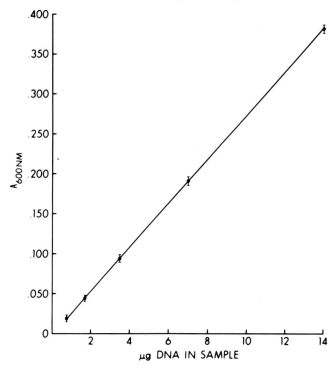

Fig. 2.   A standard curve for DNA.

Net $A_{600nm}/\mu g$ DNA).   A typical standard curve is shown in Fig. 2.   To calculate DNA content of unknowns falling on the linear part of the graph, divide the net A_{600nm} (versus the PBS blank) by the extinction coefficient.

V. COMMENTS

The assay is sensitive to 1 µg DNA or 100,000 macrophages (4). 1×10^6 murine peritoneal macrophages contain 10.1 ± 0.36 g DNA (4). The coefficient of variation between triplicate samples should be approximately ±2%. The principal problems with assaying small amounts of DNA are in complete precipitation of DNA (Section III. B, step 5), avoidance of loss of DNA (Section III. B, step 6), and complete recovery of the DNA (Section III. B, step 8). The reproducibility of the assay can be increased by using samples containing the lysate of $\cong 5.0 \times 10^5$ macrophages, but this should not be necessary if the assay is carefully performed.

Acknowledgment

Supported in part by USPHS Grant 16784.

REFERENCES

1. Z. A. Cohn and B. Benson. The differentiation of mono-nuclear phagocytes: Morphology, cytochemistry, and bio-chemistry. *J. Exp. Med. 121*: 153-169, 1965.
2. J. Schnieder and M. Baggiolini. Secretion of lysosomal hydrolases by stimulated and nonstimulated macrophages. *J. Exp. Med. 148*: 435-450, 1978.
3. D. O. Adams. Macrophages. *In* "Methods in Enzymology," Vol. LVIII, Cell Culture (W. Jakoby and I. Pastan, eds.), pp. 494-505. Academic Press, New York, 1979.
4. S. L. Cookson and D. O. Adams. A simple, sensitive assay for determining DNA in mononuclear phagocytes and other leukocytes. *J. Immunol. Methods 23*: 169-173, 1978.
5. K. Burton. A study of the conditions and mechanisms of the diphenylamine reaction for the colorimetric estimation of deoxyribonucleic acid. *Biochem. J. 62*: 315, 1956.
6. O. Warburg and W. Christian. Isolierung und Kristallisa-tion des Garungsferments Enolase. *Biochem. Z. 310*: 384-421, 1940.

36

LOWRY AND BRADFORD ASSAYS
FOR PROTEIN

Paul J. Edelson
Robert A. Duncan

I. INTRODUCTION

The Lowry and Bradford assays for protein determination
provide relatively simple methods for calculating specific
activities by standardizing enzyme activities to protein content. Both assays will conveniently detect protein in the
concentration ranges used for most of the enzyme assays in the
following chapters and may be modified to detect as little as
1 to 25 µg protein.

Both assays are colorimetric. The Lowry assay depends on
the complexing of copper with tyrosine and tryptophan residues,
whereas the Bradford method measures the binding of Coomassie
Brilliant Blue G-250 to protein. The protocols described here
are modified specifically for protein determination in Triton
lysates but may be altered for different conditions by simply
replacing Triton with the appropriate agent.

METHODS FOR STUDYING
MONONUCLEAR PHAGOCYTES

337

II. LOWRY ASSAY

A. *Reagents*

    (1). 2% Sodium carbonate in 0.1 *N* sodium hydroxide:
20 gm Na_2CO_3 (Fisher Scientific Co., Catalog No. S-263);
4 gm NaOH (Fisher Scientific Co., Catalog No. S-318).
    Dissolve in 1000 ml double distilled water. Store at
room temperature.
    (2). 2% Sodium tartrate: 2 gm Na tartrate (Fisher
Scientific Co., Catalog No. S-435).
    Dissolve in 100 ml double distilled water and store at
4°C.
    (3). 1% Copper sulfate: 1 gm $CuSO_4$ (Fisher Scientific
Co., Catalog No. C-493).
    Dissolve in 100 ml double distilled water and store at 4°C.
    (4). Lysozyme protein standard (200 µg/ml): Hen egg
white lysozyme (Worthington Chemical Co., Catalog No. 2931).
Dissolve 10 mg lysozyme in 10 ml sterile distilled water to
make a 1.0 mg/ml solution. Then, take 200 µl of 1 mg/ml solution and 9.8 ml sterile water to make a 200 µg/ml solution.
Freeze the remaining 1 mg/ml solution, and aliquot the 200 µg/
ml solution into 1-ml portions and store at -20°C.
    (5). 2% Triton: 2 ml Triton X-100 (Sigma Chemical Co.,
Catalog No. T-6878).
    Dissolve in 98 ml double distilled water.

B. *Assay Procedure*

    (1). Prepare 0.05% Triton (0.1 ml of 2% Triton X-100
diluted in 3.9 ml distilled water). The Triton solution
should be diluted fresh on the day of the assay from the 2%
stock. Lyse cells.
    (2). Prepare protein standards. See Table I.
    (3). Working assay mixture. Add in this order: 20 ml
2% Na_2CO_3 in 0.1 *N* NaOH, 0.2 ml 2% Na tartrate, 0.2 ml 1%
$CuSO_4$.
    (4) Working phenol reagent. Dilute stock Phenol Reagent
(Sigma Chemical Co., Catalog No. F-9252) 1:1 with distilled
water. The working phenol reagent must be prepared fresh on
the day of the assay.
    (5). Spectrophotometer. Set spectrophotometer to read
absorbance at 750 nm. Absorbance at 500 nm may also be used,
but this is less sensitive than 750 nm when the protein concentration is less than 125 µg/ml.

(6). Assay. Aliquot 200 µl of cell lysate into small disposable plastic test tubes (12 x 75 mm, no cap, Falcon Plastics, Catalog No. 2052). Add 1 ml of working assay mixture to each unknown and each lysozyme standard. Vortex briefly and leave at room temperature for 10 min. Add 0.1 ml working phenol reagent to each tube, vortex, and leave at room temperature for 30 min. Read absorbance at 750 nm within 30 min of the end of the second incubation.

C. Calculation of Data

The standards may be plotted on a linear graph of concentration versus absorbance, and unknown concentrations may then be read directly from the graph.

Alternatively, a straight line may be fit to the standard data by the method of least squares and the formula generated may be used to calculate unknown concentrations. This latter method is especially convenient for use with a hand-held programmable calculator.

III.   BRADFORD ASSAY

A. Reagents

(1). Diluted dye reagent. Dilute 1 volume Bio-Rad Protein Assay Dye Reagent Concentrate (Bio-Rad Laboratories, Richmond, California, Catalog No. 500-0006) with four volumes double-distilled water and filter through Whatman No.1 filter paper. This may be stored at room temperature for up to two weeks. The reagent contains methanol and phosphoric acid and should be appropriately handled.

(2). Protein standard. Add 20.0 ml sterile distilled water to Bio-Rad Protein Standard I (Bio-Rad Laboratories, Richmond, California, Catalog No. 500-0005). This yields a solution of bovine γ-globulin at approximately 1.4 mg/ml. Bio-Rad also supplies a bovine plasma albumin standard (Protein Standard II, Catalog No. 500-0007), or individual protein standards may be made to correspond most closely to the protein being measured. Reconstituted protein may be stored up to 2 months at 4°C or frozen in aliquots for long-term storage at -20°C.

(3). 0.5% Triton X-100. Dilute 1 ml 2% Triton X-100 (see section I for details) with 3 ml double-distilled water. Prepare fresh for each assay.

B. Assay Procedure

(1). Preparation of standard. To 13 x 100 mm disposable glass test tubes (Curtin Matheson Scientific, Inc., Houston, Texas, Catalog No. 339-283) add (as given in the tabulation below):

Protein standard (1.4 mg/ml)	Triton X-100 (0.5%)	Distilled water	Protein concentration (mg/ml)	Total protein (μg)
---	10 μl	90 μl	0 (Blank)	0
10 μl	10	80	0.140	14
20	10	70	0.280	28
30	10	60	0.420	42
40	10	50	0.560	56
50	10	40	0.700	70
60	10	30	0.840	84
70	10	20	0.980	98
80	10	10	1.120	112
90	10	---	1.260	126

(2). Assay. Add 5.0 ml diluted dye reagent to 100 μl of sample or standard and vortex gently but thoroughly (avoid foaming). After 5 min, read absorbance on a spectrophotometer at 595 nm (visible band) versus a reagent blank. (A high optical density for the blank, around 0.45 versus water, is usual.) The color is stable for approximately 1 hr.

(3). Interference. Strongly alkaline conditions and detergent concentrations in excess of about 0.1% cause substantial background interference. Such samples may be neutralized or diluted to minimize background, but the interfering reagent (e.g., 0.05% Triton) should be included in the blank and standard. For a more complete consideration of interfering reagents, see Bio-Rad Bulletin 1069. (This bulletin also details a microassay procedure for detecting total protein content from 1 to 25 μg.)

(4). Cleaning cuvettes. The dye reagent slowly stains cuvettes, especially quartz cuvettes. Glass cuvettes are a better choice and may be cleaned with methanol and/or 0.1 N HCl. The blank cuvette should be rinsed approximately every 10 min to avoid progressive staining of the cuvette. This problem may be avoided by using disposable cuvettes (Bolab, Inc., Derry, New Hampshire, Catalog No. 202195).

TABLE I.

Triton (0.1%)	Lysozyme (200 µg/ml)	Distilled water	Protein concentration (µg/ml)	Total protein (µg)
0.100 ml	---	0.100 ml	0	0
0.100	0.025 ml	0.075	25	5
0.100	0.050	0.050	50	10
0.100	0.075	0.025	75	15
0.100	0.100	---	100	20

C. Calculation of Data

A standard curve may be prepared in the same manner as for the Lowry assay in the preceding section. When using the least-squares calculation, a correlation coefficient approaching unity (> 0.990) is expected.

D. Critical Comments

Both the Lowry and Bradford procedures may be conveniently used for protein determination in phagocyte lysates. They both suffer from interference by detergents, but at levels below 0.1% detergent, the problems are minimal. The choice of which assay to use is usually dictated by either convenience or the amount of protein available for assay. The Bradford assay is an easy choice for convenience, since only one reagent is used and the reaction is complete in 5 min, compared to two reagents and 40 min incubation time for the Lowry assay. In addition, the protein-dye complex is stable for about an hour, thus eliminating the need for strict timing. However, if amounts of protein lower than about 15 μg are to be measured, the Bradford procedure must be modified and detergent interference may become prohibitive. The Lowry assay is therefore preferable for samples containing 1 to 20 μg protein when detergent is present. However, the Bradford procedure, as presented here, is less sensitive to other interfering reagents than the Lowry method. We routinely use the Bradford assay.

When using these assays for purified protein samples, one should be cautioned that both assays show different color responses with different proteins, depending on the proportion of various amino acids present. In such instances, and when an accurate assessment of absolute (rather than relative) protein content is needed, it is a good idea to check the protein sample with a nitrogen determination (e.g., Kjeldahl).

REFERENCES

1. M. Bradford. A rapid and sensitive method for the quantitation of microgram quantities of protein utilizing the principle of protein-dye binding. *Anal. Biochem. 72:* 248-254, 1976.
2. Bio-Rad Protein Assay. Bulletin 1069, Bio-Rad Laboratories, Richmond, California, 1979.
3. P. J. Edelson, R. Zwiebel, and Z. A. Cohn. The pinocytic rate of activated macrophages. *J. Exp. Med. 142:*1150-1164, 1975.

4. O. Folin and V. Ciocalteu. On tyrosine and tryptophane determinations in proteins. *J. Biol. Chem.* *73*:627, 1927.
5. O. H. Lowry, N. J. Rosebrough, A. L. Farr, and R. J. Randall. Protein measurement with the folin phenol reagent. *J. Biol. Chem.* *193*:265-275, 1951.

37

USE OF WRIGHT'S STAIN AND CYTOCENTRIFUGE PREPARATIONS

Monte S. Meltzer

I. INTRODUCTION

Quantitation and, therefore, identification of mononuclear
phagocytes in mixed leukocyte preparations presents an initial
problem in any study of macrophage function. This becomes especially important in studies that examine responses of different groups of cells: numbers of macrophages and not numbers
of total cells within each group should be constant. We have
found the Diff-Quik stain of cytocentrifuged cell smears to be
an accurate, reproducible, and rapid method to determine the
percentage of macrophages in mixed cell suspensions and to
study histology of various leukocytes. Excellent results can
be obtained with mouse, guinea pig, and human leukocyte suspensions from blood or peritoneal cavities. Cytocentrifugation
applies cell suspensions onto glass slides by controlled centrifugal force. With increasing force, cells appear spread and
display fine nuclear and cytoplasmic detail without significant
morphologic distortion. Diff-Quik, a series of dye solutions

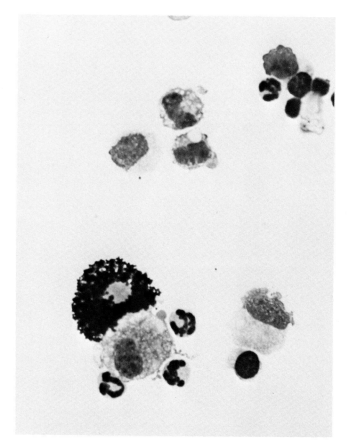

Fig. 1.   Diff-Quik stained cytocentrifuged smears of mouse resident peritoneal cell populations.   Oil immersion.

that stain leukocyte suspensions much like Wright's stain, is reproducible and fast. Diff-Quik has most of the advantages of Wright's stain without its ritual and mystery.

II. REAGENTS

Cytocentrifuge: Cytospin cytocentrifuge, Shandon Southern Instruments, Sewickley, Pennsylvania.
Diff-Quik solutions I and II and Fixative (Harleco, Gibbsville, New Jersey)

III. PROCEDURE

Cell morphology on cytocentrifuged smears is dependent upon cell concentration, suspension medium, centrifuge speed, and time. We have found the following to give optimal results:
(1) Cell concentrations of about 1×10^6 cells/ml. This cell concentration includes erythrocytes.
(2) Cells suspended in medium with 10% serum or albumin. Serum prevents cell disruption during centrifugation.
(3) Spin 0.2 ml in cytocentrifuge block at 1500 rpm for 5 min at room temperature.
(4) Cytocentrifuged cell smears are air dried and stained as follows:
(a) Diff-Quick Fixative: 15 sec. Time is not critical. Fixative solution can be reused for months.
(b) Diff-Quik solution I: 15 sec. Time is not critical. Dye solution can be reused for months.
(c) Diff-Quik solution II: 30 sec. Time is important. Care should be taken not to overstain. Dye solution should be changed every two weeks.
(d) Slides are washed repeatedly in tap water and air dried. Stained smears are examined under oil immersion lens.

IV. COMMENTS

A typical Diff-Quik stained cytocentrifuged mouse peritoneal cell population is shown in Fig. 1.

38

USE OF PHASE CONTRAST MICROSCOPY

Stanton G. Axline

I. INTRODUCTION

Phase contrast microscopy is a very useful and powerful tool for examining the morphology of mononuclear phagocytes. The power of this system lies in the ability of phase contrast illumination to enhance enormously contrast within cell tissue samples. It is particularly useful in studies of thin unstained samples in which only minimal detail can be seen by standard bright field illumination.

Much of the theoretical and practical work in developing phase contrast microscopy was performed by the Dutch physicist Zernike who first applied the principle to microscopy in 1932 (1). However, it was not until after World War II that phase contrast microscopy was developed effectively. It represented an advance in microscopy of sufficient magnitude that in 1953 Zernike was awarded the Nobel Prize for his achievement. A detailed, theoretical analysis of phase contrast microscopy is not appropriate here, but the interested reader may wish to refer to the works by Zernike (1, 2), Martin (3), Loveland (4, 5), or James (6).

In light microscopy the two important changes that occur in light passing through a specimen are changes either in amplitude or phase. For conventional bright field illumination, microscopy with stained specimens contrast within an object is brought about mainly by differences in light absorption. In phase microscopy, on the other hand, differences in refractive index within the sample cause the emitted light to be changed in phase relative to that which entered the sample. Such phase difference in light waves are then visualized as changes in light amplitude.

Illumination for phase microscopy requires a light source that is a relatively narrow line in the rear focal plane of the substage condenser. With the condenser and the objective properly focused, light waves that originate at a point in the annular source will form a parallel bundle of rays when passing through the field plane. If not affected by the object to be examined, they will be focused again by the rear focal plane of the objective to provide an image of the annular source. They will then be dispersed to cover the entire field. However, with a specimen in the field, some light will be diffracted by its optical edges including interior detail. With a specimen composed of many refracting points, the entire aperture will be filled. This system provides an extremely sensitive method of separating undeviated light waves from those that were deviated by the sample. In phase contrast microscopy the change in phase of direct versus diffracted light that emerges from the specimen makes the object visible. Changes in refractive index or light path length occur primarily at edges within a specimen, thus making the phase phenomenon an edge effect.

If the image of the specimen is darker than the field background, the system is referred to as dark phase contrast, whereas if the image is brighter than the background, the system is bright phase contrast. The shift in phase between the undeviated and diffracted light is usually designed to be ±1/6 to 1/4 of a wave length (7, 8). If the direct beam is advanced relative to the diffracted beam, the system is referred to as positive phase and dark contrast usually results. For negative phase the direct beam is retarded relative to the diffracted beam and bright contrast is usually obtained.

II. EQUIPMENT AND REAGENTS

Special features of phase contrast microscopy worthy of separate mention are the light source, condenser, phase ob-

jectives, and telescopic arrangement for viewing the phase annulus. Each will be discussed in more detail below in Sections
A through D.

A. Light Source

Kohler illumination must be used for phase contrast microscopy. This system, invented by August Kohler in 2893 (8, 9),
requires a light condenser to focus the image of the light
source on the back field plane of the microscope condenser.
The light must be shaped so that the bright portion of the
source will cover the annular aperture of the condenser.
Whether the light source is built into the microscope stand or
is separate is not important, but the light must be of high intensity to overcome the luminious inefficiency of phase microscopy. Phase contrast typically requires ten to twenty times
the light intensity used for bright field illumination. Lamps
most commonly used for phase contrast have a ribbon filament
or are "arc" lamps using zirconium, mercury, tungsten, or carbon. Open incandescent wire lamps are generally not suitable
for phase contrast.

B. Condenser

The light emitted from a phase condenser is typically annular in shape. Variables of the annular ring that will influence the quality of image produced are the diameter of the
ring, width of the band, and position of the annulus in the optical system. In phase microscopes, the annular aperture in
the substage can be centered since the image must lie within
the annulus of the phase plate. The diameter of the annulus
must be matched precisely to the diameter of the phase plate
in the objective. Therefore, most phase condensers have more
than one phase annulus in the condenser.

C. Phase Objective

The characteristic of a phase objective that separates it
from a bright field objective is the requirement for a phase
plate. The phase plate on the objective is annular in shape
and is produced by the evaporation of thin layers of magnesium
or cryolite on the back lens. The thickness of the layers affects directly the magnitude of the phase shift that will be
produced. It will determine if the direct rays are advanced
or retarded relative to the diffracted rays. The phase annulus should be imaged exactly over the phase plate near the back

of the focal point of the objective. The condenser annulus and
the phase plate of the objective should match each other precisely and thus only objectives of identical geometric and optical characteristics can be used with the same phase condenser
annulus.

D. Telescope

The image of the annulus as projected onto the phase plate
can be observed by removing the eyepiece and looking down the
tube. To provide proper adjustment, a focusing telescope is
used that can be inserted into the tube in place of the eyepiece. The centering telescope is a small instrument resembling
an eyepiece with which the image of the condenser annular diaphragm formed at the back focal plane of the objective can be
viewed under magnification. Such a device is also referred to
as an Amici - Bertrand lens. In some systems an Amici - Bertrand lens is mounted in the microscope tube that, together
with the eyepiece, forms a telescopic system.

E. Microscope Coverslips

American manufacturers have designed objectives to be used
with coverslips of 0.18-mm thickness, whereas European manufacturers typically have assumed a coverslip thickness of 0.17 mm.
Coverslips identified as No. 1 1/2 thickness have a mean thickness of 0.18 mm with 85% of this designation being ±10 μm of
0.18 mm thickness. If a thicker coverslip is used, the image
contrast will be diminished and spherical aberrations will be
produced. This is a particular problem with phase objectives
of high numerical aperature and magnification. For objectives
with a low numerical aperature no visible degradation in image
due to coverslip thickness will be produced.

F. Observation Chambers

If phase contrast observations of living cells are to be
performed, a culture vessel should be selected that has a flat
top as well as bottom and both surfaces should be of uniform
thickness. The characteristics of the vessel bottom are the
most critical. For reasons outlined above the ideal thickness
is 0.18 mm for observations requiring a high power objective.
Any deviation from this standard thickness will result in diminished quality of phase contrast. The thickness requirement

for the vessel top is less stringent but uneven thickness will
affect the apparent lamp alignment as well as the ability to
center the phase ring.

G. Reagents

1. Buffered Glutaraldehyde Fixative

Prepare 0.1 M phosphate-buffered saline at pH 7.4 (PBS) as
indicated. The following reagents are used: NaCl Crystals
Reagent Grade, 8.00 gm, KCl Crystals - U.S.P., 0.20 gm,
$Na_2HPO_4 \cdot 7 H_2O$, 2.17 gm, KH_2PO_4 Anhydrous - A.R., 0.20 gm. Add
double-distilled H_2O in volume sufficient to make 1000 ml.
Sterilize by autoclaving.
Prepare 1% glutaraldehyde solution in PBS at pH 7.4 as follows: glutaraldehyde, 8%, 10 ml, E.M. Grade aqueous glutaraldehyde in snap open vial stored under nitrogen, Polysciences,
Inc., and sterile PBS, pH 7.4, 70 ml. Store glutaraldehyde in
PBS at 4°C. Glutaraldehyde prepared in this fashion will be
slightly hypertopic with an osmolality of 330 mOsm/kg.

H. Inverted Phase Microscope

To examine living tissue culture preparations in T flasks
or petri dishes an inverted phase microscope offers many advantages. It eliminates the need to use specialized chambers
such as the Sykes-Moore (10) or Rose (11) chamber in which only
a small number of cells can be examined. Inverted phase microscopy is quite useful for checking the progress of cultures
in flasks and can be adapted readily for still photography or
cinephotomicrography. The optical principles and general considerations involved in inverted phase microscopy are identical
to those for upright phase microscopy.

III.   PROCEDURES

A. Phase Microscope Adjustment

1. The microscope light should be ignited a sufficient
time before use so that the light intensity is at its maximum
and the output is stable. This is especially important if "arc"
type lamps are used.
2. The light source, if adjustable, should first be centered. For this step the condenser should be removed and no

slide or specimen placed in the light path. A 40X objective
should be placed in the operating position and the viewing
telescope placed in the ocular tube. Focus the telescope while
moving the field diaphragm until the light spot is well centered. The light should be positioned so that the light spot
provides maximum brightness.

    3. Rotate the condenser collar until the clear aperture
is positioned in the optical axis of the microscope.

    4. Replace the telescope with a viewing eyepiece, rotate
a 10X objective into position, insert specimen, and focus the
specimen image.

    5. Move the Abbe condenser up or down until the image of
the field diaphragm is in focus through the eyepiece.

    6. Adjust the condenser until the image of the light
source is centered in the field of view. The field diaphragm
should then be opened until the border of its image just disap-
pears from the field of view.

    7. Insert a green filter into the light pathway before it
enters the condenser. A green filter should be used since contrast in phase image is enhanced by use of monochromatic light.
Microscopes used for analysis of biologic specimens are designed
to produce optimum phase quality with incident light of 543 nm
in wavelength.

    8. Change to the desired objective and rotate the condenser
ring until the annular ring matching that of the objective is in
the optical path.

    9. Recenter the condenser annulus in the light path if the
microscope being used requires separate centering for each phase
annulus.

    10. Replace one of the eyepieces with the phase telescope
and adjust the microscope until the condenser annular diaphragm
is in sharp focus.

    11. Adjust the phase condenser so that the phase plate and
the annular diaphragm of the condenser are centered precisely.

B. Macrophage Sample Preparation

    Sample preparation, important in all types of microscopy,
is especially important in phase contrast microscopy. The
sample to be examined should be quite thin for phase work (approximately 1 μm in thickness). If the sample is too thick undeviated light from one layer may be diffracted in an upper
layer and produce an image of low contrast. Macrophages maintained as monolayers on an optically clean glass surface such
as a coverslip provide the most suitable type of sample for
high magnification phase contrast microscopy.

    During *in vitro* cultivation the macrophage coverslip prepa-
ration can be maintained in tissue culture medium in a suitable

vessel. If the sample is to be fixed prior to microscopy it is convenient to maintain the coverslip preparation in a petri dish or Leighton tube. If a living macrophage preparation is to be examined, one of several tissue culture chambers such as the Sykes-Moore (10) or Rose (11) chamber is more convenient. Such chambers offer the advantage that high magnification objectives (100X) with short working distances can be used. For lower magnification microscopy in which less detail is required, macrophages can be cultured in tissue culture flasks.

C. *Fixation of Coverslip Preparation of Macrophage Monolayers*

1. Macrophages are cultured in a Leighton tube containing one 10 × 35 mm coverslip (No. 1 1/2). In this configuration 1 ml of tissue culture media is used.
2. At the time the cells are to be fixed the Leighton tube is removed from the 37°C incubator and the ti-sue culture media is aspirated immediately using a Pasteur pipette.
3. The monolayer should be rinsed once rapidly but gently with saline at 37°C.
4. A 1 ml volume of 1% glutaraldehyde in PBS at 37°C should be added to the Leighton tube.
5. The fixative should remain in place for at least 10 minutes at room temperature. The glutaraldehyde should be removed by aspiration with a Pasteur pipette and the coverslip preparation rinsed twice in 5 ml portions of distilled water.
6. The coverslip is then withdrawn gently from the Leighton tube using a hooked wire and mounted in a drop of distilled water or phase contrast mounting fluid cell side down on a clean microscope slide.
7. Care must be taken to remove all air bubbles from between the two glass surfaces. Excess water is then removed by absorbant paper from the edges and exposed surface of the coverslip.
8. The edges of the coverslip are sealed with warm paraffin wax. If the wax is applied carefully the mounted coverslip preparation will remain sufficiently moist if stored at room temperature for satisfactory phase contrast microscopy for 24 to 48 hours. Storage time can be prolonged by keeping the slide preparation in a humid chamber. Since no attempt is made to keep the coverslip preparation sterile during mounting the effective life of the sample is often limited by bacterial growth.

IV.   CRITICAL COMMENTS

A. *Köhler Illumination*

     Köhler illumination is far preferable to "critical illumi-
nation" for phase contrast microscopy. Köhler illumination by
design requires a separate condenser to project an enlarged
image of the lamp filament, and an iris or field diaphragm to
provide control over the size of the area to be illuminated.
The Köhler system does not require a homogenous light source
since the lamp condenser system provides even illumination.
An additional advantage is its ability to provide more light
from a low wattage lamp due to the ability of the system to
collect more light from the source. Of special importance in
phase contrast work is the ability of Köhler illumination to
provide higher contrast and thus yield a qualitatively better
image.

B. *Phase Contrast Versus Interference Microscopy*

     A discussion of the use of phase contrast microscopy for
the examination of mononuclear phagocytic cells would not be
complete without mention of interference microscopy. Interference microscopy is a more recent development than phase microscopy but both systems have been in widespread use for a
sufficient period of time to assess their relative roles. Theoretically, there is no fundamental difference between the two
types of microscopy. In both forms the objective is to convert
invisible phase changes of light into visible amplitude changes.
However, the optical equipment required for the two forms of
microscopy differs and consequently the images produced are not
identical. An excellent description of the similarities and
differences between phase contrast and interference microscopy
can be found in a monograph by Barer (12).
     Interference microscopy systems have the capability of vary-
ing at will the phase shift. Such flexibility is enormously
useful for studies in which quantitation of the degree of phase
shift is required. However, it represents only a modest advantage for morphologic analyses.
     Phase contrast microscopy offers the advantage that contrast
between adjacent objects within a specimen is greater than with
interference microscopy. Although the latter provides a more
true representation of phase shifts, the exaggeration of contrast at edges characteristic of phase microscopy is often a major advantage for morphologic studies. The explanation for such
differences is that phase contrast is an imperfect method of
interference contrast. A phase plate is used to separate direct

and diffracted light and thus produce phase changes. Direct
light falls on the phase annulus and diffracted light falls on
the annulus and the entire phase plate. Thus, the direct and
diffracted light are not separated completely. Incomplete separation results in images that do not quantitatively reflect
changes in phase shift. One manifestation of this effect is enhancement of contrast at zones of sharp changes in phase and
thus the production of a halo at such boundaries. In contrast,
interference microscopy produces a truer representation of phase
changes and the resultant images are characterized by the absence of a halo and diminished phase effect at boundaries. The
ability to reproduce phase changes more accurately in interference microscopy accounts for the "contoured" appearance of cells
examined by this technique.

Images produced by interference microscopy have the appearance of being three dimensional and create the impression that
surface details are being observed. In fact, the apparent increase in depth of field is an illusion. Contrast is produced
in a thin section and thus the image is free of out-of-focus details. Phase contrast systems gather light from functionally
thicker specimens than interference systems. The ability to obtain information from a thicker "section" is often an advantage
for morphologic studies. However, if the sample is too thick a
diffuse halo may result and internal detail will not be visible.
In such circumstances, interference microscopy may be more suitable than phase contrast.

Interference microscopy is quite sensitive to subtle variations in slide and coverslip thickness. Thus, frequent read-
justment may be required for different parts of the preparation.
Phase contrast microscopy, on the other hand, is much less sensitive to such variations.

C. *Phase Contrast Photomicrographs of the Macrophage*

The typical phase contrast appearance of well differentiated
mouse peritoneal macrophages are shown in Figures 1 and 2.
Cells were grown as monolayers on a coverslip in Leighton tubes
under culture conditions described previously (13, 14). Monolayers were fixed and mounted as described in this monograph
and phase contrast microscopy and photography were performed
using a Zeiss Ultraphot II. Cells shown in Figure 1a were cultured for 48 hours in 50% heat-inactivated newborn calf serum
(NBCS) in tissue culture medium 199 whereas cells shown in
Figure 1b were cultivated for the same duration of time in 5%
NBCS. Each macrophage has a single slightly indented nucleus
containing prominent nucleoli. The centrosphere region contains
abundant large phase dense secondary lysosomes which are well
demarcated from more peripheral cell regions. Note that the

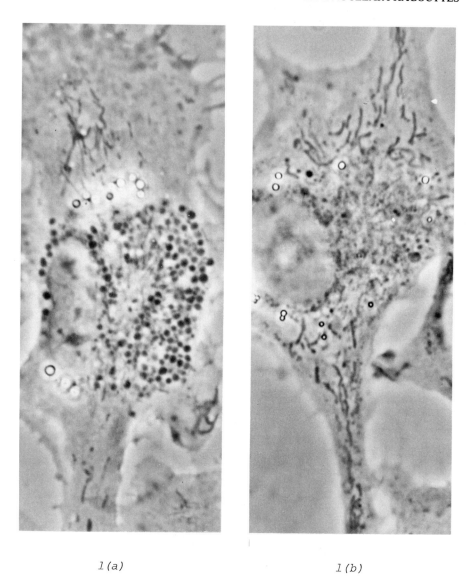

1(a)   1(b)

Fig. 1a,b. Mouse peritoneal macrophages cultivated in
Medium 199 for 48 hours (a) in 50% NBCS, (b) in 5% NBCS. Cells
were grown as monolayers on coverslips in Leighton tubes.
Phase contrast x 2500.

cell grown in a high concentration of NBCS contains much larger
and more numerous lysosomes than the cell grown in the tenfold
lower concentration of NBCS. Surrounding the lysosome contain-

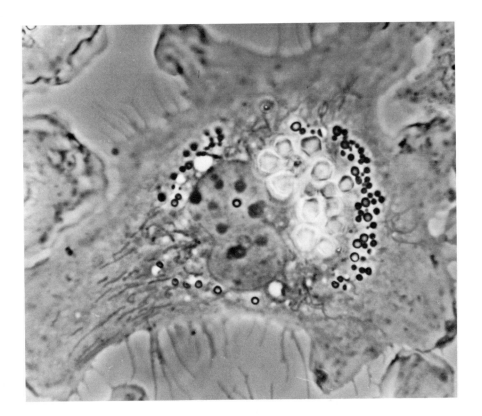

Fig. 2. Cultivated mouse peritoneal macrophage shortly after ingestion of nondigestible Amaranthus starch particles. Phase contrast x2800.

ing centrosphere region is a narrow zone containing highly refractile lipid droplets. Lipid droplets are present in even
greater abundance in the cell shown in Figure 2.

Peripheral to the centrosphere region the cytoplasm forms
a thin veil which by phase microscopy is only slightly more
phase dense than the background. In these regions of the cells
are seen phase dense mitochondria as well as pinocytic vesicles
which have the appearance of clear "punched out" areas in the
cytoplasm.

The macrophage shown in Figure 2 was cultivated in 50% NBCS
for 48 hours and then permitted to phagocytize starch particles.
The starch is irregular in shape and because of its thickness
each piece is surrounded by a halo. Phagocytized particles are
limited in distribution to the centrosphere region of the cell.
Irregularities of the cell surface at sites of attachment to the
glass substratum are particularly well seen in this cell.

D. *Glutaraldehyde*

Multiple chemicals have been used as fixatives of biologic specimens for microscopy. Among these the aldehydes have been found to be especially suitable. Formaldehyde was the first of the aldehydes to be used but, since 1963, glutaraldehyde has gained widespread acceptance. The basis for the use of glutaraldehyde for this purpose is the work of Sabatini, Bensch, and Barnett (15) who performed comparative studies of multiple aldehydes as a tissue fixative for electron microscopy. Glutaraldehyde was demonstrated to yield superior preservation of morphology as assessed by electron microscopy. Further, it has the additional advantage of preserving a substantial fraction of multiple tissue enzyme activities. Thus, glutaraldehyde-fixed samples can be used for histochemical and cytochemical studies.

Glutaraldehyde is a dialdehyde that reacts quickly with proteins, particularly the free amino groups, in a manner presumably analogous to formaldehyde. Unlike formaldehyde, however, glutaraldehyde is difunctional and can participate extensively in cross-linking of amino acids and proteins. The chemical reactions involved in the interactions of glutaraldehyde with proteins are not clearly understood. Schiff base formation has been mentioned frequently as the principle reaction. However, the assumption is not consistent with the observations that protein cross-linking by glutaraldehyde is not reversed by treatment with semicarbazide and can withstand wide variations in pH, ionic strength, and temperature (16). Whatever the mechanisms, the extreme stability of protein cross-linking represents a major advantage of glutaraldehyde over other tissue fixatives.

Glutaraldehyde penetrates rapidly into tissues and produces fixation quickly. However, to obtain optimal fixation it is important to use an excellent grade of the monomeric form of the chemical. Glutaraldehyde, like any aldehyde, is subject to oxidation when exposed to air and to self-polymerization when stored in concentrated solutions (>25%). Polymerization also occurs rapidly at an alkaline pH. From the view point of the microscopist both reactions are undesirable since the resultant compounds are less effective than monomeric glutaraldehyde as a tissue fixative and are more inhibitory to enzyme activities. Polymerization can be avoided by using E.M. Grade glutaraldehyde prepared by Polysciences, Inc. In this preparation monomeric glutaraldehyde is prepared as an aqueous solution at pH 5.0 packaged in nitrogen. This material can be stored for long periods of time at 4°C.

Acknowledgment

This work was supported by a grant from the Medical Research Service, Veterans Administration, Washington, D.C.

REFERENCES

1. F. Zernike (1935). Das Phasenkontrastverfahren bei der mikroskopischen Beobachtung. *Z. Tech Phys.* *16*: 454-457.
2. F. Zernike. Phase contrast, a new method for microscopic observation of transparent objects. Reproduced *In* "Achievements in Optics" (A. Bouwers, ed.), pp. 116-135. Elsevier, New York, 1950.
3. L. C. Martin. The microscopy of phase contrast. *In* "Theory of the Microscope" (L. C. Martin, ed.), pp. 338-407. Blackie & Son Ltd., Glasgow and London, 1966.
4. R. P. Loveland. Darkfield, stop-contrast, and phase-microscopy principles. *In* "Photomicrography," Vol. 1 (R. P. Loveland, ed.), pp. 78-91. John Wiley & Sons, New York, 1970.
5. R. P. Loveland. Phase illumination. *In* "Photomicrography," Vol. 1 (R. P. Loveland, ed.), pp. 453-460. John Wiley & Sons, New York, 1970.
6. J. James. Special techniques of image formation. *In* "Light Microscopic Technique in Biology and Medicine," (J. James, ed.), pp. 165-180. Martinus Nijhoff, The Hague, 1976.
7. R. P. Loveland. The application of phase microscopy. *In* "Photomicrography," Vol. II (R. P. Loveland, ed.), pp. 540-554. John Wiley & Sons, New York, 1970.
8. G. H. Needham. The phase-contrast microscope, the interference microscope. *In* "The Practical Use of the Microscope" (G. H. Needham, ed.), pp. 151-162. Charles C. Thomas, Springfield, Ill., 1958.
9. A. Kohler (1893). Ein neues beleuchtungsverfahren fur mikrophotographische Zwecke. *Z. Wiss. Mikr. 10*: 433-440.
10. J. A. Sykes and E. B. Moore (1959). A new chamber for tissue culture. *Proc. Soc. Exp. Biol. Med. 100*: 125-130.
11. G. Rose. (1954). A separable and multipurpose tissue culture chamber. *Texas Reports on Biol. and Med. 12*: 1074-1083.
12. R. Barer. Phase contrast and interference microscopy in cytology. *In* "Physical Techniques in Biological Research," Vol. III, Part A (A. W. Pollister, ed.), pp. 1-53. Academic Press, New York, 1966.
13. S. G. Axline and Z. A. Cohn (1970). *In vitro* induction of

lysosomal enzymes by phagocytosis. *J. Exp. Med. 131*: 1239-2360.

14. S. G. Axline and E. P. Reaven (1974). Inhibition of phagocytosis and plasma membrane mobility of the culti- vated macrophage by cytochalasin B. *J. Cell Biol. 62*: 647-659.

15. D. D. Sabatini, K. Bensch, and R. J. Barnett (1963). Cytochemistry and electron microscopy: The preservation of cellular ultrastructure and enzymatic activity by al- dehyde fixation. *J. Cell Biol. 17*: 19-58.

16. F. A. Quiocho. Immobilized proteins in single crystals. *In* "Methods in Enzymology," Vol. 44 (K. Mosbach, ed.), pp. 546-558. Academic Press, New York, 1976.

39

USE OF PEROXIDASE STAIN BY THE KAPLOW METHOD

Monte S. Meltzer

I. INTRODUCTION

Peroxidases, enzymes that catalyze the oxidation of certain organic compounds (notably benzidine derivatives) by peroxide, can be demonstrated in many cells of the mononuclear phagocyte series. The distribution and intensity of peroxidase activity, however, varies with stages of cell maturation and phagocytic activity (for review see ref. 1). Promonocytes synthesize peroxidase and store the enzyme in cytoplasmic granules, primary lysosomes. Enzyme production generally ceases at the end of the promonocyte stage. The number of granules decrease as promonocytes differentiate into monocytes and in turn distribute granules to mitotic daughter cells. Peroxidase activity may also change with phagocytosis. Peroxidase granules can fuse with phagosomes and release enzyme. Since enzyme synthesis is restricted to promonocytes, phagocytizing monocytes eventually lose their peroxidase content.

Cytochemical demonstration of peroxidase by a method modi-

363

fied from that described by Kaplow (2) can be used as a marker
for several stages of mononuclear phagocyte maturation.
Peroxidase-positive granules are most prominent in promonocytes
and cluster in the perinuclear cytoplasm. Monocytes have fewer
positive granules and these are characteristically located within the convexity of the reniform nucleus. Inflammatory macrophages, recently derived from blood monocytes, are initially
peroxidase-positive. With phagocytic activity, however, these
positive cells lose peroxidase content. In addition to cytoplasmic granules in the inflammatory macrophages, small membrane-
bound peroxidase particles can sometimes be observed at the cell
surface. Resident peritoneal macrophages and other mature tissue
macrophages have no detectable peroxidase activity by light microscopy (3, 4).

II. REAGENTS AND EQUIPMENT

   Cytocentrifuge: Cytospin centrifuge, Shandon-Southern
Instruments, Sewickley, Pennsylvania.
   Fixative: Absolute ethanol and formaldehyde mixed 9:1; can
be stored at 4°C for at least 1 yr.
   Stain: Prepare stock solutions of the following:

   (1) Benzadine dihydrochloride (practical grade 75%, Sigma
Chemical Co.). CAUTION: Benzadine derivatives are known
HUMAN CARCINOGENS and must be appropriately handled. Add 1.0 gm
benzidine to 1000 ml 0.01 M K phosphate buffer, pH 7.0. Opalescent slurry results. Adjust pH to 7.0 with NaOH. Slurry clears
to violet-brown suspension. We usually do not filter out undis-
solved benzidine. Stock can be stored at room temperature in
amber glass bottle for at least 1 yr.
   (2) Sodium nitroprusside (Fisher Chemical Co.): Add 40 gm
nitroprusside to 100 ml water. Stock saturated solution can be
stored in amber glass bottles at room temperature for at least
1 yr.
   (3) Hydrogen peroxide. 30% (Fisher Chemical Co.). Store at
4°C.

   Counterstain: Diff-Quik stain solutions I and II (Harleco,
Gibbstown, New Jersey.

III.   PROCEDURE

(1) Cell smears are prepared on glass slides by cytocentrifugation. Place 0.2 ml cell suspension (about 1×10^6 cells/ml)
in medium with 10% serum into cytocentrifuge chamber. Spin at
1500 rpm for 5 min. Remove slide and air dry.
(2) Fix cell smear in ethanol-formaldehyde for 1 min at room
temperature. Wash repeatedly in tap water and air dry.
(3) Peroxidase stain must be prepared fresh. Mix: 30 ml
benzidine stock, 0.3 ml 1/10 nitroprusside stock in water and
0.3 ml dilute H_2O_2 (0.1 ml 30% stock atn 7.6 ml water).
(4) Stain fixed smear for 90 - 120 sec at room temperature.
Wash repeatedly with tap water and air dry.
(5) Counterstain with Diff-Quik, a Wright's stainlike dye:
20 sec solution I and 30 sec solution II. Wash repeatedly in
tap water and air dry.

IV.   COMMENTS

(1) For best results, slides should be fixed and stained
as soon as possible. We have kept fixed slides at 4°C for up
to 4 hr without obvious change. Fixed slides should not be
kept overnight.
(2) Neutrophilic granulocytes serve as a built-in positive
control. These cells have very prominent peroxidase-positive
granules. Erythrocytes, which contain catalase, do not stain
by this protocol.
(3) Peroxidase-positive inflammatory macrophages can usually be differentiated from peroxidase-negative macrophages that
have phagocytized peroxidase granules of neutrophilic granulocytes. This artifact must be considered with mixed cell populations with a high percentage of granulocytes.

REFERENCES

1. W. Th. Daems, D. Roos, Th. J. C. Van Berkel, and H. J. Van
    Der Rhee. The subcellular distribution and biochemical
    properties of peroxidase in monocytes and macrophages.
    In "Lysosomes in Biology and Pathology," Volume 6 (J. T.
    Dingle and R. T. Dean, eds.). North Holland, Amsterdam,
    1979.
2. L. S. Kaplow. Simplified myeloperoxidase stain using ben-

zidine dihydrochloride. *Blood 26*: 215-218, 1965.

3. L. P. Ruco and M. S. Meltzer. Macrophage activation for tumor cytotoxicity: Increased lymphokine responsiveness of peritoneal macrophages during acute inflammation. *J. Immunol. 120*: 1054-1062, 1978.

4. R. van Furth, M. M. C. Diesselhoff-Den Dulk, and H. Mattie. Quantitative study on the production and kinetics of mononuclear phagocytes during acute inflammatory reactions. *J. Exp. Med. 138*: 6-22, 1973.

40

USE OF NONSPECIFIC ESTERASE STAIN

Glenn A. Miller
Page S. Morahan

I. INTRODUCTION

Esterases catalyze the hydrolysis of a large number of uncharged carboxylic esters:

$$R_1-\overset{\overset{\textstyle O}{\|}}{C}-O-R_2 \; + \; HOH \; \longrightarrow \; R_1-\overset{\overset{\textstyle O}{\|}}{\underset{\underset{\textstyle OH}{}}{C}} \; + \; R_2-OH$$

Esterase activity has, over the years, been used in conjunction with such activities as adherence and phagocytic tests to identify and quantitate mononuclear phagocytes (1). Esterase activity is generally demonstrated by using α-naphthyl acetate or butyrate as substrates. The naphthol liberated by the enzyme is coupled with a diazonium salt to give an insoluable, brightly colored, azo dye (2, 3).

Most esterase-staining procedures have employed cells
fixed as a smear on glass slides or as cytocentrifuged preparations (2 - 6). The adaptation of Koski *et al.* (1) using
α-naphthyl butyrate is generally reproducible and reliable;
however, it does require cell smears, freshly prepared
reagents, and a minimum of 1 hr to complete the staining procedure. Recently, modifications have been made to permit the
esterase identification of mononuclear phagocytes while the
cells are suspended in a fluid medium (7, 8). These procedures were originally developed for use in the Technicon
automated analysis Hemalog D machine. The procedure that we
shall detail is the latter and has been used as an aid for
the identification of monocytes and macrophages in the studies
of human, rat, and mouse cells (7 - 11).

II. REAGENTS

All materials used in the assay are available premixed
from Technicon Instruments Corporation, Tarrytown, New York
and include the following:

    Solution A, Sodium nitrate, 1% w/v (T01-0530)
    Solution B, Basic fuchsin, 1% w/v (T01-0529)
    Solution C, Sodium cacodylate, 7% (buffer and serum
                lipase inhibitor, T01-0678)
    Solution D, α-naphthyl butyrate (T01-0680)
    Solution E, Saponin formalin fixative (T01-1679)

These reagents are available from the Technicon Corporation,
are stable at room temperature and have a shelf life of about
1 yr.
    Note: Recently the formulas for the various Technicon
monocyte staining reagents became available (11a). It is now
possible either to use stable reagents that are available commercially or that may be prepared in the laboratory as follows:

Solution A (Mononitrite) (for 1 liter contains)
    Water, deionized
    Sodium nitride, 10.00 gm
    (adjust to pH 8 with 0.05 H HCl)
Solution B (Mono dye) (for 1 liter)
    Water, deionized
    Sulfuric acid, 41.20 gm
    Pararosaniline hydrochloride, 10.00 gm
Solution C (Mono buffer) (for 1 liter)
    Water, deionized
    Sodium cacodylate, 70.00 gm

Solution D (Mono sub) (for 1 liter)
    Diethylene glycol
    α-Naphthyl butyrate, 2.45 gm
    Methanol 200 ml
    30% Brij 35 (polyxyethylene lauryl ether)
    in water, 58 ml
Solution E (Mono fix) (for 1 liter)
    Water, deionized
    Diethylene glycol, 478.50 gm
    Formaldehyde (35%), 50 ml
    Sodium acetate, 10.90 gm
    Eserine sulfate, 0.584 gm

We must emphasize, however, that our experience stems exclusively from the use of the commercially available reagents.

III. PROCEDURE

(1) In a 12 × 75 mm disposable glass tube (Tube A) 6 drops of solution A (nitrate) and 6 drops of solution B (dye) are mixed for 1 min to form the unstable hexazonium pararosanilin.

(2) To tube A add 18 drops of solution C (buffer) and 3 drops of solution D (substrate). Set the tube aside.

(3) Add to a second 12 × 75 mm tube (tube B) 2 drops of the test cell suspension at about 10^7 cells/ml. The cell concentration is not critical but should be sufficient to permit easy counting.

(4) To tube B also add 2 drops of fetal calf serum to preserve the osmotic balance of the solution and 4 drops of solution E (fixative). Mix for 40 sec. Since fixation has been shown to influence the esterase activity of a cell population, do not mix longer than 40 sec.

(5) Add the contents of tube B to tube A, mix well and incubate in a 37°C water bath for 12 min.

(6) Fill the wells of a hemacytometer slide, add a coverslip, and count the cells which are stained deeply red.

IV. CALCULATION OF DATA

Generally 200 cells are counted in each sample to determine the percentage of esterase-staining cells.

V. CRITICAL COMMENTS

A. *Typical Reactions*

Nonspecific esterase-staining mononuclear phagocytes are
easily distinguished due to the red or reddish brown staining
pattern produced in esterase-positive cells. Cells that do
not have nonspecific esterase activity appear unstained.
There is generally a good correlation between such markers as
phagocytosis, adherence, presence of prominent lysosomes by
acridine orange fluorescence (12), and the presence of IgG-Fc
receptors in esterase containing cells. Representative results
are presented in Table I.

In Table II is shown the percentage of esterase-staining
cells in various species and under various treatment procedures.
There is good correlation between increases in the number of
cells with staining activity and elicitation procedures.

Our experience, however, has indicated that human monocytes
stain more intensely than rat macrophages that stain more intensely than mouse peritoneal macrophages. Mouse thioglycollate-elicited peritoneal macrophages stained more intensely than

TABLE I. *Correlation of Esterase Activity with Various
Macrophage Markers*

	Range of percentages of activity		
	Phagocytosis	Fc receptor	
Species	*(latex)*	*activity*	*Esterase*
Rat PEC[a]			
Unseparated	*54 – 68*	*68 – 83*	*65 – 75*
Collagen adherent cells[b]	*93 – 98*	*92 – 98*	*94 – 98*
Human PBL[c]			
After preparation			
on Ficoll-hypaque	*ND[d]*	*ND*	*11 – 18*
Nonadherent population			
after adherence of			
monocytes to plastic	*ND*	*ND*	*0.5 – 1.0*

[a]*Corynebacterium parvum-activated peritoneal exudate cells.*
[b]*Peritoneal macrophage population after adherence to collagen, removal of nonadherent cells, and recovery of adherent
cells (8).*
[c]*Peripheral blood lymphocytes.*
[d]*ND, Not determined.*

TABLE II. *Species and Treatment Procedure Variation in Esterase Staining*

		Esterase positive cells (%)		
Species	Resident	Proteose	Thioglycollate	C. parvum
Human[a]	13 - 18	ND[d]	ND	ND
Rat[b]	45 - 55	60 - 70	ND	65 - 75
Mouse[c]	20 - 30	ND	42 - 58	17 - 28

[a]Ficoll-Hypaque separated peripheral blood.
[b]Peritoneal exudate cells of Lewis, Brown Norray or Sprague
[c]Peritoneal exudate cells of CD1 mice.
[d]ND, Not determined.

resident or *Corynebacterium parvum* macrophages; positive cells in the latter groups often appear pink rather than brightly dark red. With some mouse macrophage preparations, the Koski *et al.* (1) method may be more reliable. When investigators from the Technicon Corporation tested peripheral blood of various species for esterase activity according to the method used for human blood, they concluded that only human and rabbit monocytes stained well, while staining of mouse, rat, guinea pig, and bovine monocytes was less reliable (Cremins *et al.*, unpublished observations). In our hands peritoneal macrophages of any type, elicited mouse and rabbit alveolar macrophages, and rabbit splenic macrophages, have all stained deep red.

It is important to reemphasize, however, that no single method will be optimum in identifying mononuclear phagocytes in all situations. Methods aimed at different properties of these cells will need to be tested in order to determine which is most reliable for the particular case; often more than one method will need to be routinely used.

B. *Advantages and Disadvantages*

The assay system as indicated is relatively simple to set up and should be followed as indicated in Section III. It is important to allow the hexazonium pararosanilin to form before dilution with buffer, and fixation should not be permitted to proceed too long. The availability of commercially available reagents that are stable at room temperature is a major convenience of the method. The use of cells in suspension is also an advantage.

The major disadvantage of the method is the price of the reagents. They are available from the Technicon Corporation

only in 3.8 liter quantities each and in the price range of
$750.00, with more than half of the price being attributed to
the substrate. Since such small quantities are involved in
the assay, a single laboratory would not use liter quantities
in several years. The availability of Hemalog D machines in
various cities make the reagents available locally in many
areas and negotiations can be made to acquire the small quantities of the reagents that are needed.

C. Specificity of the Reaction for Mononuclear Phagocytes

Recently, a number of reports have appeared indicating that
localized granules of esterase reaction product, in addition to
being found in mononuclear phagocytes, may also be found in
mature, resting T cells (2, 13 - 18) and in null cells (2).
B cells and lymphocytes with high-affinity Fc receptors for IgG
termed L lymphocytes) and activated T cells appeared to be
negative. There is one report, however, of activity in some
B cells with EAC rosetting capacity (19). The various positively staining cell types, however, may still be differentiated
from each other due to the variety of staining patterns seen.
Mononuclear phagocytes generally show a dotlike granular staining pattern all over the cytoplasm. T cells show a single
granule or several localized granules near the membrane, and
null cells show scattered granular staining patterns (2, 13 -
18). The identification of cells other than those of the monocyte-macrophage group by esterase activity involved an alteration of the various procedures. Time of incubation, fixation
procedure, and type and quantity of substrate all seem important, and results vary substantially from one procedure to another. It would not be surprising for other lymphoid cell types
to demonstrate positivity as variations of the procedure evolve.

REFERENCES

1. I. R. Koski, D. G. Poplack, and R. M. Blaese. A non-
    specific esterase stain for the identification of mono-
    cytes and macrophages. In "In Vitro Methods in Cell-
    Mediated and Tumor Immunity" (B. R. Bloom and J. R. David,
    eds.), pp. 359-362. Academic Press, New York, 1976.
2. K. E. Higgy, G. F. Burns, and F. G. J. Hayhoe. Discrimi-
    nation of B, T, and Null lymphocytes by esterase cytochem-
    istry. J. Haematol. 18: 437-448, 1977.
3. C. Y. Li, K. W. Lam, and L. T. Yam. Esterases in human
    leucocytes. J. Histochem. Cytochem. 21: 1-12, 1973.

4. L. T. Yam, C. Y. Li, and W. H. Crosby. Cytochemical identification of monocytes and granulocytes. *Am. J. Clin. Pathol.* 55: 283-290, 1971.

5. H. Braunstein. Esterase in leukocytes. *J. Histochem. Cytochem.* 7: 202, 1959.

6. L. Rozenszajn, M. Leiberich, D. Shoham, and J. Epstein. The esterase activity in megaloblasts, leukaemic, and normal haemopoetic cells. *Br. J. Haematol.* 14: 605-610, 1968.

7. H. Ansley and L. Ornstein. Enzyme histochemistry and differential white cell counts on the Technicon Hemalog D. *Adv. Automated Anal.* 1: 437-446, 1971.

8. S. B. Tucker and R. E. Jordan. Rapid identification of monocytes in a mixed mononuclear cell preparation. *J. Immunol. Methods* 14: 267-269, 1977.

9. M. W. Campbell, M. M. Sholley, and G. A. Miller. Macrophage heterogeneity in tumor resistance: Cytostatic and cytoxic activity of *Corynebacterium parvum*-activated proteose peptone elicited rat macrophages against Moloney sarcoma tumor cells. *Cell. Immunol.* 50: 153-168, 1980.

10. G. A. Miller, M. W. Campbell, and J. L. Hudson. Separation of rat peritoneal macrophages into functionally distinct subclasses by centrifugal elutriation. *J. Reticuloendothel. Soc.* 27: 167-174, 1980.

11. P. S. Morahan and A. M. Kaplan. Antiviral and antitumor functions of activated macrophages. *In* "Immune Modulation and Control of Neoplasia by Adjuvant Therapy" (M. A. Chirigos, ed.), pp. 447-457. Raven Press, New York, 1978.

11a. C. Lawrence and R. Grossman. Simple butyrate esterase stain for monocytes. *Stain Technol.* 54: 321-323, 1980.

12. A. C. Allison. Fluorescence microscopy of lymphocytes and mononuclear phagocytes and the use of silica to eliminate the latter. *In* "*In Vitro* Methods in Cell-Mediated and Tumor Immunity: (B. R. Bloom and J. R. David, eds.), pp. 395-404. Academic Press, New York, 1976.

13. J. Mueller, G. Brun de Re, H. Buerki, H. U. Keller, M. W. Hess, and H. Cottier. Nonspecific acid esterase activity: A criterion for differentiation of T and B lymphocytes in mouse lymph nodes. *Eur. J. Immunol.* 5: 270-274, 1975.

14. J. Mueller, H. U. Keller, G. Brun de Re, H. Buerki, and M. W. Hess. Nonspecific esterase activity in T cells. *In* "Advances in Experimental Medicine and Biology, Immune Reactivity of Lymphocytes, Development, Expression, and Control: (M. Feldman and A. Globerson, eds.), pp. 117-122. Academic Press, New York, 1976.

15. A. Ranki. Nonspecific esterase activity in human lymphocytes: Histochemical characterization and distribution among major lymphocyte subclasses. *Clin. Immunol. Immunopathol.* 10: 47-58, 1978.

16.   A. Ranki, T. H. Totterman, and P. Hayry. Identification
      of resting human T and B lymphocytes by acid α-naphthyl
      acetate esterase staining combined with rosette formation
      with *Staphylococcus aureus* strain Cowan 1. *Scand. J.
      Immunol. 5*: 1129-1138, 1976.
17.   D. A. Horwitz, A. C. Allison, P. Ward, and N. Knight.
      Identification of human mononuclear leucocyte populations
      by esterase staining. *Clin. Esp. Immunol. 30*: 289-298,
      1977.
18.   D. M. Knowles, H. T. Hoffman, M. Ferrarini, and H. G.
      Kunkel. The demonstration of acid α-naphthyl acetate
      esterase activity in human lymphocytes: Usefulness as a
      T-cell marker. *Cell. Immunol. 35*: 112-123, 1978.
19.   T. J. Yang, P. A. Jantzen, and L. F. Williams. Acid
      α-naphthyl acetate esterase: Presence of activity in
      bovine and human T and B lymphocytes. *Immunology 38*:
      85-93, 1979.

41

HISTOCHEMICAL STAINS FOR MACROPHAGES
IN CELL SMEARS AND TISSUE SECTIONS:
β-GALACTOSIDASE, ACID PHOSPHATASE, NONSPECIFIC ESTERASE,
SUCCINIC DEHYDROGENASE, AND CYTOCHROME OXIDASE

Arthur M. Dannenberg, Jr.
Moritaka Suga

I. INTRODUCTION

Mononuclear phagocytes emigrate from the bloodstream into
sites of inflammation, where they may differentiate (or
mature) into <u>activated</u> macrophages that contain high levels of
lysosomal, mitochondrial, and other enzymes. Our laboratory
uses histochemical procedures to demonstrate some of these enzymes in smears of rabbit pulmonary alveolar macrophages and
peritoneal exudate macrophages, and in frozen, paraffin-embedded
and water-soluble plastic-embedded tissue sections of rabbit
granulomas induced by tubercle bacilli (BCG).
These histochemical stains are not specific for macrophages and therefore cannot be used to differentiate them from
activated fibroblasts, activated (short-lived) lymphocytes,
and perhaps activated endothelial cells. Because BCG preferentially attracts and activates macrophages, we believe that
almost all of the heavily stained mononuclear cells in BCG
granulomas are indeed macrophages, and that many of the more

METHODS FOR STUDYING
MONONUCLEAR PHAGOCYTES

375

lightly stained cells and unstained cells are also macrophages.

Certain types of macrophage activation can be recognized
by certain histochemical stains. In rabbits our most useful
stain is for the lysosomal enzyme, β-galactosidase, which reflects the digestive capacity of these cells (1). Although
the microbicidal capacity of macrophages seems to parallel
their digestive capacity, lysosomes may not be responsible for
the former. Recent studies (2 - 6) suggest that the major
mechanism by which macrophages kill microorganisms is the production of hydrogen peroxidase, superoxide, singlet oxygen,
and hydroxyl radical. Macrophages with strong microbicidal
activity probably have high levels of mitochondrial enzymes
(cytochrome oxidase and succinic dehydrogenase) because these
enzymes are involved with oxygen transport.

In BCG granulomas, the levels of specific digestive enzymes may vary with the substance ingested by the macrophage.
In other words, the levels of acid phosphatase, but not
β-galactosidase, may be high in certain macrophages, and vice
versa (7). However, some enzymes almost always increase together, e.g., esterase and β-galactosidase (7). To obtain
these results, we used a double-staining histochemical technique that combined both naphthol and indoxyl methods (7).

With different incubation times, these methods are applicable to other animal species including man, but we have had
only limited experience with other species. Strong β-galactosidase activity seems to be an ideal marker for activated rabbit macrophages. On the other hand, strong acid phosphatase
activity is a much more satisfactory marker for activated
mouse macrophages.

Many histochemical stains exist for macrophages (see 8 -
18), but only five, which utilize synthetic substrates, are
presented in this chapter. Immunocytochemical techniques have
also been used by our laboratory, namely, specific antibody, a
"bridge", and the peroxidase-antiperoxidase complex (19) to
stain macrophage cathepsin D (20), lysozyme (unpublished), and
RNase (unpublished).

In addition, we have used the Daoust-type substrate film
techniques (21) to stain for RNase, DNase, proteinase, and
hyaluronidase (22). The localization of enzymes by this technique is not as precise as other methods, and negative results
may be due to poor association of the enzyme and substrate
rather than an absence of enzyme. This histochemical technique
is unique in that it directly demonstrates active enzymes that
hydrolyze the major macromolecular components of tissues. Immunocytochemical techniques can identify the presence of an
enzyme but cannot determine whether it is active or not.

Our laboratory has not developed the histochemical reactions herein reported but has applied them to study macrophages

in exudates and bronchial perfusates and in tissue sections of granulomatous lesions. The textbooks and original references should be consulted for the mechanisms, reliability, specificity, stability, and other characteristics of each histochemical stain.

II. GENERAL PROCEDURES

A. *Procedures for Macrophage Suspensions (23)*

1. *Rabbit Peritoneal Exudate Mononuclear Phagocytes (MN)*

MN were elicited in rabbits by the intraperitoneal injection of 35 ml of mineral oil (U.S.P.). Five to 6 days later, the animals were killed by exsanguination, and their peritoneal cavities washed with citrate-saline (0.4% sodium citrate in 0.85% sodium chloride) or Hanks' solution (24), containing 0.01% heparin. The exudate cells were filtered through gauze and collected by gentle centrifugation (2000 for 5 min). Total counts ranged from 30 to 150 million cells per exudate, with a mean of about 80 million. Differential cell counts employing Wright's stain ranged from 80 to 99% MN, with a mean of about 95%. A high percentage of the mononuclear cells were of medium size with fairly basophilic cytoplasm that sometimes contained mineral oil vacuoles. The other cells in these exudates included larger, paler MN, PMN, and occasional lymphocytes and mesothelial cells.

2. *Alveolar Macrophages*

Alveolar macrophages (AM) were obtained by a method adapted from that of Myrvik *et al.* (25). Specifically, about 35 ml of 0.85% NaCl, citrate-saline, or heparinized Hanks' solution were injected intratracheally after removal of the lungs from a recently sacrificed rabbit. The fluid was then allowed to drain out. This procedure was repeated two or more times; and the washings were pooled, centrifuged, and counted in a manner similar to that used for the peritoneal exudates. Total counts averaged about 20 million cells; differential counts averaged 98% AM and 2% PMN.

3. *Viability*

The viabilities of the exudate cells were determined by the trypan blue and eosin methods. These methods, adapted from others (26 - 29), consisted of mixing, on a microscope

slide, one drop of exudate, one drop of autologous serum, and
a third of a drop of 1% trypan blue or 0.5% eosin Y in 0.85%
NaCl solution, covering the mixture with a coverslip, and incubating it at 37°C for 10 min. Examination under the microscope revealed stained cells (dead) and unstained cells (alive).
AM and MN averaged 93 to 99% viability with trypan blue. With
eosin, the viabilities of all three types of cells appeared 5
to 10% less than with trypan blue, but the reason for this discrepancy is not known. High degrees of viability were also
found in phagocytosis studies on AM, MN, and PMN (30), which
have been shown by Tullis (31) to be a more rigorous criterion
than dye-permeability tests.

4. Cell Smears

The cells were smeared on clean glass slides, on coverslips
or Mylar strips (23). The slides sometimes were first coated
with 1% gelatin (Bacto-Gelatin, Catalog No. B143, Difco Laboratories, Inc., Detroit, Michigan 48201) to aid their sticking.
Although the results described here were made on unfixed dried
MN and AM preparations, mild fixation in cold buffered glutaraldehyde is sometimes recommended to decrease enzyme diffusion
into the incubating solutions (see Section II.B.3).

B. Procedures for Tissue Sections (32)

1. Biopsies

We have had the most experience with granulomas produced in
the skin of rabbits by the intradermal inoculation of the BCG
strain of *Mycobacterium bovis*. Four to 40 days after the onset
of the BCG lesions, biopsies were taken. Local 1% procaine
was used to encircle (but not infiltrate) the lesion. It was
cut through its center, and twice again, 3 mm to each side of
the center. The wound was then sewed with surgical silk.

2. Fixation

Various fixatives are mentioned in this report. Most seem
satisfactory, but we have not made a comparison of their relative advantages and disadvantages.

3. Frozen Sections

Biopsies of the lesions were quickly frozen in semisolid
isopentane cooled in liquid nitrogen (33). They were sealed in
Parafilm (American Can Co., Dixie/Marathon, Greenwich, Connecticut 06830) and stored at -25°C until sectioned at 6 μm in a

cryostat; the sections were collected on glass slides (subbed
with 1.0% gelatin) and stored in a desiccator over silica gel
at 4°C until used. At that time, those to be stained for
β-galactosidase, acid phosphatase, and esterase were fixed in
1.25% glutaraldehyde in 0.15 M phosphate buffer (pH 7.2) for
5 min at 4°C. This fixative was not used in our laboratory before staining for succinic dehydrogenase and cytochrome oxidase. However, after the sections were stained for each of the
five enzymes, they were fixed in 4% formaldehyde (made from
paraformaldehyde) in 0.15 M sodium phosphate buffer (pH 7.2)
for 5 min at room temperature, washed 3 times in distilled
water, and counterstained with hematoxylin (see Section II.C).

4. Paraffin-Embedded Sections

Biopsies of the BCG lesions were fixed in cold 4% paraformaldehyde in 0.15 M sodium phosphate (pH 7.2) for 24 hr at
4°C on a mechanical rocker. They were washed in two changes
of cold (4°C) 0.15 M sodium phosphate buffer (pH 7.2) each for
20 to 24 hr on a mechanical rocker. They were dehydrated at
room temperature in 80, 80, 95, 100, and 100% ethanol for 1.5
hr each. They were then placed in two changes (1 hr each) of
xylene and melted paraffin (65°C), embedded in paraffin, and
sectioned at 5 μm onto slides subbed with 1% gelatin. The
paraffin was removed by passing the sections through two
changes of xylene (5 min each), 100% ethanol (3 sec), 95%
ethanol (3 sec), 75% ethanol (3 sec), and three changes of
distilled water for 5 min each.

5. Water-Soluble Methacrylate (JB-4) Embedded Sections (32)

Biopsies were fixed in 2.0% paraformaldehyde and 2.5% glutaraldehyde in 0.02 M cacodylate buffer (pH 7.4) containing
0.025% CaCl$_2$. This is Dvorak's (34) modification of Karnovsky's
fixative (35). For histochemistry, fixation for 16 to 18 hr at
4°C is advised. For general staining (see below), 3 to 18 hr
at 23°C were used. After washing for several hours in cacodylate buffer, they were dehydrated in 75, 85, 95, 100 and 100%
ethanol for 15 min each.
     The JB-4 embedding system is supplied by Polysciences, Inc.
(Paul Valley Industrial Park, Warrington, Pennsylvania 18976)
and used according to their instructions. It contains three
components: (a) the plastic solution A (which is of unre-
vealed composition, but probably contains glycol methacrylate); (b) the polymerizer (solution B); and (c) an organic
peroxide catalyst. The dehydrated biopsies are infiltrated in
catalyzed solution A overnight with gentle rocking. They are
then transferred to plastic molds (Sorvall Division of Dupont
Instruments, Norwalk, Connecticut 06470), and covered with the

catalyzed solution A to which has been added solution B. The
rate of polymerization depends on the ratios of plastic A to
polymerizer B. Our laboratory routinely uses 40:1, which
usually hardens at room temperature overnight. When filled,
the wells are covered with metal block holders (Dupont -
Sorvall), to which the plastic adheres upon hardening. Exclusion of oxygen (e.g., sealing the mold with paraffin) hastens
hardening. Sections of the plastic blocks (1 - 2.5 µm) were
cut with glass knives on a Dupont - Sorvall JB-4 microtome.
They were mounted on clean glass slides subbed with solution A.

C. Stains

1. Counterstains

Our standard counterstain is Harris' hematoxylin (ACCRA-
LAB, Inc., Bridgeport, New Jersey 08014). Cell smears and
frozen sections from tissues that had not been already fixed
in formalin were fixed before counterstaining for 5 min in
buffered 4% formaldehyde (see Section II.B.3). Frozen sections,
deparaffinized sections, and plastic sections were stained
about 3, 5, and 8 min, respectively, washed in distilled water,
dipped in 1% HCl in 70% ethanol for 1 to 3 sec (but not the
plastic sections), washed three times in distilled water,
dipped in 0.35% $NaHCO_3$ - 2% $MgSO_4$ solution for 30 sec, washed
in distilled water, and mounted in glycerin jelly mounting
medium (Fisher Scientific Co., Fairlawn, New Jersey 07410).

2. Stains for Plastic-Embedded Sections

(a) Toluidine-blue (1% aqueous) is applied directly to the
section for 1 to 3 min. The slide is rinsed in tap water,
air-dried, and mounted in Flo-Texx (Lerner Laboratories, Stam-
ford, Connecticut 06902, available from Scientific Products,
Columbia, Maryland 21045). This stain is excellent for basophils, mast cells, and nuclear morphology.
(b) Lee's methylene blue-basic fuchsin stain is described
in "Data Sheet 123" that comes with Polyscience's JB-4 kit as
follows:

Stock solutions: (a) 0.13 grams methylene blue in 100 ml
deionized water; (b) 0.13 gm basic fuchsin in 100 ml deionized
water; (c) 0.20 M sodium phosphate buffer, pH 7.6.
Staining solution: Mix 12 ml of methylene blue solution,
12 ml of basic fuchsin solution, 21 ml of 0.2 M phosphate buffer, and 15 ml of ethanol (95% or absolute). This filtered
solution can be used for four or five days.
Staining procedure: The sections are immersed in the

staining solution for 10 - 15 sec. The slides are removed,
dipped briefly into deionized water, and blown dry with a
blast of clean, inert gas. The dried slides are mounted under
a coverslip with Flo-Texx.

This is a good general stain, although the granules of PMN are
not well stained.

   (c) Giemsa stain. A buffered Giemsa stain is our preference for sections of inflammatory lesions (36): 5 ml of stock
Giemsa solution (Harleco No. 620, Philadelphia, Pennsylvania
19143) is added to 45 ml of TRIS-maleate buffer (0.05 M, pH
5.5) containing 0.5 ml of glycerol. The solution is mixed for
10 min on a magnetic stirrer and then filtered through Whatman
No. 1 paper (or equivalent). The plastic sections are immersed in the filtered stain for 30 to 90 min. The sections
are then rinsed in water, blown dry, and mounted in Flo-Texx.
This stain is excellent for nuclear morphology, for all leukocytes, and for vascular basement membranes. Staining times
and pH levels may have to be adjusted for optimal results, depending on the type of fixation and the type of tissue. Higher
pH levels enhance basophilic staining, while lower pH levels
enhance eosinophilic staining.

   (d) Other stains. Stains including Wright's, Giemsa,
azure-eosin, and silver stains, may be used but modifications
in composition (from those used with paraffin sections) are
usually required to produce the best results.

D. *Precautions*

   1. *Specificity Controls*

Control specimens without substrate should always be run.
When specific inhibitors exist, they should be used (see
references 23, 32, and 37 for details). It is also important
to choose an incubation time in the range where both heavily
and lightly stained cells are present (23).

   2. *Stability of Reagents*

In general, the dry histochemical reagents herein described are rather stable. We store them in the refrigerator
at 4°C. Cytochrome c, however, is stored in the freezer at
-23°C. Care must be taken not to allow the various reagents
to absorb moisture when removing samples. Different lots,
obtained from the same or different manufacturers, may vary.
The time of incubation of new and old lots should, therefore,
be compared.

3. Safety

Many histochemical reagents are carcinogenic, especially the naphthyl compounds. Naphthylamines and *p*-aminodiphenylamine are classic examples that produce cancer in man. Many of the stable diazo compounds used in histochemistry may also be carcinogenic. In handling these compounds, care should be taken not to inhale them as powders or as spray while pipetting solutions. They may also be absorbed through the skin. A hood, mask, and gloves should be used if inhalation and/or contact with the skin are likely; thorough washing of hands before eating should be standard procedure.

III. β-GALACTOSIDASE

A. Introduction

The indolyl method for the histochemical demonstration of β-galactosidase was developed by Pearson (38). When liberated by enzyme action in aqueous solutions exposed to air, the substituted indolyl oxidizes to the corresponding indoxyl and self-couples to form an indigo blue derivative. This colored compound is insoluble in alcohol, xylene, and permanent mounting media. In contrast, the frequently used diazo-coupled naphthols are often soluble in organic solvents, so that an aqueous mounting medium (e.g., glycerol gelatin) is usually required. The ability of the indigo blue derivative to withstand organic solvents enabled us to stain 6 μm sections of BCG lesions for tubercle bacilli after staining the sections for β-galactosidase (33, 39). Subsequently, we could also autoradiograph these sections (33, 39) (if the macrophages had incorporated tritiated thymidine).

B. Reagents

5-Bromo-4-chloro-3-indolyl-β-D-galactoside (Catalog No. B 4252, Sigma Chemical Co., P.O. Box 14508, St. Louis, Missouri 63178)
    Potassium ferricyanide
    Potassium ferrocyanide
    Spermidine hydrochloride
    Sodium acetate buffer
    Sodium chloride
    N,N-Dimethylformamide

Potassium ferriferrocyanide (0.05 M) is made up as follows: 210 mg potassium ferrocyanide in 5.0 ml of distilled water is mixed with 165 mg potassium ferricyanide in 5.0 ml of distilled water.

For stability the reader is referred to Section II.D.2.

In regard to safety, we do not know whether or not this substituted galactoside is carcinogenic. Dimethylformamide is hepatotoxic and irritating to the skin, eyes, and mucous membranes.

C. Procedure

Unfixed cell smears and unfixed frozen sections are fixed for 5 min either in cold (4°C) 1.25% glutaraldehyde in 0.15 M sodium phosphate buffer (pH 7.2), or in cold (4°C) 4% formaldehyde in the same buffer.

5-Bromo-4-chloro-3-indolyl-β-D-galactoside (2 mg) was dissolved in 0.5 ml of dimethylformamide, and then 31 ml of 0.10 M acetate buffer (pH 5.4), 0.5 ml of 0.085% NaCl, 8 mg of spermidine hydrochloride, and 3.0 ml of 0.05 M potassium ferriferrocyanide were added. The cell exudate smears and frozen tissue sections were generally incubated at 37°C for 18 hr, although 5 hr were satisfactory. The paraffin- and plastic-embedded sections were incubated at 37°C for 24 to 48 hr. After incubation, they were rinsed with three changes of distilled water, counterstained with Harris' hematoxylin (see Section II.C), and mounted in glycerin-gelatin (see Section II.C). Alternatively they can be cleared in ascending alcohols and xylene, and mounted in permanent mounting medium (Permount, Catalog No. So-P-15, Fisher Scientific Company, King of Prussia, Pennsylvania 19406).

D. Comments

In our laboratory, this method proved to be ideal for studying the digestive-type of activation of rabbit macrophages. The blue-green color resulting from β-galactosidase activity varies from zero in unactivated macrophages to almost black in strongly activated macrophages. This color is readily distinguishable from the pure blue color of the hematoxylin counterstain.

Fixed and unfixed frozen sections and paraffin-embedded sections give satisfactory results. However, plastic-embedded sections give variable results: sometimes excellent and sometimes poor (i.e., very weak). Fixation and embedding at 4°C seems to correct this trouble.

A good stain is defined as one with a strong color, good

localization (i.e., less diffusion), and reliability (i.e., consistent results). With these criteria, β-galactosidase is our best stain for rabbit macrophages in fixed and unfixed exudate smears (23, 37) and in frozen sections (32). β-galactosidase and acid phosphatase, are equally good in paraffin sections (32), and in plastic (JB-4) sections that were fixed and embedded at 4°C.

Control cells and sections should always be run without the β-galactoside substrate, because occasionally the smears and sections contained cells that stained a granular blue-green color, apparently due to iron (Fe^{3+}) in these cells reacting with the ferrocyanide in the staining solution. [Ferricyanide is added as a catalyst to hasten the oxidation of the liberated indolyl to the insoluble indigo dye (9). Ferrocyanide is added to prevent further oxidation to a colorless dehydroindigo compound (9).]

The indolyl blue-green color resembles Prussian blue, but it is unusually diffuse and not granular. The number of false-positive cells were usually less than 3% of the number of β-galactosidase-positive cells in cell smears and in frozen and paraffin-embedded sections of BCG lesions, but varied from 0 to 20%. Many were macrophages, some were fibroblasts and dermal epithelial cells.

Three effective, specific inhibitors exist for β-galactosidase (37): (a) 1% galactose; (b) 1% 1,4-galactonolactone; and (c) 1% o-nitrophenyl-β-galactopyranoside.

IV. ACID PHOSPHATASE

A. *Introduction*

In histochemistry, acid phosphatase is the classic lysosomal enzyme. [This activity probably represents more than one enzyme (8).] It is demonstrable by Gomori's lead substitution method with glycerophosphate as the substrate (see 40, 8), as well as with naphthyl phosphate substrates and simultaneous diazo coupling, developed by Seligman and others (8). The lead substitution method has localized acid phosphatase in the phagosomes of macrophages (41, 8) and can be used for electron microscopy. Our laboratory, however, has only used Burstone's diazo coupling methods described below (42, 43, 8).

B. Reagents

Naphthol AS-BI phosphoric acid (sodium salt) (Catalog No. N2250, Sigma Chemical Co., P.O. Box 14508, St. Louis, Missouri 63178)

Fast red-violet LB salt (Catalog No. UN 1485, Verona Dyestuffs, Division of Verona-Pharma Chemical Corp., Springfield Rd., Union, New Jersey 07083)

Sodium acetate buffer (pH 5.2)

$MnCl_2$

N,N-dimethylformamide

For stability the reader is referred to Section II.D.2.
For precautions the reader is referred to Sections II.D.3 and III.B.

C. Procedure

We recommend fixation of <u>unfixed</u> cells and frozen tissue sections as in Section III.C. However, our studies with cell smears were made on dried, unfixed preparations (23) before we adopted this procedure.

Five mg of naphthol AS-BI phosphate was dissolved in 0.5 ml of dimethylformamide. Fifty ml of 0.1 M acetate buffer (pH 5.2) and 10 mg of fast red-violet LB were added and also two drops of 10% $MnCl_2$ solution as a possible activator. The somewhat opalescent solution was then filtered. The exudate cell smears and frozen tissue sections were incubated in this solution at 23°C for 10 to 60 min (23, 32). The paraffin and plastic sections were incubated at 37°C for 6 to 24 hr (32).

After incubation, the rinsing and counterstaining procedures were the same as in Section III.C. However, this azo dye product must be mounted in glycerin-gelatin, and cannot be cleared and mounted in Permount.

D. Comment

The red azo dye granules formed in <u>peritoneal exudate macrophages</u> usually were discrete, fairly uniform in size, and almost never small enough to create a diffuse appearance (23). This enzyme was rather stable, for such macrophages still showed activity after several months of storage at -25°C (23). Because of these properties, MN acid phosphatase was used to establish the granule count method (23) to quantitate time, pH, substrate concentration, and inhibitor (NaF) relationships in a relative manner. [No histochemical procedure gives quantitation in a biochemical sense, because an unknown amount of enzyme is denatured during cell and tissue preparation and incubation with diazonium salts (8).] The dye deposits in alveolar macrophages were both diffuse and granular, so they could not be as accurately quantitated. Sodium molybdate (0.005 M) and sodium fluoride (0.01 M) are effective inhibitors of macrophage acid phosphatase (23).

With unfixed exudate cells, the dye granules probably do not localize in lysosomes. However, more accurate localization (which may relate to lysosomes) can be obtained by fixing dried, smeared exudate cells for 5 min as described in Section III.C.

In unfixed and fixed frozen sections, and in fixed paraffin- and plastic-embedded sections, the diazo method usually produces a nongranular reaction product. In these sections, it is doubtful that individual lysosomes were stained. Both fixed and unfixed frozen sections showed some dye diffusion, but were satisfactory. Paraffin sections showed no dye diffusion and stained excellently. Plastic sections stained the best of all.

V. ESTERASE

A. Introduction

There are several histochemical substrates for the nonspecific esterases (9). None will identify a given enzyme because overlapping substrate specificities (as well as isozymes) exist (9). Various inhibitors help group these esterases (9) (see Section V.D). Tsuda et al. (44) found that different substrates stained different cell populations. Li et al. (45) evaluated the several histochemical esterase substrates on human granulocytes, monocytes, lymphocytes, plasma cells, mast cells, and megakaryocytes. The substrate used determined which cells stained.

We only evaluated two substrates: naphthyl AS-D acetate and indoxyl acetate (7). They both stained the same macrophage population in rabbit dermal BCG lesions. Burstone's naphthyl AS-D acetate procedure (23, 46) is presented here.

B. Reagents

Naphthol AS-D acetate (Cat. No. N2875, Sigma Chemical Co., P.O. Box 14508, St. Louis, MO 63178)

Fast garnet GBC salt (practical grade) (Cat. No. F0875, Sigma Chemical Co.)

Tris buffer: Tris(hydroxymethyl)aminomethane ("Trizma

base" reagent grade, Cat. No. T1503, Sigma Chemical Co.)
N,*N*-Dimethylformamide

For stability the reader is referred to Section II.D.2.
For precautions the reader is referred to Sections II.D.3
and III.B.

C. *Procedure*

We recommend <u>fixation</u> of unfixed cells and frozen tissue
sections as in Section III.C. However, our studies with cell
smears were made on dried, unfixed preparations (23) before we
adopted this procedure.
Naphthol AS-D acetate (5 mg) was dissolved in 0.5 ml of
dimethylformamide, and 50 ml of 0.10 *M* Tris buffer at pH 7.1
was added, followed by fast garnet GBC (10 mg). The mixture
was then filtered, and the cell exudate smears and frozen tissue sections were incubated for 3 to 40 min at room temperature (23°C). The paraffin-embedded sections were incubated
for 3 to 6 hr at 37°C. Plastic-embedded sections were incubated for 5 to 24 hr at 37°C.

D. *Comments*

With fast garnet GBC as the diazo-coupling agent, the
reaction product varies in color from a bright brown-red to a
dark brown-black. The dark color probably represents two
naphthol AS-D molecules bound to one fast garnet GBC molecule.
The reaction product may be diffuse or granular in nature.
The azo dye granules produced ranged in size. Some of
them were so small that a diffuse appearance resulted whereas
some were as large as the average bacterium. The esterase of
both intact and injured MN, PMN, and AM in smears seemed
rather stable in the deep freezer (23). AM were darkly
stained; MN and PMN were weakly to moderately stained. Macrophages and plasma cells in tissue sections frequently stained
strongly.
Sodium azide (0.01 *M*) and diisopropyl fluorophosphate
(DFP) (0.001 *M*) are effective inhibitors of the naphthol AS-D
esterase activity (23). Sodium fluoride (0.01 *M*) inhibits
PMN esterase activity and partly inhibits MN esterase activity,
but does not inhibit AM esterase activity (23). A classification of the various esterases is presented by Pearse (9). It
is based on using a variety of inhibitors. Macrophages probably contain more than one type of esterase [see Section V.A and
(44)].
In tissue sections, the pH 7.1 results in some nonspecific

background staining that can be eliminated by incubating the
substrate and diazo coupler at pH 6.0. This lower pH causes
some decrease in esterase activity. It is recommended for
plastic- and paraffin-embedded sections.

A few paraffin sections of BCG lesions were stained with
naphthol AS-D chloroacetate (Catalog No. N3000, Sigma Chemical Co.) using 0.10 M potassium phosphate buffer at pH 6.0
(instead of Tris) and fast garnet GBC at 10X the above concentrations (47). Under these conditions, rabbit PMN and perhaps
mast cells stained much more quickly and strongly than macrophages. A 3-hr incubation time was used.

VI. SUCCINIC DEHYDROGENASE

A. *Introduction*

Succinic dehydrogenase, a mitochondrial enzyme linked with
the cytochrome system, participates in the Krebs' tricarboxylic
acid cycle of aerobic metabolism. Its activity is among the
first to disappear when a cell dies (48, 49). Therefore, its
presence (detected histochemically) suggests that the cell containing it was viable at the time of biopsy.

We use the nitro blue tetrazolium (Nitro BT) method developed by the Seligman group (50, 23).

B. *Reagents*

Nitro blue tetrazolium (2,2'-di-p-nitrophenyl-5,5'-
diphenyl-3,3'-(3,3'-dimethoxy-4,4'-biphenylene) ditetrazolium
chloride (Catalog No. N6876, Sigma Chemical Co., P.O. Box
14508, St. Louis, Missouri 63178)
Sodium succinate
Ethanol
Tris buffer [Tris(hydroxymethyl)aminomethane] (Sigma
Chemical Co.)
For stability the reader is referred to Section II.D.2.
For precautions the reader is referred to Section II.D.3.
We do not know whether tetrazolium salts are carcinogenic or
not.

C. Procedure

We recommend fresh cell smears and fresh frozen sections with no fixation before staining for succinic dehydrogenase (but see Section VI.D.).

Nitro BT (10 mg) dissolved in 0.5 ml of ethanol was added to 500 mg of sodium succinate dissolved in 40 ml of 0.10 M Tris buffer at pH 7.4, and the solution was filtered. Cells and tissue sections on glass slides were incubated in this solution at 37°C for 0.5 to 3 hr. We usually use 90 min for each type of preparation. The cells and sections were then washed in saline, lightly counterstained with hematoxylin (see Section VI.D.), and mounted in glycerol gelatin.

D. Comments

1. Peritoneal and Pulmonary Alveolar Macrophages (MN and AM)

The formazan granules formed by the reduction of nitro BT are blue-black and show considerable variation in size. Morphologically intact MN and AM frequently show high succinic dehydrogenase activity, especially the AM, which have a more aerobic metabolism (23). A red product due to half-reduction or other factors may occur in areas of low enzyme activity (9), but we have never seen this in our preparations.

Nitro BT is reduced by a variety of substances in cellular oxidoreductase systems. Positive reactions may therefore occur in controls where sodium succinate has been omitted from the incubating solution. With PMN, these control reactions are often as strong as the reactions containing the succinate substrate; but with monocytes and alveolar macrophages, they are usually much weaker. Thus, this histochemical stain is not always specific for succinic dehydrogenase and caution must be exercised in stating that the cells were stained for this enzyme. In general, smears of PMN, MN, and AM stain with increasing intensities.

2. Tissue Sections

Frozen sections can be stained for succinic dehydrogenase. Minimal fixation (10 min in cold formol-calcium) is recommended by Pearse (9), but we tried 5 min in cold (4°C) buffered glutaraldehyde and found that it destroyed the succinic dehydrogenase activity of macrophages in dried cell smears and frozen tissue sections. The fixation and embedding procedures involved in preparing paraffin- and plastic-embedded sections destroy the activity of this enzyme (32). This loss of activity

is at least partly due to the extraction of mitochondrial ubi-
quinone (coenzyme Q) (9), which is probably the intermediate
electron carrier.

As with cell exudates, controls without sodium succinate
must be run in order to determine whether this oxidoreductase
reaction is specific for this substrate.

In BCG lesions, macrophages showing high succinic dehydrogenase (SD) activity may or may not be the same cells as those
showing high activity for the other four enzymes discussed in
this chapter. We did not study SD with double-staining techniques (7). In the intact tissue bordering the caseous center
of such lesions, many macrophages became rich in this enzyme,
just as many became rich in the other four enzymes (51).

Sometimes the hematoxylin counterstain obscures the blue-
black formazan color. If so, other counterstains may be
used, e.g., methyl green (9).

Sodium malonate (0.05 M) is a specific inhibitor of this
enzyme. Sodium azide (0.01 M) and sodium or potassium cyanide
(0.01 M) are the inhibitors recommended by Pearse (9).

VII. CYTOCHROME OXIDASE

A. *Introduction*

The mitochondrial enzyme cytochrome oxidase catalyzes the
terminal oxidation of metabolic hydrogen by molecular oxygen
(11). It seems to be more stable in cells and tissue sections
than succinic dehydrogenase. Since these enzymes are involved
in the oxygen metabolism of macrophages, their levels may correlate with the ability of macrophages to produce H_2O_2, O_2^-,
$^1O_2$, and $OH\cdot$, and therefore may reflect in tissue sections the
microbicidal powers of these cells (2 - 6). The Burstone
stain (52, 53, 23) described here is quite satisfactory provided cytochrome c is added (11, 12).

B. *Reagents*

8-Amino-1,2,3,4-tetrahydroquinoline (Grade II, practical,
Catalog No. A3755, Sigma Chemical Co., P.O. Box 14508, St.
Louis, Missouri 63178)

p-Aminodiphenylamine (British Drug Houses, Ltd., Poole,
England; also available as Catalog No. A5379, Sigma Chemical
Co.)

Ethanol
Tris buffer [Tris(hydroxymethyl)aminomethane] (Sigma

Chemical Co.)
Cytochrome *c* (Type II-A, practical grade, from Horse Heart,
Catalog No. C7010, Sigma Chemical Co.)
Cobalt acetate
Formalin
Sodium acetate buffer

For stability the reader is referred to Section II.D.2.
For precautions see Section II.D.3. Utmost care should be
exercised in handling *p*-aminodiphenylamine, which is the most
carcinogenic of all the compounds mentioned in this chapter.
The inhibitor NaCN is very poisonous, as is the gas HCN which
is released upon acidification of NaCN solutions. Sodium
azide (NaN$_3$) is also poisonous.

C. Procedure

Cytochrome oxidase. We recommend fixation of unfixed cells
and frozen tissue sections as in Section III.C. However, our
studies with cell smears were made on dried, unfixed preparations (23) before we adopted this procedure.

8-Amino-1,2,3,4-tetrahydroquinoline (10 mg) and *p*-aminodi-
phenylamine (10 mg) were dissolved in 0.5 ml of ethanol and
made up to 50 ml with 0.10 M Tris buffer at pH 7.4. The solution was then filtered into a Coplin jar and 10 mg of cytochrome *c* was added. Slides containing tissue sections or
smeared exudate cells were then incubated in the solution for
1/2 to 2 hr at room temperature (23°C). A blue-black color
resulted.

The preparations were then fixed for 1 hr in a solution
containing 10% of each of the following materials: cobalt
acetate, formalin (37% HCHO), and 0.20 M sodium acetate buffer
(pH 5.2). They were washed in water and covered with a glass
coverslip using glycerin-gelatin. No counterstain is used,
because this stain lightly colors most of the tissue section.

D. Comments

1. Peritoneal and Pulmonary Alveolar Macrophages (MN and AM)

Rabbit macrophages can be graded ± to 4+ in staining intensity, although this range is about one-half that of
β-galactosidase: The 4+ β-galactosidase color would be about
twice as dark as the 4+ cytochrome oxidase color. Rabbit alveolar macrophages stain intensely; peritoneal exudate macrophages, moderately; and peritoneal exudate PMN, weakly (23).

Catalase (which destroys H_2O_2) had no apparent effect on the enzyme's activity, which suggests that cytochrome oxidase, rather than peroxidase (9) is demonstrated by this reaction. NaCN (0.001 M), Na_2S (0.01 M) and NaN_3 (0.01 M) were partially inhibitory (23, 12).

2. Tissue Sections

This cytochrome oxidase stain is satisfactory for unfixed frozen sections (32), for frozen sections fixed as in Section III.C, and for JB-4 plastic-embedded sections (32) fixed for 18 hr at 4°C in 2.5% glutaraldehyde and 2.0% paraformaldehyde cacodylate buffer (pH 7.3). Standard paraffin-embedded sections show negative to weak staining (32).

Like succinic dehydrogenase (see Section VI.D), cytochrome oxidase is high in macrophages in the viable tissue at the edge of the caseous center of BCG lesions. These macrophages may or may not be the same cells as those rich in other enzymes, since we did not study cytochrome oxidase with double-staining techniques.

Acknowledgments

The techniques for staining of plastic sections were provided by Robert F. Vogt, Jr., of our laboratory. Dr. Philip L. Sannes, of our Department, and Dr. John R. Esterly, of the University of Chicago School of Medicine, critically reviewed this manuscript.

Supported by Grant HL-14153 from the National Heart, Lung, and Blood Institute, U.S. Public Health Service, for the Johns Hopkins Specialized Center on Lung; Contract DAMD-17-80-C-0102, U.S. Army Medical Research and Development Command; and Grants ES-01879 and ES-00454 from the National Institute of Environmental Health Sciences, U.S. Public Health Service.

REFERENCES

1. M. Ando, A. M. Dannenberg, Jr., M. Sugimoto, and B. Tepper. Histochemical studies relating the activation of macrophages to the intracellular destruction of tubercle bacilli. *Am. J. Pathol. 86*: 623-633, 1977.
2. R. B. Johnston, Jr., C. A. Godzik, and Z. A. Cohn. Increased superoxide anion production by immunologically activated and chemically elicited macrophages. *J. Exp. Med. 148*: 115-127, 1978.

3. C. F. Nathan, L. H. Brukner, S. C. Silverstein, and Z. A. Cohn. Extracellular cytolysis by activated macrophages and granulocytes. I. Pharmacologic triggering of effector cells and the release of hydrogen peroxide. *J. Exp. Med.* *149*: 84-99, 1979.

4. C. F. Nathan, S. C. Silverstein, L. H. Brukner, and Z. A. Cohn. Extracellular cytolysis by activated macrophages and granulocytes. II. Hydrogen peroxide as a mediator of cytotoxicity. *J. Exp. Med.* *149*: 100-113, 1979.

5. H. W. Murray and Z. A. Cohn. Macrophage oxygen-dependent antimicrobial activity. I. Susceptibility of *Toxoplasma gondii* to oxygen intermediates. *J. Exp. Med.* *150*: 938-949, 1979.

6. H. W. Murray, C. W. Juangbhanich, C. F. Nathan, and Z. A. Cohn. Macrophage oxygen-dependent antimicrobial activity. II. The role of oxygen intermediates. *J. Exp. Med.* *150*: 950-964, 1979.

7. M. Suga, A. M. Dannenberg, Jr., and S. Higuchi. Macrophage functional heterogeneity *in vivo*: Macrolocal and microlocal macrophage activation, identified by double-staining tissue sections of BCG granulomas for pairs of enzymes. *Am. J. Pathol.* *99*: 195-212, 1980.

8. A. G. E. Pearse. "Histochemistry, Theoretical and Applied," Vol. 1, 3rd ed. Little, Brown, & Co., Boston, Massachusetts, 1968.

9. A. G. E. Pearse. "Histochemistry, Theoretical and Applied," Vol. 2, 3rd ed. The Williams & Wilkins Co., Baltimore, Maryland, 1972.

10. R. D. Lillie and H. M. Fullmer. "Histopathologic Technic and Practical Histochemistry," 4th ed. McGraw-Hill, New York, 1976.

11. T. Barka and P. J. Anderson. "Histochemistry Theory, Practice and Bibliography." Harper & Row, Hoeber Medical Division, New York, 1963.

12. M. S. Burstone. "Enzyme Histochemistry and Its Application in the Study of Neoplasms." Academic Press, New York 1962.

13. J. F. A. McManus and R. W. Mowry. "Staining Methods Histologic and Histochemical." Harper & Row, Hoeber Medical Division, New York, 1965.

14. H. A. Davenport. "Histological and Histochemical Technics." W. B. Saunders Co., Philadelphia, Pennsylvania, 1964.

15. E. Gurr. "Methods of Analytical Histology and Histo-Chemistry." The Williams & Wilkins Co., Baltimore, Maryland, 1959.

16. J. D. Bancroft. "An Introduction to Histochemical Technique." Appleton-Century-Crofts, New York, 1967.

17. S. W. Thompson. "Selected Histochemical and Histopatho-

logical Methods." Charles C. Thomas, Springfield, Illinois, 1974.

18. P. R. Lewis and D. P. Knight. "Staining Methods for
Sectioned Material." North Holland, Amsterdam, 1977.

19. L. A. Sternberger. "Immunocytochemistry." 2nd ed.,
Wiley, New York, 1979.

20. O. Rojas-Espinosa, A. M. Dannenberg, Jr., L. A. Sternberger, and T. Tsuda. The role of cathepsin D in the
pathogenesis of tuberculosis. *Am. J. Pathol. 74*: 1-12,
1974.

21. R. Daoust. Histochemical localization of enzyme activities by substrate film methods: Ribonucleases, deoxy-
ribonucleases, proteases, amylase, and hyaluronidase.
Int. Rev. Cytol. 18: 191-221, 1965.

22. T. Tsuda, A. M. Dannenberg, Jr., M. Ando, O. Rojas-
Espinosa, and K. Shima. Enzymes in tuberculous lesions
hydrolyzing protein, hyaluronic acid, and chondroitin
sulfate: A study of isolated macrophages and developing
and healing rabbit BCG lesions with substrate film techniques; the shift of enzyme pH optima towards neutrality
in "intact" cells and tissues. *J. Reticuloendothel. Soc.
16*: 220-231, 1974.

23. A. M. Dannenberg, Jr., M. S. Burstone, P. C. Walter, and
J. W. Kinsley. A histochemical study of phagocytic and
enzymatic functions of rabbit mononuclear and polymorphonuclear exudate cells and alveolar macrophages. I.
Survey and quantitation of enzymes and states of cellular
activation. *J. Cell Biol. 17*: 465-486, 1963.

24. J. H. Hanks and R. E. Wallace. Relation of oxygen and
temperature in the preservation of tissues by refrigera-
tion. *Proc. Soc. Exp. Biol. Med. 71*: 196-200, 1949.

25. Q. N. Myrvik, E. Soto Leake, and B. Fariss. Studies on
pulmonary alveolar macrophages from the normal rabbit:
A technique to procure them in a high state of purity.
J. Immunol. 86: 128-132, 1961.

26. P. Rous and F. S. Jones. The protection of pathogenic
microorganisms by living tissue cells. *J. Exp. Med. 23*:
601-612, 1916.

27. H. Stähelin, E. Suter, and M. L. Karnovsky. Studies on
the interaction between phagocytes and tubercle bacilli.
I. Observations on the metabolism of guinea pig leucocytes and the influence of phagocytosis. *J. Exp. Med.
104*: 121-136, 1956.

28. R. Schrek. A method for counting the viable cells in
normal and malignant cell suspensions. *Am. J. Cancer 28*:
389-392, 1936.

29. J. H. Hanks and J. H. Wallace. Determination of cell
viability. *Proc. Soc. Exp. Biol. Med. 98*: 188-192, 1958.

30. A. M. Dannenberg, Jr., P. C. Walter, and F. A. Kapral.

A histochemical study of phagocytic and enzymatic functions of rabbit mononuclear and polymorphonuclear exudate cells and alveolar macrophages. II. The effect of particle ingestion on enzyme activity; two phases of *in vitro* activation. *J. Immunol. 90*: 448-465, 1963.

31. J. L. Tullis. Preservation of leucocytes. *Blood 8*: 563-575, 1953.

32. S. Higuchi, M. Suga, A. M. Dannenberg, Jr., and B. H. Schofield. Histochemical demonstration of enzyme activities in plastic and paraffin embedded tissue sections. *Stain Technol. 54*: 5-12, 1979.

33. K. Shima, A. M. Dannenberg, Jr., M. Ando, S. Chandrasekhar, J. A. Seluzicki, and J. I. Fabrikant. Macrophage accumulation, division, maturation, and digestive and microbicidal capacities in tuberculous lesions. *Am. J. Pathol. 67*: 159-176, 1972.

34. H. F. Dvorak, M. C. Mihm, A. M. Dvorak, R. A. Johnson, E. J. Manseau, E. Morgan, and R. B. Colvin. Morphology of delayed type hypersensitivity reactions in man. I. Quantitative description of the inflammatory response. *Lab. Invest. 31*: 111-130, 1974.

35. M. J. Karnovsky. The ultrastructural basis of capillary permeability studied with peroxidase as a tracer. *J. Cell Biol. 35*: 213-236, 1967.

36. R. F. Vogt, Jr., and N. A. Hynes. Inflammatory lesions of the skin: I. The use of Giemsa-stained glycol methacrylate embedded sections for the accurate identification of basophils and other leukocytes. (In preparation)

37. D. J. Yarborough, O. T. Meyer, A. M. Dannenberg, Jr., and B. Pearson. Histochemistry of macrophage hydrolases. III. Studies on β-galactosidase, β-glucuronidase, and aminopeptidase with indolyl and naphthyl substrates. *J. Reticuloendothel. Soc. 4*: 390-408, 1967.

38. B. Pearson, P. L. Wolf, and J. Vazquez. A comparative study of a series of new indolyl compounds to localize β-galactosidase in tissues. *Lab. Invest. 12*: 1249-1259, 1963.

39. A. M. Dannenberg, Jr., M. Ando, and K. Shima. Macrophage accumulation, division, maturation, and digestive and microbicidal capacities in tuberculous lesions. III. The turnover of macrophages and its relation to their activation and antimicrobial immunity in primary BCG lesions and those of reinfection. *J. Immunol. 109*: 1109-1121, 1972.

40. G. Gomori. "Microscopic Histochemistry," pp. 189-194. University of Chicago Press, Chicago, 1952.

41. Z. A. Cohn and E. Wiener. The particulate hydrolases of macrophages. II. Biochemical and morphological response to particle ingestion. *J. Exp. Med. 118*: 1009-1020, 1963.

42. M. S. Burstone. Histochemical comparison of naphthol AS-phosphates for the demonstration of phosphatases. *J. Natl. Cancer Inst. 20*: 601-615, 1958.

43. M. S. Burstone. Histochemical demonstration of acid phosphatases with naphthol AS-phosphates. *J. Natl. Cancer Inst. 21*: 523-539, 1958.

44. T. Tsuda, M. Ando, K. Shima, M. Sugimoto, O. Onizuka, and H. Tokuomi. Chronologic changes of activities of naphthol AS-D acetate esterase and other nonspecific esterases in the mononuclear phagocytes of tuberculous lesions. *Am. J. Pathol. 97*: 235-246, 1979.

45. C. Y. Li, K. W. Lam, and L. T. Yam. Esterases in human leukocytes. *J. Histochem. Cytochem. 21*: 1-12, 1973.

46. M. S. Burstone. The cytochemical localization of esterase. *J. Natl. Cancer Inst. 18*: 167-172, 1957.

47. P. M. Starkey and A. J. Barrett. Neutral proteinases of human spleen: Purification and criteria for homogeneity of elastase and cathepsin G. *Biochem. J. 155*: 255-263, 1976.

48. M. Wachstein and E. Meisel. Influence of experimental renal damage on histochemically demonstrable succinic dehydrogenase activity in the rat. *Am. J. Pathol. 30*: 147-165, 1954.

49. M. Wachstein and E. Meisel. A comparative study of enzymatic staining reactions in the rat kidney with necrobiosis induced by ischemia and nephrotoxic agents (mercuhydrin and DL-serine). *J. Histochem. Cytochem. 5*: 204-220, 1957.

50. M. M. Nachlas, K. C. Tsou, E. de Souza, C. S. Cheng, and A. M. Seligman. Cytochemical demonstration of succinic dehydrogenase by the use of a new p-nitrophenyl substituted ditetrazole. *J. Histochem. Cytochem. 5*: 420-436, 1957.

51. A. M. Dannenberg, Jr. and M. Sugimoto. Liquefaction of caseous foci in tuberculosis. *Am. Rev. Resp. Dis. 113*: 257-259, 1976.

52. M. S. Burstone. New histochemical techniques for the demonstration of tissue oxidase (cytochrome oxidase). *J. Histochem. Cytochem. 7*: 112-122, 1959.

53. M. S. Burstone. Histochemical demonstration of cytochrome oxidase with new amine reagents. *J. Histochem. Cytochem. 8*: 63-70, 1960.

42

USE OF TRANSMISSION ELECTRON MICROSCOPY

Martha E. Fedorko

I. INTRODUCTION

Standard methods for studying the ultrastructure of tissues are inadequate to study leukocytes in suspension, monolayers, and small clumps of cells. Leukocytes fixed with glutaralde-hyde followed by osmium tetroxide have poorly preserved cyto-plasmic granules and defined membranes. In the method of pro-cessing leukocytes described here, the basic approach involved: a new method of fixation for better cell preservation; post-fixation with uranyl acetate for enhanced definition of cell membranes, a modification of Kellenberger's method (1); a rapid method adequate for processing cells in suspension; a new tech-nique for embedding cell pellets. The method has proven to be satisfactory for human leukocytes (2), mouse monocytes (3) mouse macrophages (4), mouse and guinea pig bone marrow cells (5,7), monolayers of L cells (6), and isolated intestinal cells (8).

METHODS FOR STUDYING
MONONUCLEAR PHAGOCYTES

II. REAGENTS

   Physiologic saline (i.e., 0.15 M NaCl)
   Glutaraldehyde, 2.5 vol % (Fischer Scientific Co., Fairlawn, New Jersey) in cacodylate buffer 0.1 M, pH 7.4
   One per cent osmium tetroxide in 0.1 M cacodylate buffer,
pH 7.4
   Mixed fixative: A mixture of one part reagent 2.2 at 4°C
and two parts reagent 2.3 at 4°C, combined at 4°C within ½ hr
before use
   Uranyl acetate (0.25m%) in 0.1 M acetate buffer, pH 6.3
   Noble agar, 20 gm % in water, boiled or autoclaved and
used at 50°C

III. PROCEDURE

   A. *Standard Fixation*

   (1) Cell suspensions (5 × 10^6 cells or 5 packed cells)
are centrifuged out of dextran-plasma or suspending medium at
250 g for 10 min. About 2 ml glutaraldehyde (reagent 2.2), at
room temperature or at 37°C if filament preservation is desired,
is added to the cell pellet for 15 min. Cells are resuspended
by gentle pipetting with a Pasteur pipette. The cell suspension is transferred to a 3-ml conical centrifuge tube and centrifuged at 300 g for 2 min in a table top Clinical centrifuge
(International Equipment Co., Needham Heights, Massachusetts).
Cold, freshly prepared mixed fixative (reagent 2.4) is added to
the pellet for 10 min. Fixation, washing and poststaining are
all performed on cells in suspension. The specimen is pelleted
and a fresh aliquot of cold, mixed fixative is added for an
additional 5 min. The cells are then washed twice in physiologic saline. The cell pellet is next suspended in cold (4°C)
uranyl acetate (reagent 2.5) for 15-30 min, and followed by two
washes in physiologic saline. After the second wash, the cell
pellet is warmed to 50°C in a water bath for 5 min and then
suspended with a warm Pasteur pipette in ½ ml of warmed 2%
Noble agar. The agar is prewarmed (50°C) by boiling or autoclaving and allowed to cool to 50°C. The agar-cell suspension
is then centrifuged at about 50°C at 750 g for 2 min in carriers
partially filled with hot tap water. In an adequate centrifugation, the cells are pelleted in the agar; unsuccessful centrifugation produces a fuzzy zone of cells in agar. In the latter
event, the tube containing the cells is heated in a steam bath.
The tube is then cooled in ice to solidify the agar. 70% alcohol is added to the tube for an hour or more and the pellet is

removed by an 18-gauge needle at the tip of a 1-ml disposable syringe. The blackened cell pellet is then trimmed into small blocks for standard dehydration and embedding procedures (2).

(2) Cells in tissue culture on plastic or glass surfaces are washed once with physiologic saline at 37°C or room temperature and then exposed to warm or room temperature glutaraldehyde (reagent 2.2) for 15 min. The cell monolayer is then cooled on ice and two changes of freshly combined mixed fixative are added for another 15 min. The cells are next washed in cold physiologic saline and scraped off the dish with a rubber policeman. The cell suspension is then pelleted in a 3-ml conical centrifuge tube and processed as above through uranyl acetate postfixation and pelleting in agar.

B. Fixation for Special Studies

(1) Enzyme histochemistry can be performed on cell suspensions or cells in culture after initial glutaraldehyde fixation and then processed through mixed fixative with or without uranyl acetate. The peroxidase and acid phosphatase reactions have been performed with this method (unpublished observations).

(2) For better preservation of lipid and to minimize artifacts, cells are fixed in a solution containing 0.83% glutaraldehyde and 0.6% osmium tetroxide in 0.1 M cacodylate buffer, pH 7.4 for 1 hr in the cold. After a physiologic saline wash, postfixation with uranyl acetate (reagent 2.5) is performed and cells are processed as in Section III. A (9).

(3) For preservation of intact cells from monolayer cultures growing on plastic surfaces, the cells are fixed and poststained in situ through to alcohol, exposed to propylene oxide, and rapidly decanted when they are freed from the dish. The monolayer is then pelleted and embedded in Epon (5).

(4) Cells processed as in Section III. A can be sectioned, placed on grids but not stained with lead citrate or uranyl acetate. This method has been especially helpful in studying ferritin distribution in cells (10).

IV. INTERPRETATION OF ADEQUATE SPECIMENS AND FIXATION

The procedure described here permits obtaining an adequate sample of good cell density on a grid. Differential counts can be easily obtained on the specimen. When the cells are adequately fixed, leukocytes do not appear to have any extraction of contents and have good preservation of nuclear morphology, cytoplasmic matrix, cytoplasmic granules, and vesicles.

Use of cacodylate buffer seems to produce good preservation of mitochondria. When the initial fixation is in warm glutataldehyde, microfilaments and microtubules are well preserved.

V. CRITICAL COMMENTS

The above method has proved to be reproducible in several thousand experiments involving the fixation of leukocytes. The method is simple, rapid, and useful for leukocytes in suspension as well as for diverse cell monolayers in culture. When fixation of cells in suspension is employed, there is little problem with penetration of fixative, and therefore times of fixation can be relatively brief. Use of the Clinical centrifuge permits rapid pelleting and washing of specimens. Use of the mixed fixative produces more reproducible results than ordinary methods, with excellent preservation of small vesicles and cytoplasmic granules. Postfixation with uranyl acetate permits better definition of membranes.

Possible pitfalls in the method include use of oxidized fixative, if the mixing of glutaraldehyde and osmium is not performed in the cold or if the mixture is allowed to stand longer than 30 min. In this case the mixture will be dark or violet. Adequate centrifugation and pelleting of the cells in agar may rarely be unsuccessful. In that case, the cell-agar mixture can be reheated and pelleted again.

REFERENCES

1. E. Kellenberger, A. Ryter, and J. Sechaud. Electron microscope study of DNA-containing plasma. *J. Biophys. Biochem. Cytol. 4:*671, 1958.
2. J. Hirsch and M. Fedorko. Ultrastructure of human leukocytes after simultaneous fixation with glutaraldehyde and osmium tetroxide and "postfixation" in uranyl acetate. *J. Cell Biol. 38:*615-627, 1968.
3. M. Fedorko and J. Hirsch. Structure of monocytes and macrophages. *Semin. Hematol. 7:*109-124, 1970.
4. R. van Furth, J. Hirsch, and M. Fedorko. Morphology and peroxidase cytochemistry of mouse promonocytes, monocytes, and macrophages. *J. Exp. Med. 132:*794-812, 1970.
5. M. Fedorko. Morphologic and functional characteristics of bone marrow macrophages from Imferon-treated mice. *Blood 45:*435-449, 1975.

6. M. Fedorko, J. Hirsch, and Z. Cohn. Autophagic vacuoles produced *in vitro*. II. Studies on the mechanism of formation of autophagic vacuoles produced by chloroquine. *J. Cell Biol.* *38:*392-402, 1968.

7. R. Levine and M. Fedorko. Isolation of intact megakaryocytes from guinea pig femoral marrow. *J. Cell Biol.* *69:* k59-172, 1976.

8. M. Fedorko and P. Wiesenthal. Isolation and characterization of two duodenal epithelial cell populations in mice. Submitted for publication.

9. E. Mahoney, W. Scott, F. Landsberger, A. Hammil, and Z. Cohn. The influence of fatty acyl substitution on the composition and function of macrophage membranes. *J. Biol. Chem.* *255:*4910, 1980.

10. M. Fedorko, N. Cross, and J. Hirsch. Appearance and distribution of ferritin in mouse peritoneal macrophages *in vitro* after uptake of heterologous erythrocytes. *J. Cell Biol.* *57:*289-305, 1973.

43

PREPARATIVE TECHNIQUES FOR
SCANNING ELECTRON MICROSCOPY

Susan R. Walker
John D. Shelburne

I. INTRODUCTION

This chapter is designed primarily as an introduction to the literature for those techniques most applicable to the study of macrophages by scanning electron microscopy. Details will be given on the advantages and disadvantages of techniques used in our laboratory.

Some understanding of the scanning electron microscope (SEM) is required to select the most appropriate preparative technique. Interactions between the primary electron beam and

Acknowledgment

This work was supported in part by the Diagnostic Electron Microscopy Laboratory, Veterans Administration Medical Center, Durham, North Carolina, by NIEHS Grants No. ESHL01581, and ESO7031, and by E.P.A. Grants R805460-2 and CR807560-01.

the sample produce a variety of signals. Some primary electrons pass through the sample and are referred to as *transmitted electrons*. Others collide with the nucleus of atoms
in the sample and are deflected elastically as *backscattered
electrons*. Some of the primary electrons collide with an orbital electron within the sample. The electron is knocked out
of orbit and is called *a secondary electron*. After electrons
within the sample are excited, there is a reorganization of
atomic shells. The very low energy orbital electrons thus released are referred to as *Auger electrons*. When a secondary
electron is produced, it leaves a vacancy within an orbital
shell. An electron from a higher shell fills the vacancy and
the resulting energy loss produces an *x-ray* which has an energy and wavelength characteristic for that element. Finally,
when the excited electrons return to ground state, *photons* are
produced (cathodoluminescence).

Instrumentation developed within the last decade to collect these signals has revolutionized the field, closing the
gap between biochemists, physiologists, and morphologists.
It has also, of course, spurred the development of preparative
techniques necessary to optimize data collection.

The familiar "three-dimensional" images usually thought
of as "scanning electron micrographs" are created by collecting only the *secondary* electrons. Scanning transmission electron microscope (STEM) images utilize the transmitted electrons and hence are very similar in appearance to transmission
electron micrographs (TEM). A backscattered image generally
reflects the contrasts in atomic number within the sample, and
heavier elements appear darker. Histochemists have exploited
this mode of operation by specifically staining organelles or
enzyme sites with heavy metals (e.g., silver-stained nuclei,
tantalum-loaded phagosomes). Energy or wavelength dispersive
x-ray microanalysis (abbreviated EDX and WDX) allows identification and, on occasion, quantitation of most elements within
cells and, in some cases, within organelles. These data can
be presented as a spectrum of detected elements, a map of
specific element location, or as a total x-ray image (1).
Only those Auger electrons within the first few atomic layers
of the surface of the sample escape and are detected; therefore, surface elemental analysis is also available (2). If
appropriate fluorescent probes can be devised, cathodoluminescence may permit immunofluorescence studies to be done at
electron microscopic magnification.

The optimun results from each of these collection modes
can only be achieved by using the proper preparatory techniques. Since freezing is in general the best method for fixing ions, considerable space will be devoted to the discussion
of freezing techniques. It should be mentioned that these
same techniques can be applied to secondary ion mass spectro-

metry that presently is not widely applied to biological samples (3) but that can potentially identify all elements and
even organic compounds within cells.

While this discussion will cover only techniques for preparation of monolayers of macrophages for scanning electron
microscopy, methods have been developed for prepation of macrophages in suspension (4), which facilitate ultrathin frozen
sectioning. Frozen sections are best for elememtal analysis
and for scanning transmission microscopy.

II. CULTURE TECHNIQUES

Our experience in preparation of macrophages for scanning
electron microscopy is with two cell types: rabbit pulmonary
alveolar macrophages obtained by pulmonary lavage and mouse
peritoneal macrophages elicited with either BCG or thioglyco-
late broth. Since macrophages are avidly adherent, many supports can be utilized in the study of monolayers of these
cells. Glass coverslips have proven to be excellent supports
for studies of surface morphology of conventionally fixed
cells. In addition, we have found that macrophages readily
attach to aluminum, gold, and tantalum foils, a property which
we have exploited for surface morphology studies of freeze-
fixed macrophages. Macrophages attach well to Thermonox coverslips that, in addition to being one of the better supports
for EDX studies, can subsequently be embedded in Epon and sectioned for transmission electron microscopy. Macrophages will
also attach to Formvar-coated nylon or gold transmission electron microscope grids for STEM studies. Copper grids are toxic
to macrophages. Other supports could probably be used for
scanning electron microscopy but the toxicity of each potential
support should be tested.

The appropriate support is placed in a small petri dish.
A suspension of macrophages is then added to the dish so that
the supports are completely covered. We have found that a concentration of 7×10^6 cells/ml is sufficient to produce a monolayer on the support surfaces we have used. Approximately 1 to
2 hr are allowed for attachment. Either the top or bottom of
the support should be easily recognized macroscopically in order to orient the support properly during processing and subsequent mounting for scanning electron microscopy. For example,
if aluminum foil is the selected support, allow the macrophages
to attach to the dull side; the shiny side can then be easily
identified as the bottom during subsequent manipulations.

Monolayers of cells fixed in suspension (5,6) and monolayers of living cells (e.g., cancer cells) that are less adherent than the mature macrophages used in our laboratory (7)

can be prepared by first coating a glass substrate with poly-L lysine, which positively charges the surface and thus increases cellular yield (5). It should be noted that the surface morphology might be affected by the adherence of living cells to poly-L lysine. Proper control studies should be done if poly-L lysine is used. Alternatively, cells fixed in suspension can be harvested on membrane filters (8). Silver membrane filters (8) are conductive and thus are useful for SEM studies if no x-ray microanalysis is contemplated.

III. FIXATION

   A. *Chemical Fixation*

     The most widely used and our recommended primary chemical fixative is buffered glutaraldehyde, although many other chemical fixatives are available and some are better suited for specialized studies (9-11).
     Buffered glutaraldehyde is easy to use and tissue can be stored in it for years with little change. Fixation at room temperature is better than fixation at 4°C, since microtubule morphology is preserved. For convenience, we routinely fix overnight although for monolayers of cells 1 hr is probably more than ample for excellent fixation.
     For single cells and monolayers, several workers have argued that the osmolarity of the buffer alone has more influence on final cell volume than does the osmolarity of buffer plus fixative (12,13). This concept has recently been challenged (14). Clearly there is a need for more research in this area. We recommend 3% glutaraldehyde buffered with 0.15 M sodium cacodylate (see Appendix I). Cacodylate is an organic arsenical compound and should be used with caution, although we have had ourselves and our technicians tested and have found no detectable urinary arsenic. We have been unable to detect arsenic in tissues fixed in cacodylate buffered glutaraldehyde, subsequently dehydrated with ethanol and embedded in Epon using energy dispersive x-ray microanalysis. Presumably most of the cacodylate is removed from the tissue during dehydration. Phosphate buffers (0.1 M, pH 7.4) avoid the theoretical dangers of cacodylate, but precipitates may form. In addition, bacteria may grow in stored phosphate buffers (prior to mixing with glutaraldehyde).
     For SEM, postfixation with osmium tetroxide and *en bloc* staining with uranyl acetate are not necessary, although it has been argued that these steps improve the crispness of the SEM image.

B. Freeze Fixation

Boyde (15) has demonstrated that marked volume changes occur during chemical fixation and subsequent dehydration. It has also been well documented that even brief exposure to chemical fixatives allows translocation of ions (16-18). Chemical fixation is slow enough that it might allow some changes in surface morphology (19) before fixation is complete. Fixation by ultrarapid freezing avoids these potential drawbacks, but is associated with its own unique problems. Since we are interested in the subcellular localization of translocatable ions, we have found that for many experiments fixation by freezing is essential.

Monolayers are first rinsed in medium without fetal calf serum and "blotted" as well as possible. (The back of the support is placed on filter paper as are the edges in order to remove as much of the excess medium as possible.) Fixation is performed by rapidly plunging the monolayer of macrophages into liquid propane cooled with liquid nitrogen. As propane is explosive, extreme caution should be taken. Freezing should be performed under a hood vented directly *out of the building,* and any sparks, open flames, and ultrasonic vibrations should be avoided. Other freeze fixatives are available (18), but results obtained with propane have thus far proved the best in our laboratory.

The best supports for monolayers fixed by freezing are thin foils, although Thermonox coverslips are adequate. According to Corless and Costello (18), the metal foils permit the rapid dissipation of heat that is necessary for the fastest possible freezing rates and hence less recognizable ice-crystal damage. Thermonox and glass coverslips, on the other hand, are insulators. Depending on the orientation of the substrate to the coolant, this may be disadvantageous since cooling may be slower, allowing for ice-crystal damage.

Macrophages fixed by freezing can be freeze-dried (4,15) or freeze-substituted (4,19). If instantaneous fixation of surface morphology is desired, the method of freeze-substitution described by Barlow and Sleigh (19) using a 40% ethylene glycol/methanol mixture is suggested. In order to examine intracellular morphology as well as surface morphology, we employ a 1% osmium tetroxide/acetone mixture for freeze-substitution (4). If osmium is used as a fixative, aluminum foil cannot be used as a support, since the aluminum becomes oxidized.

IV. DRYING

A. Chemically Fixed Cells

With few exceptions, biological samples must be dry when examined with a scanning electron microscope. Traditionally, critical point drying is the technique used to avoid the distortion of the sample that occurs during air drying. The principle behind drying by this method is that at a critical point, the density of the liquid and gas phases is identical and there is no surface tension force. The critical point of water is very high and cannot be easily and safely reached. Water within the sample must therefore be replaced by a liquid with a low critical point, which will undergo the phase transition from liquid to gas, a *transition fluid*. The most common transition fluids are Freon 13 and carbon dioxide. Since these fluids are not miscible with water, an *intermediate fluid* must be employed that is miscible with water and the transition fluid. When carbon dioxide is used as the transition fluid, ethanol or acetone is used as the intermediate fluid. Freon 113 is the intermediate fluid for Freon 13. The dehydration schedule used in our laboratory appears as Appendix II. Fairly good results can be achieved without critical point drying just by lowering the surface tension forces (20,21), thereby avoiding both the cost of a critical point dryer and the possibility of an explosion that exists when a critical point dryer is misused.

If monolayers have been freeze substituted, they can be critical point dried directly from acetone or enter the schedule by transferring from acetone to 100% ethanol.

B. Cells Fixed by Freezing

Freeze-fixed cells can be dehydrated by freeze-drying. We prefer this method of drying monolayers since no manipulation of the sample after fixation is required. After cells are frozen in liquid propane, they are maintained at liquid nitrogen temperature and placed under a vacuum of greater than 10^{-2} Torr. The cells are then allowed to slowly warm in this vacuum to ambient temperature over several hours. For a thorough discussion of freeze drying, see Boyde (15).

One drawback of freeze drying is the formation of salt and protein precipitates from the medium that is adherent to the surface of the cells and substrate. These precipitates are readily visible by SEM and may obscure surface details.

C. *Treatment after Drying*

Cells that have been dried by any method should have no
contact with water vapor in the air. Therefore, all samples
should be stored and transported in a vacuum dessicator.

V. COATING

It is necessary that the surface be conductive in order
to disspiate the electrons that will bombard the monolayer in
the scanning electron microscope. If the surface is not conductive, electrons will "pile up" on the cells and will interfere with the SEM image; this is referred to as "charging."
In addition, contrast and resolution are improved by coating.
Platinum coating is recommended for optimum resolution and
carbon is recommended for microprobe studies (EDX/WDX).
The coating should be either evaporated onto a rotating
sample in a vacuum evaporator or sputtered onto the sample
using a triode sputter coater. It has been shown that diode
sputter coaters may cause heat damage to the sample (22).

LITERATURE SOURCES

R. M. Albrecht and B. Wetzell. Ancillary methods for biologi-
    cal scanning electron microscopy. *In* "Scanning Electron
    Microscopy/1979/III" (R. P. Becker and O. Johari, eds.),
    pp.203-222. SEM, Inc., AMF O'Hare, Illinois, 1979.
K. E. Carr and P. G. Toner. Scanning Electron Microscopy of
    Macrophages: A Bibliography. *Scanning Electron Microscopy/
    1979/III*, op.cit., pp.637-644.
N. A. Hayat. *Introduction to Biological Scanning Electron
    Microscopy.* University Park Press, Baltimore, 1978. This
    short book is an excellent and comprehensive review of all
    of the major techniques currently available. Many refer-
    ences are given as well.
N. A. Hayat. *Principles and Techniques of Scanning Electron
    Microscopy.* Van Nostrand Reinhold Company, New York, 1976.
    This multivolume series gives details of techniques discussed
    more briefly in the first references.
G. R. Hooper, K. K. Baker, S. L. Flegler. *Exercises in elec-
    tron microscopy: A laboratory manual for biological and
    medical sciences.* Center for Electron Optics, Michigan
    State University, East Lansing, Michigan 48824, 1979.

O. Johari (Editor): "Scanning Electron Microscopy."
IIT Research Institute, Chicago, Illinois, 1978. These
annual proceedings contain a wealth of papers on every con-
ceivable aspect of scanning electron microscopy. Since 1978
the series has been published by SEM, Inc., AMF O'Hare,
Illinois. 60666.

REFERENCES

1. P. Ingram and J. D. Shelburne. Total rate imaging with
    x-rays (TRIX) - A simple method of forming a nonprojection
    x-ray image in the SEM and its application to biological
    specimens. "Scanning Electron Microscopy/1980," pp.285-
    296. (O. Johari, ed.), SEM, Inc. AMF O'Hare, Illinois,
    60616, 1980.
2. G. B. Larrabee. The characterization of solid surfaces.
    "Scanning Electron Microscopy/1977/I," pp. 639-650.
    IIT Research Institute, Chicago, Illinois. 60616, 1977.
3. R. W. Linton, S. R. Walker, C. R. DeVries, P. Ingram, and
    J. D. Shelburne. Ion microanalysis of cells. "Scanning
    Electron Microscopy/1980/II," pp.583-596. O. Johari, ed.
    SEM, Inc. AMF O'Hare, Illinois, 60616, 1980.
4. S. K. Masters, S. W. Bell, P. Ingram, D. O. Adams, and
    J. D. Shelburne. Preparative techniques for freezing and
    freeze-sectioning macrophages for energy dispersive x-ray
    microanalysis. "Scanning Electron Microscopy/1979/III.
    (O. Johari, ed.), pp.97-110, 122. SEM, INC., AMF O'Hare,
    Illinois, 60666, 1979.
5. S. Sanders, E. Alexander, and R. Braylan. A high yield
    technique for preparing cells fixed in suspension for
    scanning electron microscopy. J. Cell Bio. 67:476-480,
    1975.
6. B. Wetzel. Cell Kinetics: An interpretative review of
    the significance of cell surface form. "Scanning Electron
    Microscopy/II/1976," pp.136-144. IIT Research Institute,
    Chicago, Illinois, 60616, 1976.
7. L. G. Koss and W. Domagala. Configuration of surfaces of
    human cancer cells in effusions. A review. "Scanning
    Electron Microscopy/1980/III." (R. P. Becker and O.
    Johari, eds.), pp.89-100. SEM, Inc., AMF O'Hare, Illinois,
    1980.
8. M. L. Saint-Guillain, B. Vray, J. Hoebeke, and R. Leloup.
    SEM Morphological studies of phagocytosis by rat macro-
    phages and rabbit polymorphonuclear leukocytes. "Scanning
    Electron Microscopy/1980/II" (R. P. Becker and O. Johari,
    eds,), pp. 205-212. SEM, Inc., AMF O'Hare, Illinois, 1980.

9. N. A. Hayat. Fixation. *In* "Principles and Techniques of Electron Microscopy. Biological Applications," Vol. I. pp.5-105. Van Nostrand Reinhold Company, New York, 1973.

10. G. Millonig. "Laboratory Manual of Biological Electron Microscopy." MarioSaviolo, Vericelli C. P. 182, Italy, 1976.

11. E. M. McDowell and B. F. Trump. Histologic fixatives suitable for diagnostic light and electron microscopy. *Arch. Pathol. Lab. Med. 100:*405-414, 1976.

12. A. Penttila, H. Kalimo, and B. F. Trump. Influence of glutaraldehyde and/or osmium tetroxide on cell volume, ion content, mechanical stability and membrane permeability of Ehrlich ascites tumor cells. *J. Cell Biol. 63:* 197-214, 1974.

13. Q. Bone and E. J. Denton. The osmotic effects of electron microscope fixatives. *J. Cell Biol. 49:*571-581, 1971.

14. J. Renau-Piqueras, A. Miguel, and E. Knecht. Effects of techniques on the fine structure of human peripheral blood lymphocytes: Effects of glutaraldehyde osmolarity. *Mikroskopie 36:*65-80, 1980.

15. A. Boyde, E. Bailey, S. J. Jones, and A. Tamarin. Dimensional changes during specimen preparation for scanning electron microscopy. "Scanning Electron Microscopy/1977/I." IIT Research Institute, Chicago, Illinois, 60616, 1977.

16. A. Dörge, R. Rick, K. Gehring, J. Mason, and K. Thurau. Preparation and applicability of freeze-dried sections for microprobe analysis of biological soft tissue. *J. Micro. Biol. Cell 22:*205-214, 1975.

17. S. W. Bell, S. K. Masters, P. Ingram, M. D. Waters, and J. D. Shelburne. Ultastructure and x-ray microanalysis of macrophages exposed to cadmium chloride. "Scanning Electron Microscopy/1979/III" (O. Johari, ed.), pp.111-121. SEM, Inc., AMF O'Hare, Illinois, 60666, 1979.

18. M. J. Costello and J. M. Corless. The direct measurement of temperature changes within freeze fracture specimens during rapid quenching in liquid coolants. *J. Microsc. 112:*17-37, 1978.

19. D. I. Barlow and M. A. Sleigh. Freeze-substitution for preservation of ciliated surfaces for scanning electron microscopy. *J. Microsc. 115:*81-95, 1979.

20. A. Liepins and E. de Harven. A rapid method for cell drying for scanning electron microscopy. "Scanning Electron Microscopy/1978/II" (R. P. Becker and O. Johari, eds.), pp. 37-43. SEM, Inc., AMF O'Hare, Illinois, 60666, 1978.

21. J. C. Lamb and P. Ingram. Drying of biological speci-
     mens for scanning electron microscopy directly from
     ethanol. "Scanning Electron Microscopy/1979/III"
     (O. Johari and R. P. Becker, eds.), pp. 459-464,472.
     SEM, Inc., AMF O'Hare, Illinois, 60666, 1979.
22. P. Ingram, N. Morosoff, L. Pope, F. Allen, and C. Tisher.
     Some comparisons of the techniques of sputter (coating)
     and evaporative coating for scanning electron microscopy.
     "Scanning Electron Microscopy/1976/I," pp.75-81. IIT
     Research Institute, Chicago, Illinois, 60616, 1976.

APPENDIX I

To make a 0.15 M sodium cacodylate buffer, add 32.10 gm
of sodium cacodylate to 1000 ml of distilled water. Adjust pH
to 7.4 with concentrated hydrochloric acid.

APPENDIX II: Preparation of Monolayers for Critical Point
              Drying

Fix in 3% buffered glutaraldehyde for at least 1 hr.
Wash in same buffer for 5 min.
Dehydrate in 50% ethanol for 5 min.
                70% ethanol for 5 min.
                95% ethanol for 5 min.
               100% ethanol, 3 changes of 5 min each.
     If tissue is to be critical point dried with carbon
dioxide as the transition fluid, ethanol or acetone can be
used as the intermediate fluid.
     For critical point drying with Freon 13, follow schedule
as above, then infiltrate with

            50/50   100% ethanol/Freon 113 for 5 min.
            30/70   ethanol/Freon 113 for 5 min.
            100% Freon 113, 3 changes of 5 min each.
Critical point dry in fresh Freon 13.

44

USE OF ULTRASTRUCTURAL HISTOCHEMISTRY

Barbara A. Nichols

I. GENERAL INTRODUCTION

Cytochemical methods for electron microscopy have the
unique capability of ultrastructurally localizing enzymes or
chemical substances. There are several requirements for
success with these methods. It is essential that the enzyme
be fixed in its native position in the tissues, yet retain
sufficient activity to be demonstrable by the cytochemical
technique subsequently used. It is essential that the substrate have access to the enzyme, and that the product which
results from the cytochemical reaction be electron dense and
remain at the site of its formation. Although there are fewer
cytochemical methods available for electron microscopy than
for light microscopy, there are nonetheless several volumes
now devoted to the discussion of them (1).

This chapter is intended to provide some practical information about the localization in mononuclear phagocytes of
peroxidase and two acid hydrolases, acid phosphatase and aryl

sulfatase, by methods that have been used successfully in our
laboratory (2 - 5). These methods have proven applicable to
all mammalian species thus far studied.

A. General Considerations

Enzymes are easily inactivated by compounds such as osmium
that are routinely used in preparing tissue for electron microscopy. Because osmium vapors are very pervasive, the histochemistry area of the laboratory must be completely separated
from rooms where osmium is used. It is also essential that the
glassware used in cytochemistry never be used in other parts of
the laboratory because of possible contamination by enzyme-
inactivating substances. Careful dish washing is also a basic
requirement of the well-run histochemistry laboratory. After
washing in Tetrox detergent, glassware should be rinsed 7
times in tap water, followed by 7 rinses in double-distilled
water.

B. Fixatives

Glutaraldehyde is the fixative of choice for most cytochemical procedures (6), although brief (5-min) fixation with
dilute Karnovsky's fixative (7) may also be used if the enzyme
to be studied is relatively stable to fixation. The purity of
the glutaraldehyde is fundamental to the success of a cytochemical experiment, since impurities lead to the inactivation
of enzymes (6, 8). The purity of commercially available glutaraldehyde greatly varies (9). Glutaraldehyde from Electron
Microscopy Sciences has been used with success in our laboratory, although that from other suppliers may be equally good.
Before glutaraldehyde is used, its purity should be established
by ultraviolet spectroscopy (8 - 10).

C. Fixation

One of the most difficult steps in cytochemical work is the
selection of a method of tissue fixation that adequately pre-
serves both tissue structure and enzymatic activity. In general, fixation must be brief if adequate amounts of enzyme are
to be preserved for cytochemical demonstration. However, tissue that has been only minimally fixed may lose structural integrity during subsequent preparation. This is particularly
true when the enzyme to be demonstrated has a pH optimum in the
acid or alkaline range. If intracellular membranes are disrupted as a result of inadequate cellular preservation, it is

clearly impossible to define the intracellular localization of
an enzyme with confidence. The best conditions of fixation
must be determined by trial and error for each tissue and each
enzyme, since enzymes differ in their susceptibility to inactivation by fixation. Optimally, biochemical analyses can be
used to determine the amounts of enzyme in tissue before and
after various fixation treatments (11-13). As an additional
cautionary note, it is highly desirable when carrying out cytochemical experiments to fix parallel samples of tissue with
formaldehyde - glutaraldehyde for optimal morphological preservation (without cytochemical incubation) to ensure that the
structural relationships observed intracellularly in the incubated specimens have not been altered by the conditions of the
cytochemical test.

D. *Collection and Handling of Tissues*

    Tissue is fixed *in situ* or as soon as possible after re-
moval from the experimental animal. For example, fixative is
used to wash cells from the lungs or peritoneal cavities as
previously described (4). To separate leukocytes from red
cells as rapidly as possible, Kaplow buffy coat tubes (The
Virtis Company, Inc., Gardiner, New York 12525) are routinely
used in our laboratory (14). Blood is drawn into a heparinized syringe (50 U heparin/ml of blood) and immediately dispensed into Kaplow tubes. The tubes are then centrifuged in
a table-top centrifuge (Sorvall GLC-2) with a swinging bucket
head at top speed for 10 min, which gives a good separation of
the buffy coat. The serum is drawn off and discarded. The
buffy coat is then drawn off and immediately dispersed in
glutaraldehyde fixative.
    Cell suspensions (i.e., bone marrow, blood leukocytes, al-
veolar or peritoneal macrophages) are centrifuged and resuspended between changes of solution until postfixation in osmium. Prior to osmication, the cell suspensions are pelleted
in a Beckman Microfuge. The resulting mass of cells is co-
herent and can be cut from the 0.4-ml plastic centrifuge tube,
chopped into 1/2-mm cubes, and handled subsequently as tissue
blocks.
    Solid tissues, such as lung or liver, must be cut after
fixation into 20- to 40-μm sections with a Smith-Farquhar
Tissue Chopper (Sorvall Instruments) (10) or an Oxford Vibra-
tome. Chopped sections can then be transferred manually
through changes of solutions, or solutions can be decanted
from the sections.
    When possible, the entire cytochemical procedure, from
fixation to embedding, should be carried out in one day to
minimize loss of enzymatic activity or loss of reaction product.

TABLE I. Reagents Used in Electron Microscopic Cytochemistry

Reagents	Source[a]	Use	Comments
3-Amino-1,2,4-triazole	Sigma	Inhibitor of catalase	Store desiccated below 0°C
Ammonium sulfide (20% solution)	Mallinckrodt	Conversion of aryl sulfatase reaction product to lead sulfide	Stable at room temperature. Evolves hydrogen sulfide, a poisonous, noxious gas. Use only in fume hood.
Barbital	Sigma	Acetate Veronal wash buffer	Stable at room temperature
Cytidine monophosphate	Sigma	Acid phosphatase substrate	Store in dark, desiccated below 0°C
3,3'-Diaminobenzidine tetrahydrochloride	Sigma	Peroxidase medium	Carcinogenic. Avoid inhalation of powder and skin contact. Store in dark, desiccated below 0°C
Glutaraldehyde (10% and 25% solutions)	Electron Microscopy Sciences	Primary fixation	Avoid inhalation of vapors or skin contact
β-glycerophosphate grade I	Sigma	Acid phosphatase substrate	Stable at room temperature

Table I (Cont'd.)

Horseradish peroxidase	Worthington Biochemical Corp.	Tracer of pinocytosis	Refrigerate desiccated
Hydrogen peroxide	Mallinckrodt	Peroxidase substrate	Unstable. Use a fresh bottle for each experiment.
p-Nitrocatechol sulfate	Sigma	Aryl sulfatase substrate	Stores well desiccated below 0°C
p-Nitrophenyl phosphate	Sigma	Acid phosphatase substrate	Stable at room temperature.
Osmium (4% solution)	Electron Microscopy Sciences	Postfixation	Extremely toxic. Avoid inhalation of vapors and skin contact. Use only in fume hood.
Potassium cyanide	Mallinckrodt	Inhibitor of peroxidase	Danger! May be fatal if swallowed. Contact with acid liberates poisonous gas.
Sodium cacodylate hydrochloride	Sigma	Wash buffer	Arsenical, carcinogen. Avoid inhalation or skin contact.
Sodium fluoride	Fisher	Inhibitor of acid phosphatase	Poison. May be fatal if swallowed. Keep bottle in plastic bag to avoid contamination of other reagents.

417

Table I (Cont'd.)

Reagents	Source[a]	Use	Comments
Sodium tartrate	Sigma	Inhibitor of some acid phosphatases	Stable at room temperature.
Spurr's Embedding medium	Ladd	Embedding of peroxidase specimens	Some ingredients reportedly are carcinogenic. Avoid skin contact. Mix in fume hood.
Trizma (Tris) base buffer	Sigma	Peroxidase medium	Store refrigerated
Trizma (Tris) maleate buffer	Sigma	Acid phosphatase medium	Very hygroscopic. Store desiccated, and refrigerated.
			Certain pH electrodes do not give accurate results with Tris-maleate buffers. See Sigma Technical Bulletin #106B dated after 1978.

[a]*Addresses of chemical companies are given in Appendix.*

E. Reagents

Many chemicals used in electron microscopic cytochemistry are health hazards (Table I). Technicians using these reagents must be informed that they are dangerous so that the appropriate care can be used in handling them. To avoid skin contamination, laboratory assistants should always wear gloves when washing glassware that has contained these chemicals.

II. CYTOCHEMICAL DEMONSTRATION OF PEROXIDASE

Cytochemical tests for peroxidase have been used extensively in the study of mononuclear phagocytes, since the enzyme myeloperoxidase is endogenous to the monocytes of some mammalian species, and since peroxidatic activity is present in the rough endoplasmic reticulum of many tissue macrophages. For a general review of these topics, consult van Furth (15). In addition, exogenous peroxidase has been used as an extracellular tracer to follow fluid uptake by pinocytosis (16). The same cytochemical incubation procedures are used to demonstrate peroxidase whether the enzyme is endogenous or exogenous.

The fixation of tissues to be incubated for peroxidase may be very brief, or may even be omitted entirely (17, 18), since the incubation is carried out at a near neutral pH, causing little tissue damage.

A. The Protocol for Peroxidase (see Appendix for formulas of solutions)

(1) Fix tissues for 10 min in 1.5% glutaraldehyde.

(2) Wash 3 times in sodium cacodylate - HCl wash buffer.

(3) Incubate in peroxidase medium at room temperature on Dubnoff shaker for 15-60 min.

(4) Wash 3 times in Michaelis wash buffer.

(5) Pellet loose cells in a Beckman Microfuge.

(6) Postfix in Palade's osmium for 1 hr at 4°C.

(7) Stain one specimen in Kellenberger's uranyl acetate stain for 10 min at room temperature.

(8) Omit the stain for an identical specimen.

(9) Dehydrate rapidly in ethanol only, according to the procedure given in the tabulation below:

70% ethanol		2 min
95% ethanol		2 min
100% ethanol	3 changes	15 min each
1:1 ethanol:Spurr's medium		
	2 changes	20 min each
100% Spurr's	2 changes	30 min each or longer

(10) Embed in fresh Spurr's medium.
(11) Cure overnight at 60°C.

B. Technical Problems

There are several technical problems associated with the demonstration of peroxidase. This enzyme is particularly vulnerable to loss of activity, which usually occurs at two points during the procedure. First, there can be loss of activity before incubation, either because of overfixation or because the briefly fixed tissues have been held overnight in buffer. Second, reaction product, once formed, can be removed from the tissues by subsequent steps of tissue processing. The reaction is diminished by uranyl acetate staining in block. Kellenberger's stain is therefore omitted, or two samples are run in parallel, one from which Kellenberger's is omitted and the other in which only a 10-min stain is used. The two samples can then be compared for the best preservation of the tissue and the reaction product. Diaminobenzidine (DAB) reaction product can also be removed by prolonged exposure to solvents. For this reason, Spurr's low-viscosity embedding medium (19) is used because dehydration can be carried out rapidly with the omission of propylene oxide. Rapid polymerization of Spurr's plastic is also an advantage because the solvent effects of liquid plastics are reduced. It should be noted, however, that this embedding material reacts with water to produce a brittle plastic, which is difficult to section. In handling it, care should be taken to avoid moisture, as with other embedding materials.

DAB penetrates tissues slowly. It is advisable to examine unstained 1-μm sections by light microscopy to determine the depth of reactive tissue before selecting an area for thin sectioning.

As a general rule for all cytochemical specimens, an unstained grid is examined by electron microscopy and compared with a stained grid to determine whether reaction product has been removed by the stain on grid. Remarkably enough, reaction product for peroxidase is removed from the plastic sections by uranyl acetate staining on grid. This poses a dilemma, since the omission of uranyl acetate both in block and on grid greatly diminishes specimen contrast, and thus makes the specimen

very difficult to examine and photograph. A further complication is that Spurr's plastic does not stain readily with lead
stains. It is essential, however, to examine a specimen not
stained with uranyl acetate to ensure that no intracellular
sites of peroxidase localization are overlooked. Later, a dip
of uranyl acetate before 30 min of Reynold's lead citrate may
be tried.

C. Interpretation of Results

As with other cytochemical procedures, tests for peroxidase
are not specific (20). Other heme proteins, such as hemoglobin
and cytochromes, can also oxidize DAB to give a positive result.
Definite identification of a given enzyme must therefore be obtained by biochemical procedures.

Considerable study has been devoted to analyzing the conditions that favor the demonstration of peroxidase over that of
catalase, and vice-versa. Several excellent review articles
thoroughly discuss this subject (17, 20 - 23).

Diffusion of reaction product occasionally poses a problem
in peroxidase cytochemistry. It is possible that the brief
fixation procedures employed in cytochemistry sometimes do not
adequately stabilize cellular membranes, so that leakage of
reaction product occurs. Generally speaking, the presence of
reaction product outside of a membrane-limited organelle should
be considered questionable.

D. Control Specimens

Incubations without substrate must be carried out as a
control for the cytochemical tests to ensure that electron-
dense components of the medium are not nonspecifically adsorbed
to cellular structures, leading to false positive results. In
control experiments in which hydrogen peroxide, the substrate
for peroxidase, is omitted from the incubation medium, some
staining may result from the presence of hydrogen peroxide in
the tissue itself. This staining can be eliminated by the use
of catalase in the control incubation medium (20). Aminotria-
zole, once considered a specific inhibitor of catalase, also
inhibits some peroxidatic activities (22). Although potassium
cyanide has no effect on the peroxidase of eosinophils, it is
an effective inhibitor of other peroxidases, including the
peroxidase of other leukocytes. The use of inhibitors is discussed fully by Essner (20).

III. CYTOCHEMICAL LOCALIZATION OF ACID PHOSPHATASE AND ARYL
      SULFATASE

        Lysosomes cannot be identified solely on the basis of their
ultrastructural appearance, for they are remarkably heterogeneous in size, shape, and content. Therefore, their identification in tissue sections depends upon the use of cytochemical
methods. Acid phosphatase is the most widely used "marker"
enzyme for cytochemical staining of lysozomes, and the assumption is generally made, and appears valid (24), that a dense
body containing acid phosphatase probably contains other acid
hydrolases as well. However, it is highly desirable to corro-
borate the localization of one enzyme with that of another enzyme in the same cells (25), since cytochemical methods lack
specificity. For example, there are not only multiple acid
phosphatase enzymes (with possibly different functions) in the
same cell (26, 27), but also many other phosphatases that have
overlapping enzymatic activities (28 - 33). Of several techniques available for the demonstration of lysosomal enzymes,
tests for acid phosphatase and aryl sulfatase have proved to
be the most useful in our hands in the study of mononuclear
phagocytes (34).

A. *The Protocol for Acid Phosphatase (see Appendix for for-*
    mulas of solutions)

        (1) Fix tissues for 10 min in 1.5% glutaraldehyde.
        (2) Wash 3 times in sodium cacodylate - HCl wash buffer.
        (3) Incubate in acid phosphatase medium on a Dubnoff
shaker for 30 - 90 min at $30° - 37°C$.
        (4) Wash 5-10 times in Michaelis wash buffer.
        (5) Pellet loose cells in a Beckman Microfuge.
        (6) Postfix in Palade's osmium at $4°C$ for 1 hr.
        (7) Stain in Kellenberger's uranyl acetate for 15 - 60 min
at room temperature.
        (8) Dehydrate according to the schedule given in the fol-
lowing tabulation:

70% ethanol		*5 min*
95% ethanol	*2 changes*	*5 min each*
100% ethanol	*3 changes*	*10 min each*
Propylene oxide	*2 changes*	*15 min each*
1:1 Epon : propylene oxide		*2-4 hr*

        (9) Infiltrate in pure Epon overnight at $4°C$.
        (10) Embed in fresh Epon.
        (11) Cure at $60°C$ for 24 hr.

B. *The Protocol for Aryl Sulfatase (see Appendix for formulas of solutions)*

    (1) Fix tissues for 10 min in 1.5% glutaraldehyde.

    (2) Wash 3 times in sodium cacodylate wash buffer.

    (3) Incubate specimens in aryl sulfatase medium at 30° - 37°C for 30-90 min in a Dubnoff shaking incubator.

    (4) Wash until clear with Michaelis wash buffer (5 - 7 rinses).

    (5) Convert reaction product with 2% ammonium sulfide in Michaelis buffer for 5 - 15 min. [In this step, the lead sulfate formed as a result of the reaction is converted to lead sulfide (35). The resulting specimen is easier to section than specimens prepared without this step.]

    (6) Wash until clear with Michaelis buffer (8 - 10 washes).

    (7) Pellet loose cells in a Beckman Microfuge.

    (8) Postfix in Palade's osmium at 4°C for 1 hr.

    (9) Stain in block for 10 - 60 min with Kellenberger's uranyl acetate stain at room temperature.

    (10) Dehydrate in ethanol and propylene oxide (see Section III.A), as for acid phosphatase.

    (11) Embed in Epon.

    (12) Cure at 60°C for 24 hr.

C. *Technical Problems*

    One of the chief technical problems in the cytochemistry of acid phosphatase and aryl sulfatase is the tissue damage that occurs during the incubation of the tissues in the cytochemical medium at an acid pH (5.0 - 5.5). Even though this problem can be anticipated, some experiments must be carried out with only very brief fixation (5-10 min) in order to obtain maximal amounts of enzyme deposits. Once the sites of reactivity are determined, slightly longer fixation times can be tried (10-30 min), with the aim of providing better tissue preservation.

    Low levels of nonspecific "background" staining in the tissues often make the specimens appear "dirty." Specimens can be "cleaned up" with Kellenberger's in block stain (36, 37), but it must be recognized that some reaction product is removed, along with the nonspecific staining, during this process. Reaction products composed of lead salts are also removed to some extent by other acid solutions during tissue processing (28). The problem of scanty reaction product may be somewhat diminished by reducing both the time of postfixation in osmium and the time of Kellenberger staining.

    Histochemical latency is one of the most difficult problems to deal with. This property of lysosomes has been

observed and analyzed extensively in cytochemical investigations (12, 25, 40) of leukocytes, in which granules known to
contain lysosomal enzymes were found to remain unreactive for
those enzymes after cytochemical tests using lead salt techniques. The granules must be disrupted using methods such as
freezing or thawing, smearing, or prolonged incubation at acid
pH to demonstrate histochemical activity with lead salts.
Since latency is not present when azo dye methods are used,
correlated light microscopy may be essential in some cases
(41).

D. *Interpretation of Results*

   There are many problems in interpreting phosphatase cytochemical activity. In most tissues there are many different
enzymes that hydrolyze a wide variety of phosphatase substrates
(28, 30, 38, 39). As mentioned previously, biochemical assays
when possible can provide essential evidence in confirming the
identity of an enzyme (40). In addition, the careful use of
selective inhibition in control cytochemical experiments can
also provide valuable information concerning the identity of an
enzyme in question (38). For example, a brief preincubation of
a specimen in buffer at an acid pH will inhibit glucose-6-
phosphatase activity (which is sensitive to acid), whereas the
activity of an acid phosphatase is unaffected (38).
   There are multiple aryl sulfatases as well as phosphatases
(42 - 44). It is significant that the genetic deficiency of
aryl sulfatase A produces a clinically different mucopoly-
saccharidosis from that produced by the genetic deficiency of
aryl sulfatase B (43). As yet, however, which of the enzymes
are demonstrated cytochemically by the Goldfischer method (42)
remains uncertain (44).

IV. CONCLUDING REMARKS

   Although cytochemistry for electron microscopy is a de-
manding technique, it is rewarding in that it provides information that cannot otherwise be obtained. These methods are of
greatest value when used to distinguish among organelles or
cell populations that could not otherwise be distinguished
(i.e., by either biochemical or morphological techniques). For
example, cytochemistry has been used successfully to identify
functionally different cells in a mixed population (45, 46) and
to distinguish between morphologically similar organelles with
different functions (3, 47, 48). Although the number of methods

available for cytochemistry remains limited, there are nonetheless many significant problems that can profitably be explored
using cytochemistry for electron microscopy.

V.   APPENDIX

A.   *Incubation Media*

    (1) Barka - Anderson Acid Phosphatase Incubation Medium
       (49) (Modified Gomori Method)

Stock solutions
    1.25% β-Glycerophosphate, Grade I (make fresh)
      (Add 125 mg β-glycerophosphate to 10 ml distilled H_2O)
      Adjust to pH 5.0 with 1 N HCl
    0.2 M Tris-maleate buffer, pH 5.0 (make fresh)
    0.2% Lead nitrate (store at room temperature)
Medium
    (a) 10 ml Tris-maleate buffer
    (b) 10 ml distilled Water
    (c) 10 ml Substrate (β-glycerophosphate)
    (d) 20 ml Lead nitrate, added dropwise with constant
        stirring
    Combine ingredients in the order listed above (a - d).
    Adjust pH to 5.0. Add 5% sucrose.
Controls
    Without substrate: Make up medium as above but substitute
      additional 10 ml buffer for the substrate solution.
    Sodium fluoride inhibition: Add 0.01 M NaF to the complete
      incubation medium.

    (2) Aryl Sulfatase Incubation Medium (42)

Stock solutions
    Acetate Veronal buffer, see Buffers, Section V.D.2.
    24% Lead nitrate (store at room temperature)
Medium
    (a) 25 mg *p*-Nitrocatechol sulfate
    (b) 5.0 ml Acetate Veronal buffer, pH 5.4
    (c) 0.16 ml 24% Lead nitrate. Add slowly with stirring.
      (Lead nitrate causes a precipitate, but it will go into
      solution at pH 5.7.) Adjust to pH 5.5 with 0.1 N HCl.
Add 5% sucrose.
Control without substrate: Make up medium as above but omit
      p-nitrocatechol sulfate. At present, a specific inhi-
      bitor of aryl sulfatase is not available.

(3) Peroxidase Incubation Medium (50)

Medium
  (a) 10 ml 0.05 M Tris-HCl buffer, pH 7.6
  (b) 5 mg 3,3'-Diaminobenzidine tetrahydrochloride
  (c) 0.1 ml Diluted hydrogen peroxide (dilute 0.3 ml 30%
      hydrogen peroxide to 10 ml). Add to medium just
      before use.
  Adjust pH to 7.6. Add 5% sucrose. All solutions used in
    the incubation medium should be made the day that they
    are used.
Controls
  Without substrate: Prepare incubation medium without hy-
    drogen peroxide.
  Inhibitors: The following inhibitors (0.01 *M* concentra-
    tion) may be useful in the interpretation of peroxidase
    cytochemistry: potassium cyanide, sodium azide, and
    amino-triazole. One hour preincubation of fixed tissues
    with inhibitors in media lacking substrate may be neces-
    sary for penetration of the inhibitors into organelles
    such as leukocyte granules. Then incubate as usual in
    the complete medium with added inhibitor.

B. *Fixatives*

  (1) 1.5% Glutaraldehyde in 0.1 *M* sodium cacodylate-HCl,
      pH 7.4 + 1% sucrose:
      30 ml 10% Glutaraldehyde (E. M. Sciences)
      100 ml 0.2 *M* Sodium cacodylate stock
      70 ml distilled H₂O. Total solution 200 ml. pH
      to 7.4. Add 2 gm sucrose. Keeps 2-4 weeks refrigerated.
  (2) Dilute Formaldehyde-glutaraldehyde (7):
      0.5 gm paraformaldehyde powder
      19 ml distilled water
      25 ml 0.2 *M* Sodium cacodylate stock
      6 ml 25% Glutaraldehyde. Total solution 50 ml. Warm
      paraformaldehyde and water for 30 min in a 70°C water
      bath with stirring. Add 4-5 drops 0.1 *N* NaOH. Swirl
      until clear and cool. Add cacodylate and glutaralde-
      hyde. pH to 7.4. Add 25 mg CaCl₂ just before use.
      Fix tissues either cold or at room temperature, usually
      1-4 hr for optimal morphology. Fix only 5 min before
      cytochemical experiments.
  (3) Palade's Osmium:
      Mix just before use
      4 ml Acetate-Veronal stock
      4 ml 0.1 *M* HCl
      2 ml distilled water. Total volume 10 ml. pH to 7.6.

Add 10 ml osmium, 2% stock solution.   Add 5% sucrose.

C. In Block Stain

Kellenberger's in Block Uranyl Acetate Stain (36)
20 ml Acetate-Veronal stock
28 ml 0.1 N HCl
52 ml distilled H_2O.   Total solution 100 ml.
Adjust pH to 6.0.   Add 0.5 gm uranyl acetate to 100 ml
of buffer.   Store in refrigerator.   Keep from light.
Add 4% sucrose to a small aliquot on day of use.

D. Buffers

(1) Acetate-Veronal (A-V) Stock
1.943 gm Sodium acetate (MW 136, formula concentration 0.14 M)
2.943 gm Sodium Veronal (MW 206.18, formula concentration 0.14 M)
Dissolve and dilute to 100 ml with distilled H_2O.
(2) Acetate-Veronal Buffer
20 ml A-V stock
20 ml 0.1 N HCl
Dilute to 100 ml with distilled H_2O.   Adjust to pH 5.4
for aryl sulfatase incubation medium.
(3) Michaelis Wash Buffer
20 ml A-V stock
20 ml 0.1 N HCl
Mix and dilute to 100 ml with distilled H_2O.   Adjust
pH to 7.4.   Add 7 gm reagent grade sucrose.
(4) 0.2 M Sodium cacodylate Stock
21.4 gm sodium cacodylate
Add distilled H_2O to make 500 ml.
(5) Sodium cacodylate-HCl Wash Buffer
50 ml 0.2 M Sodium cacodylate stock
Dilute with distilled H_2O to 100 ml.   Adjust pH to 7.4
with 0.1 N HCl.   Add 7 gm sucrose.

E. Addresses of Chemical Companies

J. T. Baker Chemical Company
Phillipsburg, New Jersey 08865
(201) 859-2151
or: VWR Scientific, Inc.

Electron Microscopy Sciences
Box 251
Fort Washington, Pennsylvania 19034
(215) 646-1566

Fisher Scientific Co.
711 Forbes Ave.
Pittsburgh, Pennsylvania 15219
(412) 562-8300

Ladd Research Industries
P.O. Box 901
Burlington, Vermont 05401
(802) 658-4961

Mallinckrodt, Inc.
P.O. Box 5439
St. Louis, Missouri 63147
(314) 231-8980
or: Scientific Products

Sigma Chemical Co.
P.O. Box 14508
St. Louis, Missouri 63178
(800) 325-3010 (Order toll-free)

Worthington Biochemical Corporation
Freehold, New Jersey 07728
(800) 631-2142 (Order toll-free)

REFERENCES

1. M. A. Hayat (ed.). "Electron Microscopy of Enzymes.
    Principles and Methods," Vols. 1-4. Van Nostrand Reinhold,
    New York, 1973-1975.
2. B. A. Nichols, D. F. Bainton, and M. G. Farquhar. Differ-
    entiation of monocytes. Origin, nature, and fate of their
    azurophil granules. *J. Cell Biol. 50*: 498-515, 1971.
3. B. A. Nichols and D. F. Bainton. Differentiation of human
    monocytes in bone marrow and blood. Sequential formation
    of two granule populations. *Lab. Invest. 29*: 27-40, 1973.
4. B. A. Nichols. Normal rabbit alveolar macrophages. II.
    Their primary and secondary lysosomes as revealed by elec-

tron microscopy and cytochemistry. *J. Exp. Med. 144*: 920-932, 1976.

5. D. F. Bainton, B. A. Nichols, and M. G. Farquhar. Primary lysosomes of blood leukocytes. *In* "Lysosomes in Biology and Pathology," Vol. 5 (J. T. Dingle and R. T. Dean, eds.), pp. 3-32. North-Holland, Amsterdam, 1976.

6. D. D. Sabatini, K. Bensch, and R. J. Barrnett. Cytochemistry and electron microscopy. The preservation of cellular ultrastructure and enzymatic activity by aldehyde fixation. *J. Cell Biol. 17*: 19-58, 1963.

7. M. J. Karnovsky. A formaldehyde-glutaraldehyde fixative of high osmolality for use in electron microscopy. *J. Cell Biol. 27*: 137A-138A, 1965.

8. H. D. Fahimi and P. Drochmans. Essais de standarisation de la fixation au glutaraldéhyde. I. Purification et détermination de la concentration du glutaraldéhyde. *J. Microsc. 4*: 725-736, 1965.

9. E. A. Robertson and R. L. Schultz. The impurities in commercial glutaraldehyde and their effect on the fixation of brain. *J. Ultrastr. Res. 30*: 275-287, 1970.

10. R. E. Smith and M. G. Farquhar. Lysosome function in the regulation of the secretory process in cells of the anterior pituitary gland. *J. Cell Biol. 31*: 319-347, 1966.

11. D. Janigan. The effects of aldehyde fixation on acid phosphatase activity in tissue blocks. *J. Histochem. Cytochem. 13*: 476-483, 1965.

12. P. M. Seeman and G. E. Palade. Acid phosphatase localization in rabbit eosinophils. *J. Cell Biol. 34*: 745-756, 1967.

13. A. Leskes, P. Siekevitz, and G. E. Palade. Differentiation of endoplasmic reticulum in hepatocytes. 1. Glucose-6-phosphatase distribution *in situ*. *J. Cell Biol. 49*: 264-287, 1971.

14. L. S. Kaplow. Buffy coat preparatory tube. *Am. J. Clin. Pathol. 51*: 806-807, 1969.

15. R. van Furth (ed.). "Mononuclear Phagocytes, Functional Aspects. Parts I and II." Martinus Nijhoff Publishers, The Hague, 1980.

16. R. M. Steinman and Z. A. Cohn. The interaction of soluble horseradish peroxidase with mouse peritoneal macrophages *in vitro*. *J. Cell Biol. 55*: 186-204, 1972.

17. F. Roels, E. Wisse, B. De Prest, and J. van der Meulen. Cytochemical discrimination between catalases and peroxidases using diaminobenzidine. *Histochemistry 41*: 281-312, 1975.

18. J. Breton-Gorius and J. Guichard. Améliorations techniques permettant de révéler la peroxydase plaquettaire. *Nouv. Rev. Fr. Hematol. 16*: 381-390, 1976.

19. A. R. Spurr. A low-viscosity epoxy resin embedding medium

for electron microscopy. *J. Ultrastr. Res. 26*: 31-43, 1969.

20. E. Essner. Hemoproteins. *In* "Electron Microscopy of Enzymes. Principles and Methods," Vol. 2 (M. A. Hayat, ed.), pp. 1-33. Van Nostrand Reinhold, New York, 1974.

21. H. D. Fahimi. An assessment of the DAB methods for cytochemical detection of catalase and peroxidase. *J. Histochem. Cytochem. 27*: 1365-1366, 1979.

22. V. Herzog and H. D. Fahimi. Intracellular distinction between peroxidase and catalase in exocrine cells of rat lacrimal gland: A biochemical and cytochemical study. *Histochemistry 46*: 273-286, 1976.

23. M. LeHir, V. Herzog, and H. D. Fahimi. Cytochemical detection of catalase with 3,3'-diaminobenzidine. *Histochemistry 64*: 51-66, 1979.

24. U. Bretz and M. Baggiolini. Biochemical and morphological characterization of azurophil and specific granules of human neutrophilic polymorphonuclear leukocytes. *J. Cell Biol. 63*: 251-269, 1974.

25. D. F. Bainton and M. G. Farquhar. Differences in enzyme content of azurophil and specific granules of polymorphonuclear leukocytes. II. Cytochemistry and electron microscopy of bone marrow cells. *J. Cell Biol. 39*: 299-317, 1968.

26. S. G. Axline. Isozymes of acid phosphatase in normal and Calmette-Guérin Bacillus-induced rabbit alveolar macrophages. *J. Exp. Med. 128*: 1031-1048, 1968.

27. R. T. Dean. Multiple forms of lysosomal enzymes. *In* "Lysosomes in Biology and Pathology," Vol. 4 (J. T. Dingle and R. T. Dean, eds.), pp. 349-382. North-Holland, Amsterdam, 1975.

28. E. Essner. Phosphatases. *In* "Electron Microscopy of Enzymes. Principles and Methods," Vol. 1 (M. A. Hayat, ed.), pp. 44-76. Van Nostrand Reinhold, New York, 1973.

29. H. Beaufay. Methods for the isolation of lysosomes. Appendix I. The nonlysosomal localization of acid (*p*-nitro)phenyl phosphatase activity in various tissues. *In* "Lysosomes. A Laboratory Handbook" (J. T. Dingle, ed.), pp. 33-35. North-Holland, Amsterdam, 1972.

30. S. Goldfischer, E. Essner, and A. B. Novikoff. The localization of phosphatase activities at the level of ultrastructure. *J. Histochem. Cytochem. 12*: 72-95, 1964.

31. A. B. Novikoff. The endoplasmic reticulum: A cytochemist's view (A Review). *Proc. Nat. Acad. Sci. USA 73*: 2781-2787, 1976.

32. C. Oliver. Cytochemical localization of acid phosphatase and trimetaphosphatase activities in exocrine acinar cells. *J. Histochem. Cytochem. 28*: 78-81, 1980.

33. S. E. Nyquist and H. H. Mollenhauer. A Golgi apparatus

acid phosphatase. *Biochim. Biophys. Acta 315*: 103-112, 1973.

34. B. A. Nichols and D. F. Bainton. Ultrastructure and cytochemistry of mononuclear phagocytes. *In* "Mononuclear Phagocytes in Immunity, Infection, and Pathology" (R. van Furth, ed.), pp. 17-55. Blackwell Scientific Publications, Oxford, 1975.

35. E. Holtzman and R. Dominitz. Cytochemical studies of lysosomes, Golgi apparatus and endoplasmic reticulum in secretion and protein uptake by adrenal medulla cells of the rat. *J. Histochem. Cytochem. 16*: 320-336, 1968.

36. E. Kellenberger, A. Ryter, and J. Séchaud. Electron microscope study of DNA-containing plasms. II. Vegetative and mature phage DNA as compared with normal bacterial nucleoids in different physiological states. *J. Biophys. Biochem. Cytol. 4*: 671-678, 1958.

37. M. G. Farquhar and G. E. Palade. Cell junctions in amphibian skin. *J. Cell Biol. 26*: 263-291, 1965.

38. M. Borgers and F. Thoné. Further characterization of phosphatase activities using nonspecific substrates. *Histochem. J. 8*: 301-317, 1976.

39. J. Hugon and M. Borgers. Fine structural localization of acid and alkaline phosphatase activities in the absorbing cells of the duodenum of rodents. *Histochemie 12*: 42-66, 1968.

40. M. G. Farquhar, D. F. Bainton, M. Baggiolini, and C. de Duve. Cytochemical localization of acid phosphatase activity in granule fractions from rabbit polymorphonuclear leukocytes. *J. Cell Biol. 54*: 141-156, 1972.

41. D. F. Bainton and M. G. Farquhar. Differences in enzyme content of azurophil and specific granules of polymorphonuclear leukocytes. I. Histochemical staining of bone marrow smears. *J. Cell Biol. 39*: 286-298, 1968.

42. S. Goldfischer. The cytochemical demonstration of lysosomal aryl sulfatase activity by light and electron microscopy. *J. Histochem. Cytochem. 13*: 520-523, 1965.

43. A. A. Farooqui and P. Mandel. Minireview. On the properties and role of arylsulphatases A, B and C in mammals. *Int. J. Biochem. 8*: 685-691, 1977.

44. V. K. Hopsu-Havu and H. Helminen. Sulfatases. *In* "Electron Microscopy of Enzymes. Principles and Methods," Vol. 2 (M. A. Hayat, ed.), pp. 90-109. Van Nostrand Reinhold, New York, 1974.

45. R. H. J. Beelen, D. M. Fluitsma, J. W. M. van der Meer, and E. C. M. Hoefsmit. Development of exudate-resident macrophages, on the basis of the pattern of peroxidatic activity *in vivo* and *in vitro*. *In* "Mononuclear Phagocytes, Functional Aspects, Part I" (R. van Furth, ed.), pp. 87-112. Martinus Nijhoff Publishers, The Hague, 1980.

46. W. Th. Daems and H. J. van der Rhee. Peroxidase and
     catalase in monocytes, macrophages, epithelioid cells
     and giant cells of the rat. *In* "Mononuclear Phagocytes,
     Functional Aspects, Part I" (R. van Furth, ed.), pp. 43-
     60. Martinus Nijhoff Publishers, The Hague, 1980.
47. D. S. Friend and M. G. Farquhar. Functions of coated
     vesicles during protein absorption in the rat vas
     deferens. *J. Cell Biol. 35*: 357-376, 1967.
48. M. E. Bentfeld and D. F. Bainton. Cytochemical localiza-
     tion of lysosomal enzymes in rat megakaryocytes and
     platelets. *J. Clin. Invest. 56*: 1635-1649, 1975.
49. T. Barka and P. J. Anderson. Histochemical methods for
     acid phosphatase using hexazonium pararosanilin as
     coupler. *J. Histochem. Cytochem. 10*: 741-753, 1962.
50. R. C. Graham, Jr. and M. J. Karnovsky. The early stages
     of absorption of injected horseradish peroxidase in the
     proximal tubules of mouse kidney: ultrastructural cyto-
     chemistry by a new technique. *J. Histochem. Cytochem.
     14*: 291-302, 1966.

45

LYSOSOMAL ENZYMES

Earl H. Harrison
William E. Bowers

I. GENERAL INTRODUCTION

Mononuclear phagocytes are very active in the uptake and intracellular digestion of a variety of biological substances. The enzymes mainly responsible for the digestion of these substances are the lysosomal acid hydrolases, and these enzymes are found in relatively large amounts in mononuclear phagocytes. The cells also secrete acid hydrolases, as well as other hydrolytic enzymes that can degrade extracellular components. The latter enzymes, including lysozyme, collagenase, proteinases, neutral caseinases, elastaselike enzymes, and plasminogen activator are discussed in detail in other chapters. This chapter focuses on the assay of a number of the lysosomal acid hydrolases.

The assays described below have been used for a number of years in our laboratory to study the acid hydrolases in a variety of tissues and cell types and should, with the appropriate precautions, be easily applicable to mononuclear phago-

cytes from any species or tissue. It is, nonetheless, advisable to carry out preliminary kinetic studies with the particular enzyme source of interest to determine the optimal
conditions for each enzyme assay. It is essential to carry
out each assay under conditions where product formation is
proportional to the time of incubation and to the quantity of
enzyme assayed.

Although the acid hydrolases act on a wide variety of
substrates, they share certain properties. The most characteristic common feature is enzyme *latency,* which results from
the localization of acid hydrolases within membrane-bounded
lysosomes. An accurate determination of the total enzyme
activity requires that the lysosomal membrane be disrupted,
which can be achieved by including the detergent, Triton X-100
(at a concentration of about 0.1%) in the enzyme reaction mixture. If desired, latency can be determined by measuring both
the total activity and the free activity simultaneously, where
the latter is determined under conditions that preserve the
integrity of the lysosomal membrane (1,2,10). Latent activity
represents the difference between the free and total activities.

Acid hydrolases are very stable enzymes and can be assayed
without loss of activity after storage of many tissue homogenates in the freezer. It is, however, advisable to determine
the stability of the enzyme in each instance. Unless stated
otherwise below, the substrate solutions used in the assay of
the hydrolases are stable for several weeks when stored in the
refrigerator. They should be discarded when the blank values
substantially increase.

II. ACID PHOSPHATASE

A. *Introduction*

Acid phosphatase (EC 3.1.3.2) is most reliably measured by
assaying the enzymic release of inorganic phosphate from β-glycerophosphate. The inorganic phosphate formed during the reaction is determined colorimetrically by the micromethod of Chen
et al. (3).

B. *Reagents*

1. *For enzyme assay*

(a). 62.5 mM β-Glycerophosphate in 62.5 mM acetate buffer,
pH 5.0, containing 0.125% (w/v) Triton X-100

(b). Bovine serum albumin, 100 mg/ml
(c). 35% Trichloroacetic acid

2. *For Phosphate Determination*
(a). 10% (w/v) Ascorbic acid (store at 4°C, stable for 1 week)
(b). 2.5% (w/v) Ammonium molybdate
(c). 6 *N* Sulfuric acid

C. *Procedure*

1. *Enzyme Assay*
To 1.6 ml of substrate mixture add 0.4 ml of enzyme. Enzyme blanks receive 1.6 ml of buffer containing Triton X-100 and 0.4 ml of enzyme. Substrate blanks receive 1.6 ml of substrate mixture and 0.4 ml of enzyme diluent. Reactions are run at 37°C for the appropriate time and then terminated by setting the tube in an ice-water bath. To each tube add 0.2 ml of bovine serum albumin (100 mg/ml), mix, and add 0.4 ml of 35% trichloroacetic acid. Wait 10 min and centrifuge the tubes at 1500 *g* for 10 min at 4°C. Remove 1 ml of supernatant for phosphate determination.

2. *Phosphate Determination*
Prepare phosphate reagent by mixing 1 volume of 6 *N* sulfuric acid with 2 volumes of water and 1 volume of 2.5% ammonium molybdate, then add 1 volume of 10% ascorbic acid and mix well. This reagent must be prepared fresh daily.
Standards are prepared containing 20-200 nmol inorganic phosphate in a final volume of 1 ml. Samples contain 1 ml of supernatant from enzyme assay. To all tubes add 2 ml of phosphate reagent and mix. Incubate tubes at 37°C for 30 min to develop color. Read absorbance at 820 nm.

D. *Calculation of Data*

Results are expressed as milliunits, i.e., nanomoles inorganic phosphate released per minute.

E. *Critical Comments*

The presence of several phosphatases in most cell types makes the assay of any one of them in crude preparations problematical. Thus, although acid phosphatase is the "classical" lysosomal acid hydrolase, its assay poses more problems than many of the other acid hydrolases. The lysosomal β-glycero-

phosphatase is characteristically completely inhibited by low
concentrations (2-5 mM) of fluoride or L-(+)-tartrate, but is
totally resistant to treatment with N-ethylmaleimide (4).
The use of substrates other than β-glycerophosphate in the
assay of acid phosphatase (e.g., the chromogenic, p-nitrophenyl phosphate, or fluorogenic, 4-methylumbelliferyl phosphate) should be avoided unless the activities responsible
for their hydrolysis can be shown to have the characteristics
of the lysosomal enzyme.

III. ACID GLYCOSIDASES

A. *Introduction*

    The acid glycosidases [N-acetyl-β-glucosaminidase
(EC 3.2.1.30), β-galactosidase (EC 3.2.1.23), α-mannosidase
(EC 3.2.1.24), etc.] can be conveniently assayed by using the
nitrophenyl or phenolphthalein derivatives of the appropriate
glycosides as substrate and determining the amount of released
chromophore by absorption spectrophotometry. Alternatively,
when high sensitivity is required, the fluorogenic 4-methyl-
umbelliferyl derivatives can be used as substrate and the
product of the reaction fluorometrically determined.

B. *Reagents*

    1. For Colorimetric Assay
    (a). 7.5 mM p-Nitrophenyl-N-acetyl-β-glucosaminide in
0.125 M citrate buffer, pH 5.0, containing 0.125% (w/v) Triton
X-100 (for other glycosidase assays use 6.25 mM o-nitrophenyl-
β-galactoside, 7.5 mM p-nitrophenyl-α-mannoside, or 1.6 mM
phenolphthalein-β-glucuronide in 0.125 M acetate buffer, pH
5.0).
    (b). Glycine buffer, pH 10.7. 133 mM glycine 83 mM
sodium carbonate, 67 mM sodium chloride adjusted to pH 10.7
with sodium hydroxide.

    2. For Fluorometric Assay
    (a). 10 mM Stock solutions of the appropriate 4-methyl-
umbelliferyl glycosides (Koch-Light Laboratories, Colnbrook,
Buckinghamshire, England) are prepared in dry methoxyethanol
(stable for 4-6 weeks at 4°C).
    (b). Substrate solutions are prepared immediately before
use by diluting the above stock solutions to 0.2 mM in 0.1 M

acetate buffer, pH 5.0, containing 0.2% Triton X-100.   Use
0.1 M citrate buffer, pH 5.0, for 4-methylumbelliferyl-N-
acetyl-β-glucosaminide.
   (c).   50 mM Glycine - 5 mM EDTA adjusted to pH 10.4 with
sodium hydroxide.

C. Procedures

1. Colorimetric Assay
   To 0.4 ml of substrate add 0.1 ml of enzyme and incubate
at 37°C for the appropriate time.   Include enzyme and substrate
blanks in assay.   Terminate reaction by adding 3 ml glycine
buffer and read absorbance of resulting solution at 400 nm
(for nitrophenyl substrates) or at 540 nm (for phenolphthalein
substrates).

2. Fluorometric Assay
   To 0.1 ml of substrate add 0.1 ml of enzyme and incubate
at 37°C for the appropriate time.   Include enzyme and substrate
blanks in assay.   Terminate reaction by adding 2 ml of glycine
buffer and determine the fluorescence emission of the resulting
solution at 460 nm with an excitation wavelength of 365 nm.

D. Calculation of Data

   For the colorimetric assays, the absorbance data are converted to nanomoles of nitrophenol or phenolphthalein by reference to standard curves constructed with 10-200 nmol of the
authentic compounds in solutions having a composition identical
to those resulting from the enzyme assay.   Results are expressed in milliunits, i.e., nanomoles product formed per minute.
   Fluorometric readings are converted to nanomoles of 4-
methylumbelliferone by reference to a standard curve constructed with solutions containing 0.1 to 1.0 nmol of 4-methylumbelli-
ferone.   Results are expressed in milliunits as defined above.

E. Critical Comments

   The ease of assay and availability of chromogenic and
fluorogenic derivatives of a large number of glycosides make
the acid glycosidases attractive enzymes for study as lysosomal enzymes. N-Acetyl-β-glucosaminidase is present in relatively high amounts in most tissues and is exclusively localized in lysosomes in all tissues studied.   However, the enzyme
is inhibited to a considerable extent by acetate (5) and must
be assayed in citrate buffer for a reliable determination of

maximal activity. High sucrose concentrations are also inhibitory for glycosidases; the effect must be determined for each enzyme. The activities of other acid glycosidases are generally lower than that of N-acetyl-β-glucosaminidase. If assayed at pH values closer to neutrality, some of the glycosides may be hydrolyzed by enzymes other than the lysosomal, acid pH optimum enzyme.

IV. ARYLSULFATASE

A. *Introduction*

Arylsulfatase (EC 3.1.6.1) is assayed by incubation of enzyme with p-nitrocatechol sulfate and spectrophotometric determination of released p-nitrocatechol.

B. *Reagents*

(a). 25 mM p-Nitrocatechol sulfate in 62.5 mM acetate buffer, pH 5.0, containing 0.125% Triton X-100
(b). 2.2% Trichloroacetic acid
(c). 3.5 N Sodium hydroxide

C. *Procedure*

To 0.4 ml of substrate add 0.1 ml of enzyme and incubate at 37°C for the appropriate time. Include enzyme and substrate blanks in the assay. Reaction is terminated by adding 1.5 ml of ice-cold 2.2% trichloroacetic acid, after which each tube is placed in an ice-water bath (for 15 min). To develop the color, remove each tube from the ice bath and add 1.0 ml of 3.5 N NaOH. After 10 min read absorbance at 540 nm.

D. *Calculation of Data*

Absorbance measurements are converted to nanomoles of p-nitrocatechol by reference to a standard curve constructed with solutions containing 10-200 nmol of p-nitrocatechol. Activities are expressed in milliunits, i.e., nanomoles p-nitrocatechol released per minute.

E. Critical Comments

In rat spleen homogenates, the ionic strength of the reaction mixture affects the activity of arylsulfatase; optimal
activity was obtained in the presence of 0.2 *M* KCl (1). To
minimize hydrolysis of the substrate that occurs under acid
conditions, tubes are placed in ice after the enzyme reaction
is stopped by the addition of trichloroacetic acid.

V. ACID NUCLEASES

A. Introduction

Acid deoxyribonuclease (EC 3.1.22.1) and acid ribonuclease
(EC 3.1.27.5) are assayed by spectrophotometric quantitation
at 260 nm of enzymically produced acid-soluble nucleotides.

B. Reagents

1. For Acid Deoxyribonuclease
(a). DNA is denatured by heating for 3-5 min at 95°C,
cooling rapidly, and then dialysing overnight at 2°C against
either 0.1 *M* acetate buffer, pH 5.0, or against distilled
water.
(b). Substrate solution contains 3.125 mg/ml denatured
DNA in 62.5 m*M* acetate buffer, pH 5.0, 0.25 *M* KCl, and 0.125%
Triton X-100.
(c). 10% (w/v) Perchloric acid
(d). 0.01% Triton X-100

2. For Acid Ribonuclease
(a). RNA is dialyzed overnight at 2°C against 0.1 *M* acetate buffer, pH 5.0.
(b). Substrate solution contains 5.625 mg/ml RNA in 62.5
m*M* acetate buffer, pH 5.0, and 0.125% Triton X-100.
(c). 10% (w/v) Perchloric acid containing 0.25% uranyl
acetate.
(d). 0.01% Triton X-100.

C. Procedures

1. Acid Deoxyribonuclease
To 0.8 ml substrate solution add 0.2 ml enzyme. Incubate
at 37°C for the appropriate time. Terminate reaction by adding
1 ml of ice-cold 10% perchloric acid. Blanks are run in an

identical manner except that the incubation is stopped after
2 min. Keep mixture on ice for 15 min and filter in the cold.
An aliquot of the filtrate is made up to 3 ml with 0.01%
Triton X-100 and the absorbance of the resulting solution is
measured at 260 nm.

2. Acid Ribonuclease

To 0.8 ml substrate solution add 0.2 ml enzyme. Incubate
at 37°C for the appropriate time. Terminate reaction by adding 1 ml of ice-cold 10% perchloric acid containing 0.25%
uranyl acetate. Blanks are run in an identical manner except
that the incubation is stopped after 2 min. Mixtures are kept
on ice for 1 hr before being filtered. Readings are made as
described above for acid deoxyribonuclease.

D. Calculation of Data

For both acid deoxyribonuclease and acid ribonuclease,
results are expressed as nanomoles of mononucleotides released
per minute, assuming an extinction coefficient of 8.5×10^6
cm^2/mol at 260 nm (6).

With acid deoxyribonuclease, a sigmoidal relationship is
observed between the amount of acid-soluble nucleotides released and enzyme concentration (1,6). Thus, each sample must
be assayed at 4 or 5 enzyme concentrations and activity calculated from those in the linear range.

E. Critical Comments

With both rat spleen and liver, the optimal rate for acid
deoxyribonuclease occurs when 0.2 M KCl is present in the reaction mixture (1,6). The acid ribonuclease of rat spleen also exhibits marked increases in activity in the presence of
high salt concentrations (1). Under conditions of higher salt
concentrations, however, the enzyme activity versus time curve
shows considerable deviation from linearity. Reducing the
ionic strength to that of buffer alone results in linear kinetics for both enzyme activity versus time and for enzyme
activity versus enzyme concentration.

VI. CATHEPSIN D

A. Introduction

Cathepsin D (EC 3.4.23.5) is assayed by incubation of enzyme with 2% denatured hemoglobin followed by quantitation of
acid-soluble proteolytic products. The latter is accomplished

either by: (1) reaction of the Folin-Ciocalteau reagent with
aromatic peptides or (2) the reaction of fluorescamine with
the free amino group of peptides and amino acids to yield a
fluorescent product (7).

B. *Reagents*

   1. *For Enzyme Assay*
   (a). Preparation of substrate solution: Prepare 120 ml
of 14% bovine hemoglobin by adding water slowly to hemoglobin.
This procedure is carried out with thorough mixing so as to
avoid clumping of hemoglobin.   Dialyze solution extensively
against distilled water at 4°C, and after dialysis add 200 ml
of water.   Add 83.7 ml of 1 M lactate buffer, pH 3.6, and 41.8
ml of 2% Triton X-100.   Let solution stand at 37°C for 1 hr.
Add enough lactic acid to bring pH to 3.6.   Bring to a final
volume of 725 ml with H_2O.   Substrate solution is stored frozen and is indefinitely stable.
   (b). 35% Trichloroacetic acid.
   2. For colorimetric determination of acid soluble products:
   (a). Folin-Ciocalteau reagent
   (b). 0.44 N sodium hydroxide

   3. For fluorometric determination of acid soluble products:
   (a). Fluorescamine (Fluram, Hoffman-LaRoche Inc., 4-phenyl-
spiro [furan-2(3)H, 1'-phthalan]-3,3'-dione), 0.1 mg/ml in
acetone
   (b). 0.2 M borate buffer, pH 8.5, containing 0.1% Triton
X-100.

C. *Procedures*

   To 0.9 ml of substrate add 0.1 ml of enzyme and incubate
at 37°C for the appropriate time.   Blanks of identical composition (including enzyme) are incubated for 10 min.   Terminate
reaction by adding 5 ml of ice-cold 3.5% trichloroacetic acid,
mix well, and keep on ice for 20 min.   Centrifuge at 1500 g
for 10 min and use an aliquot of the supernatant for subsequent
assay.
   For the colorimetric assay, a 2 ml aliquot of the supernatant is mixed with 1 ml of Folin-Ciocalteau reagent.   5 ml of
0.44 N Sodium hydroxide is added, and after 10 min the absorbance at 660 nm is determined.
   For the fluorometric assay, a 0.2 ml aliquot of the supernatant is diluted to 0.4 ml with water.   After addition of 1.0
ml of borate buffer, 1.0 ml of the fluorescamine reagent is

Table I.   Studies on Lysosomal Acid Hydrolases in Mononuclear Phagocytes

Ref.	Species	Macrophages Studied	Enzymes Studied
(10)	Mouse	Resident peritoneal macrophages	Acid phosphatase N-Acetyl-β-glucosaminidase β-Glucuronidase α-Galactosidase α-Mannosidase
(11)	Mouse	Resident peritoneal macrophages Thioglycollate peritoneal macrophages Proteose-peptone peritoneal macrophages Cell Wall (strep A) peritoneal macrophages	Acid phosphatase N-Acetyl-β-glucosaminidase β-Glucuronidase α-Mannosidase Cathepsin D
(12)	Mouse	Resident peritoneal macrophages	Acid phosphatase N-Acetyl-β-glucosaminidase β-Glucuronidase β-Galactosidase Cathepsin D
(13)	Mouse	Resident peritoneal macrophages Thioglycollate peritoneal macrophages Endotoxin peritoneal macrophages	N-Acetyl-β-glucosaminidase Cathepsin D
(14)	Mouse	Thioglycollate peritoneal	N-Acetyl-β-glucosaminidase β-Glucuronidase β-Galactosidase Cathepsin D
(15)	Mouse	Resident peritoneal macrophages LPS peritoneal macrophages	Acid phosphatase β-Glucuronidase Acid ribonuclease Cathepsin D

Substrate	Studies Conducted
4-MU-phosphate[a] 4-MU-2-acetamido-2-deoxy-β-glucose 4-MU-β-glucuronide 4-MU-α-galactose 4-MU-α-mannose	Enzyme kinetics, inihibitors, activators, and latency. Complete analytical fractionation using isopycnic centrifugation and marker enzymes for various organelles. Effect of in vitro culture (72 hr) on enzyme activities, release of enzymes, and density of lysosomes and other organelles.
4-NP-phosphate[b] 4-MU-2-acetamido-2-deoxy-β-D-glucose 4-MU-β-D-glucuronide 4-MU-α-D-mannose Iodinated hemoglobin	Cellular content and secretion of enzymes during 10 days in culture. Distribution of enzymes after differential centrifugation. Stability of enzyme activities in culture medium. Other constituents studied were lysosome, plasminogen activator, lactate dehydrogenase.
α-Naphthylphosphate o-NP-2-acetamido-2-deoxy-β-D-glucose Phenolphthalein-β-D-glucuronide o-NP-β-D-galatose Hemoglobin	Cellular content and release of enzymes during 72 hr in culture in the presence or absence of streptococci type-specific polysaccharide and peptidoglycan (PPG). Other constituents were leucine-2-naphthylamidase and lactate dehydrogenase.
p-NP-2-acetamido-2-deoxy-β-D-glucose Denatured hemoglobin	Enzyme levels before and during latex ingestion. Major focus of study was on fibrinolysin and plasminogen activation.
p-NP-2-acetamido-2-deoxy-β-D-glucose Phenolphthalein-β-glucuronide p-NP-β-galatose Denatured hemoglobin	Cellular content of thioglycollate-stimulated macrophages after 2, 24, and 72 hr of culture. Major focus was on lysosome synthesis and secretion.
β-Glycerophosphate Phenolphthalein-β-glucuronide Yeast RNA Denatured hemoglobin	Cellular content of enzymes over 6 days in culture.

[a] 4-MU; 4-methylumbelliferyl.

[b] NP; nitrophenyl

Table I. (cont.)

Ref.	Species	Macrophages Studied	Enzymes Studied
(16)	Mouse	Resident peritoneal macrophages	Acid phosphatase β-Glucuronidase Cathepsin D
(17)	Mouse	Resident peritoneal macrophages	Acid phosphatase β-Glucuronidase Cathepsin
(18)	Rabbit	Mineral oil peritoneal macrophages Alveolar macrophages BCG-induced alveolar macrophages	Acid phosphatase β-Glucuronidase Acid ribonuclease Cathepsin
(19)	Rabbit	BCG-induced alveolar macrophages	Acid phosphatase β-Glucuronidase Acid ribonuclease Cathepsin

Substrate	Studies Conducted
β-Glycerophosphate Phenolphthalein-β-glucuronide Denatured hemoglobin	Effects of inhibitors of protein and nucleic acid synthesis on production of lysosomal enzymes by cultured macrophages.
β-Glycerophosphate Phenolphthalein-β-glucuronide Denatured hemoglobin	Effects of various sources and concentrations of serum on production of acid hydrolases.
β-Glycerophosphate Phenolphthalein-β-glucuronide Yeast RNA Denatured hemoglobin	Content and subcellular distribution of hydrolases after differential or isopycnic centrifugation of macrophage homogenates. Studies on enzyme latency.
β-Glycerophosphate Phenolphthalein-β-glucuronide Yeast RNA Denatured hemoglobin	Effects of phagocytosis of particles on content and release of lysosomal enzymes.

added while the contents are thoroughly mixed. The fluorescence emission at 475 nm is determined with an excitation
wavelength of 390 nm.

D. Calculation of Data

For the colorimetric assay, activity is expressed as described by de Duve *et al.* (2). The unit is defined as the
chromogenic equivalent of 1 mg/ml of bovine serum albumin assayed under identical conditions. Thus, standards (2 ml total
volume) containing 20 to 100 µg of bovine serum albumin are
included in each assay.

For the fluorometric assay, leucylleucine is used as a
standard in the range of 1-20 nmol. Enzyme activity is expressed in milliunits, one milliunit being the amount of enzyme that yields per minute a fluorescence equal to that of
1 nmol of leucylleucine.

E. Critical Comments

A potential problem in assaying cathepsin D with the Folin
reagent procedure is that the time course of the reaction is
not linear until 5-10 min after initiation of the reaction.
Thus it is extremely important that appropriate blanks be run
with each assay. The nonlinear kinetics occur because the enzyme in its initial attack on the hemoglobin molecule releases
large trichloroacetic acid-soluble peptides that are subsequently degraded without significantly increasing the amount of Folin
reactive soluble material. The fluorescamine reagent in reacting with primary amino groups is not subject to this error and
leads to more nearly linear time courses.

Other assays for cathepsin D activity that utilize radioactive hemoglobin substrates have also been described (8,9).

VII. CONCLUDING REMARKS

Most of the acid hydrolases described in this article have
been studied in both resident mononuclear phagocytes and in
those elicited by injection of animals with various substances.
In general, these studies have revealed differences in the content of acid hydrolases among macrophages from different tissue
sites, and differences between elicited and resident populations.
Studies have also been carried out to assess the effects of *in
vitro* culturing of macrophages for periods of up to several days

on the cellular content and secretion of acid hydrolases. Table I summarizes a number of the major studies that have been carried out on acid hydrolases in mononuclear phagocytes.

REFERENCES

1. W. E. Bowers, J. T. Finkenstaedt, and C. de Duve. Lysosomes in lymphoid tissue. I. The measurement of hydrolytic activities in whole homogenates. *J. Cell Biol.* *32*:325-337, 1967.
2. C. de Duve, B. C. Pressman, R. Gianetto, R. Wattiaux, and F. Appelmans. Tissue fractionation studies. 6. Intracellular distribution patterns of enzymes in rat-liver tissue. *Biochem. J.* *60*:604-617, 1955.
3. P. S. Chen, T. Y. Toribara, and H. Warner. Microdetermination of phosphorous. *Anal. Chem.* *28*:1756-1758, 1956.
4. M. Baggiolini, J. G. Hirsch, and C. de Duve. Further biochemical and morphological studies of granule fractions from rabbit heterophil leukocytes. *J. Cell Biol.* *45*:586-597, 1970.
5. D. Robinson, R. G. Price, and N. Dance. Separation and properties of β-glucuronidase, and *N*-acetyl-β-glucosaminidase from rat kidney. *Biochem. J.* *102*:525-532, 1967.
6. H. Beaufay, D. Bendall, P. Baudhuin, and C. de Duve. Tissue fractionation studies. 12. Intracellular distribution of some dehydrogenases, alkaline deoxyribonuclease, and iron in rat-liver tissue. *Biochem. J.* *73*: 623-627, 1959.
7. N. Yago, and W. E. Bowers. Unique cathepsin D-type proteases in rat thoracic duct lymphocytes and in rat lymphoid tissues. *J. Biol. Chem.* *250*:4749-4754, 1975.
8. J. S. Roth, T. Losty, and E. Wierbicki. Assay of proteolytic enzyme activity using ^{14}C-labeled hemoglobin. *Anal. Biochem.* *42*:214-221, 1971.
9. M. B. Hille, A. J. Barrett, J. T. Dingle, and H. B. Fell. Microassay for cathepsin D shows an unexpected effect of cycloheximide on limb-bone rudiments in organ culture. *Exp. Cell Res.* *61*:470-472, 1970.
10. P. G. Canonico, H. Beaufay, and M. Nyssens-Jaden. Analytical fractionation of mouse peritoneal macrophages: Physical and biochemical properties of subcellular organelles from resident (unstimulated) and cultivated cells. *J. Reticuloendothel. Soc.* *24*:115-138, 1978.

11. J. Schnyder, and M. Baggiolini. Secretion of lysosomal
     hydrolases by stimulated and nonstimulated macrophages.
     *J. Exp. Med. 148:*435-450, 1978.
12. P. Davies, R. C. Page, and A. C. Allison. Changes in
     cellular enzyme levels and extracellular release of
     lysosomal acid hydrolases in macrophages exposed to
     group A Streptococcal cell wall substance. *J. Exp. Med.
     139:*1262-1282, 1974.
13. S. Gordon, J. C. Unkeless, and Z. A. Cohn. Induction of
     macrophage plasminogen activator by endotoxin stimulation
     and phagocytosis. Evidence for a two-stage process.
     *J. Exp. Med. 140:*995-1010, 1974.
14. S. Gordon, J. Todd, and Z. A. Cohn. *In vitro* synthesis
     and secretion of lysozyme by mononuclear phagocytes.
     *J. Exp. Med. 139:*1228-1248, 1974.
15. Z. A. Cohn, and B. Benson. The differentiation of mono-
     nuclear phagocytes. Morphology, cytochemistry, and
     biochemistry. *J. Exp. Med. 121:*153-170, 1965.
16. Z. A. Cohn, and B. Benson. The *in vitro* differentiation
     of mononuclear phagocytes. I. The influence of inhibi-
     tors and the results of autoradiography. *J. Exp. Med.
     121:*279-288, 1965.
17. Z. A. Cohn, and B. Benson. The *in vitro* differentiation
     of mononuclear phagocytes. II. The influence of serum
     on granule formation, hydrolase production, and pino-
     cytosis. *J. Exp. Med. 121:*835-848, 1965.
18. Z. A. Cohn, and E. Wiener. The particulate hydrolases
     of macrophages. I. Comparative enzymology, isolation,
     and properties. *J. Exp. Med. 118:*991-1008, 1963.
19. Z. A. Cohn, and E. Wiener. The particulate hydrolases
     of macrophages. II. Biochemical and morphological re-
     sponse to particle ingestion. *J. Exp. Med. 118:*1009-
     1019, 1963.

46

MICROSOMAL HEME OXYGENASE

Diethard Gemsa

I. INTRODUCTION

Heme oxygenase (EC 1. 14.99.3) is a microsomal enzyme that catalyzes the oxidative degradation of heme to biliverdin IXα (1-3). Biliverdin is subsequently reduced to bilirubin IXα by the soluble biliverdin reductase (4). Both enzymes require NADPH as cofactor. In the overall conversion of heme to bilirubin, the microsomal heme oxygenase is the rate-limiting enzyme since biliverdin reductase is generally present in excess.

The assay method for microsomal heme oxygenase is based upon the conversion of heme to bilirubin, which can be measured spectrophotometrically by an increase in absorbance at 468 nm.

Microsomal heme oxygenase is most active in those tissues normally involved in the sequestration and breakdown of erythrocytes, namely, in spleen, liver, and bone marrow (2). In particular, the Kupffer cells of the liver (5) and the macrophages of the spleen (2) possess a high activity of the enzyme, whereas mononuclear phagocytes in the circulation or in the peritoneal cavity are devoid of it (6,7). However, microsomal heme oxygenase can be induced *de novo* in incompetent macrophages by an adaptive response to heme-containing compounds. This substrate-mediated enzyme induction in mononuclear phagocytes is principally regulated by the substrate load but other factors such as hormones, cyclic nucleotides, heavy metals, or lipopolysaccharides may be contributing components (7-9). Since bilirubin is the major catabolite in the degradation of hemoglobin in man and other mammals, heme oxygenase should theoretically be present or inducible in the various types of mononuclear phagocytes. However, this possibility has not yet been extensively studied.

Determination of microsomal heme oxygenase in mononuclear phagocytes may be of interest for the following reasons:

(1) It may serve as a marker enzyme for macrophages since other types of leukocytes apparently lack this ability.

(2) Regulation of the enzyme induction by heme compounds may characterize the synthetic capacity of organelles associated with microsomes.

(3) It may supplement studies concerned with degradation of erythrocytes by lysosomal enzymes.

(4) The activity of the enzyme in macrophages may serve to analyze other pathways of heme catabolism under *in vitro* conditions.

II.   REAGENTS

Potassium phosphate buffer, 0.1 M, pH 7.4

NADPH (reduced nicotinamide adenine dinucleotide phosphate), 4 mg/ml, dissolved in potassium phosphate buffer, stable 3 to 4 days at 4°C

Methemalbumin, 2.5 mM, prepared by dissolving 25 mg of hemin (Sigma Chem. Co.), 22.1 mg NaCl and 12.1 mg Tris base in 5 ml of 0.1 M NaOH. This solution is mixed with 10 ml of 1% human albumin and the pH is adjusted to 7.4 with 1.0 M HCl. Stable for 2 to 3 weeks at 4°C

III.   PROCEDURE

A.   *Assay of Microsomal Heme Oxygenase*

The standard reaction mixture (3.0 ml) contains the following solutions in a quartz cuvette (1-cm light path), equilibrated at 37°C: 0.02 ml methemalbumin, 2.4 ml potassium phosphate buffer and 0.4 ml of a 20,000 g supernatant of macrophages as enzyme source (see below). The reaction is initiated by the addition of 0.2 ml NADPH. In the simultaneously run control cuvette, NADPH is replaced by 0.2 ml potassium phosphate buffer. All constituents may be reduced proportionally to yield a final volume of 0.5 ml, or in the case of low heme oxygenase activity, the amount of the 20,000 g supernatant of macrophages may be increased at the expense of the potassium phosphate buffer. The cuvettes are placed in a recording spectrophotometer (Zeiss or Gilford), equipped with a constant temperature cuvette chamber set at 37°C. Formation of bilirubin can be determined from the increase in optical density at 468 nm, at which wavelength bilirubin absorbs maximally in the incubation mixture used here. The reaction rate is linear for 15 to 20 min. The increase in optical density should be compensated for the one in the control cuvette which, however, changes only occasionally due to nonspecific reactions such as agglomeration of microsomes.

B. Preparation of the Enzyme Source

Mononuclear phagocytes, at least 10×10^6, are suspended in 0.1 M potassium phosphate buffer, pH 7.4, at 4°C and sonicated for 10 to 20 sec at the lowest output of a sonifier tip. Sonication usually disrupts more than 95% of the cells when estimated microscopically and does not affect the activity of heme oxygenase. Macrophages, particularly when localized in tissue, may also be disrupted by using a Potter-Elvehjem homogenizer with a motor-driven Teflon pestle in a tight-fitting glass tube. Broken cell preparations are centrifuged at 20,000 g for 10 min at 4°C in order to obtain a supernatant fraction free of cell debris, nuclei, mitochondria, and lysosomes. This supernatant fraction, containing the small microsomes in suspension, serves as the enzyme source. Care has to be taken to secure a 20,000 g supernatant, which is uncontaminated by the lipid layer on top and the cell debris from the sediment. When kept on ice, the enzyme activity in the 20,000 g supernatant is stable for 3 to 4 hr.

IV. CALCULATION OF DATA

The linear increase of the optical density during the initial 15 min is used to determine the maximal reaction rate. Enzyme activity is calculated by using a millimolar extinction coefficient at 468 nm of 60 mM^{-1} cm^{-1} under the conditions described above. Results are expressed as nanomoles bilirubin formed per 10 mg supernatant protein per minute.

The millimolar extinction coefficient of bilirubin should be controlled for different conditions by using authentic bilirubin bound to albumin. Measured amounts of bilirubin, dissolved in 0.05 M NaOH, are mixed rapidly with an equimolar amount of 1% human albumin in 0.9% NaCl. Various amounts of this solution are added to supernatants to be tested and the extinction coefficient is determined at 468 nm.

V. CRITICAL COMMENTS

In order to obtain a measurable heme oxygenase activity, around 0.5 to 2.0 mg protein in the 20,000 g supernatant are required for the assay system.

In vitro induction of the enzyme by uptake of heme-containing compounds (methemalbumin, hemoglobin, erythrocytes) usually occurs after 3 to 5 hr of incubation and yields values between 0.3 to 0.6 nmol bilirubin/10 mg protein/min, depending on the experimental conditions and the amount of heme substrate load (7-9). In separate but identically performed incubations, the values for heme oxygenase activity usually differ by no more than 10% (7-9).

Convenient test systems for studying heme oxygenase induction *in vitro* consist of 50×10^6 to 150×10^6 macrophages, which have interiorized antibody-coated erythrocytes or other heme compounds. However, enzyme activity may also be successfully determined in the 20,000 g supernatant of as little as 10×10^6 mononuclear phagocytes, provided the assay system is proportionally reduced to a final reaction mixture of 0.5 ml.

Macrophages harvested from hemorrhagic exudates are not suitable for studying heme oxygenase induction *in vitro* since those cells already exhibit a high enzyme activity. When heme oxygenase induction is tested under *in vivo* conditions, enzyme activities as high as 1.30 and 2.60 nm bilirubin/10 mg protein/ min have been found in alveolar and peritoneal macrophages, respectively (6).

Modifications of the assay aystem, including determination of difference spectra or measurement of CO production, have been previously outlined (1,6).

REFERENCES

1. R. Tenhunen, H. S. Marver, and R. Schmid. The enzymatic conversion of heme to bilirubin by microsomal heme oxygenase. *Proc. Natl. Acad. Sci. 61:* 748-755, 1968.

2. R. Tenhunen, H. S. Marver, and R. Schmid. The enzymatic catabolism of hemoglobin: Stimulation of microsomal heme oxygenase by hemin. *J. Lab. Clin. Med. 75:* 410-421, 1970.

3. R. Tenhunen, H. S. Marver, and R. Schmid. Microsomal heme oxygenase. Characterization of the enzyme. *J. Biol. Chem. 244:* 6388-6394, 1969.

4. R. Tenhunen, M. E. Ross, H. S. Marver, and R. Schmid. Reduced nicotinamide-adenine dinucleotide phosphate-dependent biliverdin reductase: Partial purification and characterization. *Biochemistry 9:* 298-303, 1970.

5. D. M. Bissel, L. Hammaker, and R. Schmid. Liver sinusoidal cells. Identification of a subpopulation for erythrocyte catabolism. *J. Cell Biol. 54:* 107-119, 1972.

6. N. R. Pimstone, R. Tenhunen, P. T. Seitz, H. S. Marver, and R. Schmid. The enzymatic degradation of hemoglobin to bile pigments by macrophages. *J. Exp. Med. 133:* 1264-1281, 1971.

7. D. Gemsa, C. H. Woo, H. H. Fudenberg, and R. Schmid. Erythrocyte catabolism by macrophages *in vitro.* The effect of hydrocortisone on erythrophagocytosis and on the induction of heme oxygenase. *J. Clin. Invest. 52:* 812-822, 1973.

8. D. Gemsa, C. H. Woo, H. H. Fudenberg, and R. Schmid. Stimulation of heme oxygenase in macrophages and liver by endotoxin. *J. Clin. Invest. 53:* 647-651, 1974.

9. D. Gemsa, C. H. Woo, D. Webb, H. H. Fudenberg, and R. Schmid. Erythrophagocytosis by macrophages: Suppression of heme oxygenase by cyclic AMP. *Cell. Immunol. 15:* 21-36, 1975.

47

HISTAMINE-*O*-METHYLTRANSFERASE

Julian Melamed
Harvey R. Colten

I. INTRODUCTION

Histamine catabolism in man proceeds via two main enzymatic pathways: the oxidative deamination of histamine to imidazole acetic acid proceeds via the enzyme histaminase (diamine oxidase) and *N*-methylation of histamine to methylhistamine via histamine *O*-methyltransferase (EC 2.1.1.8). The latter enzyme activity is measured by its ability to form methylated metabolites of histamine in the presence of radio-labeled methyl donor (*S*-adenosyl-L-[methyl-^{14}C] methionine). The assay is performed in a mixture that contains an inhibitor of histaminase to prevent catabolism of histamine by the alternative mechanism.

This assay is a modification of that described originally by Taylor and Snyder (1) and later by Beaven (2). The method is applicable to the study of mononuclear phagocytes from all species.

II.   REAGENTS

Sodium/potassium phosphate, 0.1 M pH7.9 stored at 4°C

Aminoguanidine sulfate (Eastman, Rochester, New York.)
2×10^{-3} M, stored at -20°C

Histamine dihydrochloride (Sigma, St. Louis, Missouri)
2×10^{-3} M stored at -20°C

S-Adenosyl-L-[methyl-^{14}C]methionine (Amersham, Arlington,
Illinois) 0.5 mCi/mm, stored at -90°C

1 Methylhistamine (Calbiochem, La Jolla, California)
1.5 mg/ml in 0.4 N HClO$_4$ stored at -20°C

Enzyme standard: Prepared from guinea brain or rat
kidney as previously described (3,4)

Chloroform stored and dispensed in a repipette
(Laboratory Industries).

10 N and 3 N NaOH

Instagel (Packard Industries, Illinois)

III.   PROCEDURE

(1).   Mononuclear cell preparations either in suspension
following isolation by Ficoll-Hypaque or dextran sedimentation,
or mononuclear cell monolayers may be utilized. The cells are
washed twice in RPMI 1640 in the cold, and cell suspensions
are adjusted to 10^8 mononuclear cells/ml in 0.1 M phosphate
buffer, pH 7.9. For monolayers the cell number is estimated
by DNA content by a modification (5) of the method of Kissane
(6). One microgram of DNA is equal to 10^5 human mononuclear
cells.
(2).   Cell lysates are prepared by freezing and thawing
mononuclear cells 7 times or by sonication with five 5-second
bursts at 50 W at 4°C (Heat Systems Ultrasonic, Inc., Plainview, New York). Nuclear and other debris are removed by
centrifugation at 8000 g for 10 min. Lysates are stored at
-90°C until assayed.
(3).   Protein determination on cell lysates is performed
by the method of Lowry (7).

(4). The reaction mixture is made up as follows in
16 × 125 mm screw top tubes (Corning).

    (a) S-adenosyl-L-[methyl-^{14}C]methionine, 15 nCi in 25 µl
    (b)   Histamine dihydrochloride 2 × 10^{-3} M, 25 µl
    (c)   Aminoguanidine sulfate 2 × 10^{-3} M, 25 µl
    (d)   Enzyme source, 100 µl
    (e)   Phosphate buffer 0.1 M pH 7.9, 325 µl

(5). This mixture is vortexed and incubated at 37°C
for 90 min.
(6). The reaction is stopped by the addition of 200 µl
of 1 methylhistamine 1.5 mg/ml in 0.4 N HClO$_4$. The unlabeled
methylhistamine minimizes adsorption of labeled methylhistamine onto glass surfaces, and the HClO$_4$ precipitates the protein, inactivating the enzyme.
(7). Controls include

    (a) A source of highly active enzyme: rat kidney or
guinea pig brain extract.
    (b) An inactive source of enzyme such as boiled rat
kidney or guinea pig brain extract, as well as a boiled aliquot of the enzyme source to be assayed.
    (c) A blank in which the histamine is omitted.
    (d) A blank in which the radiolabeled methyl donor is
added at the end of the incubation period.

(8). The mixture is extracted as follows:

    (a) Two hundred microliters of 10 N NaOH are added to
each tube and the mixture briefly vortexed.
    (b) Four milliliters of chloroform are dispensed and
the mixture is vortexed for a full minute.
    (c) Tubes are spun at 1000 g for 5 min at room tempera-
ture. The aqueous phase (top phase) as well as any interphase
material is removed by aspiration.
    (d) One milliliter of 3 N NaOh is added, tubes vortexed
and spun at 1000 g for 5 min at room temperature. The aqueous
and interphase material is again aspirated.
    (e) Three milliliters of the chloroform phase is removed
with a glass pipette (with propipette) and added to glass
vials, which are dried under a heat lamp.
    (f) Ten milliliters of instagel are added to each vial,
which are shaken for 10 min and counted in a scintillation
spectrometer.

IV. CALCULATION OF DATA

Data are expressed in terms of nanomoles of histamine-converted/milligram of protein/hour. The number of nanomole converted is calculated by subtracting the counts per minute for the enzyme assay from the blank (all the blanks should be of approximately the same magnitude. Counts per minute are converted to nanomoles by counting an aliquot of S-adenosyl-L-[methyl-^{14}C]methionine.

V. CRITICAL COMMENTS

The assay is reproducible within an error of ±10% and is sensitive to 1.5 nmol/hr/mg protein. Histamine methyltransferase is present in human monocytes at a mean concentration of 10.08 nmol/hr/mg protein (8) (range 8.93 - 11.22 nmol/hr/mg) and in some human leukemic monocytes at a concentration of 20.87 nmol/hr/mg protein. This assay may not be accurate in the presence of other methylating enzyme systems.

This assay represents a modification of a widely utilized method of histamine determination.

While both guinea pig brain and rat kidney are highly active sources of this enzyme, the latter may be a more active and specific source of histamine methyltransferase (4).

REFERENCES

1. K. M. Taylor and S. H. Snyder. Isotopic microassay of histamine, histidine, histidine decarboxylase, and histamine methyltransferase in brain tissue. *J. Neurochem.* *19:*1343-1358, 1972.
2. M. A. Beaven, S. Jacobsen, and Z. Horáková. Modification of the enzymatic isotopic assay of histamine and its application to measurement of histamine in tissues, serum, and urine. *Clin. Chim. Acta 37:*91-103, 1972.
3. D. D. Brown, R. Tomchick, and J. Axelrod. The distribution and properties of a histamine methylating enzyme. *J. Biol. Chem. 234:*2948-2950, 1959.
4. R. E. Shaff and M. A. Beaven. Increased sensitivity of the enzymatic isotopic assay of histamine in plasma and serum. *Anal. Biochem. 94:*425-450, 1979.
5. L. P. Einstein, E. S. Schneeberger, and H. R. Colten. Synthesis of the second component of complement by long-

term primary cultures of human monocytes. *J. Exp. Med.* *143*:114-126, 1976.

6. J. M. Kissane and E. Robins. The fluorometric measure-
    ment of deoxyribonucleic acid in animal tissues with
    special reference to the central nervous system. *J. Biol.*
    Chem. 233:184-188, 1958.

7. O. H. Lowry, N. J. Rosebrough, A. L. Fara, and R. J.
    Randall. Protein measurement with the folin phenol re-
    agent. *J. Biol. Chem. 193*:265-275, 1951.

8. R. S. Zeiger, D. Y. Yurdin, and H. R. Colten. Histamine
    metabolism <u>II</u>. Cellular and subcellular localization of
    the catabolic enzymes, histaminase, and histamine methyl-
    transferase in human leukocytes. *J. Allergy Clin.*
    Immunol. 58:172-179, 1976.

48

5'-NUCLEOTIDASE ASSAY

Paul J. Edelson
Robert A. Duncan

I. INTRODUCTION

5'-Nucleotidase (5'-ribonucleotide phosphohydrolase
EC 3.1.3.5) hydrolyzes the phosphoester linkage in 5'-mono-
nucleotides, liberating a nucleoside and inorganic phosphate.
Because of its presence in a great variety of tissues, in
many species, and its localization to the plasma membrane, the
enzyme has been widely used as a convenient marker for the
plasma membrane in cell fractionation studies. It has been
identified as an ecto enzyme (1), oriented with its active
site accessible to the cell milieu in guinea pig neutrophils
(2), and subsequently in mouse peritoneal macrophages (3).
Its status in several other cell types is summarized in Table
I. Information on its presence in a variety of mouse mononuclear phagocyte cell lines has recently been published (4).
The absence of the enzyme has been used as one of several
tests for macrophage activation (5).

TABLE I. 5'-Nucleotidase Activity of Selected Cell Types

Cell type	Species	5'-Nucleotidase activity	Reference
Neutrophil	Guinea pig	Present	(2)
	Human	Absent	(8)
Monocyte	Mouse	Absent	(9)
	Human	Absent[a]	(10)
Alveolar macrophage	Mouse	Present	(9)
Peritoneal macrophage			
Resident	Mouse	Present	(11,12)
Thioglycollate-stimulated	Mouse	Absent	(12)
BCG/PPD-stimulated	Mouse	Absent	(13)
Granuloma macrophage	Mouse	Absent	(14)
Platelet	Human	Absent	(15)
Erythrocyte	Human	Absent	(15)
Lymphocyte			
B lymphocyte	Human	Present	(16)
T lymphocyte	Human	Present	(16)

[a]Activity develops over 24-48 Hr in culture.

Most assays for 5'-nucleotidase depend upon measuring the rate of appearance of one of the two products of hydrolysis of the nucleotide substrate: either the inorganic phosphate or the nucleoside. In the assay described below, the nucleotide carries a radioactive label in its nucleoside portion and the labeled nucleoside generated by the enzymatic hydrolysis is separated from the substrate and counted in a scintillation spectrometer. The method is modified from Avruch and Wallach (6).

II. REAGENTS

(1)   Tris-HCl buffer containing 54 mM Tris and 13 mM MgCl$_2$, pH 9.0 (1000 ml)   Dissolve 6.51 gm Trizma Base (Sigma Chemical Co., St. Louis, Missouri, Catalog No. T-1503) and 2.44 gm MgCl$_2$.6 H$_2$0 in suffieient distilled water to make 1 liter of solution. Adjust to pH 9.0 with 2 N HCl and store indefinitely at 4°C.

(2)   [3H]-AMP stock (25 µCi/ml in 50% ethanol) (10 ml)   Add 9.75 ml ice-cold 50% ethanol to 1 vial Adenosine-[2-^{3}H]-5'-monophosphate, ammonium salt, 250 µCi in 0.250 ml, >2000 mCi/mmol (Amersham Corp., Arlington Heights, Illinois, Catalog. No. TRK.344). [^{3}H]-AMP stock can be used for approximately four months if stored at -20°C.

(3)   0.25 M ZnSO$_4$ (100 ml)   Add distilled water to 7.19 gm ZnSO$_4$·7 H$_2$0 to make 100 ml of solution. This may be stored indefinitely at room temperature.

(4)   0.25 M Ba (OH)$_2$ (100 ml)   7.89 gm Ba(OH)$_2$·8 H$_2$0. Add distilled water to make 100 ml of solution. Ba(OH)$_2$ may be stored indefinitely at room temperature. This is a saturated solution and should be filtered through coarse paper (e.g., Whatman No. 1) immediately before use.

(5)   Substrate (25 nCi 5'-[^{3}H]-AMP/ml, 0.15 mM 5'-AMP, 6mM p-NP) (100 ml) 5.8 mg Adenosine-5'-monophosphoric acid, sodium salt, from yeast, crystalline, Type II (Sigma Chemical Corp., St. Louis, Missouri, Catalog No. A-1752) (MW=388.4); 222.6 mg p-Nitrophenyl phosphate, disodium (Sigma Chemical Corp., St. Louis, Missouri, Catalog No. 104.0); 0.1 ml [^{3}H]-AMP stock; 100 ml Tris-HCl buffer. Substrate should be prepared immediately prior to assay and kept on ice.

III. PROCEDURE

(1). Place 0.1 ml aliquots of sample (e.g., cell lysate prepared in fresh 0.05% Triton X-100 as described by Edelson, this volume) or of the appropriate enzyme blank (e.g., 0.05% Triton X-100 alone) in glass test tubes (culture tubes, disposable glass, 12 x 75 mm, Curtin, Matheson Scientific, Inc., Houston, Texas, Catalog No. 339-275) on ice.

(2). Add 0.5 ml substrate, shake well, and incubate in a 37°C water bath for 30 min.

(3). Stop the reaction by returning the tubes to an ice bath and adding 0.2 ml 0.25 M $ZnSO_4$. Vortex briefly.

(4). Add 0.2 ml freshly filtered 0.25 M $Ba(OH)_2$ and vortex thoroughly.

(5). Centrifuge at 1500 g for 20 min at room temperature (or 4°C).

(6). Add 0.5 ml supernatant to 5 ml Aquassure (New England Nuclear, Boston, Massachusetts, Catalog No. NEF-965) in 6 ml plastic minivials (Plastic Sampule liquid scintillation vials, Wheaton Scientific, Millville, New Jersey, Catalog No. 986624) and mix well.

(7). Prepare counting standards (equivalent of 100% hydrolysis) by diluting 1.0 ml substrate with 1.0 ml water. Add 0.5 ml to 5 ml Aquassure, as above.

(8). Count for 10 min in a liquid scintillation counter (Packard Instrument Co., Inc., Downers Grove, Illinois). Typical settings for ^3H for a Tricarb counter are A-B channel; 70% gain; 50-4000 gate setting; External standard off.

IV. CALCULATIONS

0.5 ml of 0.15 mM 5'-AMP substrate = 75 nm 5'-AMP per sample. Thus, specific activity can be expressed as mU/mg protein = nm 5'-AMP hydrolyzed/min/ng protein

$$\cong \frac{\dfrac{(CPM_{EXP} - CPM_{BL})}{(CPM_{STD} - CPM_{BL})} \times 75\,nm}{(30\ min) \times (mg\ protein/0.1\ ml)}$$

Protein concentration can be determined as described by Meltzer, this volume.

V. CRITICAL COMMENTS

This is a fairly simple and highly reproducible assay, with a range of sensitivity wide enough to detect activity of between 5 x 10^4 and 1 x 10^6 resident mouse peritoneal macrophages. The activity present in 5×10^5 resident macrophages is about 44.2 mU/mg protein.

This method presents a convenient alternative to spectrophotometric assays for 5'-nucleotidase or protocols using ^{32}P-labeled nucleotides. It requires no second enzyme for product conversion as some spectrophotometric protocols do, and offers the greater sensitivity inherent in assays using radioactive tracers without the hazard of using ^{32}P. It is also relatively rapid, a typical assay takes about 3 hr.

It is important to establish that the activity observed is actually due to 5'-nucleotidase, rather than a nonspecific phosphatase. p-Nitrophenyl phosphate is used here as a competitive inhibitor of other phosphatases. At pH 9.0 acid phosphatase activity is not of concern and 5 mM β-glycerophosphate may be used in place of p-Npp as an effective inhibitor of alkaline phosphatase in situations where confusion with other intracellular phosphatases (e.g., glucose-6-phosphate phosphatase) is not an issue. Tartrate (10 mM) inhibits phosphatases active at pH 5.0.

5'-Nucleotidase shows peaks in activity at pH 5.5 and 7.0, with an additional peak occurring at about pH 9.2 when $MgCl_2$ is included in the reaction mix. Removal of divalent cations with 20 mM EDTA reduces activity more than 95% at pH 9.0. Addition of 0.1 mM Zn^{2+} completely eliminates nucleotidase activity. One should be cautioned, however, that EDTA interferes with the $BaSO_4$ precipitation and a different assay method must be used (see reference 7).

5'-Nucleotidase is most effective hydrolyzing ribonucleoside 5'-monophosphates, with little or no cleavage of the corresponding 5'-deoxyribonucleotides or 5'-ribonucleoside di- or triphosphates observed. A nucleotide analog, α,β-methylene adenosine 5'-diphosphate (AOPCP), has been reported to be a very powerful inhibitor of 5'-nucleotidase, though its efficacy may vary among different species.

LITERATURE SOURCES

Much additional useful information may be found in the following:

C. C. Widnell. Purification of rat liver 5'-nucleotidase as a complex with sphingomyelin. *Methods Enzymol. 32:* 368-374, 1974.
B. L. Reimer, and C. C. Widnell. The demonstration of a specific 5'-nucleotidase activity in rat tissues. *Arch. Biochem. Biophys. 171:*343-347, 1975.

Z. A. Werb, and Z. A. Cohn. Plasma membrane synthesis
in the macrophage following phagocytosis of polystyrene
latex particles. *J. Biol Chem. 247:*2439-2446, 1972
R. M. Burger, and J. M. Lowenstein. Preparation and
properties of 5'-nucleotidase from smooth muscle of small
intestine. *J. Biol. Chem. 245:*6247-6280, 1970.

REFERENCES

1. P. J. Edelson. Macrophage ecto enzymes: Their identi-
    fication, metabolism, and control. "Mononuclear Phago-
    cytes: Functional Aspects" (R. van Furth, ed.),
    Martinus Nijhoff, The Hague, 1980.
2. J. W. DePierre and M. L. Karnovsky. Ecto enzymes of the
    guinea pig polymorphonuclear leukocyte. I. Evidence for
    an ecto adenosine monophosphatase, -adenosine triphos-
    phatase, and -*p*-nitrophyl phosphatase. *J. Biol. Chem.
    249:*7111-7120, 1974.
3. P. J. Edelson and Z. A. Cohn. 5'-nucleotidase activity
    of mouse peritoneal macrophages. II. Cellular distri-
    bution and effects of endocytosis. *J. Exp. Med. 144:*
    1596-1608, 1976.
4. P. S. Morahan and P. J. Edelson. Mouse mononuclear phago-
    cyte cell lines. *J. Reticuloendothel. Soc.* (in press).
5. C. Bianco and P. J. Edelson. Characteristics of the acti-
    vated macrophage. "Immune Effector Mechanisms in Disease"
    (M. E. Weksler *et al.,* eds.), pp. 1-8. Grune and Stratton,
    New York, 1978.
6. J. Avruch and D. F. H. Wallach. Preparation and properties
    of plasma membrane and endoplasmic reticulum fragments from
    isolated rat fat cells. *Biochem. Biophys. Acta 233:*334-347,
    1976.
7. B. Glastris and S. E. Pfeiffer. Mammalian membrane marker
    enzymes: Sensitive assay for 5'-nucleotidase and assay
    for mammalian 2',3'-cyclic nucleotide-3'-phosphohydrolase.
    *Methods Enzymol. 32:*124-131, 1974.
8. P. S. Shirley, P. Wang, L. R. DeCjatelet, and B. M. Waite.
    Absence of the membrane marker enzyme 5'-nucleotidase in
    human polymorphonuclear leukocytes. *Anal. Biochem. 64:*
    624-627, 1975.
9. E. James and P. J. Edelson. Unpublished observations.

10. W. D. Johnson, B. Mei, and Z. A. Cohn. The separation, long-term cultivation, and maturation of the human monocyte. *J. Exp. Med.* *146:*1613-1626, 1977.
11. R. L. Nachman, B. Ferris, and J. G. Hirsch. Macrophage plasma membranes. I. Isolation and studies on protein components. *J. Exp. Med.* *133:*785, 1971.
12. P. J. Edelson and Z. A. Cohn. 5'-Nucleotidase activity of mouse peritoneal macrophages. I. Synthesis and degradation in resident and inflammatory preparations. *J. Exp. Med.* *144:*1581-1595, 1976.
13. P. J. Edelson and C. Erbs. Biochemical and functional characteristics of the plasma membrane of macrophages from BCG-infected mice. *J. Immunol.* *120:*1532-1536, 1978.
14. R. J. Bonney, I. Gery, T. Y. Lin, M. F. Meyerhofer, W. Acevedo, and P. Davies. Mononuclear phagocytes from carrageenan-induced granulomas. Isolation, cultivation, and characterization. *J. Exp. Med.* *148:*261-275, 1978.
15. K. Gass and P. J. Edelson. Unpublished observations.
16. J. Schwaber and P. J. Edelson. Unpublished observations.

49

ALKALINE PHOSPHODIESTERASE I

Paul J. Edelson
Katherine D. Gass

I. INTRODUCTION

Phosphodiesterase I (EC 3.1.4.1) liberates 5'-nucleotides from polyribonucleotides or oligodeoxyribonucleotides in a step-wise manner starting from a nucleotide with a free 3'-OH group at the tail of the chain. In this assay, we use an artificial substrate in which a single nucleotide is coupled at its 5'-end to a phosphate group that is then bound to a *p*-nitrophenyl group instead of to a length of coupled nucleotides. When the 5'-mononucleotide is liberated from the *p*-nitrophenyl group, the group can be detected by its strong yellow color in alkaline solutions.

The assay may conveniently be used on cell lysates, cell fractions, or extracellular fluid. Sufficient activity is present in 10^6 resident mouse peritoneal macrophages for convenient detection.

II.   REAGENTS

Sorensen's Glycine II Buffer (with 2 mM Zinc acetate)
Solution A (0.1 M glycine + 0.1 M NaCl)
   7.5 gm glycine
   5.85 gm NaCl
Disolve in sufficient distilled water to make 1 liter of
solution.

Solution B (0.1 N NaOH):   4 gm NaOH
Dissolve in sufficient distilled water to make 1 liter
of solution.
Combine 732 ml solution A + 238 ml solution B. Add 440
mg zinc acetate to 1 liter of buffer. Adjust pH to 9.6.
Store refrigerated. Buffer can be indefinitely stored.

Substrate (1.5 mM Thymidine-5'-phosphate-p-nitrophenol)
Dissolve 8.11 mg TMP-p-NP (Calbiochem-Behring Corp.,
La Jolla, California Catalog No. 48786), MW 537.5, in 10
ml Sorensen's glycine II-Zn acetate buffer (pH 9.6).
Substrate should be stored dessicated, refrigerated, and
protected from light. Substrate solution should be prepared on the day of assay, and may be held on ice for
several hours if protected from light.

III.   PROCEDURE

(1). Place 50 μl aliquots of cell lysates (prepared in
0.05% Triton X-100 as described by Edelson, this volume.) or
Triton X-100 alone (for enzyme blank) in small disposable
glass test tubes (culture tubes, disposable glass, 12 x 75 mm,
Curtin, Matheson Scientific, Inc., Houston, Texas, Catalog
No. 339-275.)
(2). Add 0.5 ml substrate, prewarmed to 37°C.
(3). Shake briskly, cover rack with aluminum foil, and
incubate tubes in 37°C water bath for 30 min.
(4). At end of incubation, immediately place tubes on
ice, and stop reaction with 1.0 ml 0.1 N NaOH.
(5). Vortex thoroughly each tube.
(6). Read absorbance within 30 min at 400 nm.

IV. CALCULATION

One unit equals that amount of enzyme which hydrolyzes
1 μm of substrate per minute under above assay conditions.

mU/mg protein =

$$\frac{\text{absorbance (sample) - absorbance (blank)}}{1.55 \text{ ml}} \times \frac{1}{\text{protein conc (mg/ml)}} \times 6.7$$

The factor 6.7 is derived as follows:

Molar extinction coefficient of p-nitrophenol = 12 X 10^3
OD U/l M (at 400 nm).

Then, specific activity in mU/mg = nmol/min/mg protein=

$$\frac{\dfrac{\text{(absorbance)}}{\text{ml}}}{\dfrac{\text{(protein conc)}}{\text{(mg/ml)}}} \times \frac{10^3}{12} \times \frac{1}{30 \text{ min}} \times 1.5 \times 1.55 =$$

$$\frac{\dfrac{\text{(absorbance)}}{\text{ml}}}{\dfrac{\text{protein conc}}{\text{(mg/ml)}}} \times 6.7$$

V. CRITICAL COMMENTS

This is a simple, straightforward, and highly reliable
assay. Because it is based on a colorimetric measurement, it
is about an order of magnitude less sensitive than assays using radioactive substrates, but even so it readily detects the
activity present in 10^6 resident mouse peritoneal macrophages
that is about 1.43 mU/mg.

REFERENCES

1. The artificial substrate used in this assay was originally
    described in
    W. E. Razzell and H. G. Khorana. Studies on polynucleo-
    tides. III. Enzymic degradation. Substrate specificity
    and properties of snake venom phosphodiesterase. *J. Biol.
    Chem. 234:*2105, 1959.

2. The various phosphodiesterases are reviewed in
   H. G. Khorana. *In* "The Enzymes" Vol. 5 (P. D. Boyer,
   H. Lardy, and K. Myrback, eds.), pp. 79. Academic Press,
   New York, 1961. 2nd edition.
3. The assay was adapted from the protocol presented by
   H. Beaufay, A. Amar-Costesec, E. Feytmans, D. Thines-
   Simpoux, M. Wibo, M. Robbi, and J. Berthet. Analytical
   study of microsomes and isolated subcellar membranes from
   rat liver. I. Biochemical methods. *J. Cell Biol. 61*:188,
   1974.
4. An example of the application of this assay to macrophages
   is
   P. J. Edelson and C. Erbs. Plasma membrane localization
   and metabolism of alkaline phosphodiesterase I in mouse
   peritoneal macrophages. *J. Exp. Med. 147*:77, 1978.

50

QUANTITATION OF LEUCINE AMINOPEPTIDASE
OF MONONUCLEAR PHAGOCYTES

Page S. Morahan

I. INTRODUCTION

Aminopeptidase (EC 3.4.1.2) is a plasma membrane-bound
enzyme present on macrophages as well as a variety of other
cells (1,2). In human peripheral blood or bone marrow, the
enzyme is reported to be present on monocytes and granulocytes but not on lymphocytes, basophils, or promyelocytes (1).
Wachsmuth (2,8) has found the enzyme in mice in monocytes and
tissue macrophages, but not in granulocytes, lymphocytes, or
erythrocytes. The aminopeptidase in macrophages appears similar to that enzyme in the proximal kidney tubules and in the
small intestine of the mouse (3). The ecto enzyme nature has
been shown by removal of the enzymatic activity by treatment
of the cells with papain, under conditions that do not affect
cell viability (4).

The enzyme activity in cell lysates can be easily determined by measuring the hydrolysis of 1 mM leucine ρ-nitro-
anilide to ρ-nitroaniline. The method described by Wachsmuth
and Stoye (5) will be detailed.

II. REAGENTS

(1) 10 mM Leucine ρ-nitroanilide substrate (Sigma L-9125).
Prepare by dissolving 28.8 mg in 10 ml of absolute methanol. Store at 4°C and prepare fresh every week. About twice the specific activity is obtained with the substrate prepared in methanol rather than dimethylsulfoxide.

(2) 0.1 M Sodium phosphate buffer, pH 7.5.
Prepare by mixing approximately 500 ml of 0.1 M Na$_2$H PO$_4$ with 80 ml of 0.1 M KH$_2$PO$_4$ to a pH of 7.5. If filter sterilized, the buffer can be kept at 4°C for months.

(3) Standard microsomal leucine aminopeptidase enzyme
     (Sigma L-6007).
Hydrate the lyophilized enzyme in 1 ml distilled water. To prepare the stock, dilute the enzyme 1:100 in phosphate-buffered saline containing 0.1% bovine serum albumin as protein carrier. Store the material at 4°C. Do not freeze as activity will be rapidly lost. The standard remains stable for about 3 months.

(4) Macrophage cell lysates.
Plate cells to provide about 1-3 $\times$ 10^6 macrophages. Lyse the cells in 200 µl of freshly prepared 0.05% Triton X-100 in distilled water freshly prepared from a 5% stock which can be kept indefinitely. After centrifuging down the cell debris, place 100 µl of lysate in small tubes, seal with parafilm, and store at -20°C until assayed. Another sample should also be obtained for protein determination.

III. PROCEDURE

(1) Prepare the standard enzyme by placing in a small glass tube 25 µl of the 1:100 stock enzyme solution and 75 µl of 0.05% Triton X-100 in distilled water.

(2) Prepare blank tubes with 100 µl of 0.05% Triton X-100 in distilled water.

(3) Thaw the previously prepared 100 µl samples of macrophage cell lysates.

(4) To each of the above tubes, add 800 µl of the phosphate buffer. A repetitive micropipettor can be used. Warm at 37°C for 10 min.

(5) Rapidly add 100 µl of leucine ρ-nitroanilide substrate to each tube, to provide a final 1 mM concentration. A repetitive micropipettor can be used. Reincubate in 37°C water bath for 15 min.

(6) Stop the reaction by placing the tubes on ice, after
vortexing each tube. Read the concentration of ρ-nitroaniline
at 405 nm. Read within one hour.

IV. CALCULATION OF DATA

(1) The specific activity is calculated using a molar
extinction coefficient of 9600 for ρ-nitroaniline at 405 nm.
(2) The specific activity, in nmoles/mg protein/min at
37°C is calculated by

$$SA = \frac{\text{OD for the 100 } \mu l \text{ cell lysate}}{\text{mg protein in that volume}} \times \frac{1000}{\text{min of reaction} \times 9.6}$$

The SA can, of course, also be based on DNA content or number
of cells in the sample.
(3) The standard enzyme is used as a check on the sensitivity and reproducibility of the system.

V. CRITICAL COMMENTS

(1) Try to use cell numbers that produce reaction product
in the range of 0.1 to 0.7 OD. In this range of enzyme concentration and with 1 mM substrate concentration, the reaction
is linear through 20 min of incubation. At higher concentrations, artifactual product reactions can take place.
(2) The range of SA of murine resident peritoneal macrophages is usually 2-8 nmol/mg protein/min. In experiments
with resident macrophages from CD-1 female outbred mice, we
obtained a SA of 3.9 ± 0.5 SE for four determinations with
macrophages cultured for 24 hr (10). There were no significant
changes in activity between 2 and 72 hr of culture. There are
strain differences; resident BALB/c macrophages cultured for
24 hr showed a SA of 7.4 ± 0.9 SE for five determinations.
The values for resident macrophages are increased two- to fivefold in thioglycollate, carrageenan, C. parvum, or pyran-
elicited macrophages (4-7). Typical values we have obtained
with murine macrophage-like cell lines include 8.4 for WEHI-3,
19.6 for J774.1, 20.6 for PU5-1.8, 6.0 for P388D1, 16.4 for
RAW309.CR1, and 12.6 for WR19M1. The differences in these
values may reflect differentiation or maturational changes.
The murine P388 lymphoma cell line and L929 fibroblasts also
have activity.

(3) Aminopeptidase activity of individual cells in cyto-centrifuge preparations can also be measured as described by Wachsmuth and Stoye (5) using leucine-4-methoxy-2-napthylamide substrate and fast blue B salt. Other substrates, such as alanine-β-napthylamide (1) and angiotensin (9), have also been used since the enzyme sequentially cleaves amino acids from the N-terminal end of peptides relatively nonspecifically.

REFERENCES

1. G. A. Ackerman. Histochemical demonstration of amino-peptidase activity in leukocytes of blood and bone marrow. *J. Histochem. Cytochem. 8:* 386, 1960.
2. E. D. Wachsmuth. Lokalisation von aminopeptidase in gewebeschnitten mit einer neuen immunofloureszenztechnik. *Histochemie 14:* 282-296, 1968.
3. E. D. Wachsmuth and A. Torhorst. Possible precursors of aminopeptidase and alkaline phosphatase in the proximal tubules of kidney and the crypts of small intestine in mice. *Histochemistry 38:* 43-56, 1974.
4. E. D. Wachsmuth and J. P. Stoye. Aminopeptidase on the surface of differentiating macrophages: Concentration changes on individual cells in culture. *J. Reticuloendo-thel. Soc. 22:* 485-497, 1977.
5. E. D. Wachsmuth and J. P. Stoye. Aminopeptidase on the surface of differentiating macrophages: Induction and characterization of the enzyme. *J. Reticuloendothel. Soc. 22:* 469-483, 1977.
6. P. S. Morahan and P. J. Edelson. Characteristics of mouse macrophages. *J. Reticuloendothel. Soc. 27:* 233-239, 1980.
7. R. J. Bonney, I. Gery, T. Y. Lin, M. F. Meyenhofer, W. Acevedo, and P. J. Davies. Mononuclear phagocytes from carrageenan-induced granulomas. *J. Exp. Med. 148:* 261-273, 1978.
8. E. D. Wachsmuth and F. G. Staber. Changes in membrane-bound aminopeptidase on bone-marrow derived macrophages during their maturation *in vitro. Exp. Cell Res. 109:* 269-276, 1977.
9. A. B. Kurtz and E. D. Wachsmuth. Identification of plasma angiotensinase as aminopeptidase. *Nature 224:* 92-93, 1969.
10. Morahan, P. S., P. J. Edelson and K. Gass. Changes in macrophage ectoenzymes upon *in vivo* or *in vitro* activation for antitumor activity. *J. Immunol. 125:* 1313-1317, 1980.

51

HEXOSE MONOPHOSPHATE SHUNT ACTIVITY

AND OXYGEN UPTAKE

Lawrence R. DeChatelet
J. Wallace Parce

I. GENERAL INTRODUCTION

Phagocytic cells show marked alterations in oxidative
metabolism when stimulated with a suitable particle or membrane
perturbent. This phenomenon is collectively referred to as
the "respiratory burst" and has been best described in polymorphonuclear neutrophils. In those cells, phagocytosis
results in marked increases in oxygen consumption, oxidation
of glucose via the hexose monophosphate shunt, generation of
hydrogen peroxide, superoxide anion, and chemiluminescence,
and reduction of tetrazolium dyes (1).

Similar alterations have been described in other phagocytic cells, including eosinophils (2), monocytes (3), and
macrophages (4). In general, the alterations in macrophage
metabolism upon phagocytosis are qualitatively similar to

METHODS FOR STUDYING
MONONUCLEAR PHAGOCYTES

those observed in the neutrophil, but resting (basal) levels
tend to be higher and the degree of stimulation is generally
substantially less. This is a generalization and varies with
the type of macrophage as well as method of isolation and
degree of activation. The fact that the oxidation metabolism
of the cell may reflect the degree of "activation" allows
these parameters to be used to assess the immunologic status
of macrophages (5).

II. METHOD FOR MEASUREMENT OF HEXOSE MONOPHOSPHATE
     SHUNT ACTIVITY

A. *Introduction*

     The estimation of glucose oxidation via the hexose mono-
phosphate shunt relies on the ability of the cell to oxidze
preferentially [1-^{14}C] glucose over [6-^{14}C] glucose to $^{14}CO_2$
as originally described by Beck (6). Glucose specifically
labeled in the C-1 position with ^{14}C may be degraded to $^{14}CO_2$
by either the hexose monophosphate shunt or mitochondrial
(Krebs cycle) pathways. In contrast, glucose labeled in the
C-6 position with ^{14}C is essentially metabolized only via the
Krebs cycle. The difference in $^{14}CO_2$ evolved from [1-^{14}C] glucose and [6-^{14}C] glucose is thus a reasonably accurate measurement of hexose monophosphate shunt activity. The usual procedure involves incubating cells in a closed system separately
with [1-^{14}C] glucose and [6-^{14}C] glucose under resting and
phagocytizing conditions. The incubation system contains a
trap for $^{14}CO_2$ containing a strongly basic substance. Following a period of incubation at 37°C, the reaction is stopped by
the addition of acid (which releases $^{14}CO_2$ dissolved in the
medium) and the radioactivity in the base is determined with
a liquid scintillation counter.

B. *Reagents*

     1. Buffer. Dulbecco's phosphate-buffered saline (PBS)
without sodium bicarbonate or phenol red is purchased as a
10-fold concentrate from Grand Island Biological Co., Grand
Island, New York. The buffer does contain physiologic concentrations of Ca^{2+} and Mg^{2+}. To prepare the working buffer,
100 ml of the concentrate is diluted with 850 ml of deionized
water and the pH adjusted to 7.4 by the dropwise addition of
10 N NaOH, using a magnetic stirrer and pH meter. The concentrated buffer is made up at pH 5.0 to avoid precipitation of
magnesium and calcium salts; it is imperative to adjust the
pH in dilute solution. Once the pH has been adjusted to 7.4,
the solution is brought to a final volume of 1 liter by the

addition of deionized water. The dilute buffer may be stored
in the refrigerator for several weeks; it should be discarded
if it exhibits a cloudy appearance.

2. Isotopes. D-[1-^{14}C] glucose and D-[6-^{14}C] glucose are
purchased from New England Nuclear Corp., Boston, Mass. The
isotopes usually have a specific activity of 45 - 60 mCi/mmol
and are supplied in ethanol:water (9:1) solution. The exact
specific activity of the isotopes is not important, since the
assay is performed in the presence of a large excess of non-
labeled glucose. Before use, the isotopes are evaporated to
dryness under a gentle stream of nitrogen and the material
dissolved in deionized water to a final concentration of
2 μCi/ml. The isotope solutions are divided into 5.0 ml aliquots and stored frozen at -20°C. Under these conditions,
both isotopes are remarkably stable and may be kept for at
least 12 months without significant deterioration.

3. Zymosan. Zymosan is employed as a phagocytic stimulus
because we have generally observed that it is more avidly phagocytized and yields a greater degree of respiratory burst activity than other particles. It is purchased as a dry powder
from Sigma Chemical Co., St. Louis, Mo., and stored in the
refrigerator. Just prior to use, it is suspended in PBS so
that the absorbance at 525 nm is 1.00, using a Beckman spectrophotometer.

4. Serum. Pooled serum is obtained from the same species
of animal as the macrophages. The serum is stored frozen at
-70°C in small aliquots and is used as a source of both opso-
nins and unlabeled glucose in the assays; it is not heat-
inactivated. For expression of data in nmoles of glucose
oxidized, it is necessary to determine the serum glucose concentration by standard procedures. With rabbit alveolar macrophages, we commonly employ a final serum concentration of 10%;
with smaller animals where the amount of serum might be limiting, this can readily be reduced to 1%. In this case, non-
labeled glucose should be added to the assay to maintain the
desired glucose concentration.

C. Procedure

The reaction is typically performed in 50 ml erlenmeyer
flasks in a total volume of 3.0 ml. Cells are suspended in
PBS to a final concentration of 5×10^6/ml and zymosan to an
O.D. of 1.0 at 525 nm. All additions are made to the flasks
on ice with the exception of cells. The reaction is initiated
by the addition of cells and a center well containing 0.50 ml
of hyamine hydroxide is simply placed inside the flask. We
routinely use mini-scintillation vials for the center wells;
these fit very nicely within the 50 ml flasks. The center
well is most easily introduced into the flask by means of a

hemostat; the hemostat is inserted into the mouth of the mini-
vial and slight outward pressure allows easy manipulation of
the vial. Following addition of the center well, the flask
is tightly capped with a soft rubber stopper and transferred
to a 37°C shaking water bath. Flasks are started at timed
intervals and stopped in the same sequence. A typical protocol for an experiment is presented in the tabulation (Table I)
below; all numbers represent the ml of stock solution employed.

Triplicate assays are performed for each of the above
conditions. After 60 min incubation, the reactions are stopped
in timed sequence by the addition of 1.0 ml of 10% trichloroacetic acid to the main body of the flask; care must be exercised not to get acid into the center well. As soon as the
acid is added, the flask is re-stoppered and allowed to
incubate 15 - 30 min longer to ensure that all released $^{14}CO_2$
has been trapped in the hyamine. The center wells are then
removed and the outside of the wells washed with a stream of
deionized water to remove any adherent isotopes and dried with
a Kimwipe. Three ml of scintillation fluid (4.0 g Omnifluor,
New England Nuclear Corp., Boston, Mass., per liter of toluene)
are added to each mini-vial. The vials are capped and radioactivity determined directly in a liquid scintillation counter.

D. Calculation of Data

The average data obtained in the representative experiment
are given below in the tabulation (Table II).

The specific contribution of the hexose monophosphate
shunt is given by (cpm from [1-^{14}C] glucose) - (cpm from
[6-^{14}C] glucose). Thus the above data may be expressed
directly as HMS activity as follows (see tabulation below
(Table III)).

Table III.

Cell Type	HMS activity (cpm)	
	Resting	Zymosan
Normal Alveolar Macrophages	1,197	4,636
BCG-Induced Alveolar Macrophages	1,707	13,690

For most purposes, simple expression of the data as cpm is
sufficient. It is apparent from the above that resting HMS
activity is somewhat higher in BCG-induced as opposed to normal
alveolar macrophages. The activity in both cell types
increases with phagocytosis, but the increase in the activated
cells is 3-fold higher than in the normal cells.

Table I.

	A	B	C	D	E	F	G	H
PBS	1.60	0.60	1.60	0.60	1.60	0.60	1.60	0.60
[1-^{14}C] glucose (2 µCi/ml)	0.10	0.10	—	—	0.10	0.10	—	—
[6-^{14}C] glucose (2 µCi/ml)	—	—	0.10	0.10	—	—	0.10	0.10
Serum	0.30	0.30	0.30	0.30	0.30	0.30	0.30	0.30
Zymosan	—	1.00	—	1.00	—	1.00	—	1.00
Normal Alveolar Macrophages	1.00	1.00	1.00	1.00	—	—	—	—
BCG-Induced Alveolar Macrophages	—	—	—	—	1.00	1.00	1.00	1.00

Table II.

cpm in $^{14}CO_2$ from

Cell Type	[1-^{14}C] glucose		[6-^{14}C] glucose	
	Resting	Zymosan	Resting	Zymosan
Normal Alveolar Macrophages	1,436	6,326	239	1,690
BCG-Induced Alveolar Macrophages	2,047	16,147	240	2,457

In some situations, e.g. stoichiometric comparisons with oxygen uptake, it is useful to express the data as the absolute amount of glucose oxidized/5 × 10^6 cells. For this calculation, one must determine the cpm added to each flask under the same counting conditions used in the assay and must further know the absolute amount of glucose present in each flask. In the experiment illustrated above, 0.10 ml of [1-^{14}C] glucose was counted in 0.50 ml hyamine hydroxide and 3.0 ml scintillation fluid and yielded 310,000 cpm. Thus under phagocytizing conditions, the BCG-induced macrophages oxidized (13,690/310,000) × 100 or 4.4% of the available glucose. Since the glucose concentration of the serum was experimentally determined to be 80 mg/dl, the addition of 0.30 ml serum corresponds to 0.24 mg glucose/flask. Since the molecular weight of glucose is 180.2, then 1 μmol of glucose = 180.2 μg or .180 mg and the amount added/flask is 0.24/0.18 or 1.33 μmol. The amount oxidized via the HMS is 4.4% of this or (1.33 μmol)(0.044) = 0.059 μmol or 59 nmol. Similar calculations may be performed for the remaining data.

E. *Critical Comments*

There are a number of advantages to this assay. The assay is quite precise and replicate values are generally in very good agreement; further, a large number of experimental conditions may be performed simultaneously. Because of the isotopic nature of the assay, it is extremely sensitive. If cells are limiting, it may be easily scaled down simply by reducing simultaneously the number of cells and of serum while maintaining the same quantity of radiolabeled glucose. We have employed this assay with human neutrophils, monocytes, and eosinophils and with rabbit and guinea pig alveolar macrophages (both normal and activated); others have employed similar procedures with virtually every type of macrophage obtainable. As described, the assay utilizes cells in suspension; modifications have been described in which HMS activity in adherent cells can be measured (7). One disadvantage to this assay is that measurements are made at a single time point and thus rates are not directly determined. This can be overcome by stopping the reaction at various time intervals and plotting cpm versus time of incubation. Although we routinely employ zymosan as the challenge particle, a large number of different types of particles may be employed. However, if a live organism is used as the challenge particle, controls must be included in which the macrophages are omitted to account for the glucose oxidation of the organism itself.

III. MEASUREMENT OF OXYGEN UPTAKE

A. *Introduction*

   Oxygen uptake by the cells may be determined by measuring
the loss of oxygen from the suspending medium. This measurement is most readily performed by continuous polarographic
monitoring of the dissolved ocygen concentration in the suspending medium during the experiment. A Clark type polarographic electrode in conjunction with the proper electronics
produces a signal which is directly proportional to the concentration of dissolved oxygen in the suspension. This signal
may be applied to a meter which can be read at various time
points to determine the rate of oxygen uptake, or more typically, the signal is applied to a strip chart recorder to get
a continuous trace of oxygen concentration versus time.

B. *Equipment*

   The necessary equipment for performing oxygen uptake measurements consists of an oxygraph cell, circulating water bath,
magnetic stirrer, oxygen probe, and an oxygen meter. Also,
although not absolutely necessary, a strip chart recorder is
highly recommended as part of the setup. The following hybrid
of commercially available parts has been found to be the most
satisfactory setup for these measurements.

   1. Oxygraph cell. The Gilson oxygraph cell consists of a
1.8 ml water-jacketed sample chamber, a horizontal opening for
the oxygen probe, and a vertical opening with a ground glass
joint which accommodates a hollow glass plug used for making
additions to the sample during a measurement. Inlet and out-
let nipples on the water jacket fit 7 mm ID tygon tubing
(Fisher) which is connected to the circulating water bath for
temperature control of the sample.
   2. Circulating water bath. Practically any circulating
water bath will suffice. The temperature of the water bath
should be adjusted, however, to give the desired temperature
in the sample chamber as measured directly with a thermometer.
   3. Magnetic stirrer. Practically any magnetic stirrer will
suffice. In general, the stronger the magnet the better, since
the stir bar in the sample chamber is elevated above the stirrer due to the thickness of the water jacket. The best stir
for this system is the 2 × 7 mm stir bar sold by Tri-R
Instruments, Inc., Rockville Centre, New York. Carpet tape
(both sides sticky) is used to hold the oxygraph cell to the
top of the magnetic stirrer. The tape is pressed onto the top
of the stirrer and the bottom of the oxygraph cell is pressed

firmly against the tape. The adhesive on this tape (available at Sears and carpet stores) is sufficient to hold the oxygraph cell in place, and furthermore, it minimizes the distance between the stirrer and the stir bar.

4. Oxygen probe. The oxygen probe (Clark electrode) can be purchased from Yellow Springs Instruments (YSI 5331), Yellow Springs, Ohio. In addition a Standard Membrane/KCl Kit (YSI 5775) and a Membrane Mounting Kit (YSI 5350) should be purchased for probe preparation.

5. Oxygen meter. The oxygen meter (YSI 53) can also be purchased from Yellow Springs Instruments. This instrument contains two separate oxygen probe inputs, a meter, and a 100 mV output for a strip chart recorder.

6. Strip chart recorder. Any 100mV strip chart recorder will do.

C. Instrumental Setup and Calibration

1. Oxygen probe preparation. The oxygen probe consists of two silver anodes and a platinum cathode which are embedded in an epoxy matrix but exposed at the end of the probe. The cathode and anodes are separated from the sample solution by a Teflon membrane. Preparation of the probe involves cleaning of the silver anodes and application of the Teflon membrane to the end of the electrode. The probe should be placed in the probe holder such that the end with the exposed silver and platinum electrodes is pointing up. Clean the two silver (rectangular) anodes by gently rubbing with a cotton swab soaked in 50% concentration of NH_4OH solution. This should leave the silver electrodes clean (e.g., free of any tarnish or scale). If the silver does not come clean this way, a drop of "Pearl Drops" toothpaste should be placed on the end of the probe and the silver polished by gently rubbing with a fresh cotton swab. When the silver is completely clean, wipe the residual toothpaste off with a paper wiper and rinse the end of the eletrode with distilled water.

Place a sheet of Teflon membrane (handle only at edges) over the membrane holder ring and secure to holder ring by passing the large "O" ring over the membrane and onto the metal membrane holder ring. This should hold the membrane such that it is stretched taut (no wrinkles) over the end of the mem- brane holder ring. Slide the probe "O" ring (small) onto the Teflon applicator tool. Place a drop of the 50% saturated KCl solution on the end of the probe and wet the "O" ring groove on the probe with this solution as well. Pass the mem- brane holder ring (membrane end up) over the end of the probe until it is suspended by the membrane resting on the end of the probe. Firmly press the large end of the Teflon applica-

tor against the end of the probe and slide the probe "O" ring
down the applicator and onto the probe such that it secures
the Teflon membrane to the end of the probe. Remove the Teflon applicator, the large "O" ring and the membrane holder
ring, and cut away the excess Teflon membrane close to the
"O" ring with a pair of scissors. Inspect the end of the
probe to make sure that there are no holes or wrinkles in the
Teflon membrane and that there are no air bubbles in the KCl
solution between the Teflon membrane and the end of the probe.
Wet the "O" ring on the end of the probe and slide the probe
into the horizontal opening in the oxygraph cell until it
comes to the stop. Insert the plug on the other end of the
probe cable into either one of the two probe jacks (I and II)
on the back of the oxygen meter and set the probe switch on
the front panel (I or II) to the corresponding position.

   2. Oxygen meter calibration. Turn on circulating water
bath, magnetic stirrer and oxygen meter. Allow time for water
bath to reach desired temperature. Fill sample chamber with
air saturated distilled water (*caution:* freshly distilled or
deionized water may be low in oxygen content) and drop the
magnetic stir bar in. Adjust the magnetic stirrer for a
vigorous stir rate. Wait three minutes for temperature equilibration of the sample and probe. Set oxygen meter selector
switch to AMP ZERO and set meter to zero with AMP ZERO control.
Set selector switch to AIR position and adjust the meter to
100% with the appropriate PROBE control. At this point when
first setting up the system, it is advisable to properly
adjust the stir rate in the sample. Turn the magnetic stirrer
off and the reading on the meter should start dropping. Turn
the stirrer back on and slowly increase the stirring speed.
As the stirring speed is increased, the meter reading should
increase up to a point and then level off. Any stir rate
above the point at which the meter reading levels off is adequate. With the stir rate properly adjusted, readjust the
meter to 100% with the PROBE control if necessary.

   3. Recorder calibration. When using a recorder, set the
recorder to the 100mV full-scale setting. Set the oxygen
meter to AMP ZERO and adjust the recorder to read zero with
the recorder zero knob. Switch the oxygen meter to AIR and
adjust the recorder sensitivity knob to set the pen at full-
scale position. If the recorder does not have a sensitivity
control, use the RECORDER ADJUST control at the back of the
oxygen meter to set the recorder to full scale.

D. Procedure

   Remove water from the sample chamber by aspiration. Add
0.62 ml Dulbecco's phosphate-buffered saline (see Section II.
B.1), 0.18 ml serum (see Section II.B.4) and 1.0 ml of the

cell suspension at 5×10^6 cells/ml. Fit the hollow stopper
into the ground glass joint of the sample cell. All air
bubbles should rise to the top of the cell and exit via the
narrow channel through the center of the stopper. The sample
fluid should fill approximately the bottom one-third of the
hollow channel in the stopper. If the level is much higher
or lower than this, the amount of buffer which is added to the
sample chamber should be adjusted in order to give the proper
fluid height when the stopper is inserted. The volume of the
sample chamber varies slightly from cell to cell and it is,
therefore, often necessary to adjust the buffer volume to compensate for these differences. Allow three to four minutes
for temperature equilibration and then start the recorder or
begin reading and recording percent saturation at known time
intervals. Record this "resting" rate of oxygen uptake for
10 or 15 minutes or until a straight line is obtained on the
recorder trace. Inject 20 ul of a 55 mg/ml suspension of
zymosan (see Section II.B.3) in PBS into the sample chamber
with a 50 µl Hamilton syringe. Place the needle through the
channel in the hollow glass plug and make sure the tip of the
needle is all the way into the sample chamber before injecting.
Again record the rate of oxygen uptake for 10 to 15 minutes
as before the zymosan injection.

E. *Calculation of Data*

For data obtained without a recorder, the percent saturation versus time is plotted and the best straight line drawn
through the data points representing the resting and stimulated
rates of oxygen uptake. The slope of these plots or of the
recorder trace will give a number for the rate of oxygen uptake in units of precent saturation/time. Typical values for
human polymorphonuclear leukocytes will be 0.2 to 0.5%/min for
resting cells and 2 to 5%/min for stimulated cells. Air saturated water contains approximately 2.2×10^{-4} moles O_2/ml and
the volume of the sample cells is approximately 1.8 ml (see
Section III.D). Oxygen uptake would then be calculated as:

$$O_2 \text{ uptake } (\frac{\text{moles}}{\text{min}})$$

$$= \frac{[\% \, O_2 \text{ uptake } (\frac{\%}{\text{min}})] \, [\text{sample vol. (ml)}] \, [2.2 \times 10^{-4} \, (\frac{\text{moles } O_2}{\text{ml } H_2O})]}{100}$$

Typical values for resting human polymorphonuclear leukocytes
would therefore be 0.8 to 2.0 µmoles O_2/min and when stimulated
would give values in the range of 8 to 20 µmoles O_2/min. In
general, macrophages will have higher resting rates for oxygen

uptake (~ 4 times that for polymorphonuclear leukocytes) and higher rates for stimulated oxygen uptake. The ratio of the stimulated oxygen uptake rate to resting oxygen uptake rate is generally less for macrophages than for polymorphonuclear leukocytes (4). If more accurate oxygen uptake rates are necessary, the altitude of the laboratory should be ascertained and the final answer should be reduced by 3.4% for every 1000 feet above sea level. Extremes of barometric pressure in a given area, however, can change the final value by as much as ±3%.

F. Critical Comments

Measurement of oxygen uptake as outlined above is reasonably sensitive and values for the rate of oxygen uptake generally agree to within 5 to 10% error.

The system allows for addition of reagents (drugs, etc.) at any time during the experiment via a microliter syringe. When using various drugs, care should be taken to make sure that the drug is completely removed from the sample cell between runs. Many compounds adsorb to the Teflon membrane of the probe and the stir bar. When using these types of compounds, it is a good practice to wash the sample cell with water several times followed by one or two washes with methanol and an additional two washes with water. Washing is most simply performed by filling the sample cell with the wash solution and aspirating the solution immediately with a Pasteur pipette connected to a vacuum line.

This procedure may be used for macrophages from any source, but is limited to use of cells in suspension; oxygen consumption by adherent cells cannot be determined in this assay due to the requirement for vigorous stirring. The assay has the advantage of continuous measurement so that reaction rates are easily determined. A major disadvantage lies in the fact that if a single electrode is employed, only one parameter can be varied at a time. During the course of a series of experiments, the baseline can vary due to cell senescence, alterations in the characteristics of the membrane, etc. It is good practice to occasionally repeat a given set of conditions to ensure that similar results are obtained over a period of time.

REFERENCES

1. L. R. DeChatelet. Initiation of the respiratory burst in human polymorphonuclear neutrophils: a critical review. *J. Reticuloendothel. Soc. 24:* 73-91, 1978.
2. L. R. DeChatelet, P. S. Shirley, L. C. McPhail, C. C. Huntley, H. B. Muss, and D. A. Bass. Oxidative metabolism of the human eosinophil. *Blood 50:* 525-535, 1977.
3. M. J. Cline and R. I. Lehrer. Phagocytosis by human monocytes. *Blood 32:* 423-435, 1968.
4. D. Romeo, G. Zabucchi, T. Marzi, and F. Rossi. Kinetic and enzymatic features of metabolic stimulation of alveolar and peritoneal macrophages challenged with bacteria. *Exp. Cell Res. 78:* 423-432, 1973.
5. Q. N. Myrvik and D. G. Evans. Effect of Bacillus-Calmette -Guerin on the metabolism of alveolar macrophages. *Adv. Exp. Med. Biol. 1:* 203-213, 1967.
6. W. S. Beck. Occurrence and control of the phosphogluconate oxidation pathway in normal and leukemic leukocytes. *J. Biol. Chem. 232:* 271-283, 1958.
7. R. H. Michell, S. J. Pancake, J. Noseworthy, and M. L. Karnovsky. Measurement of rates of phagocytosis. The use of cellular monolayers. *J. Cell Biol. 40:* 216-224, 1969.

52

SECRETION OF SUPEROXIDE ANION

Richard B. Johnston, Jr.

I. INTRODUCTION

During the process of ingestion, phagocytic cells consume oxygen from the surrounding milieu. Most, if not all, of this oxygen undergoes enzyme-catalyzed univalent reduction to form superoxide anion (O_2^-) (1). Two O_2^- molecules, one of which may be in the form of HO_2, interact with each other in a rapid, spontaneous dismutation reaction to form the anion of hydrogen peroxide (O_2^{2-}) and oxygen (2). Thus, in the presence of protons, H_2O_2 is formed. Superoxide anion and H_2O_2 interact with each other in a cycle of reactions involving iron to form the potent oxidant, hydroxyl radical ($\cdot OH$), perhaps the most important microbicidal oxygen species (3). Contact of the phagocyte plasma membrane with any of a large number of surface-active materials, e.g., phorbol myristate acetate (PMA) and digitonin, induces this same "respiratory burst." The enzyme superoxide dismutase (SOD), present in the cytosol and mitochondria, increases the rate of the O_2^- dismutation reaction about 20,000-fold at physiologic pH (2), thereby effectively removing O_2^- and protecting the phagocyte from both O_2^- and $\cdot OH$.

Because production of O_2^- is the initial step in the conversion of oxygen to microbicidal metabolites, its measurement constitutes a relatively direct estimate of the microbicidal potential of the respiratory burst. In addition, O_2^- produced during phagocytosis or surface perturbation is largely released to the outside of the cell and, therefore, not adsorbed to cellular constituents. There it can be detected by its ability to reduce chemically an electron-accepting compound such as ferricytochrome c or nitroblue tetrazolium. Ferricytochrome c reduction by O_2^- provided the basis for the first assay of SOD activity (4), and modifications of the same assay have been particularly useful in detecting generation of O_2^- by neutrophils (5), human monocytes fresh from the blood (6) or in culture (7), or mouse or guinea pig macrophages (7,8).

Reduction of cytochrome c is accompanied by an increase in absorbance at 550 nm, and the molar involvement of O_2^- in the reduction can be calculated with an extinction coefficient (9). The reduction of ferricytochrome c is not, of course, an assay specific for O_2^-; many tissue constituents might accomplish the same reduction. The required specificity is achieved by the use of SOD, for which O_2^- is the only known substrate. Accordingly, the assay is run with and without SOD, and only SOD-inhibitable reduction of cytochrome c is used to calculate the amount of O_2^- released.

II. REAGENTS

(1). Hank's balanced salt solution (HBSS) without phenol red (Grand Island Biological Co. (GIBCO), Grand Island, New York, or Microbiological Associates, Los Angeles, California.) Since indicator is absent, the pH should be checked if reused.

(2). Krebs-Ringer phosphate buffer, pH 7.35, containing dextrose, 2 mg/ml (KRPD).

(3). Ferricytochrome c, horse heart, type III (Sigma Chemical Co., St. Louis, Missouri).

Dissolve in HBSS to a stock concentration of 1.2 mM. Filter through micropore membrane (0.45 μm pore size, Millipore Corp., Bedford, Massachusetts) and store at -20°C in airtight container in volumes sufficient for a single experiment. (Residual material can be refrozen and used again once.) This product may contain trace amounts (<0.01%) of cuprozinc SOD (2). At physiologic pH this concentration should have a negligible capacity to remove O_2^-.

(4). Superoxide dismutase (SOD) can be purified from bovine erythrocytes by the method of McCord and Fridovich (4).

Commercial preparations can contain various contaminants, including catalase. (Catalase activity can be tested by examining the preparations's capacity to modify the characteristic
light absorption of commercial hydrogen peroxide (10).) Preparations with excellent purity and high specific activity can
be purchased from Diagnostic Data, Inc., Mountain View, California (bovine) or from Diagnostic Materials, Ltd., Oxford,
England (bovine or human). The product of Miles Laboratories,
Elkhart, Indiana is satisfactory. Dissolve in water for a
stock concentration of 1-5 mg/ml, and store at -20°C. This
can be refrozen a few times without loss of activity.

   (5). Dimethylsulfoxide (DMSO; Sigma). Keep tightly
closed to exclude moisture.

   (6). Phorbol myristate acetate (PMA; Consolidated Midland
Corp., Brewster, New York). Dissolve in DMSO at 2 mg/ml and
store at -70°C in airtight polypropylene or glass tubes.
Avoid contact with aqueous solutions or vapor condensation because PMA loses its activity rapidly in water.

   (7). Fresh (complement-preserved) human serum. To preserve complement activity, venous blood from normal adults
should be allowed to clot for about 45 min at room temperature,
then centrifuged at 4°C. The supernatant serum should be pooled, then divided quickly into iced tubes and frozen at -70°C.

   (8). Zymosan (ICN Pharmaceuticals, Cleveland, Ohio).
Suspend in glass tube to concentration of 12 mg/ml in saline
and heat in boiling water bath, while mixing about every 10
min, for 1 hr. Centrifuge, wash once, and resuspend in physiologic saline or KRPD to a stock concentration of 50 mg/ml.
Opsonize by incubating 1-vol zymosan with 3-vol fresh human
serum in water bath at 37°C for 20 min, with agitation. Centrifuge at 6-8000 g for 15 min, wash once with KRPD, and resuspend
in KRPD to a concentration of 10 mg/ml.

   (9). Macrophage culture medium. Results in this assay
should not be affected significantly differently by culture of
the macrophages in any of the different standard culture media.
With mouse macrophages we have routinely used Dulbecco's modified Eagle's medium (DMEM, GIBCO) supplemented with 20% heat-
inactivated (56°C, 30 min) fetal calf serum, penicillin, 100
U/ml, and streptomycin, 100 μg/ml. With human monocytes we
have used DMEM with 1-10% autologous serum, penicillin, and
streptomycin. Mouse macrophages and human monocytes can be
cultured overnight without serum without a significant decrease
in stimulated O_2^- release.

III.   PROCEDURE

Macrophages and human monocytes cultured for this assay
should be plated at a density sufficient to yield at the time
of assay 40-100 µg of cell protein on a 35 mm-diameter plate
(7). For peritoneal exudates from mice injected intraperitoneally with inflammatory agents like thioglycollate or endotoxin, or from mice infected with BCG or listeria, this will
require in the neighborhood of 2-4 x 10^6 peritoneal exudate
cells per dish; for resident peritoneal cells, 3-6 x 10^6 cells
will be required. These are added in a volume of **approximate-**
ly 1 ml. The cell suspension should be mixed well between
each pipetting to ensure that a consistent number of cells is
plated.

On the basis of surface area (determined by πr^2) the appropriate density will require approximately one-quarter as many
cells for a 16 mm-diameter culture dish and approximately 3
times more cells for a 60 mm-diameter dish. (The diameter of
the area of the dish to which cells can adhere measures less
than the diameter of the entire plate; the latter figure is
used by the manufacturers to designate size.) The need for
concern about cell density stems from the observation that
although greater numbers of plated cells will release more O_2^-
when stimulated, the extent of release does not increase in
proportion to the increase in cell number (7). Therefore,
when expressed as specific activity (nmol/mg cell protein),
O_2^- release, in general, declines with increasing cell number.
That is, higher cell density is associated with lower *efficien-*
cy of stimulated O_2^- release.

Release of O_2^- may be quantitated with macrophages cultured
for 2 hr, overnight, or for days. The macrophages are prepared
by washing quickly twice with KRPD (kept at room temperature)
to remove nonadherent cells. Washing is accomplished here by
vigorous swirling. Immediately after removal of the second
wash, the reaction mixture is added, and the reaction is begun
by placing the dishes in an incubator at 37°C with 100% air or
with 95% air-5% CO_2. In order to avoid having the macrophages
remain long without a full cover of medium, washing and addition of the incubation mixture are usually performed with
groups of 4-6 plates each.

The reaction mixture, prepared in one large tube before
the cells are washed, should contain KRPD and cytochrome *c* to
give a final concentration of 80 µ*M* in the 1.5 ml volume added
to each 35 mm-diameter dish. If the stimulus is to be opsonized zymosan, it should be added in bulk to give a concentration of 1 mg/ml in the final reaction mixture. If the stimulus
is PMA, a volume of KRPD with cytochrome *c* sufficient for no
more than six culture dishes (up to 10 ml if 35 mm-diameter

dishes are used) should be placed in a separate tube, and PMA
should be added to give a final concentration of 0.5 µg/ml.
On addition of PMA, the reaction mixture should be mixed and
immediately added to plated cells to avoid inactivation of the
PMA before contact is made with the macrophages. The volume
of DMSO used to deliver the PMA (1 part in 4000) does not by
itself stimulate O_2^- or inhibit zymosan-stimulated O_2^- release.

   With eace stimulus, an additional reaction mixture should
be prepared that contains SOD at a final concentration of 40
µg/ml. In most cases, SOD at this concentration eliminates
all cytochrome c reduction by stimulated macrophages; autoclaving the SOD removes at least 90% of this inhibitory activity. In each experiment, "blanks" are prepared by incubating
each type of reaction mixture in tissue culture dishes without
macrophages. Each experimental determination should be run
with duplicate or triplicate cultures. Reaction mixtures must
be delivered precisely; a calibrated 1.5-ml "automatic" pipette
serves this purpose well.

   When carefully analyzed, the reduction of cytochrome c by
stimulated "activated" mouse macrophages occurs at a linear
rate for about 10 min; with resident macrophages the rate is
linear for 30-60 min (Sasada and Johnston, unpublished). The
rate is nearly linear for 60-90 min with any cell type (7),
however, and we have generally used a 60-min or 90-min incubation period with mouse macrophages and cultured human monocytes.
The incubation period should depend on the kinetics of the reaction obtained with the cell density, cell type, stimulus, and
other conditions employed.

   The reaction is stopped by transfer of the incubation mixture by Pasteur pipette to centrifuge tubes in an ice bath,
followed promptly by centrifugation at 1200 g for 10 min or
8000 g for 2 min. (The latter conditions are accomplished with
a microcentrifuge (Eppendorf), using 1.5 ml tubes.) One or two
ml of HBSS is added to the dishes to prevent drying of the cells.
The supernatant is transferred to separate tubes, and absorbance
of the supernatant at 550 nm is determined in a spectrophotometer. Reaction mixtures from dishes that did not contain macrophages are used as blanks, after absorbance of the blanks at 550
nm is compared to that of water. If the cytochrome concentration is proper and the reagents clean, the OD_{550} of the blanks
should be 0.55 to 0.65. Spectrophotometers utilizing single
prism monochrometers are not suitable for quantitative measurement of reduced cytochrome c. The spectral band width should
not exceed 1 nm or, at the most, 2 nm. If the actual wavelength
deviates from 550 by as much as 5 nm, light absorption by reduced cytochrome c will be almost completely lost.

   The cells remaining in the dish are washed three times with
HBSS. Copper tartrate reagent (11) is added directly to the
dish, and the protein content of the dish is determined by the

method of Lowry *et al.* (11) using bovine serum albumin as
standard. The dishes used as blanks give a significant Lowry
reaction, and this value must be subtracted from that of the
dishes containing cells. The extent of O_2^- release can be corrected for the protein content of each individual dish if one
is certain that cells are not dislodged during the incubation
with cytochrome or subsequent washes. Alternatively, if macrophage adherence is uniform from dish to dish, the mean of the
protein content of five dishes washed free of nonadherent cells
but not carried through the assay can be used for expression of
the extent of O_2^- release in individual dishes. Release of O_2^-
can also be expressed on the basis of cell number, using a conversion factor that equates cell protein and number (7) or,
preferably, an actual determination of cell number by counting
nuclei of disrupted cells (12).

IV. CALCULATION OF DATA

    The OD_{550} of the reaction mixtures is converted to nano-
moles of cytochrome *c* reduced using the extinction coefficient
$\Delta E_{550} = 21.0 \times 10^3 \ M^{-1}cm^{-1}$ (9). Thus, with the standard 1-cm
light path and a 1.5-ml reaction mixture, the observed OD_{550}
should be multiplied by 71.4 to yield the number of nanomoles
of O_2^- measured, since 1 mol of O_2^- reduces 1 mol of ferricytochrome *c*. For a reaction mixture of 1 ml, the conversion factor is 47.6.
    This conversion depends upon the assumption that the cyto-
chrome *c* in the blank is fully oxidized and, therefore, that
the observed OD represents the absorbance of only the reduced
product (a ΔOD, reduced -oxidized). This assumption can be
tested by fully oxidizing the reagent cytochrome *c* in solution
with a few milligrams of potassium ferricyanide, by fully reducing the cytochrome *c* with a few milligrams of sodium di-
thionite, and by comparing the OD_{550} of the untreated, oxidized,
and reduced solutions against that of water. We found that
98-99% of the ferricytochrome *c* in fresh reagent solutions is
oxidized and, therefore, for routine purposes, do not adjust
for the state of oxidation of our reagent material.

V. CRITICAL COMMENTS

    The use of SOD-inhibitable ferricytochrome *c* to quantitate
the O_2^- released from stimulated phagocytic cells has proved to
be a highly sensitive and reproducible assay. With monocytes
in suspension, problems should arise only if the cells are not

properly processed. With plated macrophages or monocytes, problems in reproducibility are not likely to derive from the assay per se but rather from irregularities in the density of cells on the culture dishes. That is, if the cell density is sparse, results are often erratic, presumably because small differences in numbers of adherent cells are magnified. In addition, protein content is more difficult to quantify accurately at lower concentrations. At higher cell densities, the efficiency of O_2^- release is decreased (7), as described above.

Macrophages elicited by injection of inflammatory agents such as endotoxin (LPS), thioglycollate, or proteose-peptone, or obtained from animals infected with an intracellular pathogen such as bacillus Calmette-Guérin (BCG), exhibit changes associated with a state of "activation." Along with these changes, the cell is primed to produce several times more O_2^- than resident macrophages when stimulated by phagocytosis or PMA (7). Other aspects of the phagocytosis-associated respiratory burst are also accentuated in elicited and infection-activated macrophages (reviewed in 13).

It is now clear that priming for enhanced O_2^- release also can be achieved during overnight culture with certain bacterial products, including LPS (14). With resident mouse macrophages cultured in medium without serum, the concentration of LPS required to prime for an increase in stimulated O_2^- release of up to fivefold is in the range of 1-10 ng/ml. These concentrations exist in most commercial preparations of fetal calf serum (14) and Ficoll and in some batches of tissue culture medium (Pabst and Johnston, unpublished). Although truly quiescent resident mouse peritoneal macrophages usually are not primed to release significantly more O_2^- by overnight culture in FCS (7), the potential effect of contaminating LPS on results in the O_2^- assay must be considered.

The expected range of values for O_2^- release by mouse resident peritoneal macrophages stimulated with PMA is 40-120 nmol/mg of cell protein in a 60-90 min incubation. PMA-stimulated release by elicited or infection-activated macrophages or by resident macrophages incubated overnight in LPS ranges from 450-750 nmol/mg in 60-90 min (7,14). The extent of O_2^- release from resident cells stimulated by phagocytosis of opsonized zymosan is about four times higher than that stimulated by PMA (150-300 nmol/mg). In contrast, O_2^- release from elicited and activated macrophages stimulated by zymosan is 60-80% as high as release elicited by contact with PMA (7). Viable candida serve as a weaker stimulus, but greater release from elicited or activated macrophages can still be demonstrated, as can greater stimulation by some candida species than others (15).

The extent of O_2^- release from cultured human monocytes varies greatly with the length of time in culture and the stimulus used but, in general, falls into the range of values shown by cultured mouse macrophages (7).

Acknowledgment

Supported by USPHS Grant AI 14148.

REFERENCES

1. R. B. Johnston, Jr. Oxygen metabolism and the microbicidal activity of macrophages. *Fed. Proc. 37*:2759-2764, 1978.
2. J. M. McCord, J. D. Crapo, and I. Fridovich. Superoxide dismutase assays: A review of methodology. *In* "Superoxide and Superoxide Dismutases" (A. M. Michelson, J. M. McCord, and I. Fridovich, eds.), pp. 11-17. Academic Press, New York, 1977.
3. R. B. Johnston, Jr., B. B. Keele, Jr., H. P. Misra, J. E. Lehmeyer, L. S. Webb, R. L. Baehner, and K. V. Rajagopalan. The role of superoxide anion generation in phagocytic bactericidal activity: Studies with normal and chronic granulomatous disease leukocytes. *J. Clin. Invest. 55*:1357-1372, 1975.
4. J. M. McCord and I. Fridovich. Superoxide dismutase: An enzymic function for erythrocuprein (hemocuprein). *J. Biol. Chem. 244*:6049-6055, 1969.
5. B. M. Babior, R. S. Kipnes, and J. T. Curnutte. Biological defense mechanisms: The production by leukocytes of superoxide, a potential bactericidal agent. *J. Clin. Invest. 52*:741-744, 1973.
6. R. B. Johnston, Jr., J. E. Lehmeyer, and L. A. Guthrie. Generation of superoxide anion and chemiluminescence by human monocytes during phagocytosis and on contact with surface-bound immunoglobulin G. *J. Exp. Med. 143*:1551-1556, 1976.
7. R. B. Johnston, Jr., C. A. Godzik, and Z. A. Cohn. Increased superoxide anion production by immunologically activated and chemically elicited macrophages. *J. Exp. Med. 148*:115-127, 1978
8. D. B. Drath and M. L. Karnovsky. Superoxide production by phagocytic leukocytes. *J. Exp. Med. 141*:257-262, 1975.
9. V. Massey. The microestimation of succinate and the extinction coefficient of cytochrome *c*. *Biochim. Biophys. Acta. 34*:255-256, 1959.

10. R. F. Beers, Jr., and I. W. Sizer. A spectrophotometric method for measuring the breakdown of hydrogen peroxide by catalase. *J. Biol. Chem.* *195*:133-140, 1952.

11. O. H. Lowry, N. J. Rosebrough, A. L. Farr, and R. J. Randall. Protein measurement with the Folin phenol reagent. *J. Biol. Chem.* *193*:265-275, 1951.

12. G. M. Shaw, P. C. Levy, and A. F. Lobuglio. Human monocyte cytotoxicity to tumor cells. I. Antibody-dependent cytotoxicity. *J. Immunol.* *121*:573-578, 1978.

13. R. B. Johnston, Jr., D. A. Chadwick, and M. J. Pabst. Release of superoxide anion by macrophages: Effect of *in vivo* or *in vitro* priming. *In* "Mononuclear Phagocytes -- Functional Aspects" (R. vanFurth, ed.), pp. 1143-11. Martinus Nijhoff, The Hague, 1981.

14. M. J. Pabst, and R. B. Johnston, Jr. Increased production of superoxide anion by macrophages exposed *in vitro* to muramyl dipeptide or lipopolysaccharide. *J. Exp. Med.* *151*:101-114, 1980.

15. M. Sasada and R. B. Johnston, Jr. Macrophage microbicidal activity: Correlation between phagocytosis-associated oxidative metabolism and the killing of candida by macrophages. *J. Exp. Med.* *152*:85-98.

53

RELEASE OF HYDROGEN PEROXIDE

Carl F. Nathan

I. INTRODUCTION

The capacity to release hydrogen peroxide is a useful biochemical correlate of macrophage activation, if the latter
term is defined as enhanced ability to destroy intracellular
microbes and extracellular tumor cells (1, 2). Thus, activated mouse peritoneal macrophages are capable of secreting
substantial amounts of H_2O_2 (2-5), while resident peritoneal
cells, or those elicited with thioglycollate broth, proteose-
peptone, or fetal bovine serum, secrete much smaller amounts
(2,3,5). Enhanced capacity to release H_2O_2 into the medium
marks macrophages activated either *in vivo* (such as by injection of BCG, *C. parvum*, *T. cruzi*, or *T. gondii* (2-5)), or *in
vitro*, by incubation in mediators from antigen- or mitogen-
stimulated lymphocytes (2,5). H_2O_2 or closely related substances have been directly implicated as both microbicidal
(4-8) and tumoricidal (9-12) factors in mononuclear phagocyte
effector function.

Several methods are available for measuring the concentration of H_2O_2 in biological systems (13). The following discussion concerns the assay based on the loss of fluorescence of scopoletin (6-methoxy-7-hydroxy-1, 2-benzopyrone, a coumarin) when the 7-hydroxyl group is oxidized to a ketone by H_2O_2 in concert with horseradish peroxidase. One mole of H_2O_2 oxidizes 1 mole of scopoletin. The method was introduced in 1955 by Andreae (14), improved by Perschke and Broda in 1961 (15), first applied to the measurement of H_2O_2 release from leukocytes by Root et al. in 1975 (16), and extended to the study of mononuclear phagocytes by Nathan and Root in 1977 (3). The method has been used with blood monocytes and tissue macrophages of man, mouse, rat, guinea pig, and rabbit (17).

There are two requirements in order to detect substantial H_2O_2 release from mononuclear phagocytes using the scopoletin method (3). First, if mouse peritoneal macrophages are employed, they must be activated. H_2O_2 release from nonactivated cells occurs but is small. However, blood monocytes can secrete copious H_2O_2 without prior exposure to activating (differentiative) stimuli (18,19). Second, the mononuclear phagocytes must be exposed to a triggering agent, that is, any of a variety of membrane-active stimuli, such as tumor promoters, antigen-antibody complexes, or phagocytic particles (4), which elicit a rapid response. In the absence of a triggering agent, extremely little if any H_2O_2 release is detected in the extracellular medium.

II. REAGENTS

A. Buffer

A variety of protein-free balanced salt solutions are suitable. Hank's balanced salt solution without phenol red is used frequently with monocytes. For mouse peritoneal macrophages, Krebs-Ringer phosphate buffer with glucose (KRPG) has been most extensively used. It is best prepared from double-distilled, glass-distilled water. The formulation is NaCl, 120 mM; KCl, 4.8 mM; CaCl$_2$, 0.54 mM; MgSO$_4$, 1.2 mM; sodium phosphate, 15.6 mM; glucose, 5.5 mM; pH, 7.30 to 7.40; tonicity, 300 mOsm.

B. Scopoletin

The fluorochrome is obtainable from Sigma Chemical Co., St. Louis, Missouri. A 1mM stock solution is prepared in buffer without glucose. Complete dissolution of the scopo-

letin usually requires 24-36 hr at 37°C. The concentration
is checked by assay against known amounts of ethyl hydrogen
peroxide (Polysciences, Inc., Warrenton, Pennsylvania). The
stock solution is stable for many months at 4°C.

C. Horseradish Peroxidase (HRP)

This may be obtained from Worthington Biochemical Corp.,
Freehold, New Jersey, or from Sigma (Type II). A solution of
200 purpurogallin U/ml is prepared in buffer without glucose
and stored in aliquots at -20°C, where it is stable for many
months. The optimal amount of each preparation should be
determined under typical assay conditions. Some preparations
are suppressive if used in amounts optimal for other preparations.

D. Phorbol Myristate Acetate (PMA)

This triggering agent (12-0-tetradecanoyl-phorbol-13-ace-
tate) is obtainable from Consolidated Midland, Inc., Brewster,
New York, or from Sigma. A stock solution of 0.3 mg/ml is
prepared in dimethylsulfoxide and stored at -80°C in the dark
in tightly capped glass tubes in aliquots of about 2 ml.
Periodically, one tube is used to prepare aliquots of about
50 µl. For convenience, one 50-µl aliquot may be stored at
-20°C for up to a week, after which the unused portion is
discarded. Under these conditions, PMA usually retains full
potency for about 1 yr. Failure of the solution to freeze at
-20°C is often a sign of deterioration. A dose-response curve
for the amount of PMA needed to trigger maximal H_2O_2 release
from macrophages or granulocytes should be performed with each
new lot of PMA, and as needed during the later period of use
of a given lot. The optimal concentration should initially be
about 10 ng/ml, and may shift with time to about 100 ng/ml.
If higher doses are required, a new lot should probably be
prepared.

PMA is an extremely potent tumor promoter. It must not
come into contact with the skin. Gloves should be worn
throughout the assay and mouth pipetting should be strictly
forbidden. Stock solutions should be tightly capped and
thawed as briefly as possible. PMA-containing solutions
should be disposed of according to institutional guidelines
for hazardous chemicals. The PMA waste bottle in the laboratory should be nonbreakable and should not be used for the
concomitant storage of carcinogens.

III.   PROCEDURES

A. *Cells in Suspension, Under Continuous or Intermittent
    Observation*

     The advantages of this approach are the following: The
number of mononuclear phagocytes in the cuvette can be determined by counting in a hemocytometer; the cells are ready to
use immediately after preparation; and the kinetics and magnitude of the response may be observed as it is evolving, permitting adjustments in assay conditions. The disadvantages
are the need for a thermostatted compartment in the fluorometer, the inability to employ surface adherence and *in vitro*
incubation to enrich for mononuclear phagocytes, limitation
of the number of samples that may be assayed at one time, according to the number of cuvettes which the fluorometer may
accommodate, usually 4, and difficulty in using high doses of
phagocytic particles as triggering agents.
     Cell suspensions should be freed of contaminating erythro-
cytes, if necessary, by hypotonic lysis. The cell pellet is
resuspended in 2 to 10 ml of 0.2% NaCl (the amount depending
on the size of the pellet), and promptly mixed with an equal
volume of 1.6% NaCl, followed by three volumes of buffer. A
5-sec exposure to hypotonic saline is sufficient to lyse erythrocytes in mouse peritoneal cells. The cells are then
washed several times by centrifugation to remove exogenous
protein. The cell number is determined with a hemocytometer,
and slides are made for differential counting.
     The choice of cell number, amount of scopoletin, and
amount of HPO for the assay depends on the activity of the
cells under study. For observations of rate of H_2O_2 release,
typical amounts are 3 x 10^6 cells, 10 to 20 nmoles of scopoletin initially and 1 purpurogallin unit (about 6 μg of Sigma
Type II) HPO in a total volume of 3 ml of buffer. With 2 x
10^5 cells, the initial amount of scopoletin could be reduced
to 1 nmole. With monocytes, higher values may be obtained by
adding 1 mM sodium azide, in order to inhibit the catabolism
of H_2O_2 by reactions dependent upon catalase and myeloperoxidase. The cells are allowed to equilibrate for 5 min at 37°C
in the thermostatted compartment of the fluorometer, such as
the Perkin-Elmer MPF 44A (Perkin-Elmer Co., Norwalk, Connecticut) connected to a circulating water bath. The recorder is
brought to the desired scale by selecting the slit widths
(usually between 2 and 10 nm) and the gain, and the spontaneous
activity is recorded for several minutes with the excitation
wavelength at 350 nm and the emission at 460 nm. (The apparent peak excitation wavelength of scopoletin may vary with
assay conditions. In KRPG, it is 380 nm. Sensitivity is re-

duced 25% by exciting at the conventional setting of 350 nm
rather than 380 nm. However, the precision of the determination of H_2O_2 concentration is unaffected.) The reaction is
started by adding the triggering agent in a small volume.
When the scopoletin has been 60% oxidized, additional scopoletin is added, taking care not to exceed full scale. The response may be observed for a predetermined time, or followed
to its completion, which is usually between 1.5 and 3.5 hr
later. If observation lasts more than 5 min, the contents of
the cuvettes should be stirred automatically, or mixed manually at intervals before each reading. An automatic indexer
and stirrer may be obtained from C. N. Wood Manufacturing Co.,
Newtown, Pennsylvania.

To confirm that the decrease in fluorescence is due to
H_2O_2, controls consist of omitting HPO, or adding catalase.

The cuvettes may be glass or quartz. Type 3H quartz
cuvettes (Precision Cells, Inc., Hicksville, New York) are a
reasonable choice, since they will serve also for most other
fluorometric purposes. Scrupulous care of the cuvettes is
advisable. Residue in cuvettes may trigger peroxide release
from the cells, which may be misconstrued as spontaneous activity. Higher amounts of residue may kill the cells. The
following method of cleaning is satisfactory. The cuvettes
are rinsed three times with water. A very dilute solution of
dishwashing detergent is prepared; for example, one drop of
Palmolive liquid is mixed with 50 ml of water in a beaker, the
contents discarded, and the beaker refilled. Using a cotton
Q-tip, the inner and outer surfaces of the cuvettes are gently
washed. The cuvettes are rinsed in five changes of warm water,
then filled briefly with Chromerge (potassium dichromate in concentrated sulfuric acid). The Chromerge is decanted, and the
cuvettes rinsed manually 20 times with distilled water, or
rinsed on a cuvetter washer (Precision Cells) with 100 ml of
distilled water each. They are drained on absorbent paper,
and the outsides dried with lint-free tissues. The cuvettes
are handled with disposable plastic gloves from which the
starch powder has been rinsed.

B. *Cells Adherent, under Continuous or Intermittent Observation*

The advantages of this method are as follows: The cells
may be enriched for mononuclear phagocytes by discarding nonadherent cells and permitting granulocytes to die over time;
lysis of erythrocytes is unnecessary; cells may be assayed
after various times in culture; phagocytic particles may be
centrifuged onto the cells before starting the assay; and the
kinetics of the response may be observed as it is evolving.

Disadvantages are the need for a thermostatted fluorometer; the restriction in the number of samples that can be assayed at one time; and the need to determine the adherent cell number by some means other than counting in a hemocytometer.

Cells are allowed to adhere to coverslips. The most useful coverslips are rectangular, with a width equal to the diagonal of the cuvette. This prevents shifts in position of the coverslip in the cuvette, which can cause artifacts in the reading. Coverslips measuring 13 x 27 x 0.1 mm (Bellco Glass, Vineland, New Jersey) are suitable with cuvettes having a 1-cm light path. The coverslips are cleaned and sterilized by soaking in 70% ethanol, dipping in absolute ethanol, touching off the excess, and passing through a flame to ignite the alcohol. After cells have adhered, the coverslip is picked up with jeweller's forceps and rinsed thoroughly in at least four beakers, each containing 100 ml of saline or KRPG, in order to remove serum proteins and nonadherent cells.

The coverslip is then placed directly in the cuvette, and the assay performed as above. Thorough mixing is important during the assay. For automatic stirring, the coverslip may be mounted above the stirring bar on a glass stirrup (see Fig. 1).

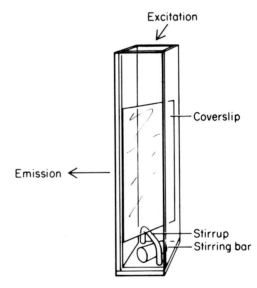

Fig. 1. A 13 x 27 x 0.1 mm glass coverslip with adherent mononuclear phagocytes is placed diagonally in the cuvette (1-cm light path) on a glass stirrup to permit the use of a magnetic stirring bar.

To use a phagocytic stimulus, the coverslips are placed in 2 ml of KRPG in a 35-mm dish on ice. The phagocytic particles, such as opsonized zymosan, are added, and the dish is centrifuged for 2 min in the cold. The slip is gently immersed in cold buffer, then transferred directly to the prewarmed reagents in the cuvette in the fluorometer. Nearly instantaneous onset of H_2O_2 release may be anticipated.

Matched coverslips should be rinsed in the same manner as above, and used to measure cellular protein or DNA. It is generally not satisfactory to use the same coverslip for both H_2O_2 release and measurement of cell number, as there is a variable loss of cells by the end of the assay.

C.   Cells Adherent with Observation at a Single Time Point

This method combines the advantages of using adherent, cultured cells with the ability to process large numbers of samples. A temperature-controlled fluorometer is not necessary. The cells may be cultured on coverslips of almost any size or shape. The disadvantage is that only one observation is made of each sample. If the amount of scopoletin added proves to be insufficient to react with all of the H_2O_2 secreted, the remainder of the H_2O_2 will be undetected. If excessive scopoletin is added, small amounts of H_2O_2 release will be difficult to measure accurately. The lag time before onset of H_2O_2 release cannot be measured, and the initial rate of secretion can only be estimated by interpolation from multiple samples.

One variant of this method will be described. Cells are cultured on 13-mm round glass coverslips (Clay-Adams, New York) in 16-mm wells in plastic multiwell plates (Costar Data Packaging, Cambridge, Massachusetts). After incubation for the desired length of time, the coverslips are rinsed in four beakers of saline or KRPG, drained briefly on absorbent paper, and transferred to a new plate, whose wells contain 1.5 ml of KRPG and the desired amounts of scopoletin, HPO, and PMA. The assay plate is then floated in a 37°C water bath for 2.5 hr. The medium in each well is transferred to a 10 x 75 mm glass test tube and allowed to come to room temperature. The tubes are then read in the fluorometer, either directly using a test-tube holder adaptor in the sample compartment, or by decanting into cuvettes. The readings are stable overnight.

Coverslips to which no cells are added are included as controls. The amount of rinsed fluid that is carried into the assay medium is thereby taken into account to avoid misinterpreting dilution of scopoletin as oxidation. In addition, these controls correct for concentration of scopoletin due to evaporation. Additional cell-bearing coverslips are saved for protein or DNA measurements.

IV.   CALCULATION OF DATA

The two most useful ways of reporting the results are in terms of the maximal rate of H_2O_2 release (nanomoles per 10^6 cells per initial 5 min) or as the total amount secreted (nanomoles per 10^6 cells, or nanomoles per microgram cell protein).

V.   CRITICAL COMMENTS

A.   *Purity of Cell Populations*

Granulocytes are potent secretors of H_2O_2 in response to the same stimuli that trigger mononuclear phagocytes.   Most preparations of freshly isolated mononuclear phagocytes contain at least a few granulocytes.   With some regimens for activating peritoneal macrophages, the proportion of granulocytes may exceed 20%.   It is necessary to determine the percentage of granulocytes in each preparation and to avoid attributing their responses to macrophages.   Granulocyte contamination can usually be eliminated by 4-18 hr incubation *in vitro*.   However, macrophage activation is reversible (2), so that with prolonged incubation, values for H_2O_2 release from activated macrophages will often decline.

B.   *Measurement of Net Extracellular Release*

The method detects only that fraction of H_2O_2 which escapes from the cell into the medium and which is not expended there in the oxidation of substances other than scopoletin. The method does *not* indicate the actual rate or amount of H_2O_2 produced by the cells; it provides a lower limit for those values.   Even in a cell-free system, in which H_2O_2 is generated enzymatically, only about 70% of the H_2O_2 is detected by the scopoletin method (20).   Cells with active catabolic pathways for H_2O_2, such as alveolar macrophages, may appear to perform poorly in the scopoletin assay.   The method reveals little regarding the rate of H_2O_2 accumulation in phagosomes, or in the zones of contact between the macrophage plasma membrane and closely adherent surfaces, such as those of tumor cells or parasites.

C. *Interference by Alternate Hydrogen Donors*

Many substances may be oxidized by H_2O_2 in competition
with scopoletin because of the wide range of substrates
for HPO (20). Thus, as little as 0.03% serum interferes with
the assay. Interference is seen with antibody-coated red
cells and tumor cells, serum-coated latex particles and starch
granules, and reducing agents such as glutathione, ascorbate,
NADPH, and NADH. The method is not well suited to the study
of cell lysates. As a related problem, H_2O_2 may be consumed
by catalase or glutathione peroxidase within the mononuclear
phagocytes themselves, or within other cells present in the
system.

D. *Influence of Triggering Agents*

The difference in rates of release of H_2O_2 from activated
and nonactivated macrophages, which is elicited by exposure to
PMA, is sometimes less marked when using phagocytic particles
as triggering agents. This shift in ratio is difficult to interpret. Activated mouse peritoneal macrophages are often
less phagocytic than nonactivated macrophages (21), and may
have less readily detectable Fc receptors (22). Phagocytic
particles themselves may interfere with the detection of
H_2O_2 release (see above). Such interference may depend in
part on the "leakiness" of the phagosome during its formation,
that is, how freely the nascent vacuole may communicate with
the extracellular space.

E. *Sensitivity to Conditions of Prior Incubation*

Activated mouse peritoneal macrophages tend to secrete
less H_2O_2 after temporary exposure to alkaline media (pH 7.8
or above). The defect may persist for some time after the pH
is corrected. During transfer of coverslips, or other operations with bicarbonate-based media performed outside the incubator, it is important to control the pH.

F. *Choice of Assay*

At least four methods are capable of recording changes in
H_2O_2 concentration of about 10^{-8} M. Three of these employ
fluorescent indicators: scopoletin, leukodiacetyldichloro-
fluorescein (LDADCF) (23-24), and homovanillic acid (25).
Assays using the latter two compounds have the advantage of
detecting an increase, rather than a decrease, in the inten-

sity of fluorescence in proportion to the concentration of H_2O_2. However, LDADCF is reacted with the cell supernatant, not with the cells themselves, which makes the assay somewhat less versatile than the scopoletin method. Homovanillic acid may oxidize spontaneously during long-term assays. All three methods share the disadvantages of dependence on HPO (see above).

The fourth assay is spectrophotometric. It is based on the shift in absorption undergone by yeast cytochrome peroxidase when it forms an enzyme-substrate complex with H_2O_2 (26). The assay is as sensitive as the fluoremetric methods when a dual-wavelength spectrophotometer is employed. The cytochrome peroxidase method is probably more accurate than the scopoletin method; it is less susceptible to interference by other hydrogen donors (20). Its disadvantages are the need for specialized equipment and the lack of commercial availability of yeast cytochrome peroxidase, which is consumed in stoichiometric amounts with the H_2O_2 detected.

The cytochrome peroxidase method will probably occupy an increasingly important role in specialized applications. The scopoletin method is likely to remain in wide use for assays with intact cells, in view of its simplicity, versatility, and the low cost of the reagents.

Acknowledgments

Some of the work reported here was supported by PHS grant CA-22090. C.N. is a Scholar of the Leukemia Society of America, and a Research Career Scientist of the Irma T. Hirschl Trust.

REFERENCES

1. Z. A. Cohn. The activation of mononuclear phagocytes: Fact, fancy, and future. *J. Immunol. 121*:813-816, 1978.
2. C. Nathan, N. Nogueira, C. Juangbhanich, J. Ellis, and Z. A. Cohn. Activation of macrophages *in vivo* and *in vitro*: Correlation between hydrogen peroxide release and killing of *Trypanosoma cruzi*. *J. Exp. Med. 149*:1056-1068, 1979.
3. C. F. Nathan and R. K. Root. Hydrogen peroxide release from mouse peritoneal macrophages: Dependence on sequential activation and triggering. *J. Exp. Med. 146*:1648-1662, 1977.

4. R. B. Johnston, Jr. Oxygen metabolism and the micro-bicidal activity of macrophages. *Fed. Proc.* *37:*2759-2764, 1978.

5. H. W. Murray and Z. A. Cohn. Macrophage oxygen-dependent antimicrobial activity, III. Enhanced oxidative metabolism as an expression of macrophage activation. *J. Exp. Med.* *152:*1596-1609, 1980.

6. H. W. Murray, C. Juangbhanich, C. F. Nathan, and Z. A. Cohn. Macrophage oxygen-dependent antimicrobial activity. II. The role of oxygen intermediates. *J. Exp. Med.* *150:*950-964, 1979.

7. C. B. Wilson, V. Tsai, and J. S. Remington. Failure to trigger the oxidative metabolic burst by normal macrophages. Possible mechanism for survival of intracellular pathogens. *J. Exp. Med.* *151:*328-346, 1980.

8. M. Sesada and R. B. Johnston, Jr. Macrophage microbicidal activity. Correlation between phagocytosis-associated oxidative metabolism and the killing of candida by macrophages. *J. Exp. Med.* *152:*85-98, 1980.

9. C. F. Nathan, L. H. Brukner, S. C. Silverstein, and Z. A. Cohn. Lysis of tumor cells by activated macrophages and granulocytes. I. Pharmacologic triggering of the effectors and the release of hydrogen peroxide. *J. Exp. Med.* *149:*84-99, 1979.

10. C. F. Nathan, S. C. Silverstein, L. H. Brukner, and Z. A. Cohn. Extracellular cytolysis by activated macrophages and granulocytes. II. Hydrogen peroxide as a mediator of cytotoxicity. *J. Exp. Med.* *149:*100-113, 1979.

11. C. F. Nathan, L. H. Brukner, G. Kaplan, J. C. Unkeless, and Z. A. Cohn. The role of activated macrophages in antibody-dependent lysis of tumor cells. *J. Exp. Med.* *152:*183-197, 1980.

12. C. F. Nathan, and Z. A. Cohn. The role of oxygen-dependent mechanisms in antibody-induced lysis of tumor cells by activated macrophages. *J. Exp. Med.* *152:*198-208.

13. B. Chance, H. Sies, and A. Boveris. Hydroperoxide metabolism in mammalian organs. *Physiol. Rev.* *59:*527-605, 1979.

14. W. A. Andreae. A sensitive method for the estimation of hydrogen peroxide in biological materials. *Nature 175:*859-860, 1955.

15. H. Perschke, and E. Broda. Determination of very small amounts of hydrogen peroxide. *Nature 190:*257-258, 1961.

16. R. K. Root, J. Metcalf, N. Oshino, and B. Chance. H_2O_2 release from human granulocytes during phagocytosis. I. Documentation, quantitation, and some regulating factors. *J. Clin. Invest.* *55:*945-955, 1975.

17. C. F. Nathan. The release of hydrogen peroxide from mononuclear phagocytes and its role in extracellular cytosis. *In* "Mononuclear Phagocytes: Functional Aspects" (R. van Furth, ed.). Martinus Nijhoff, The Hague, 1980.

18. M. Reiss, and D. Roos. Differences in oxygen metabolism of phagocytosing monocytes and neutrophils. *J. Clin. Invest.* *61:*480-488, 1978.

19. L. M. Adler, J. B. L. Gee, and R. K. Root. H_2O_2 formation and utilization by human monocytes (MONOs). *Clin. Res.* *26:*522A, 1978.

20. A. Boveris, E. Martino, and A. O. M. Stoppani. Evaluation of the horseradish peroxidase-scopoletin method for the measurement of hydrogen peroxide formation in biological systems. *Anal. Biochem.* *80:*145-158, 1977.

21. C. F. Nathan, and W. D. Terry. Decreased phagocytosis by macrophages from BCG-treated mice: Induction of the phagocytic defect in normal macrophages with BCG *in vitro*. *Cell. Immunol.* *29:*295-311, 1977.

22. C. F. Nathan, R. Asofsky, and W. D. Terry. Characterization of the nonphagocytic adherent cell from the peritoneal cavity of normal and BCG-treated mice. *J. Immunol.* *118:*1612-1621, 1977.

23. A. S. Keston, and R. Brandt. The fluorometric analysis of ultramicro quantities of hydrogen peroxide. *Anal. Biochem.* *11:*1-5, 1965.

24. J. W. T. Homan-Muller, R. S. Weening, and D. Roos. Production of hydrogen peroxide by phagocytizing human granulocytes. *J. Lab. Clin. Med.* *85:*198-207, 1975.

25. F. Rossi, B. Bellazite, A. Dobryna, T. Dri, and G. Zabucchi. Oxidative metabolism of mononuclear phagocytes. *In* "Mononuclear Phagocytes: Functional Aspects" (R. van Furth, ed.). Martinus Nijhoff, The Hague, 1980.

26. A. Boveris, N. Oshino, and B. Chance. The cellular production of hydrogen peroxide. *Biochem. J.* *128:*617-630, 1972.

54

ANTIBODY-DEPENDENT AND ANTIBODY-INDEPENDENT PHAGOCYTOSIS

Denise R. Shaw
Frank M. Griffin, Jr.

I.   GENERAL INTRODUCTION

Phagocytosis is one of the more obvious and more important functions of mononuclear phagocytes. In an effort to understand better this process, investigators have developed numerous *in vitro* assay systems, which can be divided into several groups: those which utilize a particle easily visible by light microscopy (1), those which employ radiolabeled particles and assay cell-associated label (2), those which employ particles that can be quantitated by nephelometry or spectrophotometry (3, 4), those which assess cell-associated viable bacteria by colony count determinations (5), and those which assess the metabolic consequences of phagocytosis such as O_2 uptake and chemiluminescence (6). Each of these techniques has its own inherent advantages, capabilities for providing information, pitfalls, and limitations.

METHODS FOR STUDYING
MONONUCLEAR PHAGOCYTES

II. ASSAY OF PHAGOCYTOSIS BY LIGHT MICROSCOPY

A. *Introduction*

The procedure we have used most extensively (1, 7 - 11) is a simple microscopic assay that can provide considerable information when the investigator is interested in detecting qualitative differences between the ingestibility of particles or between the abilities of various cell preparations to ingest a particle. To a reasonable extent, it can be used to determine ingestion rates. It cannot be used to detect with confidence fairly small differences in phagocytic rate or capacity.

Most of our experience has been with mouse peritoneal macrophages, but we have used the technique with human monocytes, neutrophils, and eosinophils. It can be used with any glass adherent phagocytic cell from any animal.

B. *Reagents*

1. *Particles*

To assess antibody-independent phagocytosis, any of a variety of particles that can be seen and enumerated microscopically can be used. Polystyrene latex beads and zymozan are commonly employed, and many species of nonencapsulated bacteria may likewise be used. Appropriate particle concentration is determined for each system largely by trial and error.

To assess antibody-dependent phagocytosis, again any of several particles might be used. The criteria they must satisfy are that they are ingested not at all, or only to a minimal degree, if not coated with antibody; that they are avidly ingested when coated with antibody; that they can be seen and enumerated microscopically; and that particles attached to the phagocytic cell's surface can either be removed from the cell's surface or can be readily distinguished from ingested particles. Sheep erythrocytes satisfy all of these criteria, and they are the particles with which we have the most experience. We have also used erythrocytes of other species, encapsulated pneumococci and encapsulated cryptococci. Erythrocytes in Alsever's solution may be obtained from a number of suppliers (for example, Animal Blood Center, Syracuse, New York; GIBCO, Grand Island, New York; Scott Laboratories, Fiskeville, Rhode Island. The pneumococci and cryptococci we use are clinical isolates that are passaged through mice to maintain their capsules (1).

2. Antibodies

Antisera and the IgG fraction of antisera against erythrocytes or microorganisms may be prepared in the standard fashion, using ammonium sulfate precipitation and column chromatography to prepare IgG fractions. When whole antisera are employed, they must be heat inactivated at 56°C for 30 min. Alternatively, rabbit antisheep erythrocyte IgG may be obtained from Cordis Laboratories, Miami, Florida. We have found their IgG fraction to be inexpensive and of consistent quality.

3. Tissue Culture Media

We have used minimal essential medium, medium 199, RPMI-1640, and Neuman and Tytell serumless medium, but probably any tissue culture medium can be used. When cultivating macrophages, we normally supplement medium with 10 - 20% heat-inactivated fetal bovine serum (FBS). However, whenever possible the phagocytosis assay should be performed in the absence of serum to avoid introduction of unnecessary variables.

4. Laboratory Hardware

A vacuum bottle aspirator (to facilitate washing of cultures), sterile Pasteur and serological pipettes, sterile 35-mm diameter tissue culture dishes, sterile glass or plastic test tubes, microscope slides, needle-nosed forceps, and a small paintbrush should be available.

5. Coverslips

Glass coverslips (Gold Seal, 3550) 13-mm in diameter are washed and stored in 70% ethanol. Before use they are sterilized by flaming in 95% ethanol. However, there is less spattering during flaming with 100% ethanol. The excess ethanol should be drained before flaming. Three coverslips can be conveniently arranged in the bottom of each 35-mm culture dish.

6. Glutaraldehyde Fixative

A 2.5% solution of glutaraldehyde is prepared in 0.1 M Na cacodylate buffer, pH 7.4, and stored at 4°C.

7. Paraffin-Vasoline Sealer

A convenient sealer for mounting coverslips onto microscope slides is a heated liquid mixture of 50% paraffin and 50% vasoline or quick-drying nail polish.

8. Antibodies

The optimal titer of antierythrocyte sera should be determined by a hemagglutination assay. Twofold serial dilutions of antiserum in PBS are prepared in round-bottom microtiter plate wells for a final volume of 0.1 ml/well. To each dilution of antiserum and to control wells containing 0.1 ml of PBS alone is added 0.1 ml of a 2% (v/v) suspension of erythrocytes in phosphate buffered saline (PBS). Plates are shaken gently to mix, incubated at 37°C for 30 min, and then left undisturbed at 4°C overnight. The PBS control wells and wells containing subagglutinating dilutions of antiserum should exhibit distinct "buttons" of erythrocytes that have settled to the bottom of the wells. Agglutination of erythrocytes by the antiserum results in a diffuse pellet or turbid appearance in the wells. Note that very high concentrations of antiserum may result in a "prozone" nonagglutination reaction, so that care should be taken to examine a large range of antiserum dilutions (at least 12 twofold dilutions). The amount of antiserum used to coat erythrocytes for phagocytosis assays should be no more than half the lowest agglutinating concentration, since agglutination of erythrocytes may interfere with the assay.

III. PROCEDURES

A. Macrophages

Mononuclear phagocytes may be obtained in a variety of ways from a variety of animals, as detailed elsewhere in this volume. We shall describe the plating and cultivation of mouse peritoneal macrophages, but the techniques are equally applicable to other preparations of mononuclear phagocytes and to polymorphonuclear phagocytic cells as well.

The aim in plating is to obtain a nonconfluent monolayer of cells sufficiently dense so that there are about 10 - 20 cells per oil immersion field. Such a monolayer can be obtained by inoculating each 35-mm dish with 1×10^6 macrophages. For any given cell preparation, one therefore needs to know both the total cell count and the percentage of mononuclear phagocytes.

To each 35-mm dish containing three or fewer glass cover-slips are added 2×10^6 resident peritoneal cells (50% macrophages) or 1.25×10^6 thioglycollate-elicited peritoneal exudate cells (80% macrophages) in medium-10% FBS. After a 1-hr incubation in a 5% CO_2 - 95% air incubator at 37°C and 100% humidity, dishes are washed twice with PBS to remove nonadherent cells, overlaid with medium-10% FBS, and replaced in the incubator. Studies may be performed at any time thereafter; we most often assay phagocytosis after 24 or 48 hr of *in vitro* cultivation (7).

B. Particles

1. Antibody-Independent Phagocytosis

As indicated previously, a variety of particles may be used. We shall describe a procedure using zymosan, but it is applicable to other particles as well.

A suspension of zymosan particles is prepared as described elsewhere in this volume and suspended at the desired concentration (usually about 5×10^7/ml) in medium without FBS.

2. Antibody-Dependent Phagocytosis

Again a variety of particles may be used. We shall describe a procedure using sheep erythrocytes (E) (1).

Erythrocytes are washed twice by centrifugation in PBS and suspended at a concentration of 5% (v/v) in medium. A 5% suspension is about 10^9 E/ml. An aliquot is diluted tenfold in medium (0.5% E) and placed on ice.

Another aliquot is mixed with an equal volume of anti-E IgG in medium. The exact quantity of IgG used varies with the titer of the antibody. Using rabbit anti-E IgG from Cordis Laboratories, we have found that a final concentration of between 1 and 3 μl/ml of medium is optimal. The mixture is placed in a 37°C water bath for 15 min, after which erythrocytes are washed twice in cold PBS and resuspended to 10 times the original erythrocyte volume in medium. For example, if we began with 1 ml of 5% E and added 1 ml of medium containing anti-E IgG, then we would resuspend in 10 ml of medium for a 0.5% E(IgG) suspension.

C. The Assay

(1) Macrophages are washed twice with PBS and overlaid with 2 ml of fresh medium; 0.2 ml of the particle-containing suspension is added to each dish and gently mixed.

(2) Cultures are placed for the desired time (usually
30 - 60 min) in a 37°C, humidified 5% CO_2 - 95% air incubator.

(3) Cultures are washed twice with PBS to remove non-cell
associated particles, and then covered with several milliliters
of PBS. When the particle is an erythrocyte preparation, one
coverslip is removed with needle-nosed forceps, dipped for 5
sec only into distilled water, and promptly replaced in the
culture dish. This treatment will result in the hypotonic lysis
of erythrocytes that are attached to the macrophage surface but
will not lyse either the macrophage or ingested erythrocytes.
Prolonged hypotonic treatment will damage phagocytes.

(4) PBS is removed and cultures overlaid with ice-cold
glutaraldehyde. After 10 min or longer, glutaraldehyde is removed and coverslips overlaid with distilled water. Cultures
can be stored at 4°C for several days in either glutaraldehyde
or water, as long as they are kept covered with liquid.

(5) Coverslips are mounted by inverting onto a microscope
slide, blotting dry with a Kimwipe, and then sealing the edges
using a small paintbrush to apply the heated liquid paraffin-
vasoline mixture.

(6) Mounted coverslips are examined promptly with the oil
immersion lens of a phase contrast microscope. When erythrocytes are the test particles, attachment can be scored on the
coverslip that was not subjected to hypotonic shock, while ingestion can be scored on the coverslip that was. In addition,
attachment and ingestion may be differentiated by the fact that
erythrocytes that are attached to phagocytic cells have a
bright rust-colored sheen, while ingested erythrocytes appear
dark brown or black and have no sheen. When zymosan particles
are used, distinguishing between attachment and ingestion is
more difficult. A particle that is at the cell periphery or
that is not in focus when the cell's nucleus is in focus (and
is therefore not in the same plane as the nucleus) is probably
attached but not ingested. A particle that is well within the
cell's periphery, that is in focus when the cell's nucleus is
in focus, and that is surrounded by a phase lucent area is
probably ingested. Even using these criteria, it is often difficult to be certain that a zymosan particle is ingested and
not simply attached.

D. *Calculation of Data*

Data may be expressed in a variety of ways. Many investigators count the number of phagocytic cells that have attached
or ingested even one particle and express the results as the
percentage of cells attaching or phagocytizing. Others establish some minimum cutoff (e.g., 3 particles/cell) and express
the results in a manner similar to that above. Still others

determine the number of particles ingested per cell and express the results as the percentage of cells in groups of phagocytic performance: for example, group A might be those ingesting no particles; group B, 1 to 3 particles; group C, 4 to 6; group D, more than 6.

We usually determine the percentage of cells ingesting any particles and the average number of particles ingested per cell. Our results are expressed as the phagocytic index, which is the product of the two determinations. For example, if 80% of the cells ingested an average of eight particles each, the phago-cytic index would be 640. Particle attachment can be assessed and the results similarly expressed.

E. Critical Comments

1. Pitfalls in the Performance of the Assay

There are several technical problems that may arise but which may be avoided or overcome if the investigator anticipates them.

(a) All sera used should be heat inactivated to ensure that complement is not playing an unrecognized role in the interac-tion of cells with particles.

(b) The assay of phagocytosis should, whenever possible, be performed in serum-free medium to eliminate the possibility that immunoglobulins or other serum factors are responsible for the results obtained.

(c) In assessing antibody-dependent phagocytosis, concentra-tions of antibody that result in agglutination of the particles must be avoided. Otherwise, particles will form clumps and may be unavailable for phagocytosis.

(d) When antibody-dependent phagocytosis is studied, non-coated particles should always be run as a control. Only those particles that are not significantly phagocytized in the non-coated state are suitable for studying antibody-dependent phago-cytosis.

(e) Particles, especially erythrocytes, must be handled carefully to avoid damaging them, for surface alterations will render some otherwise noningestible particles ingestible.

(f) During washing, coverslips may float and slide on top of each other. This should be recognized promptly and the coverslips moved back into their proper places. Depending upon the stage of the assay during which it occurs, failure to cor-rect this problem can lead to coverslips with no macrophages on them, to macrophage damage or death, or to markedly disparate phagocytosis results between coverslips in the same dish.

(g) If left without a layer of overlying liquid for very

long, macrophages will dry out and die. Therefore, only four
or five cultures should be washed at one time, and cultures
should be recovered with liquid as quickly as possible.

(h) When media containing bicarbonate buffers are used,
the pH can rise tremendously when dishes are left out of a CO_2
atmosphere for very long, leading to cell damage and death.
This can be recognized by the development of a purple color in
medium containing a pH indicator and should be avoided by
limiting the time cultures spend outside the incubator.

(i) Errors in washing can lead to erroneous estimates of
particle attachment. All assays of particle attachment are
dependent to some degree upon washing techniques. With inadequate washing, one can find that many cells "attach" many types
of particles. With too vigorous washing, some particles that
are specifically and fairly firmly attached can be removed.
The investigator who is beginning to use a technique that assesses particle attachment needs to develop a standard washing
procedure using particles that are known not to attach and
particles that are known to attach to the cell studied. Washing errors generally do not lead to erroneous estimates of
particle ingestion unless the washing is so vigorous that macrophages are removed from the monolayer.

(j) Exposure of cultures to hypotonic shock to remove attached erythrocytes can result in damage to or lysis of the
phagocytic cell. Therefore, it is important to limit the duration of hypotonic treatment to 5 sec.

2. *Advantages and Limitations of the Technique*

We believe that the microscopic assay of particle attachment and ingestion is simple and accurate and have found it
very useful in situations where qualitative differences are
being assessed, e.g., where the question posed is whether or
not phagocytic cells attach or ingest a given particle and, if
so, under what conditions. In such circumstances, one would
typically compare positive and negative samples demonstrating
25- to 100-fold differences in phagocytic indices, the phagocytic index for the negative sample being in the range of 10.
We have little confidence, however, in using the assay to detect relatively small differences between large phagocytic indices. There is simply too much variation in the phagocytic
indices of identically treated preparations for us to be certain that a phagocytic index of 900 is actually different from
a phagocytic index of 700, for example. This procedure also
allows assessment of heterogeneity of population of phagocytes,
unlike bulk uptake methods.

A major problem with all techniques used to study phagocytosis is that particle ingestion is difficult to distinguish
from particle attachment. Two ways to overcome this problem

are (a) to use a particle that the phagocytic cell does not
bind at all unless the particle's surface is altered, as, for
example, by being coated with antibody, and (b) to use a particle that if attached can be unequivocally removed from the
phagocytic cell's surface. Sheep erythrocytes satisfy both
conditions. Heavily encapsulated microorganisms such as pneumococci satisfy the first.

IV. ASSAY OF PHAGOCYTOSIS OF RADIOLABELED PARTICLES

A. *Introduction*

The use of radiolabeled test particles in phagocytosis assays can greatly reduce assay volumes and significantly increase the sensitivity of measurements. The assay basically
assesses the association of particle radiolabel with the mononuclear phagocyte; it can be performed with either monolayer
or suspension cultures of phagocytes from any source. Erythrocytes labeled with ^{51}Cr - Na_2CrO_4 are frequently used for
measurement of antibody-dependent phagocytosis and are especially applicable for the simultaneous measurement of ingestion and
macrophage-mediated extracellular cytotoxicity (12, 13). However, it should be noted that radioisotopes are hazardous and
regulated materials whose use demands special procedures and
equipment in the laboratory.

B. *Reagents*

1. *Particles*

In principle, any of the phagocytizable particles described
in Section II.B.1 could be employed. Major limitations include
the difficulty in separating phagocytes from radiolabeled
particles at the end of the assay, the inability to distinguish
between ingested radiolabel and label associated with particles
that are merely attached to the phagocyte, and the amount of
radiolabel that can be specifically introduced into or onto the
test particle. Erythrocytes are ideal particles since they are
readily labeled with ^{51}Cr - Na_2CrO_4 and since they can be
preferentially lysed in phagocyte cultures. Radiolabeled bacteria have also been used (14).

2. Antibodies and Assay Media

These are basically the same as described in Sections II.B.2 and II.B.3.

3. Radiolabeled Sodium Chromate

Fresh isotonic solutions of ^{51}Cr-Na$_2$CrO$_4$ (6.4 µg Na$_2$CrO$_4$/ml, 1 mCi ^{51}Cr/ml) should be obtained from the manufacturer frequently (1 - 2 times/month) since the decay products of ^{51}Cr, which accumulate in the preparations, are toxic to cells. The solutions should be stored in 4°C in a lead container. (Note: The purchase and use of radioisotopes require special licensing procedures.)

4. Lysing Solutions

A medium for lysing extracellular erythrocytes is prepared by making a 0.83% (w/v) solution of NH$_4$Cl in isotonic bicarbnate buffer, pH 7.2. Lysates of monolayer cultures of phagocytes are prepared with a 1% aqueous solution of sodium dodecyl sulfate (SDS); other detergent solutions or even prolonged treatment with water alone may also be used.

5. Laboratory Equipment and Supplies

See items listed in Section II.B.4. The use of disposable pipettes and cultureware is strongly recommended when working with radioisotopes. In addition, 24-well or 96-well flatbottom cluster tissue culture plates (Costar, Linbro), microliter-range pipettes (Eppendorf-type with disposable plastic tips), a gamma counter, and the appropriate facilities for use and disposal of radioactive materials are required.

C. Procedures

1. Phagocytic Cells in Monolayer Culture

Cells are plated, washed, and cultured basically as described in Section III.A, except that a more nearly confluent monolayer of phagocytes is desired. We routinely culture 7.5×10^5 mouse peritoneal macrophages in 1 ml of medium-10% FBS per 16 mm well of the 24-cluster plates; monolayers may also be established in the smaller wells of 96-well tissue culture plates. It is very important that phagocytes be accurately dispensed and evenly dispersed in each well.

2. *Phagocytic Cells in Suspension Culture*

For some preparations of mononuclear phagocytes, a suspension assay of phagocytosis may be conveniently performed. This is true for the continuous macrophage cell lines that are easily detached from culture vessel surfaces (12) and for other cell preparations that can be assayed without prior adherence to a surface. Suspensions of 10^6 phagocytes/ml of assay medium should be kept on ice (to prevent loss by adherence to the vessel) until added to assay tubes. Use of polypropylene tubes will also reduce sticking.

3. *Radiolabeling of Erythrocytes*

Approximately 5×10^9 sheep erythrocytes are diluted with PBS and pelleted by centrifugation. Supernatant fluid is carefully removed from the pellet, which is then suspended in about 0.2 ml of ^{51}Cr – Na$_2$CrO$_4$ solution. The mixture is incubated in a 37°C water bath for 1 – 3 hr with occasional agitation. The extent of erythrocyte radiolabeling will depend upon both the amount of radioisotope added to the erythrocyte pellet and the duration of the labeling incubation.

Erythrocytes are extensively washed after incubation (three times with 25 volumes of medium or PBS), counted in a hemacytometer chamber, and adjusted to the required concentration in the assay medium. Antibody coating of erythrocytes can be performed either before or after ^{51}Cr labeling, as described in Section III.B.2 above.

4. *Monolayer Assay of Radiolabeled Erythrocyte Phagocytosis*

(a) Monolayers of phagocytes are washed as described in Section II above and then overlaid with assay medium, using 0.5 to 1.0 ml per 24-cluster well or 0.1 ml per 96-cluster well.

(b) Labeled erythrocytes (0.1 ml) are added to each 24- or 96-cluster well and plates are gently mixed by perpendicular motions (north – south and east – west). In general, erythrocyte suspensions should be prepared so that a 0.1 ml aliquot will contain an excess of erythrocytes in relation to the number of phagocytes in each well. We routinely add 5 erythrocytes per macrophage for a 2-hr phagocytosis assay; shorter assays may call for the use of larger erythrocyte-to-phagocyte ratios.

(c) The efficiency of monolayer phagocytosis assays, especially those with short assay times, can be increased by gentle centrifugation (lowest speed, 2 – 5 min) of the culture plates to bring the erythrocytes into contact with the adherent phagocytes. Centrifuge carriers manufactured to accommodate microtiter plates (Cooke, 220-18) facilitate this centrifugation.

(d) Assay plates are incubated in a humidified, 5% CO_2 - 95% air incubator at 37°C for periods up to 2 hr.

(e) To stop the incubation, culture plates are placed on ice and washed once in ice-cold medium. Remember that this and all subsequent washings are radioactive and should be properly disposed of.

(f) Each assay well is aspirated, overlaid with NH_4Cl lysing buffer, and incubated at room temperature for 5 min.

(g) Wells are washed twice more in ice-cold medium, then the medium is carefully removed and replaced with exactly 0.5 ml (for 24-cluster) or 0.1 ml (for 96-cluster) per well of 1% SDS.

(h) After incubation at room temperature for 15 min, phagocytes are further disrupted by several direct up - down pipettings. An accurate amount of lysate from each well (e.g., 0.25 ml for 24-cluster or 0.05 ml for 96-cluster) is transferred to tubes or vials for determination of radioactivity in a gamma counter.

5. *Suspension Assay of Radiolabeled Erythrocyte Phagocytosis*

(a) Phagocyte suspension (0.1 ml) and radiolabeled erythrocytes (0.1 ml) are added to disposable plastic culture tubes (e.g., Falcon 2052). Again, the erythrocyte-to-phagocyte ratio should usually be in the range of erythrocyte excess.

(b) The assay tubes are incubated at 37°C in a humidified, 5% CO_2 - 95% air incubator, either on a rocking platform or with regular manual agitation, for the desired length of time.

(c) To stop the incubation, 2 ml of ice-cold medium is added to each tube, the tubes are shaken, and then centrifuged to pellet cells.

(d) The supernatant medium is carefully aspirated and pellets gently resuspended in 1 ml NH_4Cl lysing solution to remove extracellular erythrocytes. After incubation at room temperature for 5 min, 1 ml of ice-cold medium is added and the tubes are shaken and centrifuged.

(e) The pellets are gently resuspended in 2 ml of medium and washed once more. Supernatant medium is carefully aspirated from the final pellet, which should contain phagocytes and the labeled erythrocytes that they ingested. The pellets may be counted directly for radioactivity, or they may be resuspended in medium and transferred to vials for the gamma counter.

D. *Calculation of Data*

Results can be expressed in two ways: (a) as the radioactivity (counts per min, cpm) directly measured in the final phagocyte fraction, or (b) as the percentage of the total added radioactivity that is detected in the final phagocyte fashion. In the latter case, the radioactivity of the original erythrocyte suspension that was added to each sample must also be determined and the following calculation performed:

$$\% \text{ Phagocytosis} = \frac{\text{cpm in phagocyte fraction}}{\text{total cpm added}} \times 100$$

When only partial volumes of a sample are assayed for radioactivity (as in Section IV.C.4(h) above), appropriate corrections for total volume must be included in the above calculation.

E. Critical Comments

1. Pitfalls in the Performance of the Assay

The use of radiolabeled particles to assess phagocytic activity can yield highly reproducible results if attention is given to the following details:

(a) General precautions outlined in II.E.1 for microscopic phagocytic assays [specifically (a) - (e), (g) and (h)] are applicable to the radiolabel assay.

(b) In contrast to the microscopic assay, it is crucial when using radiolabeled particles that the concentrations of both phagocytes and particles, as well as assay volumes, be exact and accurate. Care must be taken to avoid damage to or removal of monolayer phagocytes during aspiration and pipetting.

(c) Phagocyte preparations should be checked microscopically for monolayer density and homogeneity, for possible contaminating microorganisms, and for normal cellular morphology prior to the start of the assay, since it will be difficult if not impossible to assess such parameters by the time the data are collected.

(d) When initially establishing the assay system, one should check for completeness of erythrocyte lysis after NH_4Cl treatment and for monolayer dispersal after SDS lysis of phagocytes, by microscopic examination. Ox erythrocytes may require longer NH_4Cl treatment for complete lysis. Chicken erythrocytes are also resistant to lysis and water treatment may be needed for their removal (see ref. 12 for procedure).

(e) Whenever possible, one should attempt to establish a correlation between the microscopic measurement of particle ingestion and the measured uptake of radiolabel by phagocytes. This is especially important when new particles are being tested or when assay conditions are being varied, so as to detect artifactual changes in phagocyte-associated radiolabel.

(f) The duration of incubation of radiolabeled particles with phagocytes should be limited to 4 hr, and we recommend no more than 2 hr. Some phagocyte preparations demonstrate measurable excretion of radiolabel into the assay medium, with a concommittant decrease in levels of phagocyte-associated label, after such lengths of time (authors' personal observations (12)). Therefore, prolonged incubation may result in an underestimation of the total phagocytic activity that has occurred in a sample.

(g) We routinely set up control samples in which labeled particles are added to wells (or tubes) that contain no phagocytes. Either particles themselves or radiolabel released from the particles may become nonspecifically associated with the assay vessel during incubation and be included in the final phagocyte fraction. The measured radioactivity in these control samples can be subtracted from the values for experimental samples when calculating % phagocytosis.

2. Advantages and Limitations of the Technique

The use of radiolabeled particles to measure phagocytosis enables one to make more sensitive measurements of ingestion than the microscopic assay described above and is therefore useful in determining rates of phagocytosis or for assessing the effects of antibody titers in antibody-dependent ingestion (12). The assay also makes more efficient use of cells, reagents, and manpower since assay volumes can be greatly reduced and since quantitation of phagocytosis does not require long hours at the microscope. However, there are several important limitations to its application.

First, the investigator must be trained in and usually licensed for radioisotope work and must take on the added responsibility of complying with procedures for storage, use, and disposal of radioactive materials. The special laboratory facilities and equipment that are required may be cost-prohibitive.

Second, the assay does not allow for the assessment of differential activities by cells within a population, so that in general only homogenous populations of phagocytic cells should be used.

Third, although many types of particles might be efficiently radiolabeled, most are very difficult to separate from phagocytic cells and it is therefore difficult to distinguish attachment from ingestion.

Fourth, the measurement of phagocyte-associated radiolabel can be influenced by several phenomena other than ingestion. Free or protein-bound label released from noningested particles may be nonspecifically bound to phagocytes and/or vessel surfaces, or be endocytosed by phagocytes. Also, as mentioned above, phagocytes can exocytose radiolabeled digestion products from phagocytized particles. It is difficult to adequately control for such occurrences and their possible influence must be considered when interpreting results.

V.   OTHER ASSAYS OF PHAGOCYTOSIS

A. Introduction

We shall briefly review some other techniques for measuring phagocytosis that, in general, have more limited applicability. The reader should refer to the literature cited for detailed descriptions.

B. Nephelometric and Spectrophotometric Assays of Phagocytized Particles

These assays can provide sensitive measurements of the phagocytosis of certain particles, such as latex beads (nephelometry) (3, 15), and erythrocyte or paraffin oil particles containing oil red O (spectrophotometry) (4, 16). They are especially useful in determining phagocytic rates. A major limitation is the difficulty in distinguishing between particle attachment to the phagocyte and particle ingestion.

C. Assays of Bacterial Phagocytosis by Viable Bacterial Counts

The general technique involves incubating bacteria or other microorganisms with phagocytic cells and then assessing the number of viable microbes that remain in the culture (5, 17). However, most assays of this type actually measure microbicidal activity of the phagocytic cells, since microbes attached to phagocytes may be killed but not ingested and since ingested organisms may not always be killed. Furthermore, the techniques involved are laborious and are subject to numerous artifactual variations. For example, attachment is difficult to distinguish from ingestion, although in some instances this problem can be overcome by selectively killing noningested microbes with an antibiotic that does not enter the phagocytic cell (17). In addition, clumping of bacteria may result in several bacteria being counted as one colony on the plate.

D. Metabolic Indicators as Assays of Phagocytosis

Various changes in phagocytic cell metabolism that accompany ingestion of a particle can be readily measured *in vitro* (6, 18 - 20). However, such metabolic activities can also be modulated by particle attachment alone and by other biologic or chemical stimuli. The use of metabolic indicators as an assay of phagocytosis is therefore extremely limited.

Acknowledgment

Supported by grants PCM 75-17106 from the National Science Foundation and grant IM-173 from the American Cancer Society. FMG is the recipient of Research Career Development Award AI-00135 from National Institutes of Health.

REFERENCES

1. F. M. Griffin and S. C. Silverstein. Segmental response of the macrophage plasma membrane to a phagocytic stimulus. *J. Exp. Med. 139*: 323-336, 1974.
2. R. H. Michell, S. J. Pancake, J. Noseworthy, and M. L. Karnovsky. Measurement of rates of phagocytosis. The use of cellular monolayers. *J. Cell Biol. 40*: 216-224, 1969.
3. R. A. Weisman and E. D. Korn. Phagocytosis of latex beads by *Acanthamoeba*. I. Biochemical properties. *Biochemistry 6*: 485-497, 1967.
4. T. P. Stossel, C. A. Alper, and F. S. Rosen. Serum-dependent phagocytosis of paraffin oil emulsified with bacterial lipopolysaccharide. *J. Exp. Med. 137*: 690-705, 1973.
5. O. Maaloe. "On the Relation between Alexin and Opsonin." Copenhagen, Ejnar Munksgaard, 1946.
6. R. B. Johnston, Jr., M. R. Klemperer, C. A. Alper, and F. S. Rosen. The enhancement of bacterial phagocytosis by serum: The role of complement components and two co-factors. *J. Exp. Med. 129*: 1275-1290, 1969.
7. F. M. Griffin, C. Bianco, and S. C. Silverstein. Characterization of the macrophage receptor for complement and demonstration of its functional independence from the receptor for the Fc portion of immunoglobulin G. *J. Exp. Med. 141*: 1269-1277, 1975.
8. C. Bianco, F. M. Griffin, and S. C. Silverstein. Studies of the macrophage complement receptor. Alteration of re-

ceptor function upon macrophage activation. *J. Exp. Med.* *141*: 1278-1290, 1975.

9. F. M. Griffin, J. A. Griffin, J. E. Leider, and S. C. Silverstein. Studies on the mechanism of phagocytosis. I. Requirements for circumferential attachment of particle-bound ligands to specific receptors on the macrophage plasma membrane. *J. Exp. Med.* *142*: 1263-1282, 1975.

10. F. M. Griffin, J. A. Griffin, and S. C. Silverstein. Studies on the mechanism of phagocytosis. II. Interactions of macrophages with anti-immunoglobulin IgG-coated bone marrow-derived lymphocytes. *J. Exp. Med.* *144*: 788-809, 1976.

11. J. A. Griffin and F. M. Griffin. Augmentation of macrophage complement receptor function *in vitro*. I. Characterization of the cellular interactions required for the generation of a T-lymphocyte product that enhances macrophage complement receptor function. *J. Exp. Med.* *150*: 653-675, 1979.

12. W. S. Walker and A. Demus. Antibody-dependent cytolysis of chicken erythrocytes by an *in vitro*-established line of mouse peritoneal macrophages. *J. Immunol.* *114*: 765-769, 1975.

13. R. Snyderman, M. C. Pike, D. G. Fischer, and H. S. Koren. Biologic and biochemical activities of continuous macrophage cell lines P388D$_1$ and J774.1. *J. Immunol.* *119*: 2060-2066, 1977.

14. F. Ulrich. Phagocytosis of *E. coli* by enzyme-treated macrophages. *Am. J. Physiol.* *220*: 958-966, 1971.

15. F. Ulrich and D. B. Zilversmit. Release from alveolar macrophages of an inhibitor of phagocytosis. *Am. J. Physiol.* *218*: 1118-1127, 1970.

16. T. P. Stossel, R. J. Mason, J. Hartwig, and M. Vaughan. Quantitative studies of phagocytosis by polymorphonuclear leukocytes: Use of emulsions to measure the initial rate of phagocytosis. *J. Clin. Invest.* *51*: 615-624, 1972.

17. J. W. Alexander, D. B. Windhorst, and R. A. Good. Improved tests for the evaluation of neutrophil function in human disease. *J. Lab. Clin. Med.* *72*: 136-148, 1968.

18. R. C. Graham, Jr., M. J. Karnovsky, A. W. Shafer, E. A. Glass, and M. L. Karnovsky. Metabolic and morphological observations on the effect of surface-active agents on leukocytes. *J. Cell Biol.* *32*: 629-647, 1967.

19. Z. A. Cohn and S. I. Morse. Interactions between rabbit polymorphonuclear leucocytes and staphylococci. *J. Exp. Med.* *110*: 419-443, 1959.

20. L. R. DeChatelet, M. R. Cooper, and C. E. McCall. Dissociation by colchicine of the hexose monophosphate shunt activation from the bactericidal activity of the leukocyte. *Infect. Immun.* *3*: 66-72, 1971.

55

PINOCYTIC RATE USING HORSERADISH PEROXIDASE

Paul J. Edelson

I. INTRODUCTION

Pinocytosis, or bulk interiorization of fluid, is typically assessed by measuring the cellular uptake over a fixed period of time of a marker present in a known concentration in the extracellular fluid. Clearly, the marker must not be interiorized by diffusion or specific transport, must be stable both extracellularly and intracellularly over the period of the experiment, must not be released by the cells once it has been interiorized, and must not itself affect the endogenous pinocytic rate of the cells being studied. In addition, the marker must not bind to cell surfaces, as such absorptive pinocytosis would prevent the uptake of the marker from being a true reflection of the quantity of fluid interiorized.

In addition to these requirements, it is also valuable for the marker to be detectable in very small amounts so as to reduce the number of cells necessary for the assay and for it to be possible to identify the marker electron microscopically in order to obtain structural confirmation of the inferred fate of the scout molecules.

Several marker particles, including ^{3}H-labeled sucrose, ^{14}C-labeled inulin, ^{125}I-labeled bovine serum albumin, and colloidal gold have been used to assess pinocytic rates. Although in various situations each of these markers has been useful, we have found horseradish peroxidase to have fewer drawbacks and to be more generally applicable than these alternatives. It is especially well suited to studies of adherent cells, including monocytes and macrophages from various species, with the cautions mentioned below.

II. PRINCIPLE

Horseradish peroxidase (HRP), a heme-containing protein, can catalyze the oxidation of *o*-dianisidine by hydrogen peroxide to give a dark brown product. The rate of this conversion is assessed by measuring the rate of change of absorbance of the assay solution at 460 nm on a recording spectrophotometer.

III. REAGENTS

1. *Horseradish Peroxidase*
The most satisfactory source of the enzyme for pinocytic rate measurements is Horseradish Peroxidase, Type II, Catalog No. P-8250 (Sigma Chemical Co., St. Louis, Missouri). Several more highly purified preparations have been found to give erratic results.

The enzyme may be dissolved in sterile phosphate-buffered saline (pH 7.4) at 20 mg/ml. One ml aliquots may be stored at -20°C for several months and thawed immediately before use. The enzyme deteriorates with repeated cycles of freezing and thawing.

2. *Sorensen's Phosphate Buffer (o.1M pH 5.0)*
13.446 gm KH_2PO_4
0.170 gm $Na_2HPO_4.7 H_2O$.
Dissolve in 1 liter of distilled water. Adjust pH to 5.0, store at room temperature.

3. *o-dianisidine (10 mg/ml)*

o-Dianisidine (Catalog No. D-3127, Sigma Chemical Co., St. Louis, Missouri). Dissolve 10 mg in 1 ml absolute methanol. WARNING: Gloves are mandatory when handling o-dianisidine as it is a suspected carcinogen. Vortex solution thoroughly to dissolve powder.

4. *Hydrogen Peroxide (0.3%)*

Hydrogen peroxide solution, 30% stabilized (Catalog No. 5239, Mallinckrodt Chemical Corp., St. Louis, Missouri). Dissolve 1 ml of 30% H_2O_2 in 99 ml sterile distilled water. Store refrigerated and protected from light.

5. *Substrate Solution*

To prepare assay substrate, combine reagents in these proportions, and in the following order:

6.0 ml Sorensen's phosphate buffer (0.1 M, pH 5.0)

0.05 ml o-dianisidine (10 mg/ml)

0.06 ml H_2O_2(0.3%) (add immediately before the substrate is to be used).

NOTE: Substrate must be prepared with scrupulously clean glassware, scoops, etc. The solution should be crystal clear. If it appears yellowed or muddy, discard it and prepare fresh substrate in a new container.

The substrate vessel should be wrapped in aluminum foil and kept covered. Substrate will remain usable for several hours at room temperature.

6. *Triton X-100 (0.05%)*

Triton X-100 (Sigma Chemical Co., St. Louis, Missouri). Dissolve in sterile distilled water to make a 5% stock solution. This solution may be stored indefinitely at room temperature.

A working solution of Triton (0.05%) should be freshly prepared on the day of use by diluting 100 µl of the 5% stock solution in 9.9 ml of distilled water.

IV. PROCEDURES

A. *Peroxidase Uptake*

Freshly rinsed macrophage monolayers are incubated in Dulbecco's Modified Eagle's Medium (Catalog No. 320-1965, Grand Island Biological Corp., Grand Island, New York) containing heat-inactivated fetal calf serum (20%) and horseradish peroxidase (1 mg/ml), which has been warmed to 37°C.

Cells are incubated for fixed periods of time, rinsed vigorously three times with warmed tissue culture medium without serum, and then reincubated in medium containing serum for 30 min before being rinsed vigorously with phosphate-buffered saline (pH 7.4) a final three times, and then being lysed in 500 µl of Triton X-100 (0.05%). The cells should be scraped with a rubber police person and the lysate either assayed immediately or promptly stored at -20°C until assay.

B. Peroxidase Assay

1. Spectrophotometer Settings
Adjust recording spectrophotometer to measure absorbances at 460 nm. The machine should be zeroed with distilled water, and full-scale deflection should represent 0.100 absorbance units. The cycle time should be set to 15 sec.

2. Horseradish Peroxidase Standards
Dilute the incubation solution containing horseradish peroxidase (1 mg/ml) with phosphate-buffered saline containing fetal calf serum (1%) to a final concentration of 10 ng/ml, a dilution of 10^5-fold. This standard is usually sufficient, but if additional standards are desired, 5 ng/ml and 20 ng/ml are both convenient concentrations to use.

3. To Perform the Assay
Place 0.1 ml standard or unknown sample in a 1.0 ml cuvette. Add 0.9 ml o-dianisidine substrate solution. Cover cuvettes with Parafilm and quickly mix contents by inverting twice. Immediately place cuvettes in spectrophotometer and record absorbances for 1-3 min.

V. CALCULATION OF DATA

The calculation is straightforward, based on Beer's law, which states that absorbance will be proportional to concentration. In our case, since we are using the rate of accumulation of a colored product as an indicator of enzyme activity, it is the *rate of change* of absorbance that interests us. Since this is represented by the slope of the absorbance recordings, we can simply measure these, and then convert them to enzyme activities as follows:

$$
\begin{array}{l}
\text{Enzyme} \\
\text{concentration} = \dfrac{\text{Slope (unknown)}}{\text{Slope (standard)}} \times \begin{array}{l}\text{Enzyme} \\ \text{concentration} \\ \text{(standard)}\end{array} \\
\text{(unknown)}
\end{array}
$$

To obtain *specific activity,* the activity of each sample is divided by the protein content of that sample. Since we calculate our enzyme activities as *specific activities,* they should be divided by the protein *concentration.*

The final data should be reported as the volume of fluid interiorized per unit time. Since the extracellular fluid contains 1 mg/ml enzyme, 1 ng enzyme represents 1 nl fluid interiorized. The specific activities may thus be converted to fluid volumes, and then divided by the incubation time (in hours) and the protein content of 10^6 cells to give the pinocytic rate in *nanoliters per hour per 10^6 cells.*

VI. CRITICAL COMMENTS

This note will simply emphasize a few important points to keep in mind in using the assay.

The key to reproducible results is an effective procedure for washing away the extracellular HRP before the cells are assayed for the amount of enzyme ingested. A major problem is enzyme adherent to the serum protein coating the culture dish. Our approach is to rinse vigorously the dishes 3 times with medium to remove most of the soluble extracellular material. We then refeed the cultures with serum-supplemented medium and incubate them at 37°C for 30 min. This elutes the adherent enzyme, and three additional vigorous washes remove that. During washing, one must take care never to leave the dishes without medium as the cells will rapidly dry and lyse.

There are several issues to be dealt with in interpreting the results of an HRP uptake experiment:

(a) One should confirm this is really uptake by carrying out controls on ice, under which conditions no pinocytosis occurs.

(b) One should also do "dish controls" - culture dishes preincubated with medium and serum, but without cells, to assess the effectiveness of washing.

(c) If one is measuring a pinocytic *rate,* one should in fact construct a time course of uptake with points every 15-30 min for 1-2 hr. Include a t_0 sample to check washing.

(d) Check cells for endogenous peroxidase. Monocytes and neutrophils (which may contaminate some inflammatory exudates) both have lots of peroxidase.

(e) Histochemical localization of the marker, especially by EM, provides additional assurance that what you say was endocytized actually was taken up in membrane-bound vesicles.

REFERENCES

1. The basic assay is described in R. M. Steinman.
    Horseradish peroxidase as a marker for studies of pino-
    cytosis. *In "In Vitro Methods in Cell-Mediated and
    Tumor Immunity"* (B. R. Bloom and J. R. David, eds.,)
    Chapter 32, Academic Press, New York, 1976.
2. A paper giving typical values for mouse peritoneal macro-
    phages and illustrating the use of various controls is
    P. J. Edelson, R. Zweibel, and Z. A. Cohn. The pinocytic
    rate of activated macrophages. *J. Exp. Med. 142:* 1150-
    1164, 1975.

56

CHEMOTAXIS OF HUMAN AND MURINE
MONONUCLEAR PHAGOCYTES

Ralph Snyderman

I. INTRODUCTION

Mononuclear phagocytes are motile cells that are able to
sense and migrate along gradients of certain chemical substances. The ability of phagocytes to migrate unidirectionally
in response to chemical signals may be an important mechanism
by which they accumulate at sites of inflammation. Three types
of cellular motility can be defined. Random migration is cellular locomotion in the absence of any known stimulus of migration.
Chemotaxis is the unidirectional locomotion of cells along a
concentration gradient of a chemoattractant. Chemokinesis is
stimulated random migration due to substances that enhance
phagocyte locomotion but that are not present in a gradient.
In vitro assays are available, which allow the quantification
of the three different types of mononuclear phagocyte locomotion.
These methods have been extremely useful in helping to define
the physiology and pathology of mononuclear phagocyte motility.
The assays available allow the study of the locomotion of human

(1,2), murine (3,4), guinea pig (5,6), and rabbit mononuclear phagocytes (7). The most widely used assays to study leukocyte locomotion involve the migration of cells through microporous filters in response to chemical stimuli. This method involves placing cells in a compartment of a plastic chamber above a microporous filter. Substances to be tested for their effects on leukocyte motility can be placed, in varying concentrations, below and/or above the filter. The migration of cells into or through the filter is then quantified. Direct visual observation of mononuclear phagocyte motility on glass or plastic using cinematography can also be used, but quantitative data on anything other than individual cell movement is difficult to obtain with these latter procedures. This chapter will focus on motility assays employing microporous filters in modified Boyden chemotaxis chambers (8).

II. REAGENTS AND MATERIALS

   Media: RPMI-1640 (GIBCO, Grand Island, New York), pH 7.0 or Gey's Balanced Salt Solution containing 2% Bovalbumin (Flow Laboratories, McLean, Virginia) plus 10 mM HEPES pH 7.0. When medium is used to lavage peritoneal cavities to obtain macrophages, 10 u heparin/ml is added.
   Cells: Peripheral blood mononuclear phagocytes or resident or elicited peritoneal mononuclear phagocytes.
   Chemicals: Lymphoprep (Nyegaarad and Co., Oslow, Norway), Ficoll (Pharmacia Fine Chemicals, Piscataway, New Jersey or Sigma Chemical Co., St. Louis, Missouri) and Hypaque-M 90% (Winthrop Labs., New York).
   Chemotaxis filters: Polycarbonate filters; Nuclepore, 5 μm pore size, 13-mm diameter (Neuroprobe Corp., Cabin John, Maryland or Biorad Laboratories, Richmond, California; Nitrocellulose, 8 μm pore size 13-mm diameter (Millipore Corp., Bedford, Massachusetts or Sartorius Filters, Incorp., Hayward, Celifornia.
   Chemotaxis chambers: Blindwell or modified original Boyden design (Neuroprobe Corp., Cabin John, Maryland, or any competent instrument shop).
   Stains: Absolute alcohol, Meyer's hemotoxin, acid alcohol, Bluing solution (8) or Wright's Giemsa stain (Difquik, Harleco, Gibbstown, New Jersey).
   Chemoattractants: Synthetic N-formylated oligopeptides (9) (N-formyl-methionyl-leucyl-phenylalinine, N-formyl-methionyl-methionyl-methionine, Peninsula, San Carlos, California or Sigma, St. Louis, Missouri; Zymosan-activated serum (5 mg/ml zymosan incubated with autologous serum 30 min at 37°, then 30 min at 56°; centrifuge at 500 g and discard pellet), lympho-

cyte-derived chemotactic factor [LDCF, allogeneic lymphocytes stimulated with concanavalin A or phytohemaglutinin as described in (1,2)].

III. PROCEDURES

A. Collection of Cells

Mononuclear phagocytes can be obtained by peritoneal lavage of normal mice or by lavage of mice that have received inflammatory agents given intraperitoneally. The peritoneal cavities are lavaged vigorously with Gey's medium containing 10 μ of heparin per milliliter. The cells are washed once and resuspended to contain approximately 2.0×10^6 macrophages/ml. If the cells are to be used within an hour, they can be kept at room temperature; if not, they should be kept on ice but warmed to room temperature for at least 15 min before they are placed in the chemotaxis chamber. Human mononuclear phagocytes are obtained from peripheral blood that has been separated on either Ficoll-Hypaque density gradients or with Lymphroprep. Blood is drawn into syringes containing a sufficient amount of beef lung heparin to make the final heparin concentration 10 μ/ml of blood. The blood is then diluted approximately 1:4 with isotonic saline. Approximately 35 ml of the diluted blood is placed in a 50-ml polypropylene conical centrifuge tube. Ten ml of Ficoll-Hypaque or Lymphroprep is slowly delivered into the bottom of each tube using a 16-gauge spinal needle attached to a syringe that contains the aforementioned material. The cells are centrifuged at 20°C for 35 min at 400 g. The top layer of diluted plasma is aspirated to within approximately 1 cm of the buffy coat, then the buffy coat is collected with a Pasteur pipette and placed into a second polypropylene conical centrifuge tube. The cells are washed twice at 4°C with the appropriate medium. The cells are then resuspended for a cell count and differential count and adjusted to contain 1.5×10^6 monocytes/ml.

B. Preparation of Filters

Chemotaxis filters should be handled with a fine forceps, being touched only along the edges so that portions of the filters that are to be exposed to cells or chemoattractants are not touched. The filters can be numbered along their outer edge with ballpoint ink, which is found not to run when exposed to the solutions used in the chemotaxis assay. In this laboratory, all assays are performed in triplicate. In

general, two types of chemotaxis chambers are available. The
"blindwell" chamber (Fig. 1) is designed so that the solution
to be studied for chemotactic activity is placed in the lower
compartment, the filter is placed above it, a cap is screwed
into place above the filter, and cells are then placed into
the hole within the cap. The modified Boyden chamber (Fig. 2)
has the filter and cap secured in place before the chemoattractant is added below the filter in the U-shaped lower
compartment.

C. Loading of Blindwell Chemotaxis Chambers

The chemoattractant or medium to be tested is pipetted
carefully into the lower well with enough fluid being added
so that it is convex in relationship to the surface onto which

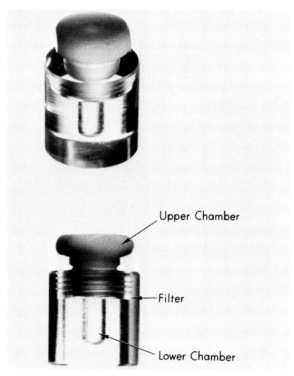

Fig. 1. Blind well chemotaxis chamber. The lower well is
filled with the appropriate material then a micropore filter
is placed above it. The top portion of the chamber is screwed
in place and cells are pipetted into the upper well.

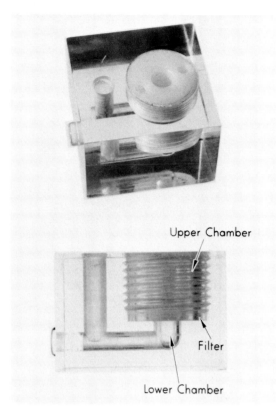

Fig. 2. Modified Boyden chemotaxis chamber. The chamber
is assembled before being filled as described in procedures.

the filter will be placed. The bottom well should not be over-
filled so that the fluid flows over the edge of the filter.
The lower chamber should not be underfilled or air bubbles
will be formed when the filter is put in place. When bubbles
are present, gradients formed will be erratic. The filter is
carefully placed in the chamber using either vacuum aspiration
or with a fine forceps; the top is screwed into place and the
chamber is inspected to see that there are no bubbles under
the filter. The cells are then pipetted into the upper well,
making sure that there are no bubbles above the filter. When
polycarbonate filters are used the dull side should always
face upwards. Cold solutions should not be placed in the
chamber unless they have been degassed since when the chambers
are warmed to 37°, bubbles will form.

D. Loading of Modified Boyden Chambers

The filter is placed in the chamber and the top is secure-
ly screwed on. The chamber is then tilted forward and with a
Pasteur pipette a small amount of the appropriate material being tested is placed in the lower compartment. At the instant
the filter is seen to moisten, the remaining fluid for the
lower compartment and the cell suspension to be added to the
upper compartment are simultaneously added. Again, care must
be taken to see that no bubbles are formed above or below the
filter.

E. Incubation of Chemotaxis Chambers

With either type of chemotaxis chamber, incubation is
carried out at 37°C in humidified air. The value of having
5% CO_2 should be determined and may vary depending on the cell
type or the medium used. The approximate incubation times
when polycarbonate filters are used are as follows: 90 min
for human monocytes, 2 hr for guinea pig macrophages, and
4 hr for mouse macrophages. For nitrocellulose filters and
the leading front assay, human monocytes 2 hr, guinea pig
macrophages, 2 hr. When nitrocellulose filters are used to
measure migration all the way through the filter, incubation
times ranging from 5 to 6 hr are generally required.

F. Staining of Filters

Following incubation, both compartments of the modified
Boyden Chambers are aspirated simultaneously; the top well of
the blindwell chamber is aspirated. The caps to the filter
are then removed and the filters are withdrawn using forceps
and placed in staining baskets. The staining sequence used in
this laboratory is as follows: isotonic saline dip, absolute
alcohol (ethanol) 15 sec, water dip, Meyer's hematoxylin 6 min,
water dip, acid alcohol 1 min, bluing solution, 1 min water
dip. When polycarbonate filters are used, at this point they
are mounted right side up on 24 × 50 mm glass coverslips.
They are air dried and then placed upside down on a glass
slide onto which a drop of immersion oil has been placed for
each filter. Nitrocellulose filters are dehydrated following
staining using 70% then 95%, then absolute alcohol for 1 min
each. The filters are placed in xylene for at least 2 min.
They should then be clear. The filters are mounted upside-
down on a glass slide with a drop of immersion oil mixed with
xylene being placed on each filter. A coverslip is then
placed over the filters. Chemotaxis is quantified using an

eyepiece grid in a microscope. With the polycarbonate filters, the average number of cells that have migrated through to the lower surface of the filter in at least 10 oil immersion fields is determined. The nitrocellulose filters permit either measurement of the cells, which have migrated all the way through to the bottom of the filter, or the distance that the leading front has migrated in a given time period. To determine the leading front, the distance from the top of the filter to the point where the two furthest cells have migrated is determined using the micrometer on the fine adjust knob of a microscope. This is done by focusing on the upper surface of the filter, noting the micrometer setting, and focusing down to the furthest migrated cell. The micrometer is then slowly moved back until two cells are in focus and the distance from the top of the filter to that level is determined. Turner has described the very useful semiautomated method for counting filters by this method (10).

IV.   CALCULATION OF DATA

     Polycarbonate filters are thin (15 μm) and have smooth linear pores. These filters allow the measurement of cells that have migrated to the lower surface. Discrimination of cells that are on the lower surface as opposed to the upper surface is best made using an oil immersion lens (1000×). Data can be expressed as the mean number of cells that have migrated per oil immersion field. Generally, 20 fields are randomly selected for counting and all experiments are performed in triplicate (Table I). It is possible to calculate the percentage of cells that have migrated as well and this is determined by measuring the diameter of the oil immersion field using a stage micrometer. The area of the field is then calculated (area=πr^2) as is the area of the filter exposed to cells and chemoattractant. To determine the number of migrated cells, one multiplies the number of cells per oil immersion field by the number of fields exposed to cells and attractant. This number is divided by the number of cells delivered to the top of the chemotaxis chamber to determine the percentage of cells that have migrated.

     Nitrocellulose filters are approximately 140 μm thick and have convoluted pores. These filters allow measurement of cells that have migrated to the lower surface of the filter. By shortening incubation times, they also allow measurement of the distance cells have migrated into the filter. This latter type of data is expressed in terms of the mean distance migrated rather than the cell number that migrated (Table II).

TABLE I. *Quantification of Chemotaxis by Measuring Migration to the Lower Surface of the Filter*[a]

Dose of chemotactic factor[b] %	Responding cell	
	Murine macrophage	Human monocyte
Medium alone		
0.1%	3.3±0.3	18.5±1
1%	10.6±2.3	nd[c]
3%	30.0±4.0	nd
5%	58.7±2.0	nd
20%	44.9±4.0	60.1±4
	nd	164.3±12

[a]Results represent the mean (±SEM) number of mononuclear phago-cytes per oil immersion field which have migrated to the lower sur-face of polycarbonate filters.

[b]Mouse serum activated by zymosan was used for murine peritoneal macrophages, LDCF was used for human monocytes (v/v in the appropriate medium).

[c]nd, not done.

TABLE II. *Quanitfication of Chemotaxis by the Leading Front Method*[a]

Dose of chemotactic factor[b] %	Responding cell		
	Guinea pig macrophage		*Human monocyte*
Medium alone	42.0±7		38.9±0.9
1%	72.3±5		nd[c]
3%	96.0±5		nd
5%	118.8±3.5		51.9±5
20%	nd		70.3±9

[a]The numbers represent the mean distance (±SEM) in micrometer
which the leading front of cells have migrated.
[b]Zymosan-activated guinea pig serum used for guinea pig peritoneal
macrophages, LDCF used for human monocytes (v/v in the appropriate
medium).
[c]nd, not done.

Differentiation of random migration, chemotaxis, and chemokinesis can be attained by placing various amounts of chemoattractant above and/or below the filter (11,12). This is
termed a "checkerboard" assay and data are reported by showing
the responses of cellular migration to the various positive
and negative gradients as well as to increasing the equal concentration of chemoattractants above and below the filter (11-
13).

V. CRITICAL COMMENTS

Each of the aforementioned methods for quantifying cellular
migration have advantages and disadvantages. The thin polycarbonate filter allows short incubation times and cellular morphology is easy to determine. The assay is somewhat less reproducible from filter to filter than is the leading front assay
and there is the danger of cells falling off the lower surface
of the filter. This latter possibility can be tested for by
counting cells in the lower compartment after the filter has
been removed. In our experience, monocytes or macrophages
rarely fall off the lower surface of polycarbonate filters.
An additional advantage of the polycarbonate filter is that
experiments can be performed in the absence of exogenous protein. The leading front technique is more reproducible from
filter to filter than is the measurement of migration through
either the polycarbonate or nitrocellulose filters. Since the
morphology of cells within the filter is difficult to determine, this method requires a homogenous cell population. An
exogenous source of protein is required for cellular migration
into nitrocellulose filters. The effects of such proteins on
the experiments being performed should be considered. Elonga-
tion of cells within the pores can contribute to errors in
leading front measurements.

The most frustrating problem with all the chemotaxis assays
yet described is day-to-day variability of responsiveness among
the cells from human or animal donors. Variability of results
from filter lot to filter lot can also be a considerable problem. All new lots of filters should be screened and compared
to those previously used. Contamination of mononuclear phagocyte cells with neutrophils adversely affects the data.

A. *Alternative Methods of Assaying Chemotaxis*

Modification of the above techniques as well as different
techniques have been developed in an attempt to measure more
quantitatively cellular motility. Gallin *et al.* (14) and

and Goetzl and Austen (15) employ a double-filter radioassay with ^{51}Cr-labeled cells. Cells are labeled with ^{51}Cr then placed above two filters in the chemotaxis chamber. Cells that migrate through the top filter into the second are counted by measuring the radioactivity in the second filter after the assay is completed. This method eliminated subjectivity, but studies only the cell population which has migrated through the upper filter. Cellular morphology cannot be distinguished so only homogeneous cell populations should be used. The assay is also more time-consuming because of longer cell preparation (1-2 hr to label cells) and longer incubation periods. The potential effects of the radiolabel, as well as the incubation time for labeling, on the chemotactic responsiveness of the cells used must be considered. A variation employing the nitrocellulose filter is measuring cellular migration at various depths within the filter. Cells are counted at 10-μm intervals throughout the filter, and may be plotted as the number of cells migrated at each interval versus the distance migrated. This allows detection of a heterogeneous cell population, e.g., a biphasic response would be obtained if two cell populations exist and migrate at different speeds. Alternatively, Maderazo and Woronick (16) devised the leukotactic index that has low reader variability, but is tedious to count unless an automatic particle counter is employed.

Another method to quantify chemotaxis is the under agarose assay, described by Nelson *et al.* (17). Briefly, series of three wells are cut into agarose that has been introduced into tissue culture plates. The center well receives the cell mixture, with the outer and inner wells receiving chemotactic factor and control medium, respectively. After incubation (10-18 hr at 37°), the plates are fixed, the agarose removed, the cells stained, and the linear distance of migration measured. This method is more useful with polymorphonuclear leukocytes, since the chemotactic factor diffuses from the well into the agarose medium during the longer incubation period required for mononuclear phagocytes. Advantages of the assay are the ability to stain the cells under agarose for enzymes, and to examine them with electron or phase microscopy.

To study cellular behavior, path direction, and morphology, visual assays of chemotaxis can be employed. These allow more rapid evaluation of cellular orientation and motility, but sample only a few cells at a given time. Zigmond's orientation assay (17) requires a minimal number of cells and is very useful for direct visualization of cellular behavior in chemotactic gradients.

REFERENCES

1. R. Snyderman, L. C. Altman, M. S. Hausman, and S. E. Mergenhagen. Human mononuclear leukocyte chemotaxis: A quantitative assay for mediators of humoral and cellular chemotactic factors. *J. Immunol. 108:*857-860, 1972.

2. L. C. Altman, R. Snyderman, J. J. Oppenheim, and S. E. Mergenhagen. A human mononuclear leukocyte chemotactic factor: Characterization, specificity, and kinetics of production by homologous leukocytes. *J. Immunol. 110;* 801-810, 1973.

3. R. Snyderman, M. C. Pike, D. McCarley, and L. Lang. Quantification of mouse macrophage chemotaxis *in vitro:* Role of C5 for the production of chemotactic activity. *Infect. Immun. 11:*488-492, 1975.

4. D. A. Boetcher and M. S. Meltzer. Mouse mononuclear cell chemotaxis: Description of a system. *J. Natl. Cancer Inst. 54:*795-801, 1975.

5. M. S. Hausman, R. Snyderman, and S. E. Mergenhagen. Humoral mediators of chemotaxis of mononuclear leukocytes. *J. Infect. Dis. 125:*595-602, 1972.

6. S. M. Wahl, L. C. Altman, J. J. Oppenheim, and S. E. Mergenhagen. *In vitro* studies of a chemotactic lymphokine in the guinea pig. *Int. Arch. Allergy Appl. Immunol. 46:*768-784, 1974.

7. P. A. Ward. Chemotaxis of mononuclear cells. *J. Exp. Med. 128:*1201-1221, 1968.

8. S. V. Boyden. The chemotactic effect of mixtures of antibody and antigen on polymorphonuclear leukocytes. *J. Exp. Med. 115:*453-466, 1962.

9. E. Schiffmann, B. A. Corcoran, and S. M. Wahl. *N*-Formylmethionyl peptides as chemoattractants for leukocytes. *Proc. Natl. Acad. Sci. USA 72:*1059-1062, 1975.

10. S. R. Turner. ACDAS: An automated chemotaxis data acquisition system. *J. Immunol. Methods 28:*355-360, 1979.

11. S. H. Zigmond and J. G. Hirsch. Leukocyte locomotion and chemotaxis: New methods for evaluation and demonstration of a cell-derived chemotactic factor. *J. Exp. Med. 137:*387-410,

12. P. C. Wilkinson and R. B. Allan. Assay systems for measuring leukocyte locomotion: An overview. *In* "Leukocyte Chemotaxis" (J. I. Gallin and P. G. Quie, eds.), pp. 1-24. Raven Press, New York, 1978.

13. R. Snyderman and M. C. Pike. Pathophysiologic aspects of leukocyte chemotaxis: Identification of a specific chemotactic factor binding site on human granulocytes and defects of macrophage function associated with neoplasia. *In* "Leukocyte Chemotaxis" (J. I. Gallin and P. G. Quie, eds.), pp. 357-378. Raven Press, New York, 1978.

14. J. I. Gallin, R. A. Clark, and H. R. Kimball. Granulocyte chemotaxis: An improved *in vitro* assay employing ^{51}Cr-labeled granulocytes. *J. Immunol. 110:*233-240, 1973.

15. E. J. Goetzl and K. F. Austen. A method for assessing the *in vitro* chemotactic response of neutrophils utilizing ^{51}Cr-labeled human leukocytes. *Immunol. Commun. 1:*421-430, 1972.

16. E. G. Maderazo and C. L. Woronick. A modified micropore filter assay of human granulocyte leukotaxis. *In* "Leukocyte Chemotaxis" (J. I. Gallin and P. G. Quie, eds.), pp. 43-55. Raven Press, New York, 1978.

17. R. D. Nelson, R. T. McCormack, and V. D. Fiegel. Chemotaxis of human leukocytes under agarose. *In* "Leukocyte Chemotaxis" (J. I. Gallin and P. G. Quie, eds.), pp. 25-42, Raven Press, New York, 1978.

18. S. H. Zigmond. A new visual assay of leukocyte chemotaxis. *In* "Leukocyte Chemotaxis" (J. I. Gallin and P. G. Quie, eds.), pp. 57-66. Raven Press, New York, 1978.

57

SECRETORY FUNCTIONS OF MONONUCLEAR PHAGOCYTES:
OVERVIEW AND METHODS
FOR PREPARING CONDITIONED SUPERNATANTS

Philip Davies

I. INTRODUCTION

The utilization of well-controlled tissue culture conditions has led to the identification and characterization of a
variety of secretory products synthesized by cells of the
mononuclear phagocyte system. It is now apparent that the
spectrum of products released by various mononuclear phagocyte populations into their culture medium is markedly dependent on the source of the cells as well as the kind of stimuli
to which they are exposed *in vivo* or in tissue culture. These
variations depend on complex cellular regulatory mechanisms by
which mononuclear phagocytes respond to their pericellular environment. Such modulation is triggered in part through a
number of plasma membrane receptors and high affinity binding
sites that interact with various ligands in the pericellular
environment. Such recognition leads to the initiation of a
complex series of biochemical events, which among other things,
induce and stimulate the secretory activity of the cells.

METHODS FOR STUDYING
MONONUCLEAR PHAGOCYTES

549

II. SECRETORY PRODUCTS OF MONONUCLEAR PHAGOCYTES

It is not intended to provide an extensive account of these products here as this has been done elsewhere (1-3). Table I provides a summary of some of the secretory products of mononuclear phagocytes. These include a large group of hydrolytic enzymes (for review see ref. 4), which can be distinguished from each other by the conditions under which they are secreted. Lysozyme, released on a constitutive basis by mononuclear phagocytes, is little affected by the source of cells or the kinds of stimuli brought into their environment *in vivo* or in culture. On the other hand, the release of both neutral proteinases and lysosomal acid hydrolases is markedly dependent upon the environment from which the cells are obtained and also the nature of the stimuli added to cultured cells. While resident cells secrete minimal amounts of neutral proteinases, mononuclear phagocytes elicited by inflammatory stimuli secrete these enzymes in significant amounts over periods of several days without further stimulation. Also, such secretion can be initiated in resident cells in culture by certain inflammatory stimuli, or enhanced further in elicited populations. Lysosomal acid hydrolases are secreted at a low rate in both resident and elicited populations (37). Such re-

TABLE I. *Some Secretory Products of Mononuclear Phagocytes*[a]

Product	Reference
Hydrolytic enzymes	
Lysozyme	*(5)*
Collagenase	*(6)*
Elastase	*(7)*
Plasminogen activator	*(8)*
Proteoglycan degrading enzyme	*(9)*
Factor D	*(10)*
Neutral caseinase	*(11)*
Lysosomal acid hydrolases	*(4)*
Arachidonic acid oxygenation products	
Prostaglandin E_2	*(12)*
Prostaglandin $F_{2\alpha}$	*(12)*
6-Ketoprostaglandin $F_{1\alpha}$	*(13)*
Thromboxane B_2	*(14)*
12-Hydroxyeicosatetranoic acid	*(15)*
SRS	*(16)*

TABLE I. (cont.)   *See also section by Humes*
Modulators of cellular behavior

Stimulant of stem cell proliferation	*(17)*
Thymic maturation factor	*(18)*
T Lymphocyte mitogen	*(19)*
B Lymphocyte mitogen	*(20)*
Inhibitor of T lymphocyte proliferation	*(21)*
Inhibitor of fibroblast proliferation	*(21)*
Stimulant of collagen synthesis	*(21)*
Stimulant of angiogenesis	*(22)*
Antagonist of steroid induction of hepatic phosphoenolpyruvate carboxykinase	*(23)*
Low molecular weight chemotactic factor for polymorphonuclear leukocytes	*(24)*

Substances cytostatic or cytotoxic to infectious agents and eukaryotic cells

Interferon	*(25)*

Oxygen metabolites

Hydrogen peroxide	*(26)*
Hydroxyl radicals	*(27)*
Superoxide	*(28)*
Listericidal factor	*(29)*
Vitamin B_{12}-binding protein	*(30)*
Arginase	*(31)*
Cytotoxic proteinase	*(11)*

Complement components

C1q	*(32)*
C2	*(33)*
C3	*(32)*
C4	*(33)*
Factor B	*(34)*
Factor D	*(10)*

Others

Pyrogen (also known as interleukin 1)	*(35)*
Tissue thromboplastin	*(36)*

---

[a]*This table is not intended to provide detailed documentation of the secretory products of mononuclear phagocytes. Only one reference is given for each product. These do not account fully for the different types of mononuclear phagocytes secreting that product; the reader is referred to the other sections of this monograph dealing with specific products and to reviews of the subject referred to in the text for detailed information.*

lease can be greatly increased by introduction of certain
types of phagocytic stimuli possessing chronic inflammatory
potency such as antigen-antibody complexes or zymosan particles. Such activity has also been ascribed to components of
the complement system such as C3b (38) and C5a (39) as well
as a number of other soluble substances that have the common
property of being activators of the alternative pathway of
the complement system (40). In contrast, phagocytic stimuli
such as carbon particles, latex beads or erythrocytes, which
lack chronic inflammatory potency, do not stimulate the selective release of lysosomal hydrolases.

It is now established that mononuclear phagocytes from
various sources synthesize a broad range of arachidonic acid
oxygenation products (for review see ref. 41). Prostaglandin
E_2 and prostaglandin $F_{2\alpha}$ were the first such products to be
discovered. Subsequently other products such as prostacyclin,
thromboxane A_2, as well as hydroxy fatty acid products of the
lipoxygenase pathway have been described.

Recent studies in a number of laboratories (see chapter by
Colten, this volume) have established that mononuclear phagocytes secrete many of the components that constitute the alternate and classical pathways of the complement system.

Mononuclear phagocytes secrete diverse substances that
affect the proliferative and differentiated functions of cells
found in their immediate environment (see Table I). In many
instances, the biochemical and physical properties of these
substances have not been established. In some cases, the biological activities by which they have been characterized may
well be shared by one molecule. An example of this is the
possible identity of a T lymphocyte-activating factor and pyrogen released by human peripheral blood monocytes (42). It
is entirely possible that other macrophage secretory products
identified by biological assay may be single molecular entities.

Since one of the primary functions of mononuclear phagocytes is the mediation of host defense mechanisms, it is to be
expected that several of the products that they release into
their environment should inhibit the growth or be cytotoxic to
a variety of infectious agents as well as eukaryotic cells
(Table I). Such molecules range from low molecular products
of oxygen metabolism to macromolecules, such as interferon,
and factors interfering with the growth of intracellular parasites and bacteria.

We have already mentioned the proteinases secreted by mononuclear phagocytes; it is notable that these cells also secrete
α_2-macroglobulin (43), which is an inhibitor of these enzymes.
Also mononuclear phagocytes secrete a tissue factor-like molecule (36) which initiates the blood coagulation cascade. Since
plasminogen activator has as its substrate the zymogen of the

enzyme responsible for fibrin degradation, it is apparent that
mononuclear phagocytes secrete products that can (a) trigger
the activity of a humoral system, blood coagulation, (b) remove
the product of its activation, fibrin, as well as (c) produce
an endogenous inhibitor (α_2-macroglobulin) of the numerous
proteinases involved in the sequential steps leading to fibrin
formation.

The physiological and pathological significance of these
secretory activities of mononuclear phagocytes remains to be
established. Obviously the appropriate use of systems for measuring secretory activities of mononuclear phagocytes can aid
greatly in answering such questions.

III. PREPARATION OF CONDITIONED MEDIUM

Since other contributors to this section will deal with
specific details concerning individual products, we shall con-
fine ourselves to general points concerning the requirements
for maintaining mononuclear phagocytes in culture and preparing
conditioned culture medium for measurement of products.

A. *Monitoring Viability of the Cultures*

An essential prerequisite for any systematic study of the
secretory activity of mononuclear phagocytes is that the cultured cells be fully viable for the duration of the experiment.
This requirement can be ascertained in a number of ways. Cell
cultures should be monitored microscopically, preferably by
phase contrast optics, to ensure that cells show a morphology
consistent with that expected of the cell population being
studied. Any irregularity in the morphologic appearance of the
cells immediately suggests potential problems of two kinds:
(a) that the donor of the cells has a pathological abnormality
or an infection that is being expressed by direct effect on the
cultured mononuclear phagocytes, or (b) that the procedures for
preparing the cells have not been properly conducted.

Specific biochemical approaches can be used to monitor the
viability of cell cultures.

Starting cell populations should be counted and adjusted to
a constant number to give a regularly plating density. The precise number of cells can be determined by measuring the DNA content of the culture. This can be readily determined by the use
of fluorometric methods such as that described by Setaro and
Morley (44), which we have regularly utilized in the laboratory.
In primary cultures of macrophages, which do not normally show
mitotic activity, the maintenance of DNA levels in cell cultures

is a good indicator of the retention of cell viability, although it does not necessarily indicate full maintenance of cellular function. Protein content of cells of cultures thoroughly washed in serum-free medium can also be determined by conventional techniques. We have also made a practice of estimating the distribution of the cytoplasmic enzyme lactate dehydrogenase between cells and their culture medium. This assay is a particularly useful one when the effect on the secretory activities of mononuclear phagocyte cultures of stimuli of unknown cellular toxicity is examined. Several cautions need to be made in relation to measurements of this enzyme. The absence of elevated levels of lactate dehydrogenase in culture medium is not necessarily a definitive indication of a lack of toxicity. This enzyme is relatively unstable, being readily inactivated at low concentrations on glass and other surfaces, particularly in the absence of other proteins. (It is to be noted also that lactate dehydrogenase is destroyed by freezing.) Therefore, cellular levels of the enzyme should also be estimated with levels of enzyme equal to or greater than those at the beginning of the experiment being a reasonable indicator of cell viability.

In many instances, the rate of secretion of a given mononuclear phagocyte product is dependent on the *in vivo* environment from which the cells are obtained. This has been particularly well established in the case of mouse peritoneal macrophages. As has been described by Edelson and Duncan (this volume) 5'-nucleotidase and leucine aminopeptidase are useful markers that can be readily assayed to indicate whether cells exhibit activities commensurate with the environment from which they are obtained. Further relevance can be given to these measurements when they are related to the DNA or protein contents of the cells.

In studies of secretory activities, it is particularly useful to be able to relate this to that of a constitutive secretory activity of mononuclear phagocytes, such as lysozyme. Such measurement is useful not only for measuring constitutive secretory function coordinate with that of another product but also as a subsequent indicator of the functional viability of the cells after exposure to any given stimulus.

The assay of the parameters, described above at the beginning and during the course of an experiment during which secretion of a given product is determined, provides not only a baseline for quantitative measurement of the product but also an indicator of the viability of the cells during the course of the experiment.

B.   Preparation of Conditioned Media

One of the primary objectives of preparing conditioned,
culture medium is that the secretory product be recovered
in quantitative amounts. The difficulties encountered in
achieving this objective are several: (a) instability of the
secretory product in the culture medium; (b) degradation of
the product by an enzyme present in the culture medium; and
(c) loss of activity due to inhibitors present in the culture
medium.
The difficulties encountered in (a) can be overcome if the
secretory product decomposes into a stable metabolite that can
be quantitated, e.g., 6-ketoprostaglandin $F_{1\alpha}$ is the stable
metabolite of prostaglandin I_2. Degradation of a secretory
product by enzymes can be overcome by culturing cells in
medium lacking sera or sera in which the enzyme has been inactivated. Difficulties with endogenous inhibitors can again
be overcome by exclusion of serum or inactivation of inhibitor.
The acid treatment of serum to destroy endogenous inhibitors
of neutral proteinases is a good example of such a procedure.
The inclusion of a radiolabeled exogenous standard can aid
in monitoring the recovery of a secreted product from conditioned media. Spontaneous breakdown of a product can be measured by inclusion of culture vessels containing medium only
to which is added a known quantity of the secretory product
being quantitated. Culture vessels containing medium only
should always be included to account for background activity
of the product being measured.

Acknowledgment

The excellent secretarial assistance of Mrs. Carolyn
Kradjel is gratefully acknowledged.

REFERENCES

1.   P. Davies and R. J. Bonney. Secretory products of mono-
     nuclear phagocytes: A brief review. *J. Reticuloendothel.*
     *Soc. 26:*37-47, 1979.
2.   S. Gordon. Lysozyme and plasminogen activator: Constitu-
     tive and induced secretory products of mononuclear phago-
     cytes. *In* "Proceedings Third Leiden Conference on Mono-
     nuclear Phagocytes- Functional Aspects" (R. van Furth, ed).
     pp. 1273-1294. Martinus Nijhoff Bv, The Hague, 1980.

3. R. C. Page, P. Davies, and A. C. Allison. The macrophage as a secretory cell. *Int. Rev. Cytol.* *52*:119-157, 1978.

4. P. Davies and R. J. Bonney. The secretion of hydrolytic enzymes by mononuclear phagocytes. *In* "Handbook of Inflammation" (G. Weissmann, ed.), Vol. 2, pp. 497-542. Elsevier North Holland, Amsterdam, 1980.

5. S. Gordon, J. Todd, and Z. A. Cohn. *In vitro* synthesis and secretion of lysozyme by mononuclear phagocytes. *J. Exp. Med.* *139*:1228-1248, 1974.

6. Z. Werb and S. Gordon. Secretion of a specific collagenase by stimulated macrophages. *J. Exp. Med.* *142*: 346-360, 1975.

7. Z. Werb and S. Gordon. Elastase secretion by stimulated macrophages. Characterization and regulation. *J. Exp. Med.* *142*:361-377, 1975.

8. J. C. Unkeless, S. Gordon, and E. Reich. Secretion of plasminogen activation by stimulation. *J. Exp. Med.* *139*:834-850, 1974.

9. P. Hauser and G. Vaes. Degradation of cartilage proteoglycans by a neutral proteinase secreted by rabbit bone marrow macrophages in culture. *Biochem. J.* *172*:275-284, 1978.

10. V. Brade, W. Pyles, U. Hadding, and C. Bentley. Synthesis of factors D and B of the alternative pathway, as well as of C3, by guinea pig peritoneal macrophages. *Fed. Proc.* *36*:1243, 1977.

11. D. O. Adams. Effector mechanisms of cytolytically activated macrophages. 1. Secretion of neutral proteases and effect of protease inhibitors. *J. Immunol.* *124*: 286-292, 1980.

12. D. Gordon, M. A. Bray, and J. Morley. Control of lymphokine secretion by prostaglandin. *Nature (London) 262*: 401-402, 1976.

13. J. L. Humes, R. J. Bonney, L. Pelus, M. E. Dahlgren, S. J. Sadowski, F. A. Kuehl, Jr., and P. Davies. Macrophages synthesize and release prostaglandins in response to inflammatory stimuli. *Nature (London) 269*: 149-151, 1977.

14. K. Brune, M. Glatt, H. Kalin, and H. Peskar. Pharmacological control of prostaglandin and thromboxane release from macrophages. *Nature (London) 274*:261-263, 1978.

15. M. Rigaud, J. Durand, and J. C. Breton. Transformation of arachidonic acid into 12-hydroxy-5,8,10,14-eicosatetraenoic acid by mouse peritoneal macrophages. *Biochim. Biophys. Acta 573*:408-412, 1979.

16. A. Capron, M. Joseph, J. P. Dessaint, G. Torpier and H. Bazin. Macrophage activation by IgE. *In* "Mononuclear Phagocytes, Functional Aspects" (R. van Furth, ed.), pp. 1539-1556. Martinus Nijhoff, The Hague, 1980.

17. F. W. Ruscetti and P. A. Chervenik. Release of colony
     stimulating factor from monocytes by endotoxin and poly-
     inosinic-polycytidylic acid. *J. Lab. Clin. Med.* *83*:64-
     72, 1974.
18. D. I. Beller and E. R. Unanue. Thymic maturation *in vitro*
     by a secretory product from macrophages. *J. Immunol.* *118*:
     1780-1787, 1977.
19. I. Gery and B. H. Waksman. Potentiation of T-lymphocyte
     response to mitogens. II. The cellular source of po-
     tentiating mediator(s). *J. Exp. Med.* *136*:143-155, 1972.
20. D. D. Wood. Mechanism of action human B-cell activating
     factor. I. Comparison of the plaque stimulating activity
     with thymocyte stimulating activity. *J. Immunol.* *123*:
     2400-2407, 1979.
21. E. R. Unanue. Secretory function of mononuclear phago-
     cytes. *Am. J. Pathol.* *83*:396-417, 1976.
22. P. J. Polverini, R. S. Cotran, M. A. Gimbrone, Jr., and
     E. R. Unanue. Activated macrophages induce vascular
     proliferation. *Nature (London)* *269*:804-806, 1977.
23. K. J. Goodman and L. J. Berry. The effect of gluco-
     corticoid antagonizing factor on hepatoma cells.
     Proc. Soc. Exp. Biol. Med. *159*:359-363, 1978.
24. R. G. Crystal, J. D. Fullmer, B. J. Baum, J. Bernado,
     K. H. Bradley, S. D. Bruel, N. A. Elson, G. A. Fells,
     V. J. Ferrans, J. E. Gadek, G. W. Hunninghake, O.
     Kawanami, J. A. Kelman, B. R. Line, J. A. McDonald,
     B. D. McLees, W. C. Roberts, D. M. Rosenberg, P.
     Tolstoshev, E. Von Gal, and S. E. Weinberger. Cells,
     collagen and idiopathic pulmonary fibrosis. *Lung* *155*:
     199-224, 1978.
25. T. J. Smith and R. R. Wagner. Rabbit macrophage
     interferons. I. Conditions for biosynthesis by virus-
     infected and uninfected cells. *J. Exp. Med.* *125*:559-577,
     1967.
26. C. F. Nathan, S. C. Silverstein, L. H. Brukner, and Z. A.
     Cohn. Extracellular cytolysis by activated macrophages
     and granulocytes. II. Hydrogen peroxide as a mediator
     of cytotoxicity. *J. Exp. Med.* *149*:100-113, 1979.
27. S. J. Weiss, G. W. King, and A. F. LoBuglio. Evidence
     for hydroxyl radical generation by human monocytes.
     J. Clin. Invest. *60*:370-373, 1977.
28. R. B. Johnston, Jr., C. A. Godzik, and Z. A. Cohn.
     Increased superoxide anion production by immunologically
     activated and chemically elicited macrophages. *J. Exp.
     Med.* *148*:115, 1978.
29. R. C. Bast, Jr., R. P. Cleveland, B. H. Littman, B. Zbar,
     and H. J. Rapp. Acquired cellular immunity extracellular
     killing of *Listeria monocytogenes* by a product of immuno-
     logically activated macrophages. *Cell Immunol.* *10*:248-
     259, 1974.

30. M. Rachmilewitz and M. Schlesinger. Production and release of transcobalamin II, a vitamin B12 transport protein by mouse peritoneal macrophages. *Exp. Hematol.* *5:*(suppl.) 2-108, 1977.

31. G. A. Currie. Activated macrophages kill tumor cells by releasing arginase. *Nature (London) 273:*758-759, 1978.

32. V. J. Stecher and G. J. Thorbecke. Sites of synthesis of human serum proteins. I. Serum proteins produced by macrophages *in vitro. J. Immunol. 99:*643-652, 1967.

33. H. V. Wyatt, H. R. Colten, and T. J. Borsos. Production of the second (C2) and fourth (C4) components of guinea pig complement by single peritoneal cells: Evidence that one cell may produce both components. *J. Immunol. 108:* 1609-1614, 1972.

34. C. Bentley, D. Bitter-Suermann, U. Hadding, and V. Brade. *In vitro* synthesis of factor B of the alternative pathway of complement activation by mouse peritoneal macrophages. *Eur. J. Immunol. 6:*393-398, 1976.

35. C. A. Dinarello and S. M. Wolff. Pathogenesis of fever in man. *N. Eng. J. Med. 298:*607-612, 1978.

36. H. Prydz, H. U. Schorlemmer, and A. C. Allison. Further link between complement activation and blood coagulation. *Nature (London) 270:*173-174, 1977.

37. J. Schnyder and M. Baggiolini. Secretion of lysosomal enzymes by stimulated and nonstimulated macrophages. *J. Exp. Med. 148:*435-450, 1978.

38. H. U. Schorlemmer, P. Davies, and A. C. Allison. Ability of activated complement components to induce lysosomal enzyme release from macrophages. *Nature (London) 261:*48-49, 1976.

39. K. McCarthy and P. M. Henson. Induction of lysosomal enzyme secretion by alveolar macrophages in response to the purified complement fragments C5a and C5a des-arg. *J. Immunol. 123:*2511-2517, 1979.

40. H. Schorlemmer, D. Bitter-Suermann, and A. C. Allison. Complement activation by the alternative pathway and macrophage enzyme secretion in the pathogenesis of chronic inflammation. *Immunology 32:*929-940, 1977.

41. P. Davies, R. J. Bonney, J. L. Humes, and F. A. Kuehl, Jr. The synthesis of arachidonic acid oxygenation products by various mononuclear phagocyte populations. *In* "Proceedings of the Third Leiden Conference on Mononuclear Phagocytes - Functional Aspects" (R. van Furth, ed.), pp. 1317-1345. Martinus Nijhoff BV, The Hague, 1980.

42. L. J. Rosenwasser, C. Dinarello, and A. S. Rosenthal. Adherent cell function in murine T lymphocyte antigen recognition. IV. Enhancement of murine T cell antigen. Recognition by human leukocytic pyrogen. *J. Exp. Med. 150:*709-714, 1979.

43. T. Hovi, D. Mosher, and A. Vaheri. Cultured human monocytes synthesize and secrete α2-macroglobulin. *J. Exp.
Med. 145:*1580-1589, 1977.
44. F. Setaro and C. Morley. A modified fluorimetric method
for determination of microgram quantities of DNA for
cell and tissue cultures. *Ana.. Biochem. 71:*313-317,
1976.

58

CHARACTERIZATION AND CLASSIFICATION OF
MACROPHAGE PROTEINASES AND PROTEINASE INHIBITORS

Zena Werb

I. PRINCIPLES

Proteolytic enzymes can be broadly classified as exopeptidases and endopeptidases (1, 2). <u>Exopeptidases</u> cleave proteins and peptides adjacent to a free amino or carboxyl terminus and may play an important role in macrophage functions. Like endopeptidases, these hydrolytic enzymes can be divided into several classes on the basis of their specificity (1). Angiotensin-converting enzyme [peptidyl dipeptidase, a zinc-dependent dipeptidase (1, 3)] and leucine aminopeptidase [also a metallopeptidase (1)] are both associated with the plasma membrane. The lysosomal peptidases, in particular carboxypeptidase A (a serine-dependent enzyme) and carboxypeptidase B (a thiol-dependent peptidase), will be of interest in some macrophage studies; e.g., macrophage lysosomes degrade proteins to peptides of less than 200 daltons that are then able to diffuse out of the lysosomes (4). In general, for recognition <u>endopeptidases</u> need the adjacent C- or N-terminal

amino acids to be blocked, usually by another amino acid.
Macrophage endopeptidases comprise a group of enzymes usually
having either broad proteolytic specificity (e.g., cathepsin D)
or highly restricted cleavage of particular proteins (e.g.,
complement proteinases).

II.   CLASSIFICATION OF MACROPHAGE PROTEINASES

     It is difficult to assign proteinases to classes based on
their specificity for various proteins or even for particular
peptides. Instead, the classification that separates these
enzymes according to the essential catalytic group of the enzyme is particularly useful (5). The four classes, carboxyl,
thiol, serine, and metallo, include the catalytic mechanisms
of virtually every known proteolytic enzyme. A newly discovered endopeptidase can be assigned to its catalytic class
by use of specific inhibitors as outlined by Barrett (1). A
simple scheme to identify proteinases is shown in Table I, and
some of the proteinases that have been attributed to macrophages are listed in Table II under the four major classifica-
tions.
     It is necessary to keep in mind that impure preparations
of enzymes give rise to special problems of classification.
The activities of several proteinases may be superimposed, endogenous inhibitors may be in the system, the specific inhibitors being used as probes may be destroyed by other components present in the mixture, or the inhibitor being tested
may act on another proteinase which is, in turn, an activator
or inactivator of the enzyme in question. Therefore, classification of proteinases should be reserved for studies with
purified enzymes, although preliminary experiments with crude
preparations can be a useful tool for further purification.
Another precaution must be taken when performing these inhibitor studies; the inhibitors should not be contaminated with
substances that may be responsible for the observed inhibition
(e.g., small amounts of reducing agents or heavy metal ions
present in some inhibitor preparations). In addition, inhibitors may be rather unstable; e.g., 4-nitrophenyl guanidinoben-
zoate is hydrolyzed rapidly in Tris buffers, and dimethyl sulfoxide, a common solvent, is a highly reactive compound in its
own right.
     Lysosomal proteinases and peptidases of macrophages, first
described by Metchnikoff (6), are considered to have major importance in the digestive functions of macrophages from a
variety of species. Cathepsins B and D have been demonstrated
to mediate digestion of exogenous proteins (7) and turnover of

TABLE I. *Use of Inhibitors to Classify Macrophage Proteinases*[a]

Inhibitor	Effective conc.	Enzyme class			
		Carboxyl 2-5[b]	Thiol 3-7[b]	Serine 7-9[b]	Metallo 7-9[b]
Pepstatin	1 μg/ml	Inhibited	–	–	–
Diazoacetylnorleucine methylester + Ca^{2+}	1 mM each	Inhibited	–	–	–
4-Chloromercuribenzoate	1 mM	–	Inhibited	–	–
5,5'-Dithiobis(2-nitrobenzoic acid)	1 mM	–	Inhibited	–	c
N-Ethylmaleimide	2 mM	–	Inhibited	–	–
Leupeptin	10 μg/ml	–	Inhibited	Inhibited	–
Diisopropyl fluorophosphate or phenylmethane sulfonyl fluoride	1 mM	–	–	Inhibited	–
Soybean, lima bean, or bovine pancreatic trypsin inhibitors	100 μg/ml	–	–	Inhibited	–
p-Nitrophenyl guanidinobenzoate	1 mM	–	–	Inhibited	–
Chloromethyl ketone derivatives of peptides	1 mM	–	Inhibited	Inhibited	–
EDTA	2 mM	–	–	–	Inhibited
Dithiothreitol	1 mM	–	Activated	–	Inhibited
1,10-Phenanthroline	1 mM	–	–	–	Inhibited
α$_2$-Macroglobulin	10 μg/ml	Inhibited	Inhibited	Inhibited	Inhibited

[a]This table is modified from Barrett (1, 2). There are exceptions to many of these generalities.
[b]Optimum pH range.
[c]Some enzymes are activated.

TABLE II. Classification of Macrophage Proteinases

Proteinase class	Enzyme	pH Optimum	References
Carboxyl (EC 3.4.23)	Cathepsin D	3 – 5	7, 8, 54 – 57
Thiol (EC 3.4.22)	Cathepsin B	4 – 7	8, 54, 55
	Cathepsin H		1
	Cathepsin L		1
	Cathepsin N (collagenolytic)		1
Serine (EC 3.4.21)	Plasminogen activator	7 – 9	1, 11, 13, 14
	C1		58, 59
	C2		12, 60
	C3		15, 59
	C5		15
	Factor B		16, 60 – 62
	Factor D		15, 16
	Casein-degrading proteinase		17, 63
Metallo (EC 3.4.24)	Collagenase (types I, II, III)	7 – 9	26 – 28
	Type V-specific collagenase		64
	Gelatinase		27, unpublished data
	Proteoglycan-degrading proteinase		29 – 34
	Macrophage elastase		29 – 34
Not classified	Thromboplastin	Neutral	39
	Amyloid-degrading proteinase	Neutral	38

564

endogenous macrophage proteins (8). Although cathepsins H, L, and N have not been shown explicitly in macrophages, these thiol proteinases are abundant in lysosomes of liver and spleen (1), which are largely of macrophage origin. Under some conditions of phagocytosis, lysosomal proteinases are secreted by macrophages (9).

Little is known about intracellular macrophage proteinases active at neutral pH. A neutral proteinase associated with chromatin (10), a group-specific proteinase with elastaselike esterase activity from human bone marrow cells (1), and a Ca^{2+}-activable thiol proteinase (2, 8) have been described.

Secreted and cell-associated serine esterases have been described for macrophages. The best-characterized serine proteinases are plasminogen activator and the complement proteinases. Although the assays for these proteinases are unambiguous, considerable confusion exists about them because (a) their production is modulated by lymphocyte products (11, 12), (b) mononuclear phagocytes in different stages of differentiation make varying amounts of these enzymes (13), (c) large species differences exist in the quantity and ease of demonstration of these enzymes (13, 14 - 16), and (d) the enzymes exist in various states of activation and inhibition (15). A casein-degrading serine proteinase secreted by activated mouse macrophages (17) is probably distinct from plasminogen activator or the complement proteinases. An amyloid-degrading proteinase associated with the surface of human monocytes is inhibited by diisopropyl fluorophosphate (DFP), but not by other serine proteinase inhibitors (18), and thus cannot be classified at this time. A number of DFP-binding serine esterases have been shown to be associated with, or secreted by, mononuclear phagocytes (19 - 25). These enzymes cannot be considered proteinases until endopeptidic catalytic activity has been shown unambiguously (e.g., acetylcholinesterase and carboxypeptidase A are serine esterases, but not proteinases).

Metalloproteinases have been shown to be associated with mouse, rat, rabbit, and guinea pig macrophages, but they have not yet been definitively shown in humans. At least three metalloproteinases are biosynthesized by mononuclear phagocytes, and they require calcium and zinc for their catalytic activity: (a) Macrophage collagenase is capable of degrading collagen of types I, II, and III (26 - 28). It is not yet clear whether this enzyme represents a gene product different from that biosynthesized by fibroblasts, but it is distinct from the collagenase contained in specific granules of human neutrophils. (b) Macrophage elastase is a metalloproteinase of 22,000 daltons. In addition to degrading elastin, this enzyme has a broad substrate specificity, degrading immunoglobulins, α_1-proteinase inhibitor, fibronectin, plasminogen, myelin basic protein, cartilage proteoglycans, gelatin, and fibrinogen (29 - 34). Thus, elastase may be identical to the cartilage proteoglycan-degrading metalloproteinase (35), the collagenase-activating metalloproteinase (28), and the myelin basic protein-degrading proteinase (36). (c) A type V-specific collagenase with properties of a metalloproteinase has recently been described (64).

Other proteinase or peptidase activities reportedly associated with macrophages include cell surface-associated proteinases or peptidases involved in macrophage tumor killing (37), chemotaxis (38), amyloid degradation (18), and procoagulant activities (39).

III. CRITICAL COMMENTS

A number of precautions apply to the classification of macrophage proteinases and the assignment of a putative proteolytic enzyme to macrophages. The activity of macrophage proteinases is a balance of synthesis of enzymes, activation of proenzymes, synthesis of enzyme inhibitors, complexing of enzyme with inhibitors, and degradation of one enzyme by the other proteinases. To determine whether macrophages synthesize a proteinase, it is usually necessary to demonstrate that the enzyme accumulates with time in the culture medium (in the case of secreted enzyme), that its production is blocked by inhibitors of protein synthesis, and, in the case of enzymes that have been sufficiently characterized to be purified, that the enzyme can be biosynthetically labeled and that the radiolabeled enzyme can be immunoprecipitated or specifically purified from other cell proteins. Additionally, the enzyme should be made at a constant rate as increasing numbers of contaminant cells are added, assuming that the enzyme produced is not also made by the major contaminating species.

A. *Macrophage Proteinase Inhibitors*

Macrophages have been reported to synthesize and secrete inhibitors of proteolytic enzymes as well as the enzymes themselves. Human macrophages synthesize inhibitory proteins [C3b inactivator (C3bINA) and β1H globulin] that regulate the alternative pathway of complement activation (15). Inhibitors of plasminogen activator have been described in a number of cells, including macrophages (40, 41). These plasminogen activator inhibitors are dissociated at low ionic strength (and are also destroyed by treatment of cell lysates below pH 3). In the presence of 50 mM Tris buffer, pH 8, macrophage-condi-

tioned medium and lysates can be shown to contain large amounts
of plasminogen activator; however, in the same buffer at physiologic salt concentration (0.15 M NaCl), the apparent activity
of plasminogen activator can be reduced by 40 - 99%. Therefore, it is important to determine proteinase activities under
conditions that are optimal for assay and give maximum enzyme
activities as well as under physiologic conditions, which may
more accurately reflect the amount of proteolytic activity
cells express *in vivo*.

Macrophages also secrete inhibitors of macrophage elastase
(32, 33). These inhibitors are removed by dialysis (33), enzyme purification (33), and assay in the presence of sodium
dodecyl sulfate (30, 33). The physiologically important enzyme
activity in tissues is that amount that is free in the presence
of these inhibitors (32), rather than the amount that can be
demonstrated when inhibitors are removed.

Macrophage collagenases are also secreted in an inactive
form (27, 28). It is likely that these inactive forms are
enzyme-inhibitor complexes or zymogens (42 - 44) and can be
activated by trypsin and by organomercurials.

Macrophages have also been reported to synthesize and secrete α_2-macroglobulin (45), an inhibitor of all endopeptidases
(1). α_2-Macroglobulin binds proteinases irreversibly (although
these complexes can be disrupted by chaotropic agents), and
thus could reduce macrophage enzymes available for assay. Macrophages also avidly ingest α_2-macroglobulin-proteinase complexes (46).

In addition to endogenous inhibitors, serum and tissue inhibitors may also be present in the systems used to identify
macrophage proteinases. These inhibitors include molecules,
such as α_1-proteinase inhibitor, that may be taken up by macrophages *in vivo* (47) and then possibly released after cell death
in subsequent culture.

The measurement of macrophage proteinase inhibitors is complicated by the fact that some inhibitors may be produced stoi-
chiometrically with the enzymes that they inhibit, and thus can
be measured only after dissociation from enzyme. Inhibitors
produced in excess can be measured directly or by inhibition
of purified enzyme.

B. *Validity of Assays*

Many of the assays that use peptides or protein substrates
for measuring proteolytic enzymes are subject to considerable
misinterpretation. Several of the specific proteinases, such
as plasminogen activator and the complement proteinases, are
determined by multistep cascade assays so that interference at
steps other than the catalytic event is possible. Other arti-

facts may arise with specific substrates. Although elastin is highly resistant to proteolysis by all but a small class of proteinases referred to as elastases, two proteinases together can degrade elastin quite well (e.g., trypsin plus chymotrypsin). Therefore, in crude mixtures of enzymes the presumed hydrolysis may be due to a mixture of enzymes rather than to a single enzyme. With protein substrates, it is important to distinguish proteolysis by a proteinase (i.e., endopeptidase cleavage) from activity of exopeptidases or dipeptidases, which may give the same final result of released soluble radioactivity, absorbance, fluorescence, or a change in molecular size. In view of the large variety of macrophage peptidases, this is an extremely important consideration in all assays for macrophage proteinases.

Another source of misinterpretation is possible with iodinated substrates because of deiodination mediated by myeloperoxidase, an enzyme found in monocytes and neutrophils. It is important to determine that release of soluble radioactivity from iodinated substrates is due to a proteolytic cleavage and yields monoiodotyrosine. With human monocytes, nearly 50% of the release of ^{125}I in the ^{125}I-labeled fibrin assay may be due to deiodination (14).

Because of the large variety of proteinases synthesized by mononuclear phagocytes, inactivation of one enzyme by another during the preparations for assay is a possibility. For example, plasmin generated by macrophage plasminogen activator will destroy elastase and collagenase present in the same culture medium (32). Several complement proteinases can be detected only by immunologic means and not by functional assays (15), possibly because of their inactivation by other proteinases.

Several final observations may help circumvent artifacts possible when using defined inhibitors and substrates for characterizing macrophage proteinases. One technique for evaluating substrate specificity of proteinases involves competitive inhibition studies with a single test substrate. When using this technique, it is important to check that the products of hydrolysis, such as peptides and esters, do not account for the observed effect. With chromogenic substrates it may be possible to check both D- and L-amino acid isomers and also to check the effects of substrates with different types of blocking groups.

Care should be taken in interpretation when one subpopulation of macrophage appears to synthesize an enzyme and another does not. In the latter case, the proteinase may still be produced but in a latent form. Mixing experiments involving activation with other enzymes and immunochemical identification are necessary before definitively stating the mode of modulation of the enzyme activity.

During the demonstration of proteolytic activity and inhibition of proteolytic activity, care should be taken that solvents or salts do not influence the outcome of the reaction. In addition, some substrates are highly unstable. This is particularly true of some of the ester substrates, and appropriate controls should be included in all of these assays. Stability of the enzyme during the course of the enzyme assay should also be considered by assaying for various lengths of time and with various concentrations of both enzyme and substrate. Stability of inhibitors is also important.

The time required for inhibitors to interact with enzymes may be very long. For some serine proteinases, 20 hr may be required before the binding and inhibition with DFP become irreversible, and, in the presence of an appropriate substrate, competitive binding to the substrate may decrease the efficacy of the inhibitor. The recommended procedure, therefore, is to preincubate enzyme with inhibitor; appropriate controls for the incubation with solvent must be included in every experiment.

C. Artificial Substrates in Assays for Macrophage Proteinases

With synthetic substrates, such as oligopeptide or amino acyl ester substrates, it is important to determine whether cleavage is in the correct place. This is particularly a problem with oligopeptide substrates, such as those used in assays for angiotensin-converting enzyme and with some of the synthetic substrates prepared for granulocyte elastase. Depending on the type of assay, an enzyme that is capable of recognizing and cleaving that sequence may be judged inactive because of its failure to release the appropriate chromogenic group, or hydrolysis may be seen with an enzyme that cleaves in a different place.

Particular confusion has resulted from the use of chromogenic substrates for the assay of macrophage elastase. DFP-sensitive esterases that degrade synthetic substrates have been described (21 - 25, 36), but these have not been shown to have proteolytic activity. Human alveolar macrophages have been shown to contain an enzyme that is a potent esterase when assayed with derivatives of trialanine (21, 48), but has no ability to degrade elastin. Indeed, macrophage elastase, a metalloproteinase with specificity determined by the amino acid present on the carboxyl end of the peptide (which gives rise to the new N-terminal amino acid) (33), would not recognize and cleave a chromogenic ester group that blocks a peptide at the C-terminal, although it may cleave elsewhere within the oligopeptide moiety. Although oligopeptide substrates present particular difficulties when dealing with complex mixtures of proteinases such as those synthesized by macrophages, these substrates can be very sensitive tools when dealing with purified enzymes.

D. *Macrophage-Associated Proteinases Not of Macrophage Origin*

Even when the criteria and precautions listed in Section III are followed, it is probable that a number of the enzymes described as being secreted by macrophages or associated with macrophage surfaces are not macrophage products at all. These proteinases may be released with time from the cell surface or intracellular organelles by mechanisms that may, in fact, require protein synthesis. Granulocyte elastase is avidly ingested by macrophages by a receptor-mediated mechanism (49), and it is probable that much of the elastase or elastaselike proteinase that has been reported to be associated with human macrophages is of granulocyte origin. Enzymes from granulocytes or plasma have access to macrophages during various phases of their differentiation and during preparation for culture. It is probable that such enzymes are bound to, or internalized by, macrophages by similar mechanisms.

Most proteolytic enzymes are synthesized as precursors (zymogens) or may be present in cells and extracellular fluids as enzyme-inhibitor complexes. Therefore, if a macrophage proteinase (e.g., plasminogen activator) present in small quantities (and unrelated to the proteinase being assayed) had a role in activating a latent enzyme of exogenous origin (e.g., plasminogen), the amount of the second proteinase (e.g., plasmin) would then increase with time as activation occurred. The appearance of plasmin would also be sensitive to inhibitors of protein synthesis that were decreasing production of the macrophage plasminogen activator. Another example is that the requirement for macrophages in the production of lymphokines could be a requirement for activation of precursor lymphokines by macrophages. In fact, it is possible that macrophage activation of such lymphokines, which then induce production of a proteolytic enzyme by a contaminating cell type, could give rise to the time-dependent accumulation of a proteinase in the culture medium of macrophages. This may be the explanation for some of the collagenase produced in macrophage cultures, because the mediator produced by mononuclear cells induces secretion of collagenase by stromal cells (50 - 53). Because the stromal cells can produce collagenase at 1000 times the rate of mononuclear phagocytes (27), minor contamination would be sufficient to account for all the collagenase in these cultures. If the macrophage function in inducing proteolytic enzyme production were also modulated by the functional state of the macrophage, production of the proteinase would then appear to be developmentally regulated. For proteinases produced in chemically small amounts, ultimate demonstration of macrophage origin will require molecular studies with suitable biochemical and immunologic probes.

Acknowledgment

Supported by the U.S. Department of Energy.

REFERENCES

1. A. J. Barrett (ed.). "Proteinases in Mammalian Cells and Tissues." North-Holland/Elsevier, Amsterdam, 1977.
2. A. J. Barrett. The many forms and functions of cellular proteinases. *Fed. Proc. 39*: 9-14, 1980.
3. J. Friedland, C. Setton, and E. Silverstein. Induction of angiotensin converting enzyme in human monocytes in culture. *Biochem. Biophys. Res. Commun. 83*: 843-849, 1978.
4. B. A. Ehrenreich and Z. A. Cohn. The fate of peptides pinocytosed by macrophages *in vitro*. *J. Exp. Med. 129*: 227-245, 1969.
5. B. S. Hartley. Proteolytic enzymes. *Annu. Rev. Biochem. 29*: 45-72, 1960.
6. E. Metchnikoff. "L'Immunity dans les Malade Infectieuses." Masson, Paris, 1901.
7. J. T. Dingle, A. R. Poole, G. S. Lazarus, and A. J. Barrett. Immunoinhibition of intracellular protein digestion in macrophages. *J. Exp. Med. 137*: 1124-1141, 1973.
8. R. T. Dean. Protein degradation in cell cultures: General considerations on mechanisms and regulation. *Fed. Proc. 39*: 15-19, 1980.
9. J. Schnyder and M. Baggiolini. Secretion of lysosomal hydrolases by stimulated and nonstimulated macrophages. *J. Exp. Med. 148*: 435-450, 1978.
10. Y. Suzuki and T. Murachi. A chromatin-bound neutral protease and its inhibitor in rat peritoneal macrophages. *J. Biochem. (Tokyo) 84*: 977-984, 1978.
11. J.-D. Vassalli and E. Reich. Macrophage plasminogen activator: Induction by products of activated lymphoid cells. *J. Exp. Med. 145*: 429-437, 1977.
12. B. H. Littman and S. Ruddy. Monocyte complement stimulator: A T lymphocyte product which stimulates synthesis of the second complement component (C2). *Cell. Immunol. 43*: 388-397, 1979.
13. S. Gordon, J. C. Unkeless, and Z. A. Cohn. Induction of macrophage plasminogen activator by endotoxin stimulation and phagocytosis. *J. Exp. Med. 140*: 995-1010, 1974.
14. C. G. Ragsdale and W. P. Arend. Neutral protease secretion by human monocytes. Effect of surface-bound immune complexes. *J. Exp. Med. 149*: 954-968, 1979.

15. K. Whaley. Biosynthesis of the complement components and the regulatory proteins of the alternative complement pathway by human peripheral blood monocytes. *J. Exp. Med. 151*: 501-516, 1980.

16. C. Bentley, W. Fries, and V. Brade. Synthesis of factors D, B, and P of the alternative pathway of complement activation, as well as C3, by guinea-pig peritoneal macrophages *in vitro. Immunology 35*: 971-987, 1978.

17. D. O. Adams. Effector mechanisms of cytolytically activated macrophages. I. Secretion of neutral proteases and effect of protease inhibitors. *J. Immunol. 124*: 286-292, 1980.

18. G. Lavie, D. Zucker-Franklin, and E. C. Franklin. Degradation of serum amyloid A protein by surface-associated enzymes of human blood monocytes. *J. Exp. Med. 148*: 1020-1031, 1978.

19. O. Rojas-Espinosa, P. Arce-Paredez, A. M. Dannenberg, Jr., and R. L. Kamenetz. Macrophage esterase: Identification, purification, and properties of a chymotrypsin-like esterase from lung that hydrolyses and transfers nonpolar amino acid esters. *Biochim. Biophys. Acta 403*: 161-179, 1975.

20. E. A. Levine, R. M. Senior, and J. V. Butler. The elastase activity of alveolar macrophages: Measurements using synthetic substrates and elastin. *Am. Rev. Resp. Dis. 113*: 25-30, 1976.

21. A. M. Dannenberg, Jr., and W. E. Bennett. Hydrolytic enzymes of rabbit mononuclear exudate cells. I. Quantitative assay and properties of certain proteases, nonspecific esterases, and lipases of mononuclear and polymorphonuclear cells and erythrocytes. *J. Cell Biol. 21*: 1-13, 1964.

22. L. W. Heck, E. Remold-O'Donnell, and H. G. Remold. DFP-Sensitive polypeptides of the guinea pig peritoneal macrophage. *Biochem. Biophys. Res. Commun. 83*: 1576-1583, 1978.

23. H. G. Remold. The enhancement of MIF activity by inhibition of macrophage associated esterases. *J. Immunol. 112*: 1571-1577, 1974.

24. S. Kitagawa, F. Takaku, and S. Sakamoto. Evidence that proteases are involved in superoxide production by human polymorphonuclear leukocytes and monocytes. *J. Clin. Invest. 65*: 74-81, 1980.

25. Y. Buchmuller and J. Mauel. Inhibitors of serine-esterases enhance lymphokine-induced microbicidal activity in macrophages. *R.E.S.: J. Reticuloendothel. Soc. 27*: 89-96, 1980.

26. Z. Werb. Biochemical actions of glucocorticoids on macrophages in culture. Specific inhibition of elastase, collagenase, and plasminogen activator secretion and effects

on other metabolic functions. *J. Exp. Med. 147*: 1695-1712, 1978.

27. Z. Werb. Pathways for the modulation of macrophage collagenase activity. *In* "Proceedings, Mechanisms of Localized Bone Loss" (J. E. Horton, T. M. Tarpley, and W. F. Davis, eds.), pp. 213-228. Special Supplement to Calcified Tissue Abstracts, 1978.

28. A. L. Horwitz, J. A. Kelman, and R. G. Crystal. Activation of alveolar macrophage collagenase by a neutral protease secreted by the same cell. *Nature 264*: 772-774, 1976.

29. M. J. Banda and Z. Werb. The role of macrophage elastase in the proteolysis of fibrinogen, plasminogen, and fibronectin. *Fed. Proc. 39*: 1756, 1980.

30. Z. Werb and S. Gordon. Elastase secretion by stimulated macrophages. Characterization and regulation. *J. Exp. Med. 142*: 361-377, 1975.

31. M. J. Banda and Z. Werb. Mouse macrophage elastase: Purification and characterization as a metalloproteinase. *Biochem. J. 193*: 589-605, 1981.

32. Z. Werb, M. J. Banda, and P. A. Jones. Degradation of connective tissue matrices by macrophages. I. Proteolysis of elastin, glycoproteins, and collagen by proteinases isolated from macrophages. *J. Exp. Med. 152*: 1340-1357, 1980.

33. M. J. Banda, E. J. Clark, and Z. Werb. Limited proteolysis by macrophage elastase inactivates human α_1-proteinase inhibitor. *J. Exp. Med. 152*: 1563-1570, 1980.

34. P. A. Jones and T. Scott-Burden. Activated macrophages digest the extracellular matrix proteins produced by cultured cells. *Biochem. Biophys. Res. Commun. 86*: 71-77, 1979.

35. P. Hauser and G. Vaes. Degradation of cartilage proteoglycans by a neutral proteinase secreted by rabbit bone marrow macrophages in culture. *Biochem. J. 172*: 275-284, 1978.

36. W. Cammer, B. R. Bloom, W. T. Norton, and S. Gordon. Degradation of basic protein in myelin by neutral proteases secreted by stimulated macrophages: A possible mechanism of inflammatory demyelination. *Proc. Nat. Acad. Sci. USA 75*: 1554-1558, 1978.

37. J. B. Hibbs, Jr., R. R. Taintor, H. A. Chapman, Jr., and J. B. Weinberg. Macrophage tumor killing: Influence of the local environment. *Science 197*: 279-282, 1971.

38. S. Aswanikumar, E. Schiffmann, B. A. Corcoran, and S. M. Wahl. Role of a peptidase in phagocyte chemotaxis. *Proc. Nat. Acad. Sci. USA 73*: 2439-2442, 1976.

39. H. Prydz and A. C. Allison. Tissue thromboplastin activity of isolated human monocytes. *Thromb. Haemostas. 39*: 582-

591, 1978.

40. D. J. Loskutoff and T. S. Edgington. Synthesis of a fibrinolytic activator and inhibitor by endothelial cells.
Proc. Nat. Acad. Sci. USA 74: 3903-3907, 1977.

41. J. Aggeler, J. Risch, and Z. Werb. Expression of the
catalytic activity of plasminogen activator under physiological conditions. *Biochim. Biophys. Acta,* in press,
1981.

42. J. C. Nolan, S. Ridge, A. L. Oronsky, L. L. Slakey, and
S. S. Kerwar. Synthesis of a collagenase inhibitor by
smooth muscle cells in culture. *Biochem. Biophys. Res.
Commun. 83*: 1183-1190, 1978.

43. A. Sellers and J. J. Reynolds. Identification and partial
characterization of an inhibitor of collagenase from
rabbit bone. *Biochem. J. 167*: 353-360, 1977.

44. A. Sellers, E. Cartwright, G. Murphy, and J. J. Reynolds.
Evidence that latent collagenases are enzyme-inhibitor
complexes. *Biochem. J. 163*: 303-307, 1977.

45. T. Hovi, D. Mosher, and A. Vaheri. Cultured human monocytes synthesize and secrete α_2-macroglobulin. *J. Exp.
Med. 145*: 1580-1589, 1977.

46. J. Kaplan and M. L. Nielsen. Analysis of macrophage surface receptors. I. Binding of α-macroglobulin protease
complexes to rabbit alveolar macrophages. *J. Biol. Chem.
254*: 7323-7328, 1979.

47. P. K. Gupta, J. K. Frost, S. Geddes, B. Aracil, and F.
Davidovski. Morphological identification of α-l-antitryp-
sin in pulmonary macrophages. *Hum. Pathol. 10*: 345-347,
1979.

48. R. J. Rodriguez, R. R. White, R. M. Senior, and E. A. Levine. Elastase release from human alveolar macrophages:
Comparison between smokers and nonsmokers. *Science 198*:
313-314, 1977.

49. E. J. Campbell, R. R. White, R. M. Senior, R. J. Rodriguez,
and C. Kuhn. Receptor-mediated binding and internalization
of leukocyte elastase by alveolar macrophages in vitro.
J. Clin. Invest. 64: 824-833, 1979.

50. K. Deshmukh-Phadke, M. Lawrence, and S. Nanda. Synthesis
of collagenase and neutral proteases by articular chondrocytes: Stimulation by a macrophage-derived factor.
Biochem. Biophys. Res. Commun. 85: 490-496, 1978.

51. D. A. Newsome and J. Gross. Regulation of corneal collagenase production: Stimulation of serially passaged
stromal cells by blood mononuclear cells. *Cell 16*: 895-
900, 1979.

52. G. Huybrechts-Godin, P. Hauser, and G. Vaes. Macrophage-
fibroblast interactions in collagenase production and cartilage degradation. *Biochem. J. 184*: 643-650, 1979.

53. Z. Werb and J. Aggeler. Proteases induce secretion of

collagenase and plasminogen activator by fibroblasts. *Proc. Nat. Acad. Sci. USA 75*: 1839-1843, 1978.

54. R. T. Dean. Macrophage protein turnover. Evidence for lysosomal participation in basal proteolysis. *Biochem. J. 180*: 339-345, 1979.

55. T. Kato, K. Kojima, and T. Murachi. Proteases of macrophages in rat peritoneal exudate, with special reference to the effects of actinomycete protease inhibitors. *Biochim. Biophys. Acta 289*: 187-193, 1972.

56. M. H. McAdoo, A. M. Dannenberg, Jr., C. J. Hayes, S. P. James, and J. H. Sanner. Inhibition of the cathepsin D-type proteinase of macrophages by pepstatin, a specific pepsin inhibitor, and other substances. *Infect. Immun. 7*: 655-665, 1973.

57. Z. A. Cohn and E. Wiener. The particulate hydrolases of macrophages. I. Comparative enzymology, isolation, and properties. *J. Exp. Med. 118*: 991-1008, 1963.

58. W. Muller, H. Hanauske-Abel, and M. Loos. Biosynthesis of the first component of complement by human and guinea pig peritoneal macrophages: Evidence for an independent production of the Cl subunits. *J. Immunol. 121*: 1578-1584, 1978.

59. R. F. M. Lai A Fat and R. van Furth. *In vitro* synthesis of some complement components (Clq, C3, and C4) by lymphoid tissues and circulating leukocytes in man. *Immunology 28*: 359-368, 1975.

60. R. G. Medicus, O. Gotze, and H. J. Muller-Eberhard. The serine protease nature of the C3 and C5 convertases of the classical and alternative complement pathways. *Scand. J. Immunol. 5*: 1049-1055, 1976.

61. Y. Kawamoto, M. Ueda, H. Ichikawa, and A. Miyama. Complement proteins and macrophages. I. Quantitative estimation of factor B produced by mouse peritoneal macrophages. *Microbiol. Immunol. 23*: 987-995, 1979.

62. C. Bentley, D. Bitter-Suermann, U. Hadding, and V. Brade. *In vitro* synthesis of factor B of the alternative pathway of complement activation by mouse peritoneal macrophages. *Eur. J. Immunol. 6*: 393-398, 1976.

63. D. O. Adams, K.-J. Kao, R. Farb, and S. V. Pizzo. Effector mechanisms of cytolytically activated macrophages. II. Secretion of a cytolytic factor by activated macrophages and its relationship to secreted neutral proteases. *J. Immunol. 124*: 293-300, 1980.

64. C. L. Mainardi, J. M. Seyer, and A. H. Kang. Type-specific collagenolysis. A type V collagen-degrading enzyme from macrophages. *Biochem. Biophys. Res. Commun. 97*: 1108-1115, 1980.

59

GROWTH OF MACROPHAGES ON COLLAGEN-, ELASTIN-, AND
GLYCOPROTEIN-COATED PLATES AS A TOOL FOR
INVESTIGATING MACROPHAGE PROTEINASES

Peter A. Jones
Zena Werb

I. GENERAL INTRODUCTION

The breakdown of the extracellular matrix is of fundamental importance in many normal and pathological situations.
Macrophages often congregate at sites of tissue breakdown and
are thought to play a significant role in the enzymatic hydrolysis of connective tissue elements. The connective tissue proteins include glycoproteins, collagen, elastin, and proteoglycans in various combinations, and their breakdown is likely to
be a complex event. Macrophages have, therefore, been cultivated in contact with collagen (1,2), fibrin (3), and elastin
(4,5) so that the enzymology of the hydrolytic process can be
better understood. In this chapter, we shall discuss the methods for preparing collagen substrates and also describe·the
use of extracellular matrices produced by cultured connective
tissue cells as substrates for stimulated macrophages. The extracellular matrices produced by cultured cells possess many
of the structural characteristics of tissues and may therefore

METHODS FOR STUDYING
MONONUCLEAR PHAGOCYTES

577

be considered representative of the insoluble proteins that
might be encountered by macrophages in the animal. In this
regard, it is obviously important to study the degradation of
mixtures of proteins in addition to working with purified substrates because the proteins may interact in a manner which
modifies their accessibility to and degradation by proteolytic
enzymes. These methods have yielded data with mononuclear
phagocytes from man, mouse, guinea pig, and rabbit, as well as
established lines of macrophages (1-7), and related data have
been obtained with fibroblasts and other cells (2,6,8).

II.   METHOD FOR PREPARATION OF NATIVE COLLAGEN GELS

A.   Introduction

     Labeled collagen films provide a useful substrate for
investigating macrophage collagenolytic activity.

B.   Reagents

     1. Materials for Acetylating Collagen
     Collagen may be prepared from guinea pig skin by standard
procedures (9) or purchased as soluble bovine skin collagen
from Sigma, St. Louis, or Collagen Corporation (Vitrogen 100;
2455 Faber Place, Palo Alto, California 94303; also available
from Flow Laboratories, McLean, Virginia). [^{3}H]Acetic anhydride
(500 mCi/mmol) is purchased from Amersham, Arlington Heights,
Illinois, ^{14}C-labeled collagen is available from New England
Nuclear, Boston, Massachusetts.

     2. Materials for Culture of Macrophages on Collagen Gels
     Tissue culture supplies are obtained from standard sources
such as GIBCO. Enzymes used in analysis of collagenolysis and
for activating collagenase are obtained from sources listed below.

C.   Procedures

     1. Acetylation of Collagen with [^{3}H]Acetic Anhydride
     The aim of this procedure is to label cold collagen by
acetylating free amino groups of lysine (10). Lyophilized
collagen (100 mg) is dissolved in 0.1 M acetic acid at 2 mg/ml.
Immediately prior to the addition of the [^{3}H]acetic anhydride,
the pH of the collagen solution is brought to pH 8.9 by the
addition of 1 M K$_2$HPO$_4$. The acetic anhydride (2 mCi) in ben-

zene (2-3 ml) is added dropwise over a 2 hr period. The reaction is carried out on ice and the pH maintained at 8.0 with
1 N NaOH using a pH meter. After all the acetic anhydride is
added, the solution is left to stir for 1 hr in ice. The pH
is then adjusted to 4.0 with glacial acetic acid and the benzene is removed. The acetylated collagen is dialysed against
0.5 M acetic acid and then against distilled H_2O with at least
five changes to remove unincorporated label and tritiated acetic acid, which is a by-product of the reaction. The product
is then dialysed against 0.1 M acetic acid. The labeled collagen is lyophilized and stored at -20°C. The final product
should have a specific activity of approximately 1 µCi/mg collagen. To reduce the background, it may be necessary to re-
purify the collagen by trichloroacetic acid/ethanol precipi-
tations followed by ultracentrifugation by the methods described by Glimcher *et al.* (9). Alternatively, collagen may
be labeled by the method of Means and Feeney (11).

2. *Preparation of Native Reconstituted Fibers from
    Radioactive Collagen*
    The aim of this procedure is to prepare dried films of
radioactive collagen that are resistant to nonspecific proteinases at physiological temperatures, pH, and ionic strength
(2). The collagen plates are prepared with acid-soluble collagen labeled as described above. The ^3H-labeled collagen is
redissolved at 4 mg/ml in 0.1 M acetic acid and then dialysed
against 0.05 M Tris buffer pH 7.6, containing 200 mM NaCl,
after which it is clarified by ultracentrifugation (60 min,
50,000 g). The collagen solution is diluted by addition of
five volumes of sterile distilled water and 300 µl aliquots
placed immediately in 16-mm diameter culture wells. The collagen is allowed to form fibrils at 37°C for 2 hr and dry to
completion for 48 hr in a dry incubator at 25°C under vacuum.
The clear collagen layers are washed six times with sterile
Hanks' balanced salt solution and stored in 1-ml sterile Hanks'
balanced salt solution containing antibiotics at 35°C until
use (within 10 days).

3. *Culture of Macrophages on Collagen Films*
    Before use, the radioactive collagen layers are again
washed twice with Hanks' solution and the cells plated onto
the collagen layer. Usually 5-10 × 10^5 macrophages are plated
on the collagen in Dulbecco's medium containing 10-20% fetal
calf serum (with or without 60 µg soybean trypsin inhibitor
per milliliter for 24-48 hr. Medium is monitored by counting
100 µl aliquots in a scintillation counter to check for any
collagen degradation. For the experiments, cell layers are
washed six times with Hanks' then 1 ml of Dulbecco's medium
supplemented with 0.2% lactalbumin hydrolysate. For assays of

collagenolysis, the liberation of radioactive peptides into
the supernatant culture medium is observed. Cell-free control
wells and samples containing trypsin (10 μg/ml) or bacterial
collagenase (50 μg/ml) are used in every assay to measure
blank counts, proteinase-sensitive counts, and total radioactivity present in the system.

Two procedures are used: (a) Secreted collagenase is
accumulated on collagen and in medium for 24-72 hr at 37°C, an
aliquot is counted, and the enzymes are then activated by the
addition of 10 μg trypsin/ml (i.e., 10 μl of 1 mg/ml) at 37°C
for 10 min, followed by soybean trypsin inhibitor (10 μl of
5 mg/ml). The activated collagenase is then followed by removal of 50-μl aliquots at intervals of 1-6 hr. If desired,
further synthesis of collagenase by the cells can be inhibited
by the addition of cycloheximide (2 μg/ml) to the culture at
the time of activation. This reaction should give linear release. (b) Trypsin (10 μg/ml), plasminogen (1-200 nM), or
other proteinases are added at the beginning of the experiments
and aliquots (50-100 μl) removed at intervals for scintillation
counting.

III. METHOD FOR PREPARATION OF EXTRACELLULAR MATRICES

A. *Introduction*

The extracellular matrices produced by cultured cells
contain mixtures of connective tissue proteins and are, therefore, useful tools in studying the total destruction of these
proteins as it occurs in tissues.

B. *Reagents*

1. *Ascorbic Acid*
Commercially available ascorbic acid is not pure and it
may be necessary to purify it by recrystallization. A saturated solution of ascorbic acid is made in boiling ethanol and
filtered while hot through a fluted filter paper. The solution
is then cooled to room temperature and concentrated to 75% of
its original volume under a stream of nitrogen. The solution
is filtered after standing overnight at -80°C and the crystals
obtained are air-dried and stored in a desiccator at -20°C.
A stock solution of ascorbic acid in phosphate-buffered saline
(PBS) is made at a concentration of 5 mg/ml and stored at -20°C
after dispensing in small aliquots.

2. *Enzymes for Matrix Analysis*

All incubations with enzymes are carried out in 0.1 M Tris-HCl buffer pH 7.6 containing 10 mM $CaCl_2$. Trypsin (Sigma, Type III) is dissolved in buffer at 200 μg/ml at 0°C and treated with 5 μg/ml elastin for 5 min to adsorb any possible elastase contamination. The elastin is removed by centrifugation for 2 min at 2000 rpm followed by filtration through a 0.45-μm Millipore filter. Elastase (Worthington, Type ESFF) is also stored frozen at -80°C at a concentration of 200 μg/ml, but bacterial collagenase (Worthington, Type CLSPA) does not keep well as a frozen solution and is normally made up fresh for each experiment. Plasminogen is prepared by affinity chromatography of plasma on lysine-Sepharose columns (12). (see Chapter 61.)

3. *Radiochemicals*

Radiochemicals such as L-[^{3}H]proline (30 Ci/mmol) and L-[^{3}H]fucose (3 Ci/mmol) are obtained from New England Nuclear, Boston, Massachusetts, or Amersham, Arlington Heights, Illinois, and diluted with tissue culture medium before addition to matrix-producing cells. Tissue culture supplies are obtained from the usual suppliers.

C. *Procedures*

1. *Derivation of Rat Smooth Muscle Cells*

Twelve hearts obtained from 3-day-old rats are excised and cut into small pieces with a pair of scissors. These pieces are washed twice in calcium- and magnesium-free phosphate-buffered saline (PBS) and trypsinized at room temperature in freshly prepared 0.1% trypsin (1:250; Difco, Detroit, Michigan). The first harvest of cells, obtained after 10 min, is discarded. The next four successive 30-min harvests are collected and the cells obtained by centrifugation. They are cultured in Eagle's minimal essential medium containing 10% calf serum or fetal calf serum, 10% tryptose phosphate broth (Difco), penicillin (100 U/ml), and streptomycin (100 μg/ml). The cells are seeded into 75-cm^2 tissue culture flasks (Falcon) at 4-5 × 10^6 cells/flask and incubated in a CO_2 incubator (95% air/5% CO_2) at 37°C for 90 min. The supernatant medium is poured off, the attached cells are washed once, and fresh medium added. The cultures are passaged shortly before confluence at a ratio of 1:4, and the secondary cultures trypsinized and frozen in liquid nitrogen at approximately 1.5 × 10^6 cells/ 2/ ml vial in medium containing 10% dimethylsulfoxide. Each vial is used to establish one 75-cm^2 flask and the cultures derived from the frozen stock cultures are then used for the production of ex-

tracellular matrix over the next eight passages. Although the
rat smooth muscle cells appear to have a long life-span in culture, there is, in general, a decrease in the amount of elastin
produced with increased passage level (13).

2. *Derivation of Endothelial Cells*

Detailed methodologies for the culture of endothelial
cells from human umbilical cord (14-16) and bovine aorta (17,
18) have been described. Although these are the two most common sources of endothelium, endothelial cells have also been
obtained from adult rat lung (19), swine aorta (20), bovine
cornea (21), rabbit vessels (22), and guinea pig vessels (23).
Endothelial cells are normally obtained by enzymatic treatment
of the vessel with collagenase and/or trypsin solutions. Alternatively, they may be scraped off the vessel with a swab or
scalpel blade.

The most common contaminants of such preparations are
smooth muscle cells that are distinguishable from endothelial
cells by their growth pattern. Endothelial cells grow as flat
cells with a characteristic "cobblestone" pattern, whereas
smooth muscle cells tend to be more spindle-shaped and to pile
up on each other. Since bovine endothelial cells grow well
when seeded at cloning densities, primary cultures may be trypsinized and the cells seeded into 60-mm dishes at 100 cells/
dish. Colonies of cells growing with the characteristic cobblestone morphology may then be ring-isolated and cultured for
matrix production. The cells should be identified as being of
endothelial origin by the presence of Factor VIII antigen (14),
which is considered to be a good marker for the phenotype. The
endothelial cells may then be stored in liquid nitrogen and
used for the production of basement membranes when required.

3. *Fibroblasts*

Cultures of human skin fibroblasts are generally available from tissue culture laboratories or medical genetics departments. Fibroblasts from other primary origins such as
mouse and hamster are easily established by standard techniques. Alternatively, it is possible to use cell lines such
as 3T3 for the production of extracellular matrix. All of
these cell types may be cryopreserved in liquid nitrogen to
ensure consistency of the matrix preparation.

4. *Production of Extracellular Matrices*

The extracellular matrix may be prepared in 16-mm tissue
culture wells (Costar, Cambridge, Massachusetts), 35- or 60-mm
culture dishes (Corning, or Falcon) or, alternatively, on 15-
or 25-mm plastic discs (Lux Scientific, Newberry Park, California). To date we have experienced some difficulty in preparing
matrices from cells growing on glass. The producer cells are

seeded into the required culture vessels at approximately 3×10^4 cells/cm^2 in the appropriate culture medium. Twenty-four hours after seeding, daily treatments with ascorbic acid (25-50 µg/ml) are begun and medium is subsequently changed twice a week. Daily additions of ascorbic acid are essential for the appearance of insoluble collagen in the extracellular matrix. The unused ascorbic acid stock solutions should be kept at -20°C to prevent oxidation of the vitamin. Radioactive precursors such as [^{3}H]proline or [^{3}H]fucose are normally added to the growth medium 3-5 days after seeding at concentrations of 0.3 - 2 µCi/ml and replenished with each medium change.

Most cell types produce an extracellular matrix within 14-16 days after seeding. It is then necessary to remove the producer cells and leave the connective tissue proteins anchored to the bottom of culture dishes. This may be achieved by lysis with nonionic detergents such as NP-40 (24), sodium deoxycholate (25), chelating agents (26), or ammonium hydroxide (7). Matrices prepared by sodium dodecyl sulfate treatment are not suitable for use as substrates for other cell types because the detergent can become strongly bound to connective tissue proteins and is subsequently detrimental to the newly added cells. We have also found that nonionic detergents such as Triton X-100 or chelating agents such as EDTA are ineffective in the removal of cells from the dense multilayers of "tissue" formed by cultured smooth muscle cells. Therefore, whilst these methods may well be of value for cells which do not form such extensive quantities of matrix, we have concentrated on the use of 0.25 M NH$_4$OH as a means of removing producer cells. Ammonium hydroxide (0.25 M) has a pH of approximately 10.6 so that it rapidly causes cell lysis and because it is volatile it has the added advantage that it is easily and *completely* removed from the matrix preparations. Therefore, this method is described in detail.

Cell layers and associated matrix are washed twice with PBS and the cells lysed by the addition of 0.25 M NH$_4$OH for 30 min at room temperature. The lysate is removed by aspiration with a Pasteur pipette linked to a vacuum reservoir and the matrix washed extensively with a stream of distilled water followed by 70% (v/v) ethanol. The matrix is then allowed to dry at 37°C and stored at room temperature of 4°C.

The matrix produced by rat smooth muscle cells and human fibroblasts remains firmly anchored to plastic so that it is possible to wash it vigorously with a stream of water and ethanol. However, the basement membrane produced by many clones of bovine endothelial cells tends to float off the culture dish bottom following cell lysis with NH$_4$OH. One can either select another clone in which the membrane does remain anchored to the plastic, or alternatively the endothelial cells can be grown on the matrix proteins previously produced by smooth muscle cells.

This increases the adhesion of the basement membrane to the bottom of the dish allowing its easy isolation.

5. *Production of Glycoprotein-Depleted Matrices*

Connective tissue glycoproteins and contaminating cellular proteins may be removed from the matrix preparations by pretreatment with trypsin. Matrices are washed with PBS and then incubated with 20 μg/ml trypsin (prepared as outlined in Section III. B. 2) in 0.1 *M* Tris-HCl pH 7.6 containing 10 m*M* CaCl$_2$. Incubations are for 5 hr at 37°C in a humid atmosphere, which is achieved in a desiccator containing a 100 mm Petri dish of water in the base. The progress of hydrolysis of radiolabeled matrices may be followed, if necessary, by removing aliquots of the supernatant fluid at various times for radioactivity determinations. The dishes are removed after 5 hr, washed thoroughly with distilled water and air-dried at 37°C.

6. *Compositional Analysis of Matrix Preparations*

The composition of radiolabeled extracellular matrices produced by cultured cells may be easily determined by sequential enzymatic hydrolysis with trypsin, elastase, and collagenase. The importance of this technique is that it allows quantification of not only the composition of the starting material, but also the composition of residual matrices at the end of an experiment, from which one can determine which components were digested from complex substrates. Matrices are treated sequentially with trypsin, elastase, and collagenase in 0.1 *M* Tris-HCl pH 7.6 containing 10 m*M* CaCl$_2$ (see Section III. B. 2) at 37°C in a humid environment. Usually 2 ml of enzyme solution are used per 35-mm dish and the final enzyme concentration is 10 μg/ml. An aliquot (50-100 μl) of the supernatant liquid is taken for radioactivity determinations after each 3 hr incubation and the matrix washed four times with PBS before the addition of the next enzyme.

The residual matrix remaining after collagenase digestion is dissolved by overnight incubation in 2 *M* NaOH at 37°C and the radioactivity present in the supernatant determined after neutralization of a 100 μl aliquot with HCl. The residual radioactivity should be less than 5% of the total radioactivity present and should always be determined to ensure the efficiency of the earlier enzyme treatments. The total radioactivity present is calculated by summation of the amounts solubilized by each enzyme and by NaOH.

It is also possible to determine directly the amount of protein solubilized by each enzyme by the method of Lowry *et al.* (27). For these experiments, PBS pH 7.6 containing 1 m*M* CaCl$_2$ is used instead of the 0.1 *M* Tris-HCl/10m*M* CaCl$_2$ buffer, which interferes with the colorimetric reaction. The matrix is

treated sequentially with trypsin, elastase, and collagenase
(10 µg/ml) in 1 ml of buffer. Samples (500 µl) of the supernatants obtained after 3 hr incubation at 37°C with each enzyme are assayed. A blank containing enzyme alone at 10 µg/ml
is run in each case. Bovine serum albumin incubated for 24 hr
at 37°C with 10 µg/ml trypsin serves as a standard for the
trypsin release; bovine *Ligamentum nuchae* elastin and rat tail
collagen incubated with their respective degradative enzymes
under the same conditions are used as standards for the elastase and collagenase release.

7. *Culture of Macrophages and Other Cells on Matrix*
    Preparations

Matrices are sterilized by allowing them to stand in 70%
ethanol for 10 min at room temperature followed by four washes
with sterile PBS. Macrophages or other cell types are then
added in the required growth medium and allowed to attach to
the matrix preparations. If necessary, the nonadherent cells
may be washed off after 3 hr and fresh medium added. The progress of matrix hydrolysis is followed by determining the a-
mount of radioactivity present in 50 µl samples of the supernatant medium withdrawn at various times after plating. It
may also be necessary to change the culture medium every 48-72
hr in long-term experiments.

At the end of the experiment, the medium is withdrawn and
the macrophages washed once with PBS and then lysed by the addition of 1-2 ml of 0.25 M NH$_4$OH for 30 min at room temperature. The lysate is aspirated off and the residual matrix
washed with distilled water, 70% ethanol, and air-dried at
37°C. The composition of the residual matrix may then be determined by sequential enzyme digestion and compared with a
control matrix that has been incubated with medium without
added cells.

IV.   CALCULATION OF DATA

A. *Sequential Release Data*

Assuming that the rate of proteinase secretion is linear,
that the enzyme is activated immediately, that it is stable
throughout the experiment, and that it has a linear rate of
hydrolysis, then the rate of release of radioactive peptides
by macrophages growing on collagen or matrix is expressed by

cpm released = kt^2

where k is a constant related to secretion rate and t is time
of incubation. Equivalent hydrolysis should then be obtained

for continuous hydrolysis by secreting cells (e.g., 48 hr) and for accumulated enzyme (e.g., 48 hr) if in the latter case the activated enzyme is incubated with substrate for a time of $t/2$ (i.e., 24 hr).

If multiple aliquots are removed, then the following corrections are necessary to determine total cpm (minus background). If 50 μl samples are removed from a starting volume of 1 ml, then (see tabulation) the total release at

t	Net cpm/50 μl	Total cpm
1	100	$100 \times 1000/50 = 2000$
2	200	$(200 \times 950/50) + 100$ cpm removed at $t_1 = 3900$
3	400	$(400 \times 900/50) + 200 + 100 = 7500$
i	X_i	$\{X_i \times [1000 - 50(i - 1)]/50\} + \sum\limits_{1}^{i} X_i$

where i is the ith sample removed at time t_1.

B. Calculation of Matrix Composition

The composition of the extracellular matrix produced by cultured cells may be expressed in terms of the amount of radioactive precursor incorporated into each component that is subsequently sensitive to trypsin, elastase, and collagenase. For example, it might be stated that 37% of the proline radioactivity present in the matrix produced by smooth muscle cells is trypsin-sensitive, 31% elastase-sensitive, and 31% collagenase-sensitive. This type of calculation is adequate for many experiments, since it allows for the determination of the percentage of each component digested by degradative cells during a defined period.

However, it does not allow one to calculate the absolute amount of each component present because of the variable amino acid compositions of the relevant proteins. The calculation of the relative masses of each component requires a knowledge of the amino acid composition of the proteins. This may be obtained from the literature or by direct measurement of the composition of material released by the enzymes. The absolute specific radioactivity present in each component may also be determined by radioactivity and protein determinations of the material released by each enzyme.

The kinetics of hydrolysis of matrix preparations are relatively easily followed by the appearance of radioactivity in the supernatant medium. The residual radioactivity present in the matrix at the end of the incubation is also determined and, therefore, the results may be expressed as a percentage of the total radioactivity released as a function of time. If more detailed analysis is required, the absolute quantities of each component digested may be calculated as outlined above.

V. CRITICAL COMMENTS

The use of an extracellular matrix film for studying proteolytic capacity of cells has many advantages, including the capacity to compare live cells under physiological conditions with purified enzymes produced by those cells. It is possible to evaluate extracellular, pericellular, and intracellular phases of the degradative events by manipulations of the systems including proximity of the cells to the matrix and the use of enzyme and metabolic inhibitors and activators.

The collagen film procedure is interesting because it can be applied to other types of collagen, including basement membrane and cartilage collagens. Its disadvantage is the rather small amounts of collagenase produced by macrophages.

The use of cultured cells to produce a radioactive extracellular matrix that can be used as a substrate for degradative cells has the following advantages:

(1). Connective tissue proteins rarely occur as single components *in vivo* so that it is important that their digestion from mixtures be studied.

(2). Many different connective tissue cell types have been successfully cultured so that it is not difficult to prepare a variety of extracellular matrices for comparative studies.

(3). The ability to introduce the radioactive label biosynthetically rather than postsynthetically results in very high specific activities.

(4). Specific components in mixtures may be labeled and the total degradation of the connective tissue proteins to the level of amino acids may be followed.

(5). The use of sequential enzyme digestion to analyze the matrix proteins means that more quantitative studies can be done.

(6). Large numbers of identical samples may be prepared from cryopreserved producer cells.

(7). Since the conditions of matrix production may be varied (e.g., by altering the addition schedule for vitamin C), the effects of such variations on the resistance of the matrix to hydrolysis may be easily approached.

(8). The matrices may be prepared on plastic discs that may be floated above test cells so that the rate of digestion may be compared to that obtained when the cells are growing in direct contact with the matrix.

The disadvantages of the system are as follows:

(1). It is not always easy to assess quantitatively and qualitatively the degree of contamination of the matrix preparations with intracellular components. The matrix prepared from smooth muscle cells contains about 1 μg of DNA/200 μg of matrix proteins, although this can be removed by treatment with DNase if necessary. We do not know the level of contamination by other cellular components such as RNA or lipids, but large-scale contamination by intracellular proteins does not seem likely since little radioactivity is solubilized from the matrices by exhaustive extraction with SDS in the presence of mercaptoethanol and little cytoskeleton can be seen by scanning electron microscopy or immunofluorescence. If trypsin-pretreated matrices are used, contamination with other proteins is even less likely.

(2). The exact characterization of the connective tissue glycoproteins in the matrices has not yet been accomplished.

(3). Since some cultured cells, particularly chondrocytes, change the type of collagen synthesized with increased passage, it may be necessary to define the types of collagen present in the matrix.

(4). The drying of the matrices may not be suitable for some experiments, especially scanning electron microscopy; however, this is not a necessary step in the preparative procedure and matrices may be stored wet in PBS until use.

(5). The matrices do not appear to contain proteoglycans and are, therefore, deficient in one of the important constituents of the extracellular matrix.

In spite of these reservations, the extracellular matrices produced by cultured cells should prove to be valuable in studies of connective tissue degradation. In general, the results are reproducible and duplicates do not usually vary from each other by more than 5%. One source of inaccuracy is that some of the collagenase-sensitive radioactivity becomes trypsin-sensitive after long incubations. This is presumably due to collagen denaturation and is usually compensated for by running appropriate controls.

Acknowledgment

This work was supported by Research Grant CD-18 from the American Cancer Society and by the U. S. Department of Energy.

REFERENCES

1. Z. Werb. Pathways for the modulation of macrophage collagenase activity. *In* "Mechanisms of Localized Bone Loss" (J. E. Horton, T. M. Tarpley and W. R. David, eds.), pp. 213-228. Calcif. Tiss. Abstr. Suppl. 5, 1978.

2. Z. Werb, C. L. Mainardi, C. A. Vater, and E. D. Harris, Jr. Endogenous activation of latent collagenase by rheumatoid synovial cells. Evidence for a role of plasminogen activator. *N. Eng. J. Med. 296:*1017-1023, 1977.

3. J. C. Unkeless, S. Gordon, and E. Reich. Secretion of plasminogen activator by stimulated macrophages. *J. Exp. Med. 139:*834-850, 1974.

4. Z. Werb, M. J. Banda, and P. A. Jones. Degradation of connective tissue matrices by macrophages. I. Proteolysis of elastin, glycoproteins, and collagen by proteinases isolated from macrophages. *J. Exp. Med. 152:* 1340-1357, 1980.

5. P. A. Jones and Z. Werb. Degradation of connective tissue matrices by macrophages. II. Influence of matrix composition on proteolysis of glycoproteins, elastin, and collagen by macrophages in culture. *J. Exp. Med. 152:* 1527-1536, 1980.

6. G. Huybrechts-Godin, P. Hauser, and G. Vaes. Macrophage-fibroblast interactions in collagenase production and cartilage degradation. *Biochem. J. 184:*643-650, 1979.

7. P. A. Jones and T. Scott-Burden. Activated macrophages digest the extracellular matrix proteins produced by cultured cells. *Biochem. Biophys. Res. Commun. 86:*71-77, 1979.

8. Z. Werb and J. Aggeler. Proteases induce secretion of collagenase and plasminogen activator by fibroblasts. *Proc. Natl. Acad. Sci. USA 75:*1839-1843, 1978.

9. M. J. Glimcher, C. J. Francois, L. Richards, and S. Krane. The presence of organic phosphorus in collagens and gelatins. *Biochim. Biophys. Acta 93:*585-602, 1964.

10. M. T. Gisslow and B. C. McBride. A rapid sensitive collagenase assay. *Anal. Biochem. 68:*70-78, 1975.

11. G. E. Means and R. E. Feeney. Reductive alkylation of amino groups in proteins. *Biochemistry 7:*2192-2201, 1968.

12. D. G. Deutsch and E. T. Mertz. Plasminogen purification from human plasma by affinity chromatography. *Science* *170*:1095-1096, 1970.

13. P. A. Jones, T. Scott-Burden, and W. Gevers. Glycoprotein, elastin and collagen secretion by rat smooth muscle cells. *Proc. Natl. Acad. Sci. USA 76*:353-357, 1979.

14. E. A. Jaffe, L. W. Hoyer, and R. L. Nachman. Synthesis of antihemophilic factor antigen by cultured human endothelial cells. *J. Clin. Invest. 52*:2757-2764, 1973.

15. E. A. Jaffe, R. L. Nachman, C. G. Becker, and C. R. Minick. Culture of human endothelial cells derived from umbilical veins. Identification by morphologic and immunologic criteria. *J. Clin. Invest. 52*:2745-2756, 1973.

16. M. A. Gimbrone, Jr., R. S. Cotran, and J. Folkman. Human vascular endothelial cells in culture; growth and DNA synthesis. *J. Cell Biol. 60*:673-684, 1974.

17. F. M. Booyse, B. J. Sedlak, and M. E. Rafelson, Jr. Culture of arterial endothelial cells. Characterization and growth of bovine aortic cells. *Thrombos. Diathes. Haemorrh. 34*:825-839, 1975.

18. D. Gospodarowicz, J. Moran, D. Braun, and C. Birdwell. Clonal growth of bovine vascular endothelial cells: Fibroblast growth factor as a survival agent. *Proc. Natl. Acad. Sci. USA 73*:4120-4124, 1976.

19. M. S. Parshley, J. M. Cerreta, I. Mandl, J. A. Fierer, and G. M. Turino. Characteristics of a clone of endothelial cells derived from a line of normal adult rat lung cells. *In Vitro 15*:709-722, 1979.

20. L. W. Hayes, C. A. Goguen, A. L. Stevens, W. W. Magargal, and L. L. Slakey. Enzyme activities in endothelial cells and smooth muscle cells from swine aorta. *Proc. Natl. Acad. Sci. USA 76*:2532-2535, 1979.

21. D. Gospodarowicz, G. Greenburg, and J. Alvarado. Transplantation of cultured bovine corneal endothelial cells to rabbit cornea: Clinical implications for human studies. *Proc. Natl. Acad. Sci. USA 76*:464-468, 1979.

22. D. J. Loskutoff and T. S. Edgington. Synthesis of a fibrinolytic activator and inhibitor by endothelial cells. *Proc. Natl. Acad. Sci. USA 74*:3903-3907, 1977.

23. S. H. Blose and S. Chacko. *In vitro* behavior of guinea pig arterial and venous endothelial cells. *Dev. Growth Differ. 17*:153-165, 1975.

24. L. B. Chen, A. Murray, R. A. Segal, A. Bushnell, and M. L. Walsh. Studies on intercellular LETS glycoprotein matrices. *Cell 14*:377-391, 1978.

25. K. Hedman, M. Kurkinen, K. Alitalo, A. Vaheri, S. Johansson, and M. Hook. Isolation of the pericellular matrix of human fibroblast cultures. *J. Cell. Biol. 81:* 83-91, 1979.

26. L. A. Culp and H. Bensusan. Search for collagen in substrate adhesion site of two murine cell lines. *Nature 273:*680-682, 1978.

27. O. H. Lowry, N. J. Rosebrough, A. L. Farr, and R. J. Randall. Protein measurement with the folin phenol reagent. *J. Biol. Chem. 193:*265-275, 1951.

28. Y. A. DeClerck and P. A. Jones. The effect of ascorbic acid on the nature and production of collagen and elastin by rat smooth muscle cells. *Biochem. J. 186:*217-225, 1980.

29. P. D. Benya, S. R. Padilla, and M. E. Nimni. Independent regulation of collagen types by chondrocytes during the loss of differentiated function in culture. *Cell 15:* 1313-1321, 1978.

60

NEUTRAL PROTEASES
BY ^{3}H-LABELED CASEIN

D. O. Adams

I. PRINCIPLE

Macrophages secrete a variety of proteases, which include
enzymes such as collagenase that react only with specific substrates. It may on occasion, however, be of use to the investigator to quantify either multiple proteases in one assay or
proteases that have a wider range of reactivity. These goals
can be achieved by quantifying lysis of casein, which is a
broadly reactive substrate hydrolysed by a wide variety of
proteases (1). Supernatants of macrophages have been shown to
split azo dyes from casein (2). The development of a highly
sensitive assay employing ^{3}H-labeled casein as a substrate has
made studies of caseinases quite easy (3). By use of the [3]H-
labeled casein substrate, lysates and supernatants of murine
peritoneal macrophages can be shown to contain serine, metallo,
and thiol proteases (4). Supernatants of macrophages contain
at least five peaks of caseinolytic activity of greater than
approximately 10,000 daltons when the supernatants are parti-

tioned by molecular gel filtration (5). These observations
suggest the assay for caseinolytic activity, when applied to
macrophages, determines the action of *multiple proteases*.

The assay quantifies the release of TCA-soluble, ^{3}H-label-
ed peptides cleaved from ^{3}H-labeled casein by macrophage-derived proteases.

The secreted and intracellular proteases of macrophages
are often labile, adherent to glass, and present in relatively
low amounts (4,6). These factors dictate the strategy for
preparation of supernatants. Medium is conditioned by several
hours to several days of culture over purified populations of
mononuclear phagocytes. Since serum contains inhibitors of
hydrolases (particularly of neutral proteases), cultures are
generally conducted in the absence of serum. The cultures,
which are washed free of serum before the conditioning, are
maintained in medium treated with acid to remove α_{-2}-macroglo-
bulin, in medium containing no serum and supplemented with
lactalbumin hydrolysate, or in a designed serumless medium
such as that of Neumann and Tytell (Grand Island Biological
Co., Grand Island, New York.) (4,6). Siliconized glassware or
plasticware and pipettes may be useful in harvesting and collecting supernatants, because many of the secreted proteases
of macrophages adhere to glass (4). The conditioned medium is
rapidly collected with Siliclad pipettes into previously chilled (4°C) Siliclad containers and freed of cells by centrifugation (10,000 g for 10 min at 4°C). The conditioned medium is
assayed immediately or stored at -20°C. If the desired product
is present in low concentration, the conditioned medium can be
concentrated by lyophilization or dialysis against an adsorbent
(i.e., Aquacide II, Calbiochem, San Diego, California). We
have found concentration at 4°C in a stirred cell against an
appropriately sized UM membrane (Amicon, Inc., Lexington,
Massachusetts.) to be the most satisfactory method (4).

II. REAGENTS

(1). Labeled substrate. Tritiated casein is prepared by
acetylation of casein with ^{3}H by the method of Levine *et al.*
(3). Briefly, casein nach Hammersten (EM Chemical, Elmsford,
New York) is dissolved in distilled water at a concentration
of 50 mg/ml. To aid in dissolution, the pH is adjusted to 7.4
with 0.1 *M* NaOH. [^{3}H]acetic anhydride (New England Nuclear,
Boston, Massachusetts) is added with vigorous stirring and the
solution is incubated at 4°C for 1 hr. After acetylation, the
solution is exhaustively dialyzed against buffer (0.1 *M* sodium
phosphate, pH 7.5, containing 0.14 *M* NaCl, 0.02 *M* KCl, and
0.05 *M* sodium acetate) until the activity in the dialysate for

24 hr is less than 10^5 cpm/ml of dialysate. Background release of the dialyzed substrate should be less than 100 cpm in the final assay. The specific activity (i.e., radioactivity per microgram casein) of the labeled casein is determined. Each newly prepared batch of substrate is checked at multiple times (5 min to 2 hr) toward multiple concentrations of trypsin to ensure linearity of release. Dilute the substrate in distilled water such that a 20 μl aliquot containing 5 μg of casein yields ∫ 50,000 cpm (10,000 cpm/μg casein). Store in small aliquots at -20°C.

(2). Unlabeled substrate. Unlabeled casein (EM Labs, Elmsford, New York, Catalog No. 2242) is dissolved in distilled water, 30 mg/ml. To aid in dissolution, adjust the pH of the mixture to approximately 7.5 with NaOH. Store at -20°C.

(3). TCA: 6% trichloroacetic acid (TCA) in water. Store at 4°C.

(4). Buffer: 0.1 M phosphate buffer, pH 7.3.

(5). Stock A: 0.1 M KH_2PO_4, anhydrous monopotassium dihydrogen phosphate (FW 136) 27.2 gm/liter. Stock B: 0.1 M Na_2HPO_4 anhydrous disodium hydrogen phosphate (FW 142) 28.4 gm/liter. Mix 23 parts of A to 77 parts of B. Check pH. Adjust pH to 7.3 by addition of A or B.

(6). Standards: Use freshly prepared solution of trypsin (Worthington Biochemical). Make a stock solution containing 1.0 μg/ml. For each assay, standards of 1, 5, 10, and 20 ng of trypsin in 20 μl of stock are tested.

(7). Do not use HCl to adjust the pH of any reagent, or premature precipitation of proteins may occur.

III. PROCEDURE

(1). Prepare samples, standards, and blanks in triplicates.

(2). In each 400 μl microfuge tube (No. 46/6P, Walter Sarstedt, Princeton, New Jersey), combine 20 μl of buffer, 20 μl of sample (or buffer for blank), and 20 μl of labeled casein.

(3). Flick all liquids down in the tube. Incubate at 37°C for 1½ hr. Halt the reaction with 50 μl unlabeled casein. Add 100 μl cold 6% TCA to precipitate proteins.

(4). Centrifuge for 10 min in a Beckman Microfuge B centrifuge. Use of this centrifuge is facilitated by employing Beckman tube racks No. 338751 and 9-hole slides No. 338742 throughout the assay.

(5). Put an aliquot of 20 µl of the supernatant into a scintillation vial containing a suitable liquid scintillation cocktail (e.g., Aquasol II, New England Nuclear, Boston, Massachusetts). Place in a liquid scintillation counter and count after chilling in the dark overnight.

IV. CALCULATION OF DATA

The assay performed as described is linear with respect to concentration of protease added or with time (Figs. 1 & 2). It is independent of substrate concentration (3).

Subtract the background (release of label in the buffer blank) from each unknown to give net released counts. If the net released counts are less than 100, the standard errors of the sample and the buffer blank should be carefully compared to ensure differences are statistically meaningful. Multiply by 2/3 to give counts per minute released in one hour. Then, divide by 100 to give enzyme unit per sample.

One EU can be defined as 100 net released counts of TCA-soluble peptides over background per hour. By using the specific activity of the substrate, an EU should be further defined in terms of microgram casein hydrolyzed per hour. One enzyme unit should be roughly equivalent to the activity of 1 to 2 ng of trypsin prepared and tested as described above. The assay is reported as EU secreted per unit number of macrophages or unit of macrophage protein per unit of time.

V. COMMENTS

It is worth reemphasizing that casein is a broadly reactive substrate. This breadth of reactivity, the ease of the assay, and the stability of the reagents make this assay useful in many circumstances. Supernatants of macrophages should be harvested into siliconized tubes at 4°C and concentrated. The present assay may be more sensitive than the spectrophotometric assay for azocaseinases.

Acknowledgment

Supported in part by USPHS Grant CA-16784.

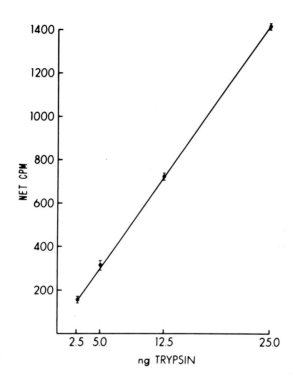

Fig. 1. The net counts per minute released at 90 min by various amounts of trypsin.

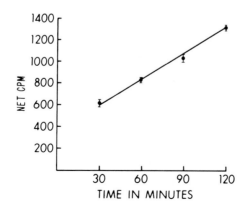

Fig. 2. The net counts per minute released by 50 ng of trypsin at various times.

REFERENCES

1. E. H. Reimerdes and H. Klostermyer. *In* "Advances in Enzymology," Vol. 45 (S. Colowick and M. Kaplan, eds.), pp. 26-28. Academic Press, New York, 1970.

2. S. Gordon and Z. Werb. Secretion of macrophage neutral proteinase is enhanced by colchicine. *Proc. Natl. Acad. Sci. USA 73*:872-876, 1976.

3. N. Levine, V. B. Hatcher, and G. S. Lazarus. Proteinases of human epidermis: A possible mechanism for polymorpho-nuclear leukocyte chemotaxis. *Biochem. Biophys. Acta 452*:458-467, 1976.

4. D. O. Adams. Effector mechanisms of cytolytically acti-vated macrophages. I. Secretion of neutral proteases and effect of protease inhibitors. *J. Immunol. 124:286,* 1980.

5. D. O. Adams, K. J. Kao, R. Farb, and S. V. Pizzo. Effector mechanisms of cytolytically activated macrophages. II. Secretion of a cytolytic factor by activated macro-phages and its relationship to secreted neutral proteases. *J. Immunol. 124*:293, 1980.

6. D. O. Adams. Macrophages. *In* "Methods in Enzymology," Vol. LVIII, Cell Culture (W. Jakoby and I. Pastan, eds.), pp. 494-505. Academic Press, New York, 1979.

61

PLASMINOGEN ACTIVATORS BY USE OF ^{3}H-LABELED CASEIN SUBSTRATE

S. V. Pizzo
J. G. Lewis

I. INTRODUCTION

Interest in plasminogen activator was originally restricted to its important role in fibrinolysis (1). However, plasminogen activators are also secreted by neoplastic cells and
macrophages, and its role in transformation and macrophage
function are topics of intense investigation (2). Detailed
structural comparisons of plasminogen activator from normal
vessel wall, neoplastic cells, and macrophages are as yet unavailable. In fact, the best studied activator is urokinase,
purified from human urine and derived from the kidney (1).
Apparent molecular weights for these activators range from -
28,000 to - 80,000 daltons (3). Despite this heterogeneity,
the function of all these enzymes appear to be identical, and
all human activators catalyze the conversion of single-chain
plasminogen to two-chain plasmin (1). Plasminogen activators
are extremely specific and show little proteolytic activity
against other substrates. Assays of plasminogen activators

METHODS FOR STUDYING
MONONUCLEAR PHAGOCYTES

599

have generally been indirect and dependent upon generation of plasmin. The plasmin can be assayed in several ways including proteolysis of fibrin plates (4), ^{125}I-labeled fibrin plates (5) or casein (6).

The fibrin plate assay has several disadvantages since proper plate preparation involves some care, and plates can only be stored for a limited period of time. On the other hand, casein is a soluble substrate that can be stored for long periods of time. Moreover, the method to be described below (8) utilizes ^{3}H-labeled casein, resulting in greatly increased sensitivity over unlabeled casein, together with a long shelf life.

II. REAGENTS

[3]H-labeled casein, see caseinolytic assay, (see chapter by Adams, this volume)
Unlabeled casein, see caseinolytic assay, (see chapter by Adams, this volume)
6% TCA, see caseinolytic assay, this volume, Chapter 60
Liquid scintillation cocktail, see caseinolytic assay, (chapter by Adams, this volume)
Buffer, 0.1 M NaPO$_4$, pH 8.0
Purified human plasminogen

Plasminogen is purified from fresh frozen human plasma by affinity chromtography as described by Deutsch and Mertz (7) and stored as a precipitate in H_2O at 4°C at a concentration of 1.7 mg/ml.

Lyophilized streptokinase (Lederle Pharmaceuticals). It is reconstituted in buffer, diluted to a concentration of 5000 U/ml and stored at -20°C in 0.5 ml aliquots.

Conditioned serumless media, see caseinolytic assay, (see chapter by Adams, this volume)

III. PROCEDURE

1. Labeled casein and plasminogen are diluted in buffer to working stocks of 1.3 mg/ml and 2.8 μg/ml, respectively. Appropriate dilutions, depending on amount of activator present, are made of the test sample. We have found that dilutions of 1/4-3/4 and full strength are sufficient for monolayers of thyoglycolate stimulated macrophages which have been allowed to condition serumless medium for 48 hr.

In 400 μl microfuge tubes add 40 μl of labeled casein, 20 μl of sample, and 40 μl of plasminogen solution. Reagents should be added immediately one after another, and in such an order as to prohibit activator and plasminogen being together without the presence of labeled casein. Controls of buffer and labeled casein, sample and labeled casein, plasminogen and labeled casein, and a positive control of 10^{-2} Ploug units/ml of streptokinase are prepared. Briefly spin the tubes to force all of the liquid to the bottom of the tubes and incubate at 37°C in a water bath for 4-16 hr depending on the amount of activator present.

At the end of the incubation period, the samples are harvested in the same manner as in the caseinolytic assay. Fifty μl of unlabeled casein is added to each tube followed by 120 μl of ice cold 6% w/v TCA. The tubes are spun for 10 min in a Microfuge (Beckman) and 20 μl of the clear supernatant is placed into 3 ml of scintillation cocktail.

2. Some practical considerations are as follows: If commercially prepared plasminogen is to be used, it must be free of plasmin contamination. If plasminogen and activator are incubated together in the absence of labeled casein for 10 min, the activity can be reduced by over 50%. If substrate limitation is encountered, it is usually the labeled casein that is the limiting ingredient. If over 50% of the counts are being released, casein will certainly be the limiting factor. While sterile technique is not necessary, grossly contaminated samples will contain very high activities. If labeled casein is stored for over 2 yr radialysis may be necessary to remove non-TCA precipitable material.

IV. CALCULATION

Direct caseinolytic activity, if present, is determined by subtracting the buffer or plasminogen control from the test sample control. Fibrinolytic activity is determined by subtracting the highest control value from the test samples. Because the reaction rates of activators in macrophage supernatants, tumor cell supernatants, and in the euglobulin fraction of human plasma are different from streptokinase, it is not possible to generate a streptokinase normal curve and express activities in common Ploug units; therefore, we arbitrarily define one unit of fibrinolytic activity as 100 net·count release of acid-soluble acyl peptides over background. This is equivalent to the lyses of 0.01 μg of casein.

V. CRITICAL COMMENTS

As little as 8×10^{-3} units/ml of streptokinase can be measured with 2 hr of incubation with this assay. When working in this range, the assay is linear to 1 U/ml giving a 125-fold linear range. This is the theoretical limit of the assay using partially purified activator, plasminogen and casein. In actual usage, the activator will be assayed under conditions where it is only a minor constituent of the solution. Thus, we find it necessary to incubate for up to 16 hr when macrophage-conditioned media are tested. If the media are conditioned for 48 hr by thyoglycolate-stimulated macrophages, the time can be as short as 4 hr. Many tumor lines produce sufficient activator such that 2-hr incubation times can be used. We have found very little activity in unconcentrated media from resident macrophage cultures.

REFERENCES

1. A. P. Kaplan, F. J. Castellino, D. Collen, B. Wiman, and F. B. Taylor. Molecular mechanisms in fibrinolysis in man. *Thrombos. Haemostas. (Stuttg.) 39*:263-283, 1978.
2. E. Reich. Plasminogen activator: Secretion by neoplastic cells and macrophages. *In* "Proteases and Biological Control," (E. Reich, D. B. Rifkin, and E. Shaw, eds.), pp. 333-341. Cold Spring Harbor Conferences on Cell Proliferation, Vol. 2. Cold Spring Harbor Laboratory, New York, 1975.
3. A. Granelli-Piperno and E. Reich. A study of proteases and protease-inhibitor complexes in biological fluids. *J. Exp. Med. 148*:223-234, 1978.
4. P. M. Permin. Properties of the fibrinokinase-fibrinolysin system. *Nature (Lond) 160*:571-572, 1947.
5. J. C. Unkeless, A. Tobia, L. Ossowskic, J. P. Quigley, D. B. Rifkin, and E. Reich. *J. Exp. Med. 137*:85-111, 1973.
6. D. L. Kline, and K. N. N. Reddy. Proactivator and activator levels of plasminogen in plasma as measured by caseinolysis. *J. Lab. Clin. Med. 89*:1153-1158, 1977.
7. D. G. Deutsch, and E. T. Mertz. Plasminogen: Purification from human plasma by affinity chromatography. *Science 170*:1095-1096, 1970.
8. J. G. Lewis, S. V. Pizzo, and D. O. Adams. A simple and sensitive assay employing stable reagents for quantifications of plasminogen activator. Submitted for publication to *Am. J. Clin. Pathol.*, in press, 1981.

62

ELASTINOLYTIC ENZYMES

Michael J. Banda
H. F. Dovey
Zena Werb

I. GENERAL INTRODUCTION

The detection and quantification of macrophage-derived elastinolytic enzymes are important considerations when studying model systems designed to evaluate the impact of macrophage secretory proteinases on lung and vascular elastin. In this chapter, elastase activity refers only to the ability of a proteinase to degrade mature, insoluble, cross-linked elastin into soluble peptides. This type of degradation parallels the biologically important destruction of the mechanical and structural properties of an elastin matrix. Only by employing an elastin substrate can one be certain of assaying elastase activity. Several nonelastin artificial substrates have been reported in the literature, such as succinyl-L-alanyl-alanyl-L-alanine-*p*-nitroanilide (SLAPN) (1) and *t*-BOC-L-alanine-*p*-nitrophenylester (NBA) (2). These substrates are based on elastin-like amino acid sequences, and it is assumed that the cleavage of these sequences is indicative of elastase activity. How-

ever, there is no guarantee that the same proteinases that
readily degrade the soluble elastinlike sequences *in vitro*
could, to any degree of biological importance, bind to or degrade the severely hydrophobic, cross-linked mature elastin.
More important, macrophage elastase will not degrade many of
these substrates (3). The techniques outlined here use elastin as a substrate so that ambiguity is avoided in determining
the nature of the proteolytic activity.

It should also be noted that, in addition to degrading
elastin, macrophage elastase can also degrade other proteins
(4-6). Therefore, assays with elastin substrates will unambiguously define an elastase but will not define the exclusive
activity of the enzyme.

Three mammalian enzymes will degrade elastin. The two
serine proteinases, pancreatic elastase (7) and granulocyte
elastase (8-10), are distinct from the macrophage elastase, a
neutral metalloproteinase (4). It is critical that the exact
source of elastase be determined, especially in the heterogeneous cell populations that are often obtained from lung and
peritoneal lavages. In the mouse and in the rabbit, purified
macrophage elastase has been shown to be catalytically distinct
from mouse and rabbit pancreatic and granulocyte elastases (unpublished observations). When constructing assays, the difference between the two serine enzymes and the macrophage metallo
enzyme can be exploited to distinguish the source of the elastase. A most convenient and biologically significant characteristic of macrophage elastase is its resistance to inhibition
by α_1-proteinase inhibitor (Worthington Biochemical Corp.,
Freehold, New Jersey) at concentrations in the assay of 1.0
mg/ml, whereas the two serine elastases are fully inhibited
(10). Soybean trypsin inhibitor (Sigma Chemical Co., St. Louis,
Missouri) at 1.0 mg/ml will not inhibit macrophage elastase but
will inhibit granulocyte elastase (10). The tri- and tetrapep-
tide chloromethyl ketone inhibitors of the serine elastases (11,
12) are ineffective against the macrophage elastase. Diisopropyl fluorophosphate and phenylmethanesulfonyl fluoride will inhibit the serine elastases but not the purified macrophage elastase (4). However, the solvents of these inhibitors, dimethyl
sulfoxide and isopropanol, can inhibit purified macrophage elastase. Thus, great care must be taken when using these inhibitors to determine the source of elastase activity, especially
from crude conditioned medium.

The inhibitor most useful in distinguishing macrophage
elastase from granulocyte elastase is 1.0 mM EDTA at pH 7.8 to
8.0, the pH optimum for macrophage elastase. The macrophage
metallo-elastase requires 5.0 mM Ca^{2+} for full activity. The
granulocyte serine elastase would not be affected by the chela-
tion of Ca^{2+} from the assay buffer, whereas macrophage elastase
would be fully inhibited. Although pancreatic elastase is not

a metalloproteinase, it does require Ca^{2+} and can be inhibited by 10 mM EDTA. However, unless specifically instilled by the investigator, pancreatic elastase would not be a contaminant of most cell populations obtained by lavage.

Unless native elastin is radiolabeled or coupled to a conveniently detected dye, its degradation is difficult to detect and quantify. Elastin is naturally fluorescent, but assays exploiting this feature (13) proved to be relatively insensitive and not as reliable as assays using labeled elastin. Scissions in the native elastin can be quantified by monitoring the appearance of free amino terminals by an increase in ninhydrin reactivity (14). This method is useful for analytic studies but not appropriate for routine assays of elastase activity, especially in culture media rich in amino acids.

Several investigators have used particulate elastin imbedded in agarose as the basis for an assay (15,16). The sample to be tested is placed in a well punched in the agarose-elastin layer, and elastinolysis is determined by measuring the area of a zone of clearing. This technique, though simple and direct, lacks flexibility and sensitivity and frequently requires several days of incubation. In addition, it is inappropriate for inhibitor studies.

The two assay systems described in detail below are relatively simple and sufficiently sensitive to allow detection and quantification of macrophage elastase from crude culture medium as well as from purified material. Both assays use commercially purified insoluble elastin. The first is based on the recovery of radioactivity in the soluble phase, and the second is based on the recovery of fluorescent peptides in the soluble phase.

II. CULTURE OF MACROPHAGES FOR DETECTION OF ELASTASE

This procedure is specifically used for the collection and tissue culture of mouse peritoneal macrophages. Unless otherwise stated, these macrophages are considered resident cells. Elastase has been detected from rat, rabbit, and guinea pig macrophage-conditioned medium. The harvest and culture conditions may have to be modified for each experimental system.

The basis of this procedure is described elsewhere. In brief, approximately 5.0 ml of PBS-heparin (700 U/ml) is injected into the peritoneum of each adult mouse. Macrophages are gently dislodged from the viscera by agitating the peritoneum (e.g., by tapping with a sterile Pasteur pipette). The PBS-heparin is withdrawn into a Pasteur pipette and transferred to a sterile centrifuge tube. The cell suspension is centrifuged and resuspended. Cells are plated at a density of

$5 \times 10^5/\text{cm}^2$ in 0.5 ml of Dulbecco's modified Eagle's medium
(DME) (GIBCO, Inc.) with 10% FCS. After incubation for 2-4
hr, the cells are washed twice with DME. The remaining adherent cells are highly enriched in macrophages.

After washing, the medium is replaced with DME containing
0.2% lactalbumin hydrolysate (GIBCO). Conditioned medium can
be collected after 24 hr and assayed for elastase activity or
frozen at or below -20°C for future assay.

For accurate comparative data, elastase activity should
be expressed as units per cell number or units per milligram
cell protein. If uniform culture conditions are maintained,
expression of activity as units per milliliter of conditioned
medium is convenient.

It is important to culture macrophages in serum-free medium when the conditioned medium will be used in elastase assays. Mouse macrophages can be maintained quite satisfactorily
in DME-LH. Rabbit alveolar macrophages should be cultured directly in DME-LH. A culture system free of exogenous inhibitors is necessary for accurate interpretation of elastase assays.

The intraperitoneal injection of 1 ml of Brewer's thioglycollate (DIFCO, Detroit, Michigan) (3%) 4 days before lavage
will increase the elastase secretion of macrophages (3,17).
Similar treatment with Freund's complete adjuvant (DIFCO) will
also increase elastase secretion. The activity of 10^6 stimulated macrophages is approximately 3.0 ± 0.2 (SD) U/24 hr,
whereas 10^6 resident cells will secrete 1.0 ± 0.3 U/24 hr.
Similar activities can be obtained from rabbit alveolar macrophages (17). Stimulation of rabbit alveolar macrophages can
be conveniently achieved with an intravenous injection of 0.1
ml of Freund's complete adjuvant 2 weeks before lavage.

Several mouse macrophage-like cell lines have been reported
to secrete elastase. Marginal activity has been detected from
J774.1, PU5-1.8, and RAW 264, and considerable activity from
WEHI-3 (18). P388D1 is a well-defined elastase-secreting cell
line (19). All cell lines develop variants quite easily and
may acquire or lose their reported phenotype. The P388D1 line
yields 0.9 ± 0.1 U/10^6 cells/24 hr.

Colchicine (Worthington) has been shown to differentially
modulate the secretion of neutral proteinases by macrophages in
culture (4,20). When mouse peritoneal macrophages are cultured
in DME-LH + 2 μM colchicine, elastase secretion can increase
five- to tenfold. Treatment with colchicine will also decrease
the secretion of plasminogen activator and lysozyme. The specific role of colchicine is not understood. Morphologically, the
mouse macrophages respond to colchicine by becoming round and
more mobile. Removal of colchicine reverses the effects.

III. [^{3}H]ELASTIN ASSAY

A. *Introduction*

The [^{3}H]elastin assay is representative of the more sensitive radioactive elastin assays (16,21,22). It is about threefold more sensitive than the rhodamine assay (see Section IV) and takes advantage of the ability of the aldol, isodesmosine, and desmosine cross-links to be reduced and labeled with [^{3}H]NaBH$_4$. These cross-links are distributed throughout the elastin structure and retain the label even after autoclaving and thus can be used in culture if necessary. The solubilization of label from these cross-links is a reliable indication of proteolytic degradation of elastin.

B. *Preparation of [^{3}H]Elastin Substrate*

1. *Reagents*
NaBH$_4$, nonradioactive, 250 mg
0.1 N NaOH, 0.003 N NaOH, approximately 100 ml each
[^{3}H]NaBH$_4$, 25 mCi (New England Nuclear, Boston, Massachusetts).
pH paper, wide range (3-10)
Antifoam B emulsion (Sigma Chemical Co., St. Louis, Missouri)
2.5 gm < 400 mesh elastin (E60 from Elastin Products Co., St. Louis, Missouri). This elastin is prepared from bovine ligamentum nuchae.
Glacial acetic acid

2. *Procedure*
(1) Because ^{3}H gas is a reaction by-product, all work must be carried out in a well-ventilated fume hood.
(2) The reaction vial should be a 500-ml Erlenmeyer flask, preferably placed in a clear, nonbreakable 2-liter plastic beaker. The flask and beaker assembly should be placed on a magnetic stirring plate in the fume hood.
(3) Suspend 2.5 gm elastin in 50 ml of distilled H$_2$O in a 500-ml Erlenmeyer flask. (Wet the elastin powder with ethanol before mixing with H$_2$O.)
(4) Adjust pH to 9.2 with NaOH.
(5) Dissolve [^{3}H]NaBH$_4$ in a minimal volume of 0.003 N NaOH and add to the elastin.
(6) After 10 min, add 250 mg nonradioactive NaBH$_4$ dissolved in a minimal volume of 0.003 N NaOH.
(7) Allow to mix in hood for 2 hr.

(8) Adjust pH to 3 by carefully adding glacial acetic acid. Check pH with paper. Be careful of foaming; a few drops of antifoam B emulsion will suppress foaming. If the flask must be removed from the beaker, wait until foaming has stopped.

(9) Mix for an additional 30 min.

(10) Collect the elastin by centrifuging at 10,000 xg for 30 min and wash repeatedly by resuspending in cold H_2O and recentrifuging until the activity of the supernatant is 1800-2000 dpm/100 µl. It is advisable to pool the elastin into one 50-ml centrifuge tube after the first two or three washes. If the labeling procedure is carried out in the early afternoon, four or five washes can be done and the elastin then left in the 50-ml tube stirring on a magnetic stirrer overnight at 4°C. This will allow much of the unreacted radioactivity to leach out of the elastin particles.

(11) Resuspend the elastin in H_2O at 16 mg/ml, stirring constantly on a magnetic stirring plate. Aliquot 5 ml (80 mg) into 50-ml sterile screwcap tubes (Corning 50-cc tubes) and keep frozen at -80°C until needed. Use a pipette with a wide mouth when aliquoting the elastin. DO NOT PIPETTE BY MOUTH.

3. Calculation of Data

Determination of specific radioactivity. Degrade a measured portion of the [^{3}H]elastin with pancreatic elastase (Sigma) at an enzyme:substrate ratio of 1:100 in 0.1 M Tris, pH 8.0, with 0.05 M $CaCl_2$. Allow the reaction to proceed at 37°C until all of the substrate is degraded, usually 3-4 hr for 100 to 300 µg. The total radioactivity incorporated should be about 600-1000 dpm/µg.

Determination of nonspecific labeling. Any nonelastin protein contamination of the [^{3}H]elastin substrate can be a substrate for nonspecific proteinases. To determine nonspecific labeling, incubate the elastin for 16 hr (overnight) with trypsin-TPCK (Worthington) in 0.05 M Tris-HCl buffer, pH 8.1, containing 0.012 M $CaCl_2$ at an enzyme:substrate ratio of 1:100. After 16 hr the released radioactivity should not exceed 2% of the total available radioactivity.

4. Critical Comments

[^{14}C]- and [^{125}I]Elastin. Alternative radioactive labeling procedures for elastin are available. Labeling of the elastin amino groups with [^{14}C]formaldehyde via reductive alkylation (23,24) yields stable substrates that can be used in a radioactive assay similar to that described below. The tritiated substrate is less complicated to prepare. Both [^{3}H]- and [^{14}C]elastin assay substrates are sensitive and specific

if purified elastin is used as the starting material. An [125I]elastin assay couples radioactive soluble elastin to CNBr-activated Sepharose 4B (Pharmacia). Although this system uses soluble elastin, it has been reported that only elastase will cleave the substrate from the Sepharose (25). This substrate may be useful in detailed rate analysis of elastase activity because a single clip in the elastin could release detectable radioactivity. Because a gamma emitter is used, this substrate eliminates the need for liquid scintillation counting, but in turn requires a gamma counter. One potential problem with ^{125}I-labeled elastin is artificial deiodination by myeloperoxidase (26), an enzyme that could be present in macrophage cultures.

C. Procedure for Assay

1. Reagents

3X Assay buffer. 0.3 *M* Tris-HCl buffer containing 0.015 *M* CaCl$_2$ and 0.02% NaN$_3$ (as a bacteriostat).

Pancreatic elastase. From porcine pancreas (E-1250, Sigma).

Substrate. Thaw a tube of [^{3}H]elastin (see B.2.11), resuspend in 10 ml of H$_2$O, and centrifuge at 2000 *xg* for 15-20 min. Discard the supernatant and resuspend to 40 ml with 3X assay buffer. This will give 2 mg/ml of [^{3}H]elastin substrate.

2. Assay

(1) Reagent blank. To a 400 µl microfuge tube, add 200 µl of DME-LH or appropriate solvent. Add 100 µl of substrate suspension in 3X assay buffer (see E.1).

(2) Total lysis control. To a 400-µl microfuge tube, add 200 µl of DME-LH or appropriate solvent plus 2 µl of pancreatic elastase. Add 100 µl of substrate suspension in 3X assay buffer (see E.1).

(3) Sample tubes. To a 400-µl microfuge tube, add up to 200 µl of sample (e.g., conditioned medium). Adjust volume to 200 µl with solvent (DME-LH) if necessary. Add 100 µl of substrate suspension in 3X assay buffer (see E.1).

(4) Cap or cover all tubes and incubate at 37°C for 16 hr. If a large number of tubes are being assayed, it may be more convenient not to cap the tubes, but simply to cover the entire rack of tubes with cellophane or Parafilm.

(5) After incubation, centrifuge for 3 min in a Beckman Microfuge (or equivalent). Remove 100 µl of supernatant from each tube to a scintillation vial. Add scintillant and count. A counting time of 1 min is usually sufficient.

D. Calculation of Data

   Units of activity. For this and the fluorometric assay
(see Section IV), a unit of elastinolytic activity is defined
as the amount of enzyme that degrades 1.0 µg of elastin/hr.
In each assay there is an internal set of controls to determine nonenzymatic release of radioactivity (blank) and the
total counts in 200 µg (100 µl) of elastin. If

   cpm_{PE} = cpm of pancreatic elastase degradation - cpm of
blank

   hr = assay time in hr
   cpm_S = cpm of sample - cpm of blank,

   then,
   200 µg/cpm_{PE} × cpm_S/hr = µg/hr = UNIT

   Units per Milliliter. Frequently, the expression of activity as units per milliliter is desirable. Using the definitions given above, if

   $µl_S$ = µl of sample assayed
   then,
   200 µg/cpm_{PE} × cpm_S/hr × 1/$µl_S$ × 1000 µl/ml = UNIT/ml.

E. Critical Comments

   1. Dispensing Elastin Substrate
   When dispensing particulate elastin substrate of any
kind, be certain that the suspension is constantly stirring
on a magnetic stirring plate. When pipetting aliquots of the
suspension, use a Gilson Pipetman P-200, or equivalent, which
has had 1-2 mm cut from the end of the disposable plastic
tip. This will enlarge the bore of the tip, preventing ob-
struction of the tip and inadvertent sieving of the elastin
particles.

   2. Reagent Blank
   Care must be taken to maintain low radioactivity in the
reagent blank. Should the activity of the blank exceed approximately 1-2% of the total radioactivity (determined with
pancreatic elastase), the elastin should be centrifuged,
washed once with H_2O, recentrifuged, and reconstituted in
fresh 3X assay buffer. Generally, high blank values are the
result of either insufficient washing after the labeling procedure or enzymatic contamination during sampling.

   3. Substrate Concentration
   The maximum substrate concentration, determined from
double reciprocal plots, suggests the use of several milligrams of elastin per assay tube. This would prove to be quite

impractical and rather expensive. The assay as described is
sufficiently sensitive not to warrant the routine use of higher substrate concentrations. The use of an insoluble substrate does not permit the Michaelis-Menten-type interpretation of kinetic data and thus the assignment of an absolute
substrate optimum.

4. The Effect of Sodium Dodecyl Sulfate on Elastase Activity

The use of sodium dodecyl sulfate (SDS) has been reported
by others (16,21,27,28). In the [^{3}H]elastin assay, SDS will
enhance elastase activity two- to tenfold, depending on the
source and treatment of the sample. Typically, the SDS-elastin assay will give elastase activity of 6-8 U/10^5 cells for
resident macrophages, 15-20 U/10^6 cells for thioglycollate-
elicited macrophages, and 5-11 U/10^6 cells for P388D1. Although the precise ratio of SDS:elastin (w/w) must be determined for each batch of elastin substrate by a dose-response
experiment, we found the optimal ratio to be 0.2.

The mechanism of SDS enhancement is not clear. Some investigators have suggested that SDS changes the conformation
of the molecule and renders the substrate more accessible to
degradation (21), whereas others suggest that SDS increases
the binding of enzyme to substrate (27,28). Another possible
role of SDS is to interfere with the action of an endogenous
elastase inhibitor (unpublished observations). Whatever the
mode of action, care must be taken when interpreting data
collected with the SDS-elastin assay. For example, macrophage-
conditioned medium has an eight- to tenfold increase in elastase activity when SDS is included in the elastin assay. When
the medium is first dialyzed against 10 mM NH$_4$HCO$_3$, there is
no change in activity in the SDS-elastin assay. However, in
the non-SDS-elastin assay, dialysis enhances the activity up
to eightfold. Thus, some effects are masked by SDS. We suggest that, for each investigation, dialyzed and nondialyzed
conditioned medium be assayed with SDS and non-SDS modified
substrate to determine the most informative assay for the particular study. SDS-elastin is especially useful in the detection of low-level elastase activity from crude conditioned
medium.

We strongly recommend that elastin without SDS be used
for the evaluation of biological inhibitors of elastase. In a
non-SDS-elastin assay, α_2-macroglobulin will readily inhibit
macrophage elastase. However, with SDS-elastin, α_2-macroglo-
bulin does not inhibit (4). The free SDS concentration (99
µg/ml; ratio of bound to free is 0.34) of an SDS:elastin ratio
of 0.2 is sufficient to dissociate α_2-macroglobulin-enzyme
complexes. Again, careful interpretation of SDS-elastin assay
data is in order.

If the SDS-elastin assay blank shows increased radioactivity, it should be discarded because the addition of fresh SDS assay buffer will change the ratio of bound to free SDS.

5. Effect of Sample Volume and Assay Time

In comparative studies of elastase from mouse macrophage-conditioned medium, it is important always to assay the same volume of sample. Frequently, the relationship between volume assayed and activity is not linear. An assay volume of 25 µl will indicate more units per milliliter than 200 µl of the same material (Banda, Takemura, and Dovey, unpublished observations). We interpret these observations to be the possible dilution of an uncharacterized proteinase inhibitor.

Elastase activity is linear with time through 18 hr. A minimum assay time of 8 hr is recommended for active samples.

IV.   RHODAMINE-ELASTIN ASSAY

A. Introduction

Elastin labeled with the fluorochrome rhodamine (29) is a refinement of several elastase assays using elastin dyed with stains such as Congo red (30), orcein (31), or remazol-brilliant blue (32,33). A distinct advantage of the rhodamine-elastin assay is its increased sensitivity over other dye assays (two- to fourfold over the Congo red or orcein assays) and its chemical stability. Unlike the ionically bonded Congo red and orcein stains, which can be removed nonspecifically from the elastin by proteins such as albumin (32,34), the covalently bonded rhodamine is less likely to give pseudo-elastase activity. A critical comparison of dye-labeled elastin assays was presented by Huebner (29).

B. Reagents

All reagents are obtained from Sigma Chemical Co., St. Louis, Missouri, unless otherwise noted.

(1) Assay buffer.   0.3 M Tris, pH 8.0, 0.015 M $CaCl_2$, 0.02% NaN_3 is prepared by dissolving 15.9 gm Trizma base, 26.64 gm Trizma HCl, 1.66 gm $CaCl_2$ (J. T. Baker Chemical Co., Phillipsburg, N. J.), and 200 mg NaN_3 in 1 liter of distilled H_2O.

(2) Elastin-rhodamine suspension. Elastin-rhodamine
(particle size <400 mesh) can be purchased from Elastin Products Co., St. Louis, Missouri, or it can be made by the method of Huebner (29). A 2 mg/ml suspension in assay buffer is
prepared by wetting a weighed quantity of elastin-rhodamine
with a minimal amount of ethanol. The wetted powder is then
suspended to 2 mg/ml with assay buffer and stirred with a
magnetic stirring bar to yield a homogeneous suspension.

(3) EDTA - Tris buffer. 300 mM EDTA, 100 mM Tris-HCl,
pH 8.0, is prepared by dissolving 107.5 gm/liter EDTA (tri-
sodium salt) in 100 mM Tris, pH 8.0 (5.3 gm Trizma base, 8.9
gm Trizma-HCl/liter of H_2O).

(4) Pancreatic elastase. From porcine pancreas
(E-1250, Sigma).

C. Procedures

(1) To prepare reagent blanks and standards, add 200 µl
of DME-LH for each replicate to a 12 × 75 mm disposable glass
tube.
(2) For each unknown sample, add 200 µl of conditioned
medium or an equal volume of diluted conditioned medium to a
12 × 75 mm disposable glass culture tube.
(3) Withdraw 100 µl elastin-rhodamine (200 µg) from a
vigorously stirring suspension at room temperature using a
Pipetman P-200 pipette, and add it to each assay tube including
blanks and standards. (See precaution in III. E.1.)
(4) Add 2 µl of pancreatic elastase to each standard tube,
being careful not to introduce it into any other assay tube.
This is a very concentrated elastase preparation, and even a
minute quantity has considerable elastinolytic activity compared to the usual activities of macrophage elastase found in
conditioned medium.
(5) Vortex all tubes and seal with Parafilm.
(6) Incubate at 37°C for 16-18 hr. Although the time
course of the reaction is linear for at least 26 hr, this incubation time allows convenient overnight incubation and gen-
erates sufficient fluorescence to be easily detected. However,
for extremely high or low elastase activities, the incubation
time can be modified as required.
(7) To stop the reaction and dilute fluorescence to a
workable range, add 1.7 ml of EDTA-Tris buffer to all tubes
using a repeating reagent dispenser (Glenco Scientific, Inc.,
Houston, Texas) and vortex briefly.
(8) Centrifuge all tubes at 250 *xg* for 10 min.

(9) Being careful not to disturb the elastin-rhodamine pellet, remove tubes from the centrifuge and measure the fluorescence of all samples directly in the same tubes using a spectrofluorometer (e.g., model 430, Turner Associates, Palo Alto, California) with the excitation frequency set at 550 nm and emission frequency at 570 nm. The standards, containing 200 μg of completely solubilized elastin-rhodamine, are used to calibrate the instrument to achieve a direct readout of micrograms of elastin-rhodamine solubilized per assay.

D. Calculation of Data

(1) Units of activity. A unit of elastinolytic activity for macrophage elastase is the degradation of 1.0 μg of elastin/hr. If

F = assay fluorescence - blank fluorescence
hr = incubation time in hours,
then
F/hr = UNIT.

(2) Units per milliliter. To calculate activity as units per milliliter the volume of the sample must be considered. If

μl_S = μl of sample assayed,
then
$(F/hr)/\mu l_S \times 1000$ μl/ml = UNIT/ml.

E. Critical Comments

(1) All of the comments and precautions for the [3H]-elastin assay are pertinent to the rhodamine-elastin assay. Therefore, before considering this assay for use in a particular investigation, read Sections III.E.1 through III.E.5. The comments on the use of SDS and on varying assay volumes pertain to the nature of macrophage elastase rather than to peculiarities of the assay substrate.

(2) This assay offers a convenient alternative to the radioactive assays. In addition to avoiding the use of radioactive reagents and associated paraphernalia, it is a one-tube assay that uses a convenient, commercially available substrate. Although slightly less sensitive than the radioactive assay, the rhodamine-elastin assay is sufficiently sensitive for routine use with macrophage cultures. The use of a fluorometer is not absolutely necessary. The rhodamine color can be detected at lesser sensitivity with a spectrophotometer.

V. CONCLUDING REMARKS

We have summarized two assay systems for the detection
of macrophage elastase from medium conditioned by macrophages
of various species. The assay of choice is the [^{3}H]elastin
assay because of its specificity and sensitivity. The fluorescently labeled elastin assay has been outlined for those
investigators who do not wish to deal with radioactive reagents
or do not have access to appropriate detection equipment. Whatever the choice of assay, considerable thought must be given to
the type of information desired from the assay. The addition
of the SDS-elastin substrate is useful for amplifying low-level
elastase activity, but probably not appropriate for the study
of biological inhibitors. In mouse macrophage systems, the nonlinearity of activity with assay volume must be considered. It
is most important to consider the source of the elastase activity when heterogeneous cell populations are investigated. In
particular, the possible uptake of granulocyte elastase by
macrophages (35) and its subsequent release during culture (26)
must be taken into consideration in interpreting elastase data.
The further intriguing possibility that mononuclear phagocytes
produce and store a granulocyte type of elastase at the time of
synthesis of azurophil granules by promonocytes remains to be
determined.

Acknowledgments

Supported by the U.S. Department of Energy and by an
NIH Fellowship (No. 1F32 HLO5998-01) to MJB.

REFERENCES

1. J. Bieth, B. Spiess, and C. G. Wermuth. The synthesis and
    analytical use of a highly sensitive and convenient sub-
    strate of elastase. *Biochem. Med. 11*:350-357, 1974.
2. L. Visser and E. R. Blout. The use of *p*-nitrophenyl *N*-
    tert-butyloxycarbonyl-L-alaninate as substrate for
    elastase. *Biochim. Biophys. Acta 268*:257-260, 1972.
3. Z. Werb and S. Gordon. Elastase secretion by stimulated
    macrophages. Characterization and regulation. *J. Exp.
    Med. 142*:361-377, 1975.
4. M. J. Banda and Z. Werb. Mouse macrophage elastase:
    Purification and characterization as a metalloproteinase.
    Biochem. J. 193:589-605, 1981.

5. M. J. Banda, E. J. Clark, and Z. Werb. Limited proteolysis by macrophage elastase inactivates human α_1-pro-
teinase inhibitor. *J. Exp. Med. 152:*1563-1570, 1980.

6. M. J. Banda and Z. Werb. The role of macrophage elastase in the proteolysis of fibrinogen, plasminogen and
fibronectin. *Fed. Proc. 39:*1756, 1980.

7. D. M. Shotton. Elastase. *Methods Enzymol. 19:*113-140,
1970.

8. A. Janoff. Neutrophil proteases in inflammation.
*Annu. Rev. Med. 23:*177-190, 1972.

9. P. M. Starkey and A. J. Barrett. Neutral proteinases
of human spleen. Purification and criteria for homogeneity of elastase and cathepsin G. *Biochem. J. 155:*
255-263, 1976.

10. P. M. Starkey and A. J. Barrett. Human lysosomal elastase. Catalytic and immunological properties. *Biochem.
J. 155:*265-271, 1976.

11. J. C. Powers and P. M. Tuhy. Active-site specific inhibitors of elastase. *Biochemistry 12:*4767-4774, 1973.

12. W. Ardelt, A. Koj, J. Chudzik, and A. Dubin. Inactivation of some pancreatic and leukocyte elastases by peptide chloromethyl ketones and alkyl isocyanates. *FEBS
Lett. 67:*156-160, 1976.

13. R. S. Quinn and E. R. Blout. Spectrofluorometric assay
for elastolytic enzymes. *Biochem. Biophys. Res. Commun.
40:*328-333, 1970.

14. H. Rosen. A modified ninhydrin colorimetric analysis
for amino acids. *Arch. Biochem. Biophys. 67:*10-15,
1957.

15. G. F. B. Schumacher and W. -B. Schill. Radial diffusion
in gel for micro determination of enzymes. II. Plasminogen activator, elastase, and nonspecific proteases.
*Anal. Biochem. 48:*9-26, 1972.

16. S. Gordon, Z. Werb, and Z. A. Cohn. Methods for the detection of macrophage secretory enzymes. *In "In Vitro*
Methods in Cell-Mediated and Tumor Immunity" (B. R. Bloom
and J. R. David, eds.), pp. 341-352. Academic Press,
New York, 1976.

17. R. White, H. -S. Lin, and C. Kuhn, III. Elastase secretion by peritoneal exudative and alveolar macrophages.
*J. Exp. Med. 146:*802-808, 1977.

18. P. Ralph, H. E. Broxmeyer, M. A. S. Moore, and I.
Nakoinz. Induction of myeloid colony-stimulating activity in murine monocyte tumor cell lines by macrophage
activators and in a T cell line by concanavalin A.
*Cancer Res. 38:*1414-1419, 1978.

19. Z. Werb, R. Foley, and A. Munck. Interaction of gluco-
     corticoids with macrophages. Identification of gluco-
     corticoid receptors in monocytes and macrophages. J.
     Exp. Med. 147:1684-1694, 1978.
20. S. Gordon and Z. Werb. Secretion of macrophage neutral
     proteinase is enhanced by colchicine. Proc. Natl. Acad.
     Sci. USA 73:872-876, 1976.
21. S. Takahashi, S. Seifter, and F. C. Yang. A new radio-
     active assay for enzymes with elastolytic activity using
     reduced tritiated elastin. The effect of sodium dodecyl
     sulfate on elastolysis. Biochim. Biophys. Acta 327:138-
     145, 1973.
22. P. J. Stone, G. Crombie, and C. Franzblau. The use of
     tritiated elastin for the determination of subnanogram
     amounts of elastase. Anal. Biochem. 80:572-577, 1977.
23. D. R. Bielefeld, R. M. Senior, and S. Y. Yu. A new
     method for determination of elastolytic activity using
     [^{14}C] labeled elastin and its application to leukocytic
     elastase. Biochem. Biophys. Res. Commun. 67:1553-1559,
     1975.
24. S. Y. Yu and A. Yoshida. Amorphous [^{14}C]elastin as a
     substrate for assaying elastolytic enzyme in cellular
     and tissue extracts. Biochem. Med. 21:108-120, 1979.
25. D. B. Rifkin and R. M. Crowe. A sensitive assay for
     elastase employing radioactive elastin coupled to Sepha-
     rose. Anal. Biochem. 79:268-275, 1977.
26. C. G. Ragsdale and W. P. Arend. Neutral protease secre-
     tion by human monocytes. Effect of surface-bound immune
     complexes. J. Exp. Med. 149:954-968, 1979.
27. H. M. Kagan, G. D. Crombie, R. E. Jordan, W. Lewis, and
     C. Franzblau. Proteolysis of elastin-ligand complexes.
     Stimulation of elastase digestion of insoluble elastin
     by sodium dodecyl sulfate. Biochemistry 11:3412-3418,
     1972.
28. H. M. Kagan. Changes in the state of ionization of
     carboxyl groups in elastin in response to the binding
     of sodium dodecyl sulfate. Connect. Tiss. Res. 6:167-
     169, 1978.
29. P. F. Huebner. Determination of elastolytic activity
     with elastin-rhodamine. Anal. Biochem. 74:419-429,
     1976.
30. M. A. Naughton and F. Sanger. Purification and speci-
     ficity of pancreatic elastase. Biochem. J. 78:156-163,
     1961.
31. B. Robert and L. Robert. Studies on the structure of
     elastin and the mechanism of action of elastolytic en-
     zymes. In "Chemistry and Molecular Biology of the Inter-
     cellular Matrix," Vol. 1 (E. A. Balazs, ed.), pp. 665-670.
     Academic Press, New York, 1970.

32. H. Rinderknecht, M. C. Geokas, P. Silverman, Y. Lillard, and B. J. Haverback. New methods for the determination of elastase. *Clin. Chim. Acta 19:*327-339, 1968.

33. J. Bieth, M. Pichoir, and P. Metais. Pseudo-zero order solubilization of remazol-brilliant blue elastin by elastase. *Anal. Biochem. 70:*430-433, 1976.

34. I. Banga and W. Ardelt. Studies on the elastolytic activity of serum. *Biochim. Biophys. Acta 146:*284-286, 1967.

35. E. J. Campbell, R. R. White, R. M. Senior, R. J. Rodriguez, and C. Kuhn. Receptor-mediated binding and internalization of leukocyte elastase by alveolar macrophages *in vitro*. *J. Clin. Invest. 64:*824-833, 1979.

63

MICROTITER ASSAY FOR ANTIVIRAL EFFECTS
OF HUMAN AND MURINE INTERFERON
UTILIZING A VERTICAL LIGHT PATH PHOTOMETER
FOR QUANTITATION

Lois B. Epstein
Nancy H. McManus
Samuel J. Hebert
Judith Woods-Hellman
Diane G. Oliver

I. INTRODUCTION

Much effort has been made by many investigators to define
the cellular origin of interferon produced in response to many
diverse agents. Our own studies have demonstrated that human
lymphocytes are the source of interferon produced in response
to mitogens and antigens (1) and that macrophages enhance such
interferon production by the lymphocytes (2). The type of interferon produced by stimulated lymphocytes was formerly called
type II, or immune interferon and, now by the new nomenclature
for interferon, IFN-γ (3). Human IFN-γ is antigenically different from other types of interferons and distinguishes itself
further by virtue of its greater lability on exposure to low pH
and heat. The other types of interferon were formerly known as
type I or classical interferons or as leukocyte or fibroblast
interferon, and now are designated as IFN-α and IFN-β, respectively. The comparative biology of the various types of interferons has been reviewed (4). Macrophages, in addition to

METHODS FOR STUDYING
MONONUCLEAR PHAGOCYTES

lymphocytes, can produce interferon (5-9), but the interferon
produced is usually of the α or β variety.

The microtiter assay for the antiviral effects of human
and murine interferon that we employ in our laboratory is rapid,
sensitive, and economical. It represents a modification of
previously reported techniques (10-13), combined with a totally
new approach for quantitating the assay. Fibroblasts are exposed to interferon containing samples and the cells are then
challenged with bovine vesicular stomatitis virus (VSV). Interferon protection conferred upon the cells is reflected by
the degree of inhibition of virus-induced cytopathic effect.
By staining the monolayer, qualitative and quantitative assessments of protection can be made. Qualitative results can be
obtained within 72 hr of cell seeding. Quantitative results
are obtained within this same period by utilizing the Titertek
Multiskan, an automated vertical light path photometer that
permits the reading and recording of the optical density of a
96-well flat bottom microtiter plate in less than 1 min. The
Titertek Multiskan also makes it possible for the entire assay
to be performed in the original microplate.

II.   REAGENTS

A.   Cells

The fibroblasts employed in this assay for human interferon
are derived from human skin biopsy or fetal tissue specimens
that we possess in our own laboratory. Alternatively, normal
human fibroblasts may be obtained from HEM Research, Inc.,
Rockville, Maryland and Microbiological Associates, Bethesda,
Maryland, or human foreskin fibroblasts may be prepared as detailed by Epstein and McManus (14). As fibroblasts of patients
with trisomy 21 (Down syndrome) have been shown to be three to
ten times more sensitive to the antiviral effects of interferon
as compared to matched diploid cells (15,16), we prefer to use
these in our assay, especially when low levels of interferon
are anticipated. Cells from such individuals may be obtained
commercially from the Human Genetic Mutant Cell Culture Facility, Camden, New Jersey or prepared directly, as we do, from
tissue specimens.

L 929 cells used for the assay of murine interferon were
kindly supplied by Dr. Werner Rosenau. These cells may be obtained commercially from American Type Culture Collection
(Catalog No. CCL-1), from Flow Laboratories, Inc., McLean,
Virginia, or from microbiological Associated, Bethesda, Maryland.

B. *Tissue Culture Reagents*

Dulbecco's modified Eagle Medium (3 gm glucose/liter) (DME) is supplemented with fetal calf serum (FCS), as indicated in the procedure, and 100 U/ml penicillin and 100 µg/ml streptomycin. For subculturing, the cells are trypsinized with a solution of saline A containing 0.05% trypsin and 0.02% ethylenediaminetetraacetate [Cell Culture Facility, University of California, or Grand Island Biological Co., (GIBCO), Santa Clara, California]. The DME is stored at 4°C; trypsin solution is stored at -20°C until use, then at 4°C.

C. *Laboratory and International Interferon Reference Standards*

A human internal laboratory standard for interferon is prepared as outlined in Epstein and McManus (14) and is calibrated against the International Reference Standard for leukocyte interferon (IFN-α), (G-023-901-527), which is available from the Viral Resources Branch, National Institutes of Allergy and Infectious Diseases (NIAID), Bethesda, Maryland 20205. Our internal laboratory standard for mouse interferon was obtained from the laboratory of the late Dr. Kurt Paucker and is calibrated against the International Reference Standard for mouse interferon (G-002-904-511), also available from NIAID.

To date no International Reference Standard for human or mouse immune interferon (IFN-γ) is available, and the other available human and mouse interferon standards are used as substitute reagents. The use of such international reference standards and the reporting of interferon in international units allows for the comparison of results from numerous laboratories.

D. *Virus*

The Indiana strain of bovine vesicular stomatitis virus is propagated on chick-embryo fibroblasts, and plaque-forming units (PFU) per milliliter are determined for human and mouse cells as described by Epstein and McManus (14).

E. *Stain and Reagent for Elution*

Qualitative results of cytopathic effect (CPE) are visualized by staining the monolayer with a dye-fixative solution containing 0.5% crystal violet (MC/B Manufacturing Chemists, Norwood, Ohio), 5% formalin (v/v), 50% ethanol (v/v) and 0.85% NaCl. Quantitation of CPE is accomplished by eluting the stain

with ethylene glycol monomethyl ether (Sigma Chemical Co.,
St. Louis, Missouri, (10). This is stored at room temperature
in the dark; inhalation of fumes should be avoided.

III. PROCEDURE

A. *Maintenance and Culture of Cell Lines*

    Culture and maintain the human fibroblasts in 75-cm^2 Falcon
flasks (Becton, Dickerson & Co., Oxnard, California) in Dulbecco's modified Eagle Medium (3 gm glucose/liter) (DME) supplemented with 10% FCS in a water-jacketed incubator (NAPCO,
National Appliance Co., Scientific Products, Menlo Park, California) at 37°C in a humidified atmosphere containing 5% CO_2.
Culture and maintain L 929 cells in the same manner using DME
+ 5% FCS.

B. *Microassay for Interferon*

    Seed the cells used in the assay into a 96-well tissue
culture plate (Linbro Division, Flow Laboratories, Inc.,
McLean, Virginia) in a 0.2-ml DME + 10% FCS-well, using a 1-ml
serological pipette. The cell concentration for human fibroblasts is 2.5 x 10^4 cells/well; the concentration for L 929
cells is 1 x 10^4 cells/well. Warm the microplates and medium
to 37°C before use. To facilitate obtaining a homogeneous
monolayer for uniform staining qualities, place the microplates
on a Micromix (Hyperion, Inc., Cordis Corp., Miami, Florida)
for 5 min immediately after seeding, after which they are incubated at 37°C in a 5% CO_2 humidified atmosphere for approximately 24 hr. At this time the monolayers should be greater
than 95% confluent. Make serial dilutions of the samples to be
tested in DME + 5% FCS and, in parallel, make serial dilutions
of an interferon preparation of known concentration that has
been calibrated against the appropriate international standard.
Remove the medium from each well by careful aspiration with a
finely tapered Pasteur pipette that has been bent to a 90° angle. Add the interferon samples in a 0.1-ml volume/well.
Eight wells, reserved for both cell and virus controls, receive
fresh medium. Incubate the plates under the above standard
culture conditions for 20-24 hr.
    Aspirate the interferon samples and control media. Add 0.1
ml DME (containing 2% FCS at 37°C for human cells, and 5% FCS
for mouse cells) to each monolayer and reincubate the plates.
Dilute bovine vesicular stomatitis virus (VSV), containing approximately 0.5 PFU/cell, in cold DME with FCS concentrations

for cells as indicated above, and add 0.1 ml to each test and virus control well after aspiration of the wash medium. Aspirate the medium from wells that serve as cell controls and reapply 0.1 ml DME + 2% FCS at this time. Reincubate the cultures under the above standard culture conditions for 20 hr to obtain 3+-4+ CPE.

At the conclusion of the VSV challenge, aspirate the supernatant fluids into a virus decontamination waste container, gently wash the monolayers twice with 0.85% NaCl and stain for 20 min with 0.1 ml dye-fixative solution. Remove excess stain by aspiration, wash the monolayers three times with distilled water and allow the plates to thoroughly air dry. At this stage in the assay, the degree of protection can be qualitatively assessed by comparing the staining intensity of the cell and virus controls with the interferon-treated monolayers. This is facilitated by the use of a microtiter plate reading mirror (Flow Laboratories, Inc., McLean, Virginia). In addition, if desired, the plates may be stored at room temperature in the dark for several weeks prior to quantitation.

To quantitate the amount of interferon protection, elute the stain by the addition of 0.2 ml ethylene glycol monomethyl ether to each well, using a Titertek 12-channel variable pipetter (Flow Laboratories, Inc., McLean, Virginia). Place the plates on a vertical vibrator (A. H. Thomas Co., Philadelphia, Pennsylvania) to hasten total stain elution. Elution time is empirically determined and ranges from 10-40 min. Elution time should be long enough to elute dye from the darkest wells. The samples should be read immediately after total elution of dye, to minimize the progressive fading of the dye with time. After blanking the instrument with a Linbro plate, in which the eight wells in the first row contain 0.2 ml eluting fluid, the optical density of the eluate contained in each well is quantitated in a Titertek Multiskan, a vertical light path photometer (Flow Laboratories, Inc., McLean, Virginia) at 550 nm. The optical density of the 96 wells is automatically read and printed out within 1 min.

IV. CALCULATION OF DATA

Convert the optical density of the eluted stain to percentage dye uptake by use of the following equation:

$$\% \text{ Dye uptake} = \frac{\text{OD test - OD virus control}}{\text{OD cell control - OD virus control}} \times 100$$

Plot the percentage dye uptake against the log of the interferon concentration. Using linear regression analysis of

points that fall between 15-85% dye uptake, calculate the 50%
protection point for each unknown sample. Do the same for the
interferon standard run in parallel. The concentration of interferon contained in the dilution of the unknown sample producing 50% protection is equated with the concentration (in
International Units per milliliter) of the standard producing
50% protection. By taking into account the dilution factor of
the unknown sample, the concentration of interferon in the
original unknown sample is calculated. A sample calculatiion
is provided below.

The mean OD of eight cell controls (CC) from a given assay
is 0.627, and the mean OD of eight virus controls (VC) is
0.329. The mean OD of three wells exposed to the human interferon standard known to contain 10 U/ml is 0.602. Thus, using
the above formula,

$$\% \text{ Dye uptake} = \frac{0.602 - 0.329}{0.627 - 0.329} = \frac{0.273}{0.298} = 92\%$$

Similar calculations made for other known concentrations of
the human interferon standard give the following data (see the
tabulation below):

Concentration of human interferon standard (IU/ml	OD	Dye uptake (%)
10.0	0.602	92
5.0	0.538	70
2.5	0.464	45
1.0	0.400	24
0.5	0.365	12

Using the values between 15 and 85%, the linear regression is
calculated. The IFN_{50} is obtained from the linear regression
data and is 2.6 IU/ml. Let us assume that one unknown sample
at a 1/100 dilution gave 50% dye uptake. Then the original
concentration of the unknown sample would be 260 IU/ml.

V. CRITICAL COMMENTS

One of the most crucial aspects of this assay, especially
to obtain excellent reproducibility when quantitated on the
Titertek Multiskan, is a homogeneous and well-stained monolayer in each well. The cells employed in our laboratory for
this assay have excellent sensitivity to interferon. The mean
±SE of IFN_{50} from seven experiments with the human trisomy 21

fibroblasts was 2.9 ± 0.3 IU/ml; that of diploid human fibroblasts in eight experiments was 7.3 ± 0.8 IU/ml; that of mouse
L cells in 15 experiments was 5.3 ± 0.9 IU/ml. However, the
fact that these human cell lines can become extremely dense
and that the mouse L cell line does not exhibit contact inhibition posed potential problems in the sloughing off of the
monolayers. This was overcome by paying careful attention to
keeping constant the conditions of cell maintenance (i.e., cell
splitting, time of cell splits, and percentage of fetal calf
serum employed). Also, the choice of a 20-hr virus challenge
minimizes time for overgrowth, and careful aspiration of fluids
during the assay minimizes disturbance of the cell layer. The
most reproducible monolayers well-to-well and assay-to-assay
were obtained by the use of either a 1.0-ml or 2.0-ml serological pipette for initial seeding and were far superior to those
obtained by seeding with an automatic pipetter. The coefficient
of variation of the optical density of cell controls was <10%
for human fibroblasts and <13% for L cells using the serological
pipettes.

We also observed that there is an unevenness of monolayer
growth within the wells around the periphery of the microplate
as compared with the interior of the plate. Thus we pay particular attention to obtaining uniform air flow, temperature, and
high humidity in our CO_2 incubator, so that this uneveness is
avoided. The reader is referred to the work of Martuza *et al.*
(17) and Duvall *et al.* (13) for further discussion of the causes
and suggestions for correction of uneven humidity and gas exchange.

The Titertek Multiskan allows the quantitation of a 96-well
flat bottom microplate in 1 min, an incredibly short time as
compared with other methods of automatic quantitation that employ horizontal light path spectrophotometers (10-12), especially those which involve manual transfer of each sample to a
cuvette for reading optical density.

As the Titertek Multiskan is a vertical light path photometer, measurement of the optical density is in cuvettes with
their longitudinal dimension parallel to the light beam. As
the path length is dependent on the total volume, variation in
the volume changes the light path by the same amount, but the
absorbance is constant (18). Thus the OD readings are independent of the volume of eluate, and this feature counteracts possible pipetting errors in the elution of stain from the monolayers. These are minimal, however, as use of the 12-channel
Titertek pipetter for adding eluate permits a coefficient of
variation of <2% in replicate sampling.

As we recognized that the absorbance is independent of the
volume of eluate, we naturally explored the possibility of reading the plates dry, without eluate, in the Titertek Multiskan,

to eliminate the time necessary for dye elution. However, we found that this was not feasible for the reason given below.

In the Titertek Multiskan with a 550-nm filter, the concentration of eluted crystal violet is linear within the OD range of 0.2 - 1.7, and our assay conditions are designed to fall within the linear range. In the case of the virus control wells and wells containing samples in which there are low levels of interferon and thus minimal antiviral protection, the OD readings frequently fall below an OD of 0.2. This is because in such wells there is more central than peripheral destruction of each well by virus, and a rimming phenomenon occurs. The light beam sees only the central portion of each well. Despite attempts to minimize the rimming phenomenon by using Linbro plates, which give less rimming than Nunc or Falcon microtiter plates, the rimming phenomenon cannot be eliminated. Therefore in order to get accurate results it is necessary to use solvent to elute all the dye from each well.

For many years in our laboratory we employed a macro virus plaque reduction technique for the assay of interferon (19). We find the present microassay to be far superior because of considerable economy of time and materials and ease in quantitation of the assay.

Acknowledgments

This work was supported by NIH grant CA 27903 and grant 6-126 from the March of Dimes Birth Defects Foundation. The authors are indebted to Flow Laboratories, McLean, Virginia for making available a Titertek Multiskan and 550-nm filter for use in the development of this assay. We also thank Mary Evelyn Rose for typing the manuscript.

REFERENCES

1. L. B. Epstein. Mitogen and antigen induction of interferon *in vitro* and *in vivo*. *Tex. Rep. Biol Med. 35*:43-56, 1978.
2. L. B. Epstein. The ability of macrophages to augment *in vitro* mitogen- and antigen-stimulated production of interferon and other mediators of cellular immunity by lymphocytes. *In* "Immunobiology of the Macrophage" (D. S. Nelson, ed.), pp. 201-234. Academic Press, New York, 1976.
3. W. E. Stewart II *et al*. Interferon nomenclature. *J. Interferon Res. 1*:vi, 1981.

4. L. B. Epstein. The comparative biology of classical (Type I) and immune (Type II) interferon. *In* "Biology of the Lymphokines" (S. Cohen, J. Oppenheim, and E. Pick, eds.), pp. 443-514. Academic Press, New York, 1979.

5. D. O. Lucas and L. B. Epstein. Interferon and macrophages. *In* "The reticuloendothelial System: A Comprehensive Treatise, Vol. 4: Physiology" (J. P. Filkens and S. M. Reichard, eds.). Plenum, New York, 1981.

6. N. Maehara and M. Ho. Cellular origin of interferon induced by bacterial lipopolysaccharide. *Infect. Immun.* *15:*78-83, 1977.

7. H. B. Fleit and M. Rabinovitch. Production of interferon by *in vitro* derived bone marrow macrophages. *Cell. Immunol.* *57:*495-504, 1981.

8. C. Sorg, C. Neumann, V. Klimetzek, and D. Hannich. Lymphokine-induced modulation of macrophage functions. *In* "Mononuclear Phagocytes, Functional Aspects" (R. Furth, ed.), pp. 539-567. Martinus Nijhoff Publishers, The Hague, 1980.

9. R. W. Fulton and B. D. Rosenquist. *In vitro* interferon production by bovine tissues: Induction with infectious bovine rhinotracheitis virus. *Am. J. Vet. Res.* *37:*1497-1502, 1976.

10. J. A. Armstrong. Semimicro dye binding assay for rabbit interferon. *Appl. Microbiol.* *21:*723-725, 1971.

11. N. H. McManus. Microtiter assay for interferon: Microspectrophotometric quantitation of cytopathic effect. *Appl. Environ. Microbiol.* *31:*35-38, 1976.

12. E. C. Borden and P. H. Leonhardt. A quantitative semimicro, semiautomated colorimetric assay for interferon. *J. Lab. Clin. Med.* *89:*1036-1042, 1977.

13. J. Duvall, A. Khan, N. O. Hill, M. Ground, D. Muntz, and R. Lanius. A computer-assisted micro-dye uptake human interferon assay. *In* "Interferon: Properties and Clinical Uses" (A. Khan, N. O. Hill, and G. L. Dorn, eds.), pp. 529-539. Leland Fikes Foundation Press, Dallas, 1980.

14. L. B. Epstein and N. H. McManus. Macro and microassays for the antiviral effects of human and mouse interferons. *In* "Manual of Clinical Immunology" (N. R. Rose and H. Friedman, eds.), pp. 275-283. American Society of Microbiologists Publications, Washington, 1980.

15. L. B. Epstein and C. J. Epstein. Localization of the gene (AVG) for the antiviral expression of immune and classical interferon to the distal portion of the long arm of chromosome 21. *J. Infect. Dis.* *133:*A56-A62, 1976.

16. J. Weil, L. B. Epstein, and C. J. Epstein. Synthesis of interferon-induced polypeptides in normal and chromosome 21-aneuploid human fibroblasts: Relationship to relative sensitivities in antiviral assays. *J. Interferon Res.* *1*:111-124, 1980.

17. R. L. Martuza, M. R. Proffitt, M. B. Moore, and C. F. Dohan, Jr. Evaporation as a cause of positional differences in cell plating and growth in microtiter plates. *Transplantation 21*:271-273, 1976.

18. H. G. Eisenweiner and M. Keller. Absorbance measurement in cuvettes lying longitudinal to the light beam. *Clin. Chem. 25*:117-121, 1979.

19. L. B. Epstein. Assay of human interferon from lymphocyte macrophage cultures by a virus plaque reduction method. *In* "Manual of Clinical Immunology" (N. R. Rose and H. Friedman, eds.), pp. 120-128. American Society of Microbiologists Publications, Washington, 1976.

64

ENDOGENOUS PYROGEN

Charles A. Dinarello

I. INTRODUCTION

Fever is a well-recognized biological response in all
vertebrates, from fish to humans. The mechanism by which
certain infections, toxins, or immunological reactions cause
fever is through the action of a mediator called endogenous
pyrogen (EP) (1). EP is a small molecular weight protein
that is synthesized by phagocytic cells and seems to have
molecular heterogeneity (2). The substances that induce
phagocytic cells to synthesize EP are called exogenous pyrogens and, although exogenous pyrogens produce fever when injected to severel species, there is no evidence that exogenous pyrogens produce fever by acting on the hypothalamic
thermoregulatory center; rather, these pyrogens cause fever
by activating the host's phagocytic cells resulting in the
production of EP. EP is not found preformed in cells but is
newly synthesized from mRNA and released without significant
storage. *In vitro,* EP appears in the supernatant fluid with-

in 4 - 6 hr and maximal production occurs at 24 hr; thereafter, production is sharply reduced. With few exceptions, EP is not spontaneously produced by phagocytic cells in culture. These exceptions include certain murine and human tumor lines derived from histiocytic lymphomas and Hodgkin's tumors (3,4). In addition, oil-induced (5) or glycogen-induced (6) peritoneal exudate cells will spontaneously release EP into the supernatant fluid, but this is most likely due to activation *in vivo*.

To measure EP in the supernates of stimulated phagocyte cultures, one must inject the supernate into a suitable animal and record core temperature. In every species studied, from *Dispososaurus dorsalis* (desert iguana) (7) to human beings (8, 9), the injection of EP into the homologous species has resulted in a brisk rise in body temperature that follows a short latent period. This early onset fever is the basis of the biological assay for EP. Although there is a radioimmunoassay for human EP (10), it determines EP antigen and not the · biologically active molecule. Fortunately, there is considerable, although not complete, species cross-over response to the fever-inducing property of EPs (11-13). Because of its response to EPs from several unrelated species, the rabbit remains the most widely used assay animal for EP and other pyrogenic substances (14-17). Other species have also been used including the dog, cat, goat, rat, and guinea pig (18-21). Recently, the mouse has been used to assay EP from human and murine sources (22,23), but far less is known about the mouse febrile response to exogenous pyrogens and EP from other species. Table I illustrates the species cross-over response for assay of EP from various sources in different animals.

II. REAGENTS

A. *Endogenous Pyrogen*

The cell sources for the production of EP will vary. Peripheral blood monocytes are separated in sterile, pyrogenfree Ficoll-Hypaque gradients and washed several times in physiologic saline. Peritoneal exudate cells or alveolar macrophages must be carefully removed to avoid contamination by bacteria. Cells should be suspended at concentrations between 1 and 5×10^6 per milliliter in standard culture media that have been tested for sterility as well as for endotoxin in the *Limulus* amebocyte lysate (LAL) test (24). Most important all reagents, glassware, pipettes, and routine solutions must be sterile and also free of endotoxin. The LAL test re-

TABLE I. *Biological Assay of EP*[a]

Source of EP	Human	Nonhuman primates	Goat	Rabbit	Mouse	Rat	Cat	Dog	Guinea pig
Human	+	+		+	+		+		+
Nonhuman primates		+		−		−			
Goat			+	+		+			
Rabbit		+	+	+	+	+	+	−	
Mouse				−	+				
Rat				−		+			
Cat		+		+			+	+	
Dog			+	+			+	+	+
Guinea pig		+		+					+

aData compiled from refs. 11–23 and personal observations (Dinarello and Coceani, 1979).

mains the best way to check for the presence of nanogram quantities of this ubiquitous material. Commercially available
LAL test kits can be purchased from several firms. Serum
sources must also be tested for the presence of endotoxin.
Fetal calf serum may contain small quantities of endotoxin
sufficient to stimulate EP production. Levels as low as 0.1
ng/ml will stimulate EP production thus yielding positive control cultures. The importance of using endotoxin-free reagents and glassware cannot be over emphasized. Glassware
needs to be heated at 180°C for 4 hr in order to render it
endotoxin free. Disposable plastic culture plates and pipettes are endotoxin-free because of the high temperatures
used in the molding process.

B. Rabbit Assay Test for EP

There are several aspects to the rabbit assay for EP that
reduce the unavoidable drawbacks of using an animal assay.
Rabbits should be bred indoors. This allows for more consistent baseline body temperature throughout the year. The type
of rabbit preferred for pyrogen testing is the New Zealand
albino between 2.5 and 3.5 kg. Females are generally more
docile than males, but a consistent sex should be used in
testing since female and male rabbits do not respond equally
to the same dose of EP (25). The restrainers should be wood
or metal with adjustable neck enclosures. Materials like
thick plastic prevent good heat exchange, which is necessary
for rabbit thermoregulation (26). Thermistors, a multichannel
thermometer and an automatic recorder, are required for the
assay (Yellow Springs Instrument Corp. is one of several firms
which provides this equipment).

III. PROCEDURES

A. Production of EP in Vitro

Whether testing for the ability of a certain cell preparation to produce EP or investigating whether a particular substance is capable of inducing EP synthesis, one must have a
"positive" and "negative" control. There are several ways to
stimulate phagocytic cells to produce EP in vitro for a positive result (1). However, the easiest and most dependable is
phagocytosis of heat-killed staphylococci (2). Any culture
of Staphylococcus albus, washed several times, boiled for 30
min and washed in saline will suffice. The optimal concentration is 10-20 bacterial particles per phagocyte. Serum (5-

10%, stored at -70°C) must be added as a source of fresh complement. Phagocytosis is rapid (30 min) at 37°C in a shaking
water bath and can be determined by simple light microscopy.
Thereafter, the suspension can be centrifuged at 200 g and the
cell-pellet resuspended in serum-free medium. For stimulating
monolayers, the staphylococci will settle onto the cellular
layer and be phagocytosed without agitating. Under these conditions, removal of serum and excess bacteria by pouring off
the supernate also removes 25 - 50% of the monolayer. These
can be added back after centrifugation. It is not necessary
to remove the excess bacteria or serum following phagocytosis,
but doing so reduces the development of hypersensitivity to
foreign proteins in the rabbit.

Soluble activators of EP can also be used but these present
problems in the rabbit assay. If endotoxin or other large molecular weight substances are used as stimulants, these may
interfere in the rabbit assay by producing their own fever and
obscure the fever produced by EP. In any case, whatever the
activator used, cultures should be incubated at 37°C for 18 -
24 hr, centrifuged at 2000 g to remove cells and cellular
debris, and stored at 4°C or frozen at -20°C before testing.
Crude EP is stable at 4°C for several months. It is advisable
to add 0.02% sodium azide during storage at 4°C to prevent bacterial contamination.

If the stimulant is dialysable, then it should be removed
before testing for EP in rabbits (27). For dialysis, routine
dialysis tubing should be autoclaved for 30 min in pyrogen-
free water and the inside rinsed with sterile, pyrogen-free
water. Supernates from stimulated cultures can be dialysed
against 0.15 M NaCl or other suitable isotonic buffers at 100
volume excess for 24 hr at 4°C. The material can be removed
from the bag with a sterile needle and syringe through the air
sac of the dialysis membrane. Before testing in rabbits, all
supernates should be cultured for possible bacterial contamination.

B. Rabbit Assay

Rabbits must be trained for 2 - 3 days before being used
for the assay of EP. For each day of training, the rabbits
should remain restrained for periods of 4 - 5 hr and then on
the 3rd or 4th day, rectal probes can be inserted and baseline
temperature recorded. It is best to insert the rectal probe
6 - 8 cm by marking this distance with a centimeter-wide band
of tape on the thermistor. The tape serves as both a marker
for the distance and as an anchor point for fixation to the
tail. Elastic bands or soft wire can be used to fix the thermistor to the tail. The room in which the rabbit assay is to

be performed should be the same temperature and humidity as
the room in which they are housed. The test room should be
quiet and used for testing only. After 2 days of stable baseline temperature, pyrogen-free saline should be injected intravenously into a lateral ear vein to ensure that the rabbits
are well trained and do not get spurious fevers from a non-
pyrogenic substance. All pyrogen testing should be done at
approximately the same time each day. Morning testing (10 AM
- Noon) of rabbits produces more consistent results than late
afternoon (28); this has been observed in other species as
well (11). All injections should be as a rapid bolus and not
exceed 5 ml for a 2.5 kg rabbit. The ideal volume is 1.0 ml;
using larger volumes, it is necessary to warm the sample to
37°C to prevent injection hypothermia. The reproducibility of
the test depends upon the accuracy of the thermometer, placement of the thermistors, function of the recorder, the proper
training of the rabbits, and environmental control of the test
room. In addition, the skill of the person injecting the
rabbit plays a role. Rabbits with unstable baseline temperatures, i.e., varying more than 0.3°C for 1 hr should not be
used, and rabbits with baseline rectal temperatures greater
than 39.6° or less than 38.0°C should also not be used. Normal rabbit rectal temperatures vary between these points for
indoor bred rabbits.

IV. CALCULATION OF DATA

     Individual rabbit response are calculated as a function of
temperature versus time. It is important to record rectal
temperature at least every 15 min. Depending on the time interval of the recording device, body temperatures are plotted
for 1 hr before and 3 hr after the injection of the material.
There are two ways to calculate the amount of fever: Integration of the area under the fever curve or determination of the
peak rise above baseline temperature. Several studies have
shown that there is a direct correlation between the peak rise
and the area under the fever curve (28) and clearly the latter
is faster and less likely to yield technical errors. A recorder which registers rectal temperature more often will clearly
yield the best data, because it is likely to record the peak
temperature when it occurs although intervals of 12 min are
acceptable.
     In order to quantitate the amount of EP in a particular
supernate, a dose response curve must be obtained. Rabbits,
like other mammals, have a thermal ceiling and increasingly
larger amounts of EP do not produce more fever. There is a
sensitive section of the dose-response curve in rabbits to EP

from either human, rabbit or guinea pig sources. Peak temperature levels (peak fever) above baseline between 0.4° and
0.8°C fall on the straight or proportional section of the
dose-response curve. Peak fevers above 1.0°C should not be
used to quantitate EP. Between six and eight rabbits need to
be employed for a two-point dose-response curve. In this assay, the rabbits are divided into two groups: one set receives an established volume and the other set half or double
that quantity. A sensible concentration in an unknown sample
is the supernate from 5×10^6 mononuclear cells. It is advisable to report data as the amount of fever produced from the
supernate of a specified number of cells and not the volume.
If the mean fever peak of one of the two groups of rabbits
lies between 0.4° and 0.8°C, then quantitation is possible.
Otherwise, the amount of EP injected must be increased or reduced until the febrile responses lie in the sensitive portion
of the dose-response curve. For example, if two different
stimulants are being tested for their ability to induce EP
production from monocytes, then the data are expressed as the
mean fever peak produced in 3 - 4 rabbits, injected with supernates from substance "X" as compared to the mean fever peak
produced with the supernate from "Y" for the same number of
cells. If there is a difference between the potency of these
two activators, then the mean peak fever can be submitted to
statistical analysis comparing the means from each group given
the standard error of the mean. See Fig. 1 as an example.

V. BIOASSAY: CRITICAL COMMENTS

     The rabbit pyrogen test is subject to individual differ-
ences in rabbit responses to the same quantity of EP. This is
partially overcome by using at least 6 - 8 rabbits in a two-
point dose-response curve. Aspects of this bioassay, which
decreases its reproducibility, include traumatic injections,
extravasation of injected materials, a rectal thermistor which
slips out, and more than one injection per day. Other factors,
however, yield data which are uninterpretable. These include
injection of contaminated materials, the presence of pyrogenic
activators that were not removed or not degraded, and development of hypersensitivity to the injected serum and cellular
products. These interfere with the fever produced by EP. Hypersensitivity reactions, endotoxin, and other exogenous pyrogens produce their own characteristic fevers. Thus, part of
the critical assessment of this assay is observation of the
individual fever curve itself. EP produces a rapid-onset
fever, which peaks 45 - 60 min following injection and temperature returns to baseline after 1.5 to 2 hr after its peak

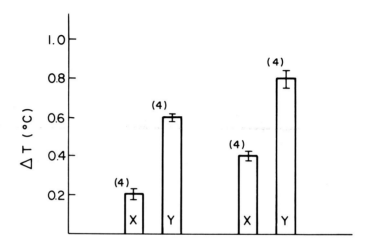

Fig. 1. Mean fever peaks above baseline (± SEM) in rabbits intravenously injected with the supernates from 5×10^6 human mononuclear cells incubated with either activator X or Y. The numbers in parentheses indicate the number of rabbits injected.

elevation. Endotoxin contamination or other pyrogenic materials in the supernate produce a superimposed fever (by inducing the rabbits's own EP production), which peaks 90 min after injection and often is biphasic with a second peak occurring after 3 hr (29). Rabbits which develop hypersensitivity to the cellular or serum proteins from other species will also develop fever (30). Like endotoxin fever, this is also a delayed fever. Figure 2 illustrates a typical EP fever, an endotoxin fever, and hypersensitivity fever to human serum albumin. The presence of either of these other febrile responses would clearly interfere with the quantitation of EP.

Acknowledgment

The author wishes to thank Dr. Sheldon M. Wolff for his helpful comments. Supported by NIH Grant RO1 AI 15614.

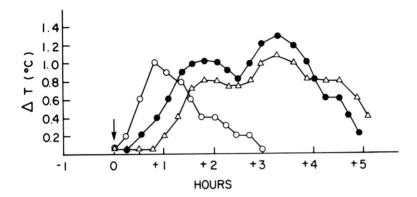

Fig. 2. Mean fever in rabbits injected with various pyrogens: (o——o), EP, (●——●), 5 ng E. Coli endotoxin; (Δ——Δ), human serum albumin in rabbits sensitized to this protein.

REFERENCES

1. C. A. Dinarello and S. M. Wolff. Pathogenesis of fever in man. *N. Engl. J. Med. 298:*607-612, 1978.
2. C. A. Dinarello, N. P. Goldin, and S. M. Wolff. Demonstration and characterization of two distinct human leukocytic pyrogens. *J. Exp. Med. 139:*1369-1381, 1974.
3. P. Bodel. Spontaneous pyrogen production by mouse histiocytic and myelomonocytic tumor cell lines *in vitro. J. Exp. Med. 147:*1503-1516, 1978.
4. P. Bodel. Pyrogen release *in vitro* by lymphoid tissue from patients with Hodgkin's disease. *Yale J. Biol. Med. 47:*101-112, 1974.
5. H. H. Hahn, D. C. Char, W. B. Postel, and W. B. Wood, Jr. Studies on the pathogenesis of fever. XV. The production of endogenous pyrogen by peritoneal macrophages. *J. Exp. Med. 126:*385-394, 1967.
6. P. B. Beeson. Temperature-elevating effect of a substance obtained from polymorphonuclear leucocytes. *J. Clin Invest. 27:*524, 1948.

7. H. A. Bernheim and M. J. Kluger. Endogenous pyrogen-like substance produced by reptiles. *J. Physiol.* *267:* 659-666, 1977.

8. W. I. Cranston, F. Goodale, Jr., E. S. Snell, and F. Wendt. The role of leukocytes in the initial action of bacterial pyrogens in man. *Clin. Sci.* Vol. 15, 219-226, 1956.

9. E. S. Snell, F. Goodale, Jr., F. Wendt, and W. I. Cranston. Properties of human endogenous pyrogen. *Clin. Sci.* *16:*615-626, 1957.

10. C. A. Dinarello, L. Renfer, and S. M. Wolff. Human leukocytic pyrogen: Purification and development of a radioimmunoassay. *Proc. Natl. Acad. Sci. USA* *74:*4624-4627, 1977.

11. M. Perlow, C. A. Dinarello, and S. M. Wolff. A primate model for the study of human fever. *J. Infect. Dis.* *132:*157-164, 1975.

12. J. M. Lipton, C. A. Dinarello, and J. I. Kennedy. Fever produced in the squirrel monkey by human leukocytic pyrogen. *Proc. Soc. Exp. Biol. Med.* *160:*426-428, 1979.

13. C. A. Dinarello, L. Renfer, and S. M. Wolff. The production of antibody against human leukocytic pyrogen. *J. Clin. Invest.* *60:*465-472, 1977.

14. P. Bodel and E. Atkins. Human leukocyte pyrogen producing fever in rabbits. *Proc. Soc. Exp. Biol. Med.* *121:*943-946, 1966.

15. E. Atkins and L. Francis. Pathogenesis of fever in delayed hypersensitivity: Factors influencing release of pyrogen-inducing lymphokines. *Infec. Immun.* *21:*806-812, 1978.

16. D. L. Bornstein and J. W. Woods. Species specificity of leukocytic pyrogens. *J. Exp. Med.* *130:*707-721, 1969.

17. D. Borsook, H. Laburn, and D. Mitchell. The febrile responses in rabbits and rats to leukocyte pyrogens of different species. *J. Physiol.* *279:*113-120, 1978.

18. T. Fukuda and K. Nurata. Species difference in the febrile and the leukocytic response to endotoxin: Endogenous hepatic pyrogen in dogs. *Jpn. J. Physiol.* *15:*169-179, 1965.

19. A. S. Van Miert and A. Atmakusuma. Fever induced with leukocytic or bacterial pyrogen in young and adult goats. *J. Comp. Pathol.* *81:*119-127, 1971.

20. R. F. Kampschmidt and H. F. Upchurch. Some effects of endotoxin and leukocytic pyrogen on the body temperature of rats. *Proc. Soc. Exp. Biol. Med.* *131:*864-867, 1969.

21. C. M. Blatteis. Comparison of endotoxin and leukocytic pyrogen pyrogenicity in newborn guinea pigs. *J. Appl. Physiol.* *42:*355-361, 1977.

22. P. Bodel and H. Miller. Pyrogen from mouse macrophages causes fever in mice. *Proc. Soc. Exp. Biol. Med.* *151:* 93-96, 1976.

23. R. J. Falk. The isolation of a mouse leukocytic pyrogen demonstrating its effect on the circadian temperature cycle of conditioned mice. *Lab. Invest.* *15:*1761-1767, 1966.

24. R. J. Elin and S. M. Wolff. Nonspecificity of the *Limulus* amebocyte lysate test: Positive reactions with polynucleotides and proteins. *J. Infect. Dis.* *128:*349-352, 1973.

25. J. M. Lipton and C. B. Ticknor. Influence of sex and age on febrile responses to peripheral and central administration of pyrogens in the rabbit. *J. Physiol.* *295:*263-272, 1979.

26. R. W. Hill and J. H. Veghte. Jackrabbit ears: Surface temperature and vascular responses. *Science 194:*436-438, 1976.

27. C. A. Dinarello, R. J. Elin, L. Chedid, and S. M. Wolff. The pyrogenicity of synthetic adjuvants muramyl dipeptide and two structural analogues. *J. Infect. Dis.* *138:*760-767, 1978.

28. E. S. Allison, W. I. Cranston, G. W. Duff, R. H. Luff, and M. D. Rawlins. The bioassay of human endogenous pyrogen. *Clin. Sci. Mol. Med.* *45:*449-458, 1973.

29. S. M. Wolff, J. H. Mulholland, and S. B. Ward. Quantitative aspects of the pyrogenic responses of rabbits to endotoxin. *J. Lab. Clin. Med.* *65:*268-276, 1965.

30. R. K. Root and S. M. Wolff. Pathogenetic mechanisms in experimental immune fever. *J. Exp. Med.* *128:*309-323, 1968.

65

PROSTAGLANDINS

John L. Humes

I. GENERAL INTRODUCTION

Mononuclear phagocytic cells synthesize and release a
series of arachidonic acid (AA) oxygenation products. We
have reported that resident mouse peritoneal macrophages,
when exposed to inflammatory stimuli in cell culture, synthesize and release prostaglandins (PG), principally PGE_2 and
6-keto-$PGF_{1\alpha}$, the stable metabolite of PGI_2 (1, 2). Other
AA oxygenation products, including $PGF_{2\alpha}$, thromboxanes, and
hydroxy fatty acids, have also been reported to be produced
by these cells (3, 4, 5).

The deacylation of cellular phospholipids to liberate free
AA initiates the synthesis of these various AA oxygenation
products. The subsequent oxygenation of this fatty acid proceeds by two independent pathways now termed the AA cascade
(Fig. 1). The cyclooxygenase branch of the cascade results
in the formation of the stable primary PGs, i.e., PGs of the
E, F, and D series. In addition, thromboxane B_2 (TXB_2) and

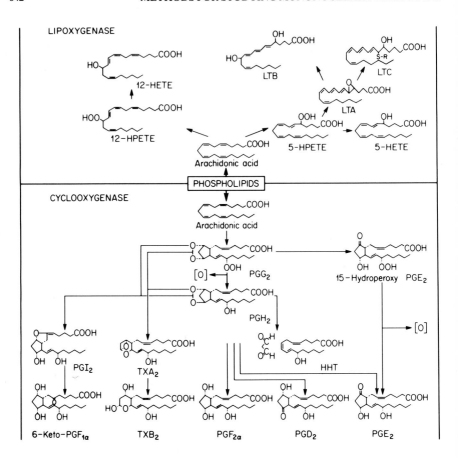

Fig. 1.   The arachidonic acid cascade.

6-keto-PGF$_{1\alpha}$, the stable metabolites of labile TXA$_2$ and PGI$_2$, respectively, are formed through this pathway. All of these products arise from two labile endoperoxide intermediates, PGG$_2$ and PGH$_2$. Nonsteroidal antiinflammatory drugs, such as aspirin and indomethacin by interacting with the cyclooxygenase-peroxidase, inhibit the formation of these intermediates and thereby inhibit the synthesis of the primary PGs, 6-keto-PGF$_{1\alpha}$, and TXB$_2$. Also, an oxygen-centered radical [O] is concomitantly produced in the peroxidatic conversions of PGG$_2$ to PGH$_2$ or 15-hydroperoxy-PGE$_2$ to PGE$_2$ (6).

In contrast, AA can also be oxygenated by indomethacin/aspirin insensitive lipoxygenase pathways. One lipoxygenase branch of the AA cascade results in the synthesis of 12-L-hydroperoxy-5,8,10,14-eicosatetranoic acid (12-HPETE) and the corresponding 12-hydroxy fatty acid (12-HETE). Recently, 12-HETE has been shown to be chemotactic for polymorphonuclear leukocytes (7). Alternatively, AA can be oxidized by another indomethacin/aspirin insensitive lipoxygenase to yield a series of 20-carbon fatty acids with one or two oxygen moieties and containing three conjugated double bonds (8). The term leukotriene has recently been proposed for these compounds (LTA, LTB, and LTC) (9). Recently, SRS-A has been shown to be leukotriene C, with R being the thioester of reduced glutathione (10).

A discussion of the physiological, pathological, modulatory, and pharmacological effects of the stable oxygenation products of the AA cascade is beyond the scope of this article. However, the reader should appreciate that the stable products have been shown in many cases to be less active than their corresponding labile precursor(s). As an example, PGI_2 is quite unstable with a 1/2 life of <5 min at $37°C$ and pH 7.4, yet this compound is extremely potent in preventing platelet aggregation. Its stable metabolite 6-keto-$PGF_{1\alpha}$ is without effect. Similarly, TXA_2, with a 1/2 life of 0.5 min, is a potent inducer of platelet aggregation, whereas TXB_2, its stable metabolite, is devoid of this activity.

These various AA oxygenation products released by cells in culture can be measured in one of several ways: (1) bioassays; (2) gas - liquid chromatography mass spectrometry; (3) release of radiolabeled products; and (4) radioimmunoassay. Only the bioassay methods allow an estimation of the labile, and thus perhaps most interesting, components. The principal advantage of bioassays is that they measure a definite physiological activity and thus can measure the labile intermediates formed in the AA cascade. It was only by the use of bioassay techniques that the discoveries of TXA_2 and PGI_2 were made (11, 12). Most of these methods are based on the potent muscle contractile/ relaxant properties of these compounds. In addition, platelet aggregation has been used as a bioassay technique for products of AA metabolism. Many of these preparations are quite sensitive and require only submicrogram amounts of the test substances. The specificity can be markedly improved by assaying the test substance on a combination of preparations, each having a different reaction to the known standard compounds. In addition, various pharmacological receptor antagonists, notably antihistamines, α- and β-adrenergic antagonists, and cholinergic antagonists, are added to further increase specificity. However, the overwhelming disadvantage of these methods is their low sample capacity. The reader is directed to an excellent review of various bioassay techniques for AA metabolites (13).

The combination of gas - liquid chromatography coupled with mass spectrometry permits the most definite statement of compound structure. However, relatively large quantities of sample, i.e., >10 μg, are generally needed and the actual sample capacity is limited. Sample preparation is also time consuming since they must first be extracted, partially separated, and subsequently derivatized. Also deuterium-labeled PGS, used as internal standards, are not readily available and must be prepared.

This report will detail the radiorelease (the release of radiolabeled products from radiolabeled cells) and radioimmunoassay methods as used in our laboratory. Both of these techniques are especially applicable for the detection and quantitation of PGs in cell culture. The former method allows the identification but not quantitation of a broad spectrum of radioactive AA metabolites. The latter method is complimentary to the former in that it allows precise quantitation of the individual AA oxygenation products.

II. RADIORELEASE METHOD

[^{3}H] or [^{14}C]AA is efficiently incorporated into cellular phospholipids of a variety of cells and tissue preparations. Resident mouse peritoneal macrophages, the cells used in these studies, incorporate considerable amounts of [^{3}H]AA over 3 - 4 hr incubation periods in cell culture (2). Other cellular preparations including platelets, lymphocytes, fibroblasts, as well as intact rabbit hearts and kidneys, have been shown to incorporate useful amounts of either [^{14}C] or [^{3}H]AA into cellular phospholipids for subsequent ^{14}C- or ^{3}H-labeled product synthesis and release (14 - 17). The primary advantage of this method is that it measures *de novo* synthesis of an AA oxygenation product and not the absolute amount of the product. In many cases this measurement of the change in *de novo* product synthesis is of greater magnitude than the corresponding measurement of the total amount of product. In addition, this method evaluates the synthesis from endogenous, and thus relevant, substrate pools.

Another advantage of the radiorelease method is its high sample capacity. In our laboratory, we find that the radiorelease method has a greater sample through-put than corresponding analysis by radioimmunoassay. In addition, the investigator can conveniently quantitate more than one AA oxygenation product as the product derived from both the cyclooxygenase or lipoxygenase enzymic pathways and can be separated one from the other in a variety of chromatographic systems. Clearly the flexibility of being able to monitor conveniently more than one product is an advantage not easily attained by the other assay methods. As the identification of the released radiolabeled product is assessed by comparing its mobility with authentic standards, this method is not an absolute criteria of product identification. The nature of the product should be further verified by other independent assay methods, such as radioim-

munoassay. Positive structure identification must be proven
by mass-spectral analysis when sufficient quantities of the
product are available.

A. Reagents

Male SW/ICR specific pathogen-free mice are purchased from
Hilltop Lab Animals, Inc., Scotdale, Pennsylvania, and maintained on a standard pellet diet and water ad libitum.

The cell culture reagents are purchased from Grand Island
Biological Co., Grand Island, New York. The porcine serum is
inactivated by heating at 56°C for 30 min (HIPS). Zymosan is
from ICN/K and K Labs, Plainfield, New York. The zymosan particles are suspended in phosphate-buffered saline (PBS), boiled,
and centrifuged 3 times. The final pellet is suspended in PBS
at a concentration of 20 mg/ml and stored frozen. The stock solution is diluted in culture medium (usually 1:10) and sonicated
immediately before addition to the cell cultures. Nunclon culture dishes, 60 mm, are from Vangard International, Inc., Neptune, New Jersey. Gentamicin is from the Schering Corp.,
Kenilworth, New Jersey.

[5,6,8,9,11,12,14,15-^{3}H]arachidonic acid, specific activity
62 Ci/mmol, is obtained from New England Nuclear Corporation,
Boston, Massachusetts. The hexane solution, 100 µCi/ml, is
stored under N_2 at -20°C and is stable for at least four weeks.

Reagent grade solvents from J. T. Baker, Phillipsburg, New
Jersey are used for extractions and chromatography. The
chromatography is routinely performed on Whatman SG-81 silicic
acid impregnated chromatographic paper from Ace Scientific,
Linden, New Jersey. The sheets, 46 × 57 cm, are cut into
2 × 28 cm strips. PGE_2, $PGF_{2\alpha}$ (Ono Pharmaceuticals, Osaka,
Japan), and arachidonic acid (Sigma, St. Louis, Missouri) are
used as internal chromatographic standards. A methanol solution
of these standards containing 3 mg PGE_2, 3 mg AA, and 5 mg PGE_2
per ml is prepared and stored at -20°C.

B. Procedures

1. Cell Culture

Resident mouse peritoneal macrophages are collected by peritoneal lavage from untreated pathogen-free mice and cultured as
previously described (2). Briefly, the lavaging medium is M 199
containing 1% heat-inactivated porcine serum (HIPS), 100 U of
penicillin and streptomycin/ml and 20 U heparin/ml. The cells
are plated at approximately 5 × 10^6 cells/50 mm culture dish and
incubated for 2 hr at 37°C in 5% CO_2 in air. The nonadherent

cells are removed by washing the adherent cell sheets with five 5-ml volumes of phosphate-buffered saline (PBS) using a mechanized cell washing apparatus designed by P. D. Wightman of this laboratory. The adherent cells are maintained overnight in 4-ml M 199 containing 10% HIPS and 100 µg gentamicin/ml.

2. Prelabeling Macrophage Phospholipids with [^{3}H]AA

After the overnight incubation, the cells are washed with PBS as described above and then incubated for 4 hr with 1 µCi [^{3}H]AA in 4 ml M 199 containing 1% HIPS. This medium is prepared by evaporating the [^{3}H]AA hexane stock solution to dryness under nitrogen and dissolving the material in DMSO at 1000 times the desired concentration. The DMSO solution is subsequently diluted 1:1000 in M 199 containing 1% HIPS to yield the desired concentration of 1 µCi/4 ml. This amount of DMSO, 0.1% has no effect in this system. Under these conditions the incorporated [^{3}H]AA is primarily found in cellular phospholipids (phosphatidylcholine and phosphatidylethanolamine) and triglycerides (2).

3. [^{3}H]PG Release

After 4 hr the adherent cells are washed as previously described to remove unincorporated [^{3}H]AA. Two ml of M 199 devoid of serum but containing the various stimuli, such as zymosan, is added. Under these conditions, the release of [^{3}H]PGE$_2$ and [^{3}H]6-keto-PGF$_{1\alpha}$ is linear for 6 - 8 hr. At the termination of the experiment, usually 4 hr, the media are collected.

4. Extraction and Chromatography of [^{3}H]AA Oxidation Products

The culture media are acidified to 0.03 M with citric acid and PGE$_2$ (50 µg), PGF$_{2\alpha}$ (30 µg), and AA (30 µg) are added (10 µl of the methanolic stock solution). The acidified media are then extracted with three successive 3-ml aliquots of chloroform/methanol (2:1, v:v). The combined organic phases are washed with two successive 2-ml aliquots of methanol water (2:1, v:v) and evaporated to dryness under a stream of N$_2$ at 45°C. The residue is dissolved in 50 µl of ethylacetate/methanol (3:1, v:v) and quantitatively applied to 2 × 28 cm strips of SG-81 paper. The strips are developed by descending chromatography with ethyl acetate/acetic acid (99:1, v:v). In some experiments, after the chromatograms are developed in this system, the strips are redeveloped in the same direction with n-hexane/diethyl ether/acetic acid (75:25:1 by vol.). The internal PG and AA standards are detected by exposure to I$_2$ vapor.

In some experiments the radioactivity profile of the entire chromatogram is determined by scanning with a Packard 7201 radiochromatogram scanner. An alternative is to cut the chromatogram with scissors into 0.5-cm segments. The radioactivity of each individual segment is determined by counting the segment in 10-ml Aquasol in a Packard 3225 liquid scintillation spectrometer. In most experiments the area corresponding to PGE_2 standard is cut out and counted. In a similar manner, other areas of the chromatogram, defined by their relative mobility to the added internal standards (PGE_2, $PGF_{2\alpha}$, AA) are cut out and counted.

D. Radioscan of [^3H]Arachidonic Acid Oxygenation Products

Resident mouse peritoneal macrophages are labeled with [^3H]AA for 4 hr. As shown in Fig. 2b, the addition of 50 µg zymosan/ml for 4 hr caused the release of a variety of ^3H-labeled components. The major ^3H-components synthesized were [^3H]PGE_2 and [^3H]6-keto-$PGF_{1\alpha}$ (6KF). Smaller amounts of labeled components cochromatographic with HETE, as well as other unidentified components more polar than this hydroxy fatty acid are also formed. Indomethacin, 10 µg/ml, completely inhibited [^3H[PGE_2 and [^3H]6-keto-$PGF_{1\alpha}$ synthesis (Fig. 2c). In the absence of zymosan no defined [^3H]AA oxygenation products are released from the cells (Fig. 2a).

III. RADIOIMMUNOASSAY

The first application of radioimmunoassay (RIA) techniques for measuring PGs was introduced by Levine and VanVunakis in 1970 (18). Since that time the use of this method has increased and a large literature now exists on the use of RIA to measure PGs and PG metabolites from a variety of cells, tissues, and body fluids. The reader is directed to the excellent review by Granström and Kindahl describing the use of RIA for measuring PGs and other AA oxygenation products (19).

RIA are exquisitively sensitive having limits of detection as low as 100 pg. In addition, these techniques have a large sample capacity. However, the poor specificity of RIA as applied to PG measurements continue to be a major drawback. Although the specificity of the antibody is usually very high with respect to the cross-reactivity with known PGs, the data obtained with RIA techniques suggest that unknown substances in the samples may interfere. In many cases the absolute values obtained by RIA techniques have been considerably greater than

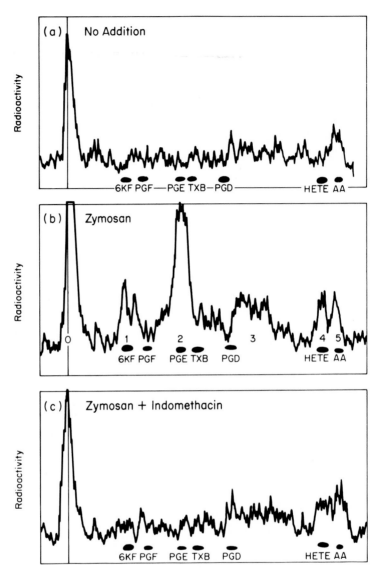

*Fig. 2. Radioscan of released arachidonic acid oxygenation
products. The organic extracts of the culture media are
chromatographed on SG-81 paper with ethyl acetate/acetic acid
(99:1, v:v). The papers are dried and then rechromatographed
in the same direction with n-hexane/diethyl-ether/acetic acid
(75:25:1 by vol.). The entire chromatogram is scanned with a
Packard 7201 radiochromatogram scanner. Reproduced from
Bonney et al. (2) with permission.*

corresponding values obtained by gas - liquid chromatography/
mass spectrometry.

To achieve a high degree of reproducibility, it is obliga-
tory to use exclusively disposable labware and Nanograde or
spectrograde solvents for extractions. To achieve utmost accuracy, the samples should be purified on silicic acid volumes
or thin-layer chromatography prior to the RIA. Every conceiv-
able control incubation (i.e., medium alone and test substances,
etc.) should be analyzed. By appreciating these specificity
pitfalls, due to the high sensitivity of the RIA technique, one
can obtain useful and meaningful PG mass analysis.

Many radioactive ligands are commercially available. Tri-
tiated PGE_1, PGE_2, $PGF_{1\alpha}$, $PGF_{2\alpha}$, TXB_2, and 6-keto-$PGF_{1\alpha}$ with
high specific activity are available from New England Nuclear,
Boston, Massachusetts. Antisera and in some cases complete
kits for analysis of primary PGs can be purchased from various
suppliers.

A. Reagents

Nanograde methanol, acetone, and ethyl acetate are from
Mallinkrodt, St. Louis, Missouri. Silica gel thin layer
chromatography plates 250 μm are from Analtech, Newark, Delaware. The plates are prewashed with ethyl acetate immediately
prior to use. Antiserum to PGE_2, lot 61-335, is from Miles
Laboratories, Elkart, Indiana. The lyophilized preparation is
reconstituted with 8 ml PET buffer containing 0.1% gelatin.
The PET buffer is 10 mM potassium phosphate, pH 7.3, containing
1 mM ethylenediaminetetraacetic acid disodium salt and 0.25 mM
thimerasol.

$[5,6-^3H]PGE_2$, specific activity 80-100 Ci/mmol, was obtained from New England Nuclear Corp., Boston, Massachusetts.
A $[^3H]PGE_2$ trace solution containing approximately 20,000
cpm/0.1 ml PET buffer containing 0.1% gelatin is prepared.
Unlabeled PGE_2 standards are prepared in methanol so that 50 μl
aliquots will contain 50 - 1000 pg.

Norit A charcoal is from Ace Scientific, Linden, New Jersey
and Dextran T-70 was from Pharmacia, Sweden. The dextran-
coated charcoal suspension is prepared as previously described
(20). Briefly, 3 gm Norit A charcoal is suspended in 100 ml
0.25% Dextran T-70 in PET buffer. The charcoal is allowed to
settle out of solution and the supernatant fluid is removed by
aspiration. This settling process is repeated two additional
times and the charcoal finally suspended in 20 ml PET buffer.
This stock solution is subsequently diluted with PET buffer
(usually a 1:10 dilution) so that 1 ml of the diluted suspension
will remove >95% of the unbound $[^3H]PGE_2$ without appreciably removing the $[^3H]PGE_2$ bound to the antibody.

B. Procedures

  1. Cell Culture

   Resident mouse peritoneal macrophages are isolated and
maintained in cell culture as previously described except that
the [^{3}H]AA is omitted. At the termination of the experiment
the media are collected.

  2. Extraction and Purification of PGs for RIA

   The culture medium is acidified to 0.03 M with citric acid
and ∿5000 cpm [^{3}H]PGE$_2$ is added as a recovery standard. The
samples are extracted with three successive 3-ml aliquots of
ethyl acetate. The combined organic phases were backwashed
with two successive 1-ml aliquots of water and evaporated to
dryness under a stream of nitrogen at 40°C.
   The sample residues are dissolved in 50 μl ethyl acetate/
methanol (3:1) and quantitatively applied to 1 cm lanes of a
silica gel thin layer chromatographic plate. On separate lanes,
well separated from the lanes containing the samples, 10 μg each
of PGE$_2$ and PGF$_{2\alpha}$ are spotted. The plate is developed 15 cm
with ethyl acetate/acetone/acetic acid (90:10:1). The lanes
containing the samples are covered with glassine paper and the
exposed lanes containing the PG standards are sprayed with a
solution of 2% KMnO$_4$ in 1% Na$_2$CO$_3$ to visualize the PG standards.
The silica gel from the area corresponding to the standard is
removed and added to 0.5 ml water. The silica - gel - water
mixture is extracted with two successive 2-ml aliquots of ethyl
acetate and the combined ethyl acetate phase is evaporated to
dryness under nitrogen at 45°C. The residues are dissolved in
methanol for radioimmunoassay. An aliquot is counted for the
recovery of the added [^{3}H]PGE$_2$ standard. The recovery through
this procedure is routinely 50 - 70%.

  3. Radioimmunoassays

   The radioimmunoassays for PGE are performed by the method
of Orczyk and Behrman (21). Briefly, aliquots of the methanolic
sample solutions as well as aliquots of the methanolic PGE$_2$
standards are evaporated to dryness under nitrogen. The samples
and standards are incubated 30 min with 0.1 ml of the antisera
solution at room temperature. The [^{3}H]PGE$_2$ trace solution,
0.1 ml, is then added and the mixtures incubated overnight at
4°C. The separation of antibody-bound [^{3}H]PGE$_2$ from the unbound [^{3}H]PGE$_2$ is achieved by adding 1 ml of the diluted
dextran-coated charcoal suspension. The charcoal suspension
and assay tubes are maintained at 4°C for this operation. The
assay tubes are mixed, incubated for 5 min at 4°C, and then

centrifuged at $4°C$ at 4000 g for 15 min. The supernatant phases, containing the antibody-bound-PGE, are decanted into 9-ml Aquasol and the radioactivity determined by liquid scintillation spectrophotometry. The resultant data are analyzed by Scatchard analysis on a Wang 2200 computer.

IV. CONCLUDING REMARKS

Cultures containing 5×10^6 resident peritoneal macrophages are prelabeled with [^{3}H]AA and subsequently challenged for 4 hr with zymosan as described in Section II. Sister cultures are maintained in an identical fashion except that [^{3}H]AA was omitted. The medium is collected and analyzed for PGE_2 by both radiorelease and RIA techniques. As shown in Table I, the zymosan induced increase in PGE_2 synthesis and release was approximately equal as evaluated by both methods.

Macrophages maintained in cell culture constitute a useful model in which to study the AA cascade at the cellular level. Resident mouse peritoneal macrophages synthesize and release large amounts of PGE_2 when exposed in culture to various inflammatory stimuli such as zymosan, phorbol myristate acetate, and antigen-antibody complexes (1, 22, 23). The synthesis and release of PGE_2, as well as the other stable cyclooxygenase products elicited by these agents, is inhibited by both nonsteroidal and steroidal antiinflammatory agents. The nonsteroidal drugs inhibit the cyclooxygenation of AA, whereas the steroidal agents inhibit the deacylation of AA from phospholipid stores.

It has been clearly demonstrated that PGs of the E series modulate both lymphocyte function and proliferation (24, 25). Consistent with these observations, inhibitors of cyclooxygenase have been shown to stimulate mitogen-driven thymidine incorporation in unfractionated spleen cell suspensions. Thus it would appear that cyclooxygenase-derived products from adherent macrophages may act alone or in concert with other soluble mediators to modulate and control immune function.

In addition to the products derived from the cyclooxygenase pathways, products derived from the lipoxygenase pathways are becoming of increasing biological interest. 12-HETE has been shown to be chemotactic for human leukocytes and is produced by mouse peritoneal macrophages (5, 7). It is reasonable to speculate that other lipoxygenase products with interesting biologic activities will be found to be produced by mononuclear phagocytic cells.

In our laboratory we find the radiorelease method to be especially useful as it has large sample capacity and evaluates

TABLE I. *Zymosan Stimulates PGE Synthesis and Release from Resident Mouse Peritoneal Macrophages as Evaluated by Both Radiorelease and RIA Methods[a]*

	Radiorelease (cpm µg DNA)	-Fold increase	(ng/µg DNA)	-Fold Increase
No additions	18 ± 2	1	0.19 ± 0.09	1
Zymosan 50 µg/ml	349 ± 22	19	4.8 ± 0.7	25
Zymosan 300 µg/ml	1053 ± 56	58	9.5 ± 1.1	50

[a]*The DNA content was 17 µg/culture. The incubation was for 4 hr.*

de novo product synthesis. The method is particularly suitable for pharmacological studies concerning the regulation of the AA cascade. However, this method does not yield absolute product amounts or the definite proof of structure. Thus to further characterize the PGE_2 released by resident mouse peritoneal macrophages, we employ RIA to quantify the mass of PGE as well as gas - liquid chromatography mass spectrometry to prove the structure of this component. Only by such a combination of various analytical techniques will the regulation, identity, and function(s) of the various products of the AA cascade be fully appreciated.

REFERENCES

1. J. L. Humes, R. J. Bonney, L. Pelus, M. E. Dahlgren, S. Sadowski, F. A. Kuehl, Jr., and P. Davies. Macrophages synthesize and release prostaglandins in response to inflammatory stimuli. *Nature 269*: 149-151, 1977.
2. R. J. Bonney, P. D. Wightman, P. Davies, S. J. Sadowski, F. A. Kuehl, Jr., and J. L. Humes. Regulation of prostaglandin synthesis and of the selective release of lysosomal hydrolases by mouse peritoneal macrophages. *Biochem. J. 176*: 433-442, 1978.
3. D. Gordon, M. A. Bray, and J. Morley. Control of lymphokine secretion by prostaglandins. *Nature 262*: 401-402, 1976.
4. K. Brune, M. Colatt, H. Kalin, and B. A. Peskar. Pharmacological control of prostaglandin and thromboxane release from macrophages. *Nature 274*: 261-263, 1978.
5. M. Rigaud, J. Durand, and J. C. Breton. Transformation of

arachidonic acid into 12-hydroxy-5,8,10,14-eicosatetraenoic acid by mouse peritoneal macrophages. *Biochim. Biophys. Acta 573*: 408-412, 1979.

6. R. W. Egan, J. Paxton, and F. A. Kuehl, Jr. Mechanism for irreversible self-deactivation of prostaglandin synthetase. *J. Biol. Chem. 251*: 7329-7335, 1976.

7. E. Goetzl and R. R. Gorman. Chemotactic and chemokinetic stimulation of human eosinophil and neutrophil polymorphonuclear leukocytes by 12-L-5-8-10-heptadecatrienoic acid (HHT). *J. Immunol. 120*: 526-531, 1978.

8. P. Borgeat and B. Samuelsson. Metabolism of arachidonic acid in polymorphonuclear leukocytes. *J. Biol. Chem. 254*: 7865-7869, 1979.

9. B. Samuelsson, P. Borgeat, S. Hammarström, and R. C. Murphy. Introduction of a nomenclature: Leukotrienes. *Prostaglandins 17*: 785-787, 1979.

10. S. Hammarström, R. C. Murphy, B. Samuelsson, D. A. Clark, C. Mioskowski, and E. J. Corey. Structure of leukotriene C identification of the amino acid part. *Biochem. Biophys. Res. Commm 91*: 1266-1272, 1979.

11. M. Hamberg, J. Svensson, and B. Samuelsson. Thromboxanes: A new group of biologically active compounds derived from prostaglandin endoperoxides. *Proc. Nat. Acad. Sci. USA 72*: 2994-2998, 1975.

12. S. Moncada, R. Gryglewski, S. Bunting, and J. R. Vane. An enzyme isolated from arteries transforms prostaglandin endoperoxide to an unstable substance that inhibits platelet aggregation. *Nature 263*: 663-665, 1976.

13. S. Moncada, S. R. Ferreira, and J. R. Vane. Bioassay of prostaglandins and biologically active substances derived from arachidonic acid. *In* "Advances in Prostaglandin and Thromboxane Research," Vol. 5 (J. C. Frölich, ed.), pp. 211-236. Raven Press, New York, 1978.

14. T. K. Bills, J. B. Smith, and M. J. Silver. Metabolism of [14C] arachidonic acid by human platelets. *Biochim. Biophys. Acta 424*: 303-314, 1976.

15. C. W. Parker, W. F. Stenson, M. G. Huber, and J. P. Kelly. Formation of thromboxane B_2 and hydroxyarachidonic acids in purified human lymphocytes in the presence and absence of PHA. *J. Immunol. 122*: 1572-1577, 1979.

16. S.-C.L. Hong and L. Levine. Stimulation of prostaglandin biosynthesis by bradykinin and thrombin and their mechanism of action on MC5-5 fibroblasts. *J. Biol. Chem. 251*: 5814-5816, 1976.

17. P. C. Isakson, A. Raz, and P. Needleman. Selective incorporation of [14C]arachidonic acid into the phospholipids of intact tissues and subsequent metabolism to [14C]prostaglandins. *Prostaglandins 12*: 739-749, 1976.

18. L. Levine and H. Van Vunakis. Antigenic activity of pros-

taglandins. *Biochem. Biophys. Res. Commun. 41*: 1171-1177, 1970.

19. E. Granström and H. Kindahl. Radioimmunoassay of prostaglandins and thromboxanes. *In* "Advances in Prostaglandin and Thromboxane Research," Vol. 5 (J. C. Frölich, ed.), pp. 119-210. Raven Press, New York, 1978.

20. H. R. Behrman, K. Yoshinaga, H. Wyman, and R. O. Greep. Effects of prostaglandins on ovarian steroid secretion and biosynthesis during pregnancy. *Am. J. Physiol. 221*: 189-194, 1971.

21. G. P. Orczyk and H. R. Behrman. Ovulation blockade by aspirin or indomethacin - *in vivo* evidence for a role of prostaglandins in gonadotrophin secretion. *Prostaglandins 1*: 3-20, 1972.

22. J. L. Humes, P. Davies, R. J. Bonney, and F. A. Kuehl, Jr. Phorbol myristate acetate (PMA) stimulates the release of arachidonic acid and its cyclooxygenase products by macrophages. *Fed. Proc. 37*: 1318, 1978.

23. R. J. Bonney, P. Naruns, P. Davies, and J. L. Humes. Antigen-antibody complexes stimulate the synthesis of release of prostaglandins by mouse peritoneal macrophages. *Prostaglandins 18*: 605-615, 1979.

24. H. R. Bourne, L. M. Lichtenstein, K. L. Melmon, C. S. Henney, Y. Weinstein, and G. M. Shearer. Modulation of inflammation and immunity by cyclic AMP. *Science 184*: 19-28, 1974.

25. J. S. Goodwin, R. P. Messner, and G. T. Peake. Prostaglandin suppression of mitogen-stimulated lymphocytes *in vitro*. *J. Clin. Invest. 62*: 753, 1978.

66

QUANTITATION OF SELECTED COMPLEMENT COMPONENTS

F. Sessions Cole
David J. Gash
Harvey R. Colten

I. GENERAL INTRODUCTION

Most of the serum complement proteins are produced primarily in liver, but monocytes and macrophages constitute an important source of extrahepatic production of many complement components. Local production of complement at tissue sites of inflammation may be of considerable importance in host defenses and immunopathological reactions. The synthesis and secretion of complement proteins by mononuclear phagocytes in culture have been measured functionally, immunochemically, and by hemolytic plaque assay. The hemolytic (functional) assay is used to monitor biologically active complement proteins secreted by mononuclear phagocytes in culture. The immunochemical assay is used for estimating the amount, size, and subunit structure of newly synthesized intracellular as well as secreted protein. The hemolytic plaque assay is used to estimate the percentage of macrophages that secrete functional complement proteins, i.e., suitable for measurement of complement production by

single cells. With these techniques, several different levels
of control of complement synthesis can be explored. Changes in
rate of translation, posttranslational modification, and secretion can be defined. This approach has been applied to studies
of complement biosynthesis in human, mouse, rat, and guinea pig.
Production of complement by cells from other species can be
measured so long as suitable functional assays and specific antibodies to the individual complement proteins are available.

II. FUNCTIONAL ASSAYS

A. Reagents

The source and preparation of buffers, partially purified
complement proteins, and indicator cell intermediates are described in detail by Rapp and Borsos (1).

B. Procedure

The functional assays for individual complement components
are based on the one-hit theory of immune lysis. The one-hit
theory states that a single effective site, resulting from the
sequential action of antibody and the nine complement components, is a necessary and sufficient condition for lysis of the
erythrocyte. As a consequence, from the Poisson distribution,
it is possible to calculate on a molecular basis the concentration of hemolytically active specific complement components
present in a given sample. More detail on the theoretical and
practical aspects of these assays can be found in Rapp and
Borsos (1). As an example of the procedure, the hemolytic
assay of the fourth component of the complement pathway (C4)
will be described.
In the hemolytic assay for C4, a sample is mixed with a cell
intermediate consisting of erythrocytes sensitized with antibody and containing the first component of complement (EAC1).
After a suitable incubation period, the cells are exposed to
the remaining complement components (C2, C3, C5 - 9) in excess
leading to lysis of the erythrocytes. The extent of lysis (the
amount of hemoglobin released) is measured spectrophotometrically, and from this the absolute number of active C4 molecules in
the sample can be calculated. Because of the sensitivity (picogram range) and specificity of these measurements, the biologically active complement components can be detected in complex
mixtures (e.g., tissue culture media) without fractionating or
concentrating the sample (2).

Procedures for hemolytic assays of the individual components and several of the regulatory complement proteins may be found in Rapp and Borsos (1). Hemolytic assays utilizing serum deficient in an individual complement component have also been described for guinea pig, human, and mouse C4 (3, 4), mouse C2 (5), and C5 (6). These assays are both sensitive and specific and do not require partial purification of individual complement components. However, sera deficient in specific components are not widely available, and species incompatibilities may interfere with the assays.

C. *Calculation of Data*

The calculation of the percentage of lysis, the application of the Poisson distribution, and the determination of the number of molecules of the active component are described in Rapp and Borsos (1).

D. *Critical Comments*

The hemolytic assays for individual complement components are extremely sensitive and specific (2). Less than nanogram quantities of the biologically active component can be detected in complex mixtures (2). However, the hemolytic assays for individual complement components vary with respect to efficiency. For example, whereas a single molecule of Cl is sufficient to generate a hemolytic site (7), as many as 300 C3 molecules on the red cell surface are required for one lytic site (8). Therefore, even discounting other potential problems of stability of the component in various tissue culture media and efficiency of uptake of the components on the indicator cells, certain components are more easily detected with this method. Direct comparison of rates of synthesis of the individual components must take these differences into account. Moreover, these measurements do not detect hemolytically inactive complement proteins, nor do they permit a distinction between preformed and newly synthesized protein. Other biological activities of complement components, such as immune adherence and chemotactic activity, may be used for quantitation of biosynthesis, but these have had only limited use in synthesis studies because of lack of specificity and/or sensitivity.

III. HEMOLYTIC PLAQUE ASSAY

A. *Reagents*

Agarose (Seakem HGTP, Marine Colloids, Rockland, Maine) is dissolved in a solution consisting of equal volumes of Hank's balanced salt solution with calcium and magnesium and 0.3 *M* dextrose, and then maintained at approximately 50°C. Preparations of buffers and other reagents are similar to those described for the hemolytic assays (1).

B. *Procedure*

The procedure described below may be used to estimate the number of C2 and C4 producing macrophages from guinea pig alveolar or peritoneal lavage (9). The indicator cells are sensitized with a high multiplicity of C1 (400 effective molecules per cell). Eight-tenths ml of the agarose solution (final concentration 0.5%), 0.08 ml of indicator cells (10^9/ml), and 0.1 ml of macrophage cell suspension are added in rapid succession to plastic tubes in a 37°C water bath. A uniform suspension, prepared by quickly vortexing the mixture, is poured into plastic tissue culture dishes. After the agarose mixture solidifies, the dishes are incubated at 37°C in a humidified 5% CO_2/95% air atmosphere. Based on preliminary kinetic experiments, C2 hemolytic plaques are developed after 1 hr incubation, and C4 plaques are assayed after 2 hr incubation (9). Hemolytic plaques are developed by successive addition of 1 ml of guinea pig C2 (3×10^{10} effective molecules/ml) and 1 ml of rat serum in EDTA (0.01 *M*) for C4, or 1 ml of rat serum in EDTA (0.01 *M*) for C2.

C. *Calculation of Data*

Plaques are counted by visual inspection and recorded as the number of complement producing macrophages per total number of macrophages in each dish. Additional details of the procedure are given in ref. (9).

D. *Critical Comments*

Other forms of agarose such as Seaplaque (Marine Colloids, Rockland, Maine) were not suitable for these experiments because of their anticomplementary effects (9).
The plaque assay allows assessment of the number of comple-

ment producing cells in a heterogeneous cell population.
Plaque formation requires the lysis of approximately 200 - 400
indicator cells (10) and is therefore a sensitive and specific
indicator of C2- and C4-producing cells. Length of incubation
and reagents must be individualized for mononuclear phagocytes
from different species and different tissues based upon the
rate of secretion, viability of the mononuclear phagocytes in
agarose, and stability of indicator cell intermediates.

IV. IMMUNOCHEMICAL DETERMINATION OF COMPLEMENT PROTEINS

A. *Reagents*

   Monospecific antisera to specific complement proteins are
raised by immunization of suitable animals with purified or
partially purified complement proteins (11 - 13). Other
reagents used are described by Hall and Colten (14).

B. *Procedure*

   For each antibody-antigen combination, the zone of equivalence should be defined. The reagents are used in a ratio that
will result in twice antibody excess and the precipitation of
approximately 30 µg of protein (14).
   Radiolabeled extracellular media or intracellular lysates
are divided into two aliquots. One aliquot is precipitated
with a test antibody-antigen combination and the other with
a control antibody-antigen combination (e.g., antivalbumin-
ovalalbumin) to correct for precipitation of nonspecific labeled
protein. The reaction, carried out in 1.0% deoxycholate-Triton
X-100 and Tris-KCl in the presence of 2 mM PMSF, is incubated
for 2 hr at room temperature (14). The precipitates are then
washed three times with 0.5% deoxycholate-Triton X-100, twice
with 0.15 M NaCl, once with acetone, and dried under vacuum.
Total specific radioactivity is measured, or the precipitates
may be subjected to sodium dodecyl sulfate polyacrylamide gel
electrophoresis (SDS-PAGE) for assessment of size and subunit
structure of the newly synthesized proteins (Fig. 1).

C. *Critical Comments*

   The choice of isotope precursor depends upon the specific
protein and question being examined. While S35 methionine is
of high specific activity, some complement proteins do not con-

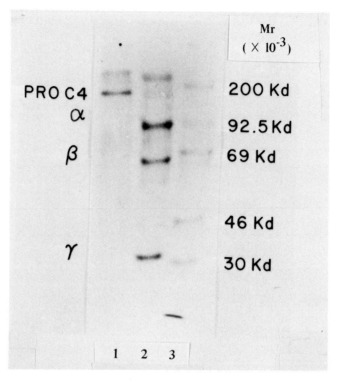

Fig. 1. SDS PAGE analysis of guinea pig Pro-C4 and native C4 synthesized by peritoneal macrophages in culture; radio-autograph of ^{35}S-labeled C4 antigen. Slot 1: Intracellular C4 antigen. Slot 2: C4 antigen secreted into medium. Slot 3: Molecular weight markers. All samples electrophoresed under reducing conditions. Control immunoprecipitates contained no detectable radiolabeled bands.

tain enough methionine to be adequately studied with this labeled amino acid (e.g., Clq) (15). For these proteins, other individual amino acids (e.g., proline for Clq) (15) or combinations of amino acids may be used. If elucidation of posttranslational glycosylation is being examined, labeled carbohydrates may be used (16).

Inclusion of small amounts of protease inhibitors (e.g., PMSF or EACA) into culture medium and intracellular lysates may be necessary to avoid cleavage of polypeptides. Incorporation of the radioisotope into trichloroacetic acid precipitable protein should also be assessed.

V.   TISSUE CULTURE METHODS

A. *Reagents*

If culture conditions require serum, medium may be supplemented with 10% heat-inactivated (56°C for 2 hr) fetal bovine
serum. For radiolabeling with amino acids in the presence of
serum, dialysis of heat-inactivated fetal bovine serum against
40 volumes of 0.15 M NaCl and 40 volumes of deionized water is
required. Intracellular lysates are obtained by freeze-
thawing in the presence of 0.5% deoxycholate-Triton X-100 in
Tris-KCl with 2 mM PMSF.

B. *Procedure*

After adherence, monolayers are washed with a balanced salt
solution. Aliquots of medium are removed at timed intervals,
the volume replenished with fresh medium, and the samples
maintained at -70°C until analysis.

C. *Calculation of Data*

The cell number is estimated by DNA content (17).

D. *Critical Comments*

Adherence conditions for mononuclear phagocytes of different species and of different origins must be defined. The
stability of the individual complement components under different culture conditions must be confirmed before biosynthetic
questions are examined.

VI. CONCLUDING REMARKS

The complement proteins are useful tools for elucidation of
both genetic and cellular control mechanisms of the inflammatory process. With the methods described above, secretion of
biologically active complement proteins and radiolabeled, immunochemically detectable complement proteins may be compared.
Regulation of the rate of synthesis of precursor protein or its
posttranslational modification can be assessed. In addition,
the size and subunit structure of the precursor and functional

proteins can be examined. By using the plaque assay, the subpopulation of mononuclear phagocytes that secrete functional
complement components can be estimated.

With these methods, several different levels of cellular
and genetic control of complement synthesis and secretion have
been explored. Maturation of mononuclear phagocytes into tissue macrophages may be signaled or enhanced by changes in their
capacity to synthesize and secrete biologically active complement proteins. For example, human breast milk macrophages secrete hemolytically active C2 and factor B immediately *in vitro*,
while a lag of 3 to 6 days in complement production is noted in
peripheral blood monocytes from the same women (18). Factor B
has been shown to promote spreading of mononuclear phagocytes
in serum-free medium (19). The rate of secretion of both C2
and C4 by macrophages from different tissues may be compared
by simultaneous plaque assay and tissue culture (9). While alveolar macrophages from guinea pig secrete less C2 and C4 than
peritoneal macrophages in culture, the rates of C2 and C4 secretion per complement producing alveolar macrophage are greater
than the rates per complement producing peritoneal macrophage
(9). Similarly, the response of mononuclear phagocytes to various inflammatory stimuli or pharmacologic inhibitors of inflammation can be assessed (9, 10, 20). The possibility that a
feedback mechanism may control C4 secretion has been proposed
(21). The levels of control at which these mechanisms operate
have not been defined.

Posttranslational modification of precursor proteins appears
to be an important regulatory step in the synthesis and secretion of complement proteins, as it is with other proteins
(6, 22, 23). Tunicamycin, an inhibitor of posttranslational
glycosylation, inhibits the secretion of C2 and C4 by guinea
pig macrophages (16). Examples of genetic control mechanisms
have been revealed in studies of cells from complement-deficient
animals and patients. C5 deficiency in mice appears to result
from a failure in secretion of C5 protein, not from a failure
in biosynthesis of the precursor protein (24). This defect in
posttranslational modification may be due to a primary structural abnormality in the precursor protein, lack of an enzyme to
perform the posttranslational modification, or lack of a specific transport protein (24).

Deficiency of C4 in the guinea pig has been shown to result
from a translational defect in the synthesis of C4 protein (25).
Under cell-free conditions, liver polysomes from C4-deficient
guinea pigs synthesize only nascent C4 polypeptides that remain
polysome bound. Thus, the mRNA appears to be present but not
completely translated.

Recent studies have attempted to define the structure of the
genes that code for murine C3 and C4 (26). Because the expression of the Slp protein, a hemolytically nonfunctional C4 pro-

tein, is strongly dependent on testosterone, elucidation of the murine C4 gene will afford a tool to explore the role of steroid hormones in the initiation of protein synthesis (27 - 29).

The complement proteins therefore provide tools with which to examine mechanisms of mononuclear phagocyte maturation and "activation," which in turn govern the local inflammatory response. In addition, specific transcriptional, translational, posttranslational, and secretory control of extracellular mononuclear cell products can be explored.

REFERENCES

1. H. J. Rapp and T. Borsos. "Molecular Basis of Complement Action." Appleton-Century Crofts, New York, 1970.
2. H. R. Colten. Biosynthesis of complement. *Adv. Immunol.* 22: 67, 1976.
3. T. A. Gaither, D. W. Alling, and M. M. Frank. A new one-step method for the functional assay of the fourth component (C4) of human and guinea pig complement. *J. Immunol.* 113: 574, 1974.
4. J. P. Atkinson, K. McGinnis, and D. Shreffler. Development and characterization of a hemolytic assay for mouse C4. *J. Immunol. Meth.* 33: 351, 1980.
5. J. C. Gorman, R. Jackson, J. R. Desantola, D. Shreffler, and J. P. Atkinson. Development of a hemolytic assay for mouse C2 and determination of its genetic control. *J. Immunol.* 125: 344, 1980.
6. Y. M. Ooi, D. E. Harris, P. J. Edelson, and H. R. Colten. Posttranslational control of complement (C5) production by resident and stimulated mouse macrophages. *J. Immunol.* 124: 2077, 1980.
7. H. R. Colten, T. Borsos, and H. J. Rapp. Efficiency of the first component of complement (C1) in the hemolytic reaction. *Science 158*: 1590, 1967.
8. H. R. Colten and C. A. Alper. Hemolytic efficiencies of genetic variants of human C3. *J. Immunol. 108*: 1184, 1972.
9. F. S. Cole, W. J. Matthews, J. T. Marino, D. J. Gash, and H. R. Colten. Control of complement synthesis and secretion in bronchoalveolar and peritoneal macrophages. *J. Immunol.* 125: 1120, 1980.
10. H. V. Wyatt, H. R. Colten, and T. Borsos. Production of the second (C2) and fourth (C4) components of guinea pig complement by single peritoneal cells: Evidence that one cell may produce both components. *J. Immunol. 108*:

1609, 1972.

11. B. F. Tack and J. W. Prahl. Third component of human com-
     plement: Purification from plasma and physicochemical
     characterization. *Biochemistry 15*: 4513, 1976.

12. C. Bolotin, S. C. Morris, B. F. Tack, and J. W. Prahl.
     Purification and structural analysis of the fourth compo-
     nent of human complement. *Biochemistry 16*: 2008, 1977.

13. B. F. Tack, S. C. Morris, and J. W. Prahl. Fifth compo-
     nent of human complement: Purification from plasma and
     polypeptide chain structure. *Biochemistry 18*: 1490,
     1979.

14. R. E. Hall and H. R. Colten. Molecular size and subunit
     structure of the fourth component of guinea pig complement.
     J. Immunol. 118: 1903, 1977.

15. K. M. Morris and M. A. Paz. Ascorbic acid dependent hy-
     droxylation of the Clq subcomponent of complement. Sub-
     mitted for publication.

16. W. J. Matthews, J. T. Marino, D. J. Gash, and H. R. Col-
     ten. Tunicamycin inhibits secretion of complement C4 and
     C2 by guinea pig macrophages。 *Fed. Proc. 39*: 1201, 1980.

17. L. P. Einstein, E. E. Schneeberger, and H. R. Colten.
     Synthesis of the second component of complement by long-
     term primary cultures of human monocytes. *J. Exp. Med.
     143*: 114, 1976.

18. F. S. Cole, D. Beatty, A. E. Davis, and H. R. Colten.
     Complement synthesis by human breast milk macrophages and
     blood monocytes. *Fed. Proc. 39*: 1200, 1980.

19. O. Gotze, C. Bianco, and Z. A. Cohn. The induction of
     macrophage spreading by factor B of the properdin system.
     J. Exp. Med. 149: 372, 1979.

20. J. E. Pennington, W. J. Matthews, J. T. Marino, and H. R.
     Colten. Cyclophosphamide and cortisone acetate inhibit
     complement biosynthesis by bronchoalveolar macrophages
     from guinea pig. *J. Immunol. 123*: 1318, 1979.

21. W. J. Matthews, J. T. Marino, G. Goldberger, D. J. Gash,
     and H. R. Colten. Feedback inhibition of the biosynthesis
     of the fourth component of complement. *Fed. Proc. 38*:
     1011, 1979.

22. S. Weitzman and M. D. Scharf. Mouse myeloma mutants
     blocked in the assembly, glycosylation, and secretion of
     immunoglobulin. *J. Mol. Biol. 102*: 237, 1976.

23. S. A. Hickman, A. Kulczycki, and R. G. Lynch. Studies of
     the mechanism of tunicamycin inhibition of IgA and IgE
     secretion by plasma cells. *J. Biol. Chem. 252*: 4402,
     1977.

24. Y. M. Ooi and H. R. Colten. Genetic defect in secretion
     of complement C5 in mice. *Nature 282*: 207, 1979.

25. R. E. Hall and H. R. Colten. Genetic defect in biosynthe-
     sis of the precursor form of the fourth component of com-

plement. *Science 199*: 69, 1978.

26. G. Fey, K. Odink, and H. Diggelman. Cloning of cDNAs for mouse C3 and C4. *Fed. Proc. 39*: 1201, 1980.

27. A. Ferreira, V. Nussenzweig, and I. Gigli. Structural and functional differences between the H-2 controlled Ss and Slp proteins. *J. Exp. Med. 148*: 1186, 1978.

28. H. C. Passmore and D. C. Shreffler. A sex-limited serum protein variant in the mouse: Inheritance and association with the H-2 region. *Biochem. Genet. 4*: 351, 1970.

29. H. C. Passmore and D. C. Shreffler. A sex-limited serum protein variant in the mouse: Hormonal control of phenotypic expression. *Biochem. Genet. 5*: 201, 1971.

67

LYSOZYME

Lata S. Nerurkar

I. INTRODUCTION

Lysozyme (EC 3.2.1.17, mucopeptide *N*-acetylmuramoyl hydrolase or muramidase) causes lysis of many gram-positive bacteria by its action on their cell walls. It catalyzes hydrolysis of a β(1→4)-glycosidic linkages of polysaccharide component of the peptidoglycan (mucopolymer of the bacterial cell wall), which is composed of alternating *N*-acetylmuramic acid and *N*-acetylglucosamine residues with alternating β(1→4) and β(1→6) linkages, cross-linked with peptide chains. The hydrolytic action of lysozyme gives rise to disaccharide units attached to the peptide chains called muropeptides.

This enzyme is of particular interest in the study of phagocytic cells as one of the main functions of these cells is to localize the microorganisms in the body of the host, then degrade and eliminate them. Lysozyme activity of the phagocytic cells appears to be of lysosomal origin, it is constantly synthesized by the mononuclear phagocytes (1-4), but its secretion appears to be independent of that of other hydrolases at least in case of peritoneal macrophages (1,4). Recent evidence indicates presence of distinct granules containing lysozyme in alveolar macrophages of normal and BCG-vaccinated rabbits (5). More interesting, lysozyme has been shown to have a modulating effect on the response of neutrophils (6,7), particularly suppressing their inflammatory action, and may function as an important mediator of tumoricidal function of macrophages (8).

Activity of lysozyme can be quantitated by a variety of methods, which are essentially based on bacteriolytic properties of this enzyme. Bacterial turbidity decreases when the cell walls are acted upon by lysozyme. The most commonly used method involves the measurement of the initial rate of lysis of *Micrococcus luteus* in suspension that can be followed at a suitable wavelength in the visible spectrum, i.e., 450-640 nm (method I). The other methods involve the measurement of the diameter of the lytic zone after radial diffusion (method II) (9) or electrophoresis (10) of the lysozyme into agarose gels embedded with *Micrococcus luteus*. Recently, a radioimmunoassay procedure has also been described (11), which revealed good correlation with other previously described techniques. An immunocytochemical technique has been used for cytochemical localization of lysozyme in various cells and tissues (12,13). All these techniques are applicable or can be adapted to the study of lysozyme activity in mononuclear phagocytes of any origin.

II. METHOD I: SPECTROPHOTOMETRIC ASSAY

A. *Introduction*

The spectrophotometric assay is performed according to the method of Litwack (14) with minor modifications.

B. *Reagents*

1. *0.067 M Sodium Potassium Phosphate Buffer pH 6.25*
   Stock A: 0.2 *M* KH_2PO_4, anhydrous monopotassium dihydrogen phosphate (FW 136) 27.2 gm/liter
   Stock B: 0.2 *M* Na_2HPO_4 anhydrous disodium hydrogen phosphate (FW 142) 28.4 gm/liter
   Mix 80 ml of stock A + 20 ml of stock B; adjust pH to 6.25 and dilute the mixture 1:3 with distilled water.

2. Buffered Substrate

Freeze-dried *Micrococcus luteus* (No. MO128, Sigma Chem. Co., St. Louis, Missouri) is suspended (10 mg/100 ml) in 0.067 M phosphate buffer, pH 6.25. The absorbance of this suspension at 450 nm should be between 0.6 and 0.7. Discard after use.

3. Enzyme Standard

Egg white lysozyme standard (Sigma, No. L6876) is prepared as a stock solution of concentration 2 mg/100 ml (20 µg/ml) in 0.067 M phosphate buffer, pH 6.25 and refrigerated.

Various working standards are prepared as shown in Table I.

C. Procedure

(1). The assay is conducted at room temperature.

(2). Set the full-scale absorbance of 0.1 on a given recording spectrophotometer. Set the wavelength to 450 nm. For multiple recording, use the auxillary offset control and zero the different cuvette positions at different heights on the recording chart paper.

(3). Transfer 2.5 ml of buffered substrate to a cuvette and add 0.1 ml of sample or standard at the desired dilutions. Mix and immediately read the change in absorbance for 1-3 min. A macrophage equivalent of 0.5-1 × 10^6 cells/0.1 ml/2.5 ml substrate is found to be a suitable sample.

(4). Given a 10-in. recording graph paper with 0.1 in. subdivisions, each subdivision represents 0.001 absorbance when the full scale is adjusted to 0.1A. Note down change in absorbance (ΔA)/min (slope of the regression line) for each standard or sample specimen.

TABLE I. Preparation of Working Lysozyme Standards

Final concentrations (µg/ml)	Volume of stock solution (20µg/ml) ml	Volume of buffer or medium[a] (ml)
2.0	0.1	0.9
4.0	0.2	0.8
10.0	0.5	0.5
15.0	0.75	0.25
20.0	1.0	--

[a]*If culture supernatants are assayed, use respective medium as the dilutent.*

D. Calculation of Data

Lysozyme activity can be expressed as absorbance change (Section II. D. 1) or can be converted to the equivalent of reference lysozyme standard as follows (Fig. 1; Section II. D. 2).

(1). One unit of activity is defined as that amount of enzyme that causes ΔA_{450} of 0.001 in a *Micrococcus luteus* suspension in 1 min at pH 6.25 in 2.6 ml reaction mixture and light path of 1.0 cm. To convert the absorbance change into units of lysozyme, simply multiply ΔA by 1000.

(2). Prepare standard curve by plotting ΔA_{450} readings from the initial rates against microgram of lysozyme standard (Fig. 1). Using this curve, obtain lysozyme concentrations in the sample preparations. As given in Fig. 1, 50- and 100-µl aliquots of a macrophage extract result in ΔA of 0.02, and

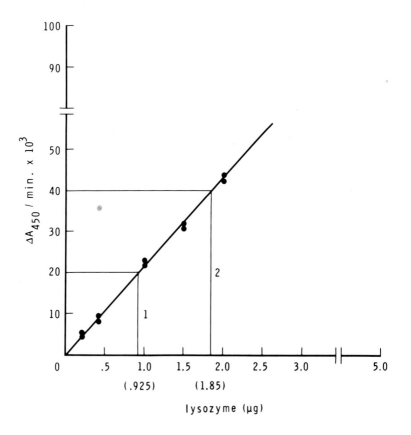

Fig. 1. Spectrophotometric method: Linear plot of egg white lysozyme standard (µg/assay) and ΔA_{450}/min.

0.04, respectively. Therefore, these aliquots contain activity equivalent to 0.925 and 1.85 μg egg white lysozyme, respectively, or 1 ml of this macrophage extract contains activity equivalent to 18.5 μg of egg white lysozyme. This activity can be further expressed as units/10^6 cells, units/mg DNA, or units/mg protein.

E. Critical Comments

1. Standard Lysozyme
Since crystalline hen egg white lysozyme is used as reference standard by many investigators, it is important to select a preparation with at least 25,000 U activity/mg dry weight. In fact, it is essential to specify the activity units of the reference standard used so that the literature values can be compared. There is some question as to the comparability of lysozyme assays expressed in absolute units (i.e., equivalent of microgram of egg white lysozyme) because the reference enzyme standards used by various investigators have ranged from 8000-50,000 U/mg. In addition, rat and human lysozymes are 2- to 3.3-fold more active, respectively, than hen egg white lysozyme (1). It is thus advisable to use reference standards from more closely related biological species (1). To overcome this problem of expression of activity units, it may be even more appropriate to express the data as absorbance change units that may be more acceptable to the system(s) recommended by the International Enzyme Commission. It is, however, essential to include several concentrations of reference standards or known serum samples into each assay to ensure within - and between - day test precision.

2. pH
A pH range of 6.0-6.5 is acceptable for most of the assays. Rabbit alveolar macrophage lysozyme has a pH optimum at 6.5 (15). The lysozyme from hen egg white and human milk have pH optima between 6.0 and 6.5, and 6.2, respectively (16). In contrast, goose lysozyme has maximal activity at acidic pH values (3.8-5.3), whereas the human plasma and leukocyte enzymes show optimal activity at pH 7.5; human urine enzyme (from acute monocytic and monomyelogenous leukemia) or chronic myelogenous leukemia leukocytes show high activity at more alkaline pH values (8.5-8.6) (16). Studies with leukemic cells have to take these properties into consideration.

3. Ionic Strength
Ionic strength of the assay medium appears to be a critical factor in the determination of lysozyme (15,17). Maximal activity for rabbit alveolar macrophage enzyme is seen at ionic strength of 0.04 and more than 50% inhibition of activity is observed at ionic strengths above 0.15 and below 0.017 (15).

It is thus necessary to prepare the test samples and reference standards in buffer or medium of identical ionic strength.

4. Inhibitors

Heparin interferes with the lysozyme assay (18) and should be used with caution especially when mononuclear cells are prepared from heparinized blood. Use of EDTA is sometimes recommended (19).

5. Wavelength

Wavelengths of 450 to 640 nm yield comparable results, though the assay is slightly more sensitive at the low wavelengths.

6. Activity Range

The method yields satisfactory results only in a narrow range of activity that may be considered as the drawback of the method. The linear increases in ΔA_{450} values are observed when lysozyme concentrations in assay are varied between 0.2–2.0 μg of egg white standard. Hence, it is necessary to dilute or concentrate properly the test samples so that the lysozyme activity can be assayed in the sensitive range.

7. Preparation of Test Samples

Dilution of samples in a buffer or medium containing 5% fetal calf serum may prevent loss of low levels of lysozyme activity. Ultrafiltration procedures may be used for concentration of culture supernatants containing low levels of lysozyme, however, preliminary trials should be performed to confirm that lysozyme activity is not lost irreversibly onto the filters due to strong electrostatic binding. Concentration by dehydration against 20,000 molecular weight polyethylene glycol (Acquacide III, calbiochem) (15) or by freeze drying (3) has been reported.

8. Advantages

The assay in our hand is fairly sensitive and reproducible with an acceptable range of variability as shown in Table II.

TABLE II. Study of Precision in Lysozyme Assay by Spectro-
           photometric Method

Lysozyme	Activity (U/mg)
Manufacturer's value	∿25,000
Laboratory value	23,785±606[a]
Coefficient of variation (CV) (%)[b]	8.5

[a]Mean ± S.E.M. of 11 determinations.
[b]$CV = 100 \times \dfrac{SD}{Mean}$.

It has an advantage of providing results on the day of testing
and it can be employed in the automated procedures.

III. METHOD II: LYSOPLATE ASSAY

A. *Introduction*

The lysoplate assay is performed according to the method
of Osserman and Lawlor (9) with minor modifications.

B. *Reagents and Materials*

(1). Petri dishes: 100 × 15 mm in diameter are obtained
from Falcon, Oxnard, California (No. 1001)

(2). Eppendorf micropipette: 10 µl micropipette
(No. P5062-10, Scientific products, McGaw Park, Illinois)

(3). Agarose: Agarose (electrophoresis grade) (No. 100267,
ICN Pharmaceuticals, Inc., Cleveland, Ohio)

(4). Gel punchers: Thin-walled gel punching tubes with
2-mm diameter can be obtained from Bio-Rad Labs., Richmond,
California (#170-4026) and used with proper template.

(5). Magnifying viewer: Calibrating viewer can be obtained
from Kallestad, Inc., Chaska, Minnesota

(6). Micrococcus luteus: See Section II. B.2.

(7). 0.067 M phosphate buffer pH 6.25: See Section II.B.1.

(8). Standard lysozyme: Stock solution: 1.0 mg/ml of
egg white lysozyme is prepared in 0.067 *M* phosphate buffer,
pH 6.25. The working standards of concentrations 5, 25, 50,
100, and 500 µg/ml are prepared by 1:200, 1:40, 1:20, 1:10,
1:2, dilutions, respectively, of the stock solution with
phosphate buffer.

C. *Procedure*

Uniform suspension of *Micrococcus luteus* is prepared in a
small volume of phosphate buffer and is added to molten (60°-
70°C) 1% agar in 0.067 *M* phosphate buffer, pH 6.25 to a final
concentration of 50 mg/100 ml. About 10-12 ml aliquots of this
agar are then poured into petri dishes (to give a depth of 3-
4 mm). The petri dishes are covered, the agar is allowed to
solidify, and kept in humid chambers for 15-20 min. The sample
wells of 2-mm diameter are then cut using gel punchers. Six-
teen sample wells (four rows of four wells) 20-mm apart can be
cut in a petri dish of the given size (100 mm). However, for
samples with high lysozyme levels, nine sample wells (three

rows of three wells) are preferred so that overlapping of the
cleared zones does not occur. The gel plates can be stored
for 2 weeks at 4°C; in that case, they have to be inverted,
kept in plastic bags to prevent evaporation, and sample wells
cut just prior to use.

Aliquots (10 µl) of the reference lysozyme standards or
the test samples are filled in the respective sample wells
using Eppendorf micropipette. The plates are left at room
temperature for 12-18 hr. Prolonged incubations (up to 20-24
hr) may be necessary in case of samples with low lysozyme
levels. As the enzyme diffuses into the gels, bacterial lysis
takes place surrounding the sample wells resulting in clear
zones. The diameters of the clear zones are then measured
directly with an enlarged viewer or after being photographed.
The former is slightly time-taking but inexpensive compared to
the latter. It is important that sample application and the
measurement of diameter of cleared zones be made as quickly as
possible. A typical lysoplate is shown in Fig. 2.

D. Calculation of Data

The diameters of the cleared zone are proportional to the
log concentration of lysozyme (µg/ml). A semilogarithmic plot
is made of diameters (mm) obtained from several reference standards against their concentrations as shown in Fig. 3 and the
concentrations in the test samples are interpolated from the
plot.

E. Critical Comments

The lysoplate method has been carefully studied and critically evaluated (20) and it appears to correlate well with the
long-used spectrophotometric method (9,21) and the recently
developed radioimmunoassay (11). However, multiple factors
seem to affect the lysoplate assay.

1. Enzyme standard
As described above, the activity differences in the reference enzyme standards obtained from different biological species can be seen in this assay. Human urine enzyme has been
shown to be more active than the hen egg white enzyme. The
ratio of activities, however, changes slightly as a function
of time (20). The usage of a standard from biologically related or similar species may at least partially resolve this
problem.

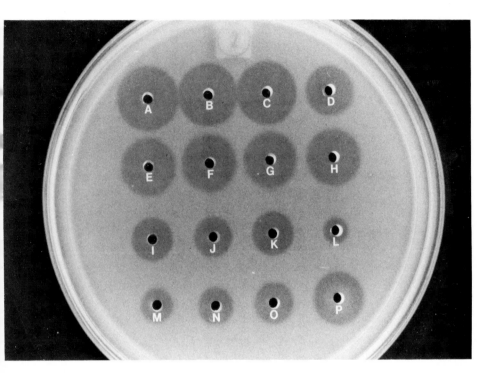

Fig. 2. Lysoplate determination of lysozyme: concentrated
(50x) human lung lavage supernatant (A-D), rabbit alveolar
macrophages homogenates (E-H), human neutrophils homogenates
(I-K), egg white lysozyme standards L = 5 μg/ml, M = 25 μg/ml,
N = 50 μg/ml, O = 100 μg/ml, P = 500 μg/ml; 10 μl samples were
used in each well.

2. pH

Unlike the spectrophotometric method, where a pH optimum
between 6-6.5 is observed for this enzyme in most instances,
the lysoplate method shows an increase in diameters of cleared
zones when pH of the system is increased from 5 to 7.5 (20).

3. Ionic Strength

Ionic strength of the gel medium influences the diameters
of cleared zones in the similar manner as in the spectrophotometric method. In the case of both human and egg enzymes,
maximum diameters were obtained when 0.1 M NaCl was added to

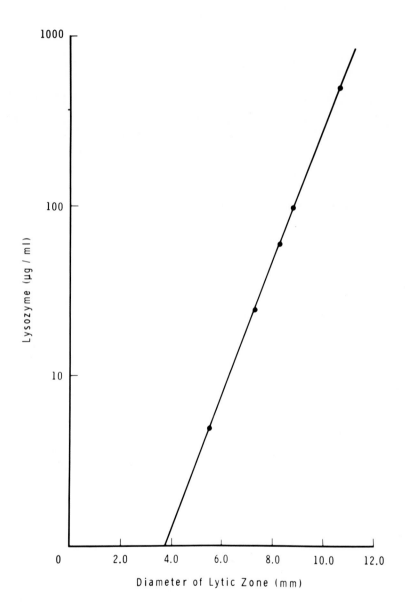

Fig. 3. Lysoplate method: Semilogarithmic plot of egg white lysozyme standard (μg/ml) and diameters in mm of the cleared zones.

0.066 M phosphate buffer, pH 6.6.   The human enzyme was more
sensitive than the hen enzyme to the further increased NaCl
concentration up to 0.4 M (20).

4. Temperature
Unlike in the spectrophotometric method where the lysozyme
activity is far depressed at low temperatures, the lysoplate
method is relatively less affected by temperature variations
(20); the effects on the latter are related to the changes in
the diffusion rate of the enzyme.

5. Activity range
The lysoplate method is applicable to a wide range of
lysozyme concentrations. A straight line semilogarithmic plot
is obtained when concentration is varied between 5-500 μg/ml
as seen in Fig. 3. Adjustment in the concentration of enzyme
in test samples may not be thus required. However, the method
is relatively less accurate for evaluating very low levels of
lysozyme compared to the spectrophotometric method.

6. Composition of Test Sample
Salt or protein content of the test sample affects the
diffusion rate of the lysozyme. Bovine serum albumin seems to
have a profound effect on diameters of clearing zone, more at
low than at high concentration of this enzyme (20). This effect is probably related to the binding of lysozyme to the
proteins (22). This may be an important factor when culture
supernatants containing serum (5-20%) are assayed for lysozyme
activity. The preparation of a standard curve in a medium
identical to the test sample may alleviate this problem.

7. Advantages
The lysoplate method is relatively simple and does not require expensive instrumentation. It can be employed where extremely accurate quantitative measures are not required. It is
widely used in clinical laboratory settings.

III. SIGNIFICANCE

Lysozyme is widely distributed throughout the body and is
particularly high in concentration in body fluids like tears
(23,24), saliva (23), and breast milk (24-26). Using immunohistochemical staining technique, this enzyme is detected in a
variety of tissues, e.g., paneth cells (12,13,27), lymph nodes,
renal tubules, respiratory tissue, stellate cells in follicle
centers, and medulla of the thymus (13), serous salivary acinar
cells, and lactating mammary tissue (27). The significance of

such wide occurrence of this enzyme is not well understood except that is is generally agreed that antibacterial action of this enzyme may complement the secretory immune system at the mucosal surfaces (25,26).

High concentration of lysozyme is found in phagocytic cells, particularly in neutrophils (28,29), monocytes (1,30), and tissue macrophages, e.g., alveolar macrophages (2,3,31-34), peritoneal macrophages (1,3,4,31), skin macrophages (3), and histiocytes (27). The neutrophils acquire their stores of lysozyme early in the cell development in bone marrow and do not synthesize it once the cells are mature. In contrast, as measured in *in vitro* cultures (1-4), mononuclear phagocytes have the capacity to synthesize actively this enzyme, which can be blocked by the inhibitors of protein synthesis (2,3). The turnover of neutrophils and monocyte-macrophages appears to contribute to the serum lysozyme activity. This is further supported by the fact that serum activity is increased in myelocytic and monocytic leukemias, (9,36,40), in infections (21), in certain granulomatous diseases, e.g., sarcoidosis, tuberculosis and Crohn's granulomata (9,27,35,47,48), and is decreased in lymphocytic leukemias (36). The cells of lymphoid or eosinophilic series show little or no lysozyme activity (3,38-40). The lysozyme content of different leukocytes is given in Table III.

Lysozyme is considered to be one of the constitutive enzymes of macrophages (1,4). It is the major secretory product and forms about 25% of the extracellularly secreted protein of macrophages. The secretion of this enzyme by monocytes and macrophages from various sources proceeds in a continuous fashion (1,2,4,44) and is unaffected by a variety of stimuli such as thioglycollate, steroids, lymphokines, and endocytosis, all of which influence the secretion of other macrophage products, e.g., plasminogen activator (4). Lysozyme secretion in culture is characterized by a large net increase in total lysozyme (1,2,4,44), 85-90% of which is excreted to the extracellular medium (1). Using ^{14}-C-labeled amino acid precursors, it has been shown that lysozyme is the major labeled protein secreted into the medium (1,3) and represents up to 2.5% of the total protein (1). The ability to secrete lysozyme appears to be one of the specific features of macrophages and is often lost after hybridization of macrophages with other somatic cells (4).

Lysozyme is a cationic polypeptide whose molecular weight is about 14,000. The primary and secondary structures of some lysozomes are well characterized. Antigenically different lysozomes are detectable as seen from the lack of cross reactivity between the rat lysozyme and antiserum to human urinary lysozyme (45). It is interesting to note that different tissues show different specificities in immunohistochemical staining procedures indicating possibility of isozymes (13). The

TABLE III. Lysozyme Concentration of Different Leukocytes

Cell type	Microgram lysozyme[a] /10^6 cells	Method of assay	Reference
Monocytes			
human	0.12[b]	I[f]	1
human	8.3	II[g]	38
Macrophages			
Mouse peritoneal	0.4	I	33
Mouse peritoneal (unstimulated)	0.35[c]	I	1
Mouse peritoneal (thioglycollate stimulated)	0.25[c]	I	1
Rabbit peritoneal	540.0[d]	I	32
Rabbit alveolar-newborn	4.0[e]	I	41
Rabbit alveolar-adult	2.2[e]	I	41
Rabbit alveolar	3.2	I	33
Rabbit alveolar	3400.0[d]	I	32
Rabbit alveolar (BCG)	9.2	I	33
Rabbit alveolar (BCG)	20.85	I	15
Human alveolar-nonsmokers	1.2	I	42
Human alveolar-smokers	2.5	I	42
Neutrophils			
human	7.2	II	38
human	7.9	I	29
human	2.87	I	43
human (smokers and nonsmokers)	2.2	I	42
Lymphocytes	0.4	II	38

[a] Hen egg white lysozyme equivalent
[b] Human lysozyme standard used
[c] Rat lysozyme standard used
[d] μg egg white lysozyme equivalent/ml of packed cells
[e] Absorbance units given in ref. (41) are converted to equivalent egg white lysozyme (μg) units (1 μg egg white lysozyme ~ 24 absorbance units)
[f] Spectrophotometric method
[g] Lysoplate method

wide occurence of lysozyme in body tissues leads one to speculate that, in addition to its antibacterial (46) and anti-in-
flammatory (6) properties, this enzyme may have more basic
function to perform through its binding to cell membranes,
changing the surface charge density and subsequently modulating
the cell function.

Acknowledgment

This work, in part, was supported by NIH Grant 5T32HD07185-
02. The author gratefully acknowledges the supply of human
lung lavage materials provided by Dr. Henry Yeager.

REFERENCES

1. S. Gordon, J. Todd, and Z. A. Cohn. *In vitro* secretion of
    lysozyme by mononuclear phagocytes. *J. Exp. Med. 139:*
    1228-1248, 1974.
2. E. R. Heise and Q. N. Myrvik. Secretion of lysozyme by
    rabbit alveolar macrophages *in vitro. J. Reticuloendothel.
    Soc. 4:*510-533, 1967.
3. D. B. L. McClelland and R. van Furth. *In vitro* synthesis
    of lysozyme by human and mouse tissues and leukocytes.
    *Immunology 28:*1099-1114, 1975.
4. S. Gordon. Regulation of enzyme secretion by mononuclear
    phagocytes: Studies with macrophage plasminogen activator
    and lysozyme. *Fed. Proc. 37:*2754-2758, 1978.
5. D. B. Lowrie, P. W. Andrew, and T. J. Peters. Analytical
    subcellular fractionation of alveolar macrophages from
    normal and BCG-vaccinated rabbits with particular reference
    to heterogeneity of hydrolase containing granules. *Bio-
    chem. J. 178:*761-767, 1979.
6. L. I. Gordon, S. D. Douglas, N. E. Kay, O. Yamada, E. F.
    Osserman, and H. S. Jacob. Modulation of neutrophil
    function by lysozyme, potential negative feedback system
    of inflammation. *J. Clin. Invest. 64:*226-232, 1979.
7. M. Klockars and P. Roberts. Stimulation of phagocytosis
    by human lysozyme. *Acta Haematol. 55:*289-295, 1976.
8. E. F. Osserman, M. Klockars, J. Halper, and R. E. Fischel.
    Effects of lysozyme on normal and transformed mammalian
    cells. *Nature 243:*331-335, 1973.
9. E. F. Osserman and D. P. Lawlor. Serum and urinary lyso-
    zome (muramidase) in monocytic and monomelocytic leukemia.
    *J. Exp. Med. 124:*921-951, 1966.

10. G. Virella. Electrophoresis of lysozyme into
     Micrococcus-containing agarose gel: Quantitative and
     analytical applications. *Clin. Chem. Acta 75*:107-115,
     1977.
11. T. L. Peeters, Y. R. Depraetere, and G. R. Vantrappin.
     Radioimmunoassay for urinary lysozyme in human serum from
     leukemic patients. *Clin. Chem. 24*:2155-2157, 1978.
12. M. Klockars, M. C. Adinolfi, and E. F. Osserman.
     Ontogeny of lysozyme in the rat. *Proc. Soc. Exp. Biol.
     Med. 145*:604-609, 1974.
13. S. S. Spicer, R. Frayser, G. Virella, and B. J. Hall.
     Immunocytochemical localization of lysozymes in respira-
     tory and other tissues. *Lab. Invest. 36*:282-295, 1977.
14. G. Litwack. Photometric determination of lysozyme acti-
     vity. *Proc. Soc. Exp. Biol. Med. 89*:401-403, 1955.
15. S. F. Carroll and R. J. Martinez. Purification and pro-
     perties of rabbit alveolar macrophage lysozyme. *Infect.
     Immun. 24*:460-467, 1979.
16. P. Jolles, I. Bernier, J. Berthou, D. Charlemagne,
     A. Faure, J. Hermann, J. Jolles, J. P. Perin, and J.
     Saint-Blancard. From lysozymes to chitinases: Struc-
     tural kinetic and crystallographic studies. *In* "Lyso-
     zyme" (E. F. Osserman, R. E. Canfield, and S. Beychock,
     eds.), pp. 31-54. Academic Press, New York, 1974.
17. R. C. Davies, A. Neuberger, and B. M. Wilson. The de-
     pendence of lysozyme activity on pH and ionic strength.
     Biochem. Biophys. Acta 178:294-305, 1969.
18. E. Kaiser. Inhibition and activation of lysozyme.
     Nature 171:607-608, 1953.
19. R. M. Bennett and T. Kokocinski. Lactoferrin content of
     peripheral blood cells. *Br. J. Haematol. 39*:509-521,
     1978.
20. T. L. Peeters and G. R. Vantrappen. Factors influencing
     lysozyme determinations by the lysoplate method. *Clin.
     Chem. Acta. 74*:217-225, 1977.
21. S. Zucker, D. J. Hanes, W. R. Vogler, and R. Z. Eanes.
     Plasma muramidase: A study of methods and clinical
     applications. *J. Lab. Clin. Med. 75*:83-92, 1970.
22. G. Virella. The electrophoretic mobility of serum
     lysozyme. *Experientia 31*:1465-1467, 1975.
23. A. Fleming and V. D. Allison. Observations on a bacterio-
     lytic substance ("lysozyme") found in secretions and tis-
     sues. *Br. J. Exp. Pathol. 3*:252-260, 1922.
24. J. Jolles and P. Jolles. Human tear and milk lysozymes.
     Biochemistry 6:411-417, 1967.
25. J. K. Welsh and J. T. May. Antiinfective properties of
     breast milk. *J. Pediat. 94*:1-9, 1979.

26. R. A. Lawrence. "Host-Resistence Factors and immunolo-
    gical Significance of human milk," pp. 73-91. The C. V.
    Mosby Co., St. Louis, Missouri, 1980.

27. D. Y. Mason and C. R. Taylor. The distribution of
    muramidase (lysozyme) in human tissues. *J. Clin. Pathol.*
    *28:*124-132, 1975.

28. J. K. Spitznagel. Advances in the study of cytoplasmic
    granules of human neutrophilic polymorphonuclear leuko-
    cytes. *In* "The Phagocytic cell in Host Resistence"
    (J. A. Bellanti and D. H. Dayton, eds.), pp. 77-85.
    Raven Press, New York, 1974.

29. L. S. Nerurkar, L. Jacob, B. J. Zeligs, J. Walser, H.
    Yeager, and J. A. Bellanti. A study of chronic granu-
    lomatous disease in adults. Submitted for publication.

30. F. Schmalzl and H. Braunsteiner. The cytochemistry of
    monocytes and macrophages. *Ser. Haematol. III:*93-131,
    1970.

31. E. S. Leake and Q. N. Myrvik. Changes in morphology and
    in lysozyme content of free alveolar cells after the
    intravenous injection of killed BCG in oil. *J. Reticulo-
    endothel. Soc. 5:*33-53, 1968.

32. Q. N. Myrvik, E. S. Leake, and B. Fariss. Lysozyme con-
    tent of alveolar and peritoneal macrophages from the
    rabbit. *J. Immunol. 86:*133-136, 1961.

33. Z. A. Cohn and E. Wiener. The particulate hydrolases
    of macrophages I. Comparative enzymology, isolation,
    and properties. *J. Exp. Med. 118:*991-1008, 1963.

34. M. E. Carson and A. M. Dannenberg, Jr. Hydrolytic en-
    zymes of rabbit mononuclear exudate cells II. Lysozyme.
    Properties and quantitative assay in tuberculous and
    control inbred rabbits. *J. Immunol. 94:*99-104, 1965.

35. S. C. Finch, J. P. Lamphere, and S. Jablon. The relation-
    ship of serum lysozyme to leukocytes and other constitu-
    tional factors. *Yale J. Biol. Med. 36:*350-360, 1964.

36. P. Jolles, M. Sternberg, and G. Mathe. The relationship
    between serum lysozyme levels and the blood leukocytes.
    *Israel J. Med. Sci. 1:*445-447, 1965.

37. R. S. Briggs, P. E. Perillie, and S. C. Finch. Lysozyme
    in bone marrow and peripheral blood cells. *J. Histochem.
    Cytochem. 14:*167-170, 1966.

38. H. J. Senn, B. Chu, J. O'Malley, and J. F. Holland.
    Experimental and clinical studies on muramidase (lyso-
    zyme). *Acta. Haematol. 44:*65-77, 1970.

39. J. L. Greenberger, A. Campos-Neto, R. Perkman, W. C.
    Moloney, A. Karpas, S. F. Schlossman, and D. S. Rosenthal.
    Immunological detection of intracellular and cell-surface
    lysozyme with human and experimental leukemic leukocytes.
    *Clin. Immunol. Immunopathol. 8:*318-334, 1977.

40. A. T. Skarin, Y. Matsuo, and W. C. Moloney. Muramidase in myeloproliferative disorders terminating in acute leukemia. *Cancer 29*:1336-1342, 1972.

41. L. S. Nerurkar, B. J. Zeligs, and J. A. Bellanti. Maturation of the rabbit alveolar macrophage during animal development II. Biochemical and enzymatic studies. *Pediat. Res. 11*:1202-1207, 1977.

42. J. O. Harris, G. N. Olsen, J. R. Castle, and A. S. Maloney. Comparison of proteolytic enzyme activity in pulmonary alveolar macrophages and blood leukocytes in smokers and nonsmokers. *Am. Rev. Resp. Dis. 111*:579-586, 1975.

43. D. G. Wright, D. A. Bralove, and J. I. Gallin. The differential mobilization of human neutrophil granules: Effects of phrobol myristate acetate and ionophore A23187. *Am. J. Pathol. 87*:273-284, 1977.

44. L. P. Einstein, E. E. Schneeberger, and H. E. Colten. Synthesis of the second component of complement by long-term primary cultures of human monocytes. *J. Exp. Med. 143*:114-126, 1976.

45. A. C. Wilson and E. M. Prager. Antigenic comparison of animal lysozymes. *In* "Lysozyme" (E. F. Osserman, R. E. Canfield, and S. Beychock, eds.), pp. 127-141. Academic Press, New York, 1974.

46. A. A. Glynn. Lysozyme: Antigen, enzyme, and antibacterial agent. *Sci. Basis Med. Ann. Rev. 31*:31-52, 1968.

47. P. T. Bodel, P. T. Major, and J. B. L. Gee. Increased production of endogenous pyrogen and lysozyme by blood monocytes in sarcoidosis. *Yale J. Biol. Med. 52*:247-256, 1979.

48. R. S. Pascual, J. B. L. Gee, and S. C. Finch. Usefulness of serum lysozyme measurement in diagnosis and evaluation of sarcoidosis. *N. Engl. J. Med. 289*:1074-1076, 1973.

68

DESTRUCTION OF *LISTERIA MONOCYTOGENES*
IN VITRO

George L. Spitalny
Robert J. North

I. INTRODUCTION

An analysis of acquired cell-mediated immunity to bacterial infection ultimately requires an investigation of the
bactericidal capacity of host macrophages *in vitro*. This
stems from the fact that there is no way of knowing whether
increased resistance *in vivo* depends on the generation of
more macrophages or macrophages more efficient at destroying
bacteria. For this reason, past investigations of acquired
resistance to tuberculosis, brucellosis, salmonellosis, and
listeriosis have involved, at some stage in the investigations,
the demonstration that animals with acquired antibacterial resistance possess macrophages that express increased bactericidal activity *in vitro* (1). It is now known that cell-mediated
antibacterial immunity, although specifically mediated by
sensitized T cells, is nonspecifically expressed, in that
macrophages of the immune host display an increased capacity
for inactivating a variety of unrelated bacteria. *Listeria*

monocytogenes is a useful organism for measuring this non-specific bactericidal activity.

A number of *in vitro* techniques have been employed to measure the increased bactericidal capacity of macrophages. Many of these have employed macrophages adherent to glass or plastic, and many have measured bactericidal activity by determining changes against time in the number of cell-associated bacteria capable of forming colonies on nutrient agar. A similar method is described here. It involves allowing peritoneal macrophages to adhere to and spread on glass coverslips, washing away all nonadherent cells, and challenging the resulting macrophage "monolayers" with an excess of *Listeria*. Phagocytosis is allowed to proceed for a short period and the bacteria not associated with cells are then thoroughly washed away. Changes against time in the number of cell-associated colony-forming bacteria are then determined by plating serial dilutions of sonicates of macrophage monolayers on nutrient agar. In this way, the rate of bacterial kill can be determined (2).

II. MATERIALS

A. *Reagents*

   1. Animals
   Mice are the most popular animals, although the procedure can be used to measure the bactericidal activity of macrophages from any animal, particularly since long-term macrophage cultures are not required.

   2. Listeria monocytogenes
   A strain must be chosen with at least moderate virulence for mice. The method for increasing virulence by repeated passage in mice is described by North and Spitalny, this volume, as is the method for obtaining a log phase culture of *Listeria* for macrophage challenge.

B. *Dissecting Materials*

   Bell jar containing chloroform-soaked surgical gauze for killing mice
   Two sterile 3-cm^3 syringes fitted with 22-gauge needles (Pharmaseal Labs, Glendale, California, #7200)
   50-ml Plastic tubes (Falcon Plastics, Oxnard, California, #2070)
   Ethanol, 70%

Blunt end, 5 1/2 in. stainless scissors (Clay Adams, Parsippany, New Jersey
    Cork board and pins
    Hemocytometer for counting peritoneal cells (Scientific Products, McGraw Park, Illinois. #B3180

C. Tissue Culture Materials

A number of 35 × 10 mm tissue culture Petri dishes (Corning Glass Works, Corning, New York, #25000, or Falcon Plastics, Oxnard, California, #3001)
    A number of 12- or 13-mm diameter circular coverslips (Clay Adams, Parsippany, New Jersey, #3350), which are cleaned and sterilized by dipping in 70% ethanol and flaming
    Small forceps for firmly holding coverslips
    RPMI 1640 medium (GIBCO, Grand Island, New York, #430-1800) containing 5% heat-inactivated (56°C for 1 hr) fetal bovine serum (RPMI-FBS) with or without 5 U/ml of preservative-free heparin (Sigma, St. Louis, Missouri, #3125)
    Incubator at 37°C supplied with humidified air containing 5% CO_2

D. Materials for Bacterial Challenge and Enumeration

Petroff-Hauser chamber for enumerating Listeria
    Sonicator set at 50% maximum output to break-up chains of bacteria and to free organisms phagocytosed by macrophages (Biosonik, Brownwill Scientific, Rochecter, New York
    Bacterial colony counter (New Brunswick Scientific, Edison, New Jersey)
    A number of 5-ml plastic tubes (Falcon Plastics, Oxnard, California, #2058) containing 0.9-ml physiological saline for serial dilutions
    Bacterial culture plates (Falcon Plastics, Oxnard, California, #1056) containing Trypticase-soy agar prepared as described by North and Spitalny, this volume.
    Plastic 15-ml tubes containing 1 ml of 0.1% WR 1339 detergent (Ruger Chemical Co., Irvington, New Jersey) in sterile distilled water
    A 2-liter aspirator bottle with outlet connected to a rubber tube fitted with adjustable clamp and hemostat. The bottle is filled with sterile saline containing 0.5% heat-inactivated fetal bovine serum.

III.   PROCEDURE

Mice are killed with chloroform vapor, their abdomens swabbed with 70% ethanol and the skin of their abdomens clipped carefully with scissors without perforating the peritoneal cavity. The clipped skin is held and pulled anteriorally to expose the peritoneal lining. A 3-cm^3 syringe with a 22-gauge needle is used to infuse 1.5 ml of heparinized RPMI-FBS into the peritoneal cavity, and the peritoneum massaged with the blunt end of a sterile pipette. The peritoneal fluid is then carefully withdrawn into a separate 3-cm^3 syringe. In spite of the fact that only 1.5 ml of culture medium are infused, it is possible, with a little practice, to withdraw most of this volume into the syringe. The small volume of RPMI-FBS is used in order to obtain a relatively large number of cells per unit volume. This avoids the need to centrifuge and resuspend the cells, a procedure that results in cell clumping. The peritoneal cells of several mice are pooled, the number of cells per unit volume determined by counting a sample with a hemocytometer, the volume adjusted to give 5×10^6 cells/ml, and 1 ml of the suspension added to each of a number of 35×10 mm petri dishes containing three 13-mm diameter circular coverslips. Since the aim is to obtain "macrophage monolayers" on the coverslips, an adequate number of cells per milliliter must be added to the petri dishes. If the number of cells per milliliter is too low, the volume added can be increased.

The macrophages are allowed to settle, adhere to, and spread on the coverslips for at least 2 hr in an incubator at 37°C with 5% CO_2. The coverslips are removed with forceps and, while being held firmly with forceps, are subjected to the shear force of a jet of saline-FBS delivered from a Pasteur pipette and fed by gravity from an overhead aspirator bottle. The rate of flow of fluid is controlled by an adjustable clamp on the connecting tubing. This washing procedure thoroughly removes all nonadherent cells. The coverslips are then placed (cells-side up) into new 35×10 mm petri dishes containing 1 ml of RPMI-FBS and incubated an additional hour at 37°C before bacterial challenge.

A sample of a log phase culture ($1-2 \times 10^8$/ml) of *Listeria* is appropriately diluted, counted with a Petroff-Hauser chamber, and the number of bacteria in the culture calculated. The culture is then diluted to 5×10^6 bacteria/ml in RPMI-FBS and subjected to ultrasound (50% maximum output) for 3 sec to break up chains of bacteria. The 1 ml of medium overlaying the macrophages on coverslips is aspirated and quickly replaced with 1 ml of medium containing the bacteria. The petri dishes

are placed in the incubator, and the macrophages allowed to
ingest bacteria for 20 min. The medium is then quickly removed and replaced with 5 ml of fresh medium to dilute the
remaining uningested bacteria and greatly reduce any further
phagocytosis. Each coverslip is then picked up with forceps
and subjected to the same washing procedure as described above
to remove nonadherent cells. This serves to remove all bacteria that are not cell-associated. The coverslips are then
placed in new 35 × 10 mm petri dishes with 1 ml of fresh RPMI-
FBS. Three coverslips from separate dishes are removed and
dropped into a 15-ml plastic tube (cell side up) containing
WR 1339 of 0.1% WRI1339 detergent in distilled water. The remaining plates are placed back in the incubator and bacterial
inactivation is allowed to proceed. The three coverslips that
were placed in the tubes represent triplicates of the T_0 time
point. Each of these coverslips are subjected to two 3-sec
bursts of ultrasound (50% maximum output) to disrupt the cells
and release intracellular bacteria. Immediately after sonication, 0.1 ml of the sonicate is subjected to 10-fold serial
dilution in 5-ml tubes containing 0.9 ml of saline, and each
dilution is plated on TSA. If the foregoing procedure is adhered to, it is only necessary to plate the undiluted, 10-fold
and 100-fold dilutions in order to obtain countable numbers of
bacterial colonies 24 hr later. Three coverslips are removed
from the incubator at 15, 30, 60, 90, 120, and 180 min and
subjected to the same procedure. These time points are designated T_1, T_2, T_3, etc.

IV. CALCULATION OF DATA

The numbers of bacterial colonies from known dilutions are
recorded and the numbers of viable bacteria in the cell sonicates for each time point calculated in triplicate. The means
are calculated and plotted against time. The data can be presented as changes against time in the $\log_{10}$ number of viable
bacteria per monolayer, or as changes in the percent bacteria
killed against time. The latter is calculated according to
the formula

$$\frac{\text{Number of colony forming units } T_1, T_2, T_3 \cdots T_n}{\text{Number of colony forming units } T_0} \times 100$$

The latter presentation is easiest to accept when two types of
macrophages are being compared, because it is not essential
that each type of macrophage be present on coverslips in equal
number. This is because the assay assures that there is no
competition for bacteria between macrophages in that the bacteria are fed uniformally to the monolayer by gravity. Conse-

quently, each macrophage should ingest and destroy bacteria without being influenced by its neighbors. This means that within limits, the percent kill will be independent of the number of macrophages doing the killing. The washing procedure assures that practically all bacteria that are not cell-associated after 20 min are washed away. This avoids the need to use antibiotics to inhibit extracellular bacterial growth. This is just as well since there is evidence (3,4) that antibiotics enter macrophages and aid in intracellular killing.

V. CRITICAL COMMENTS

An inherent problem with *in vitro* bactericidal assays is that all bacteria are not completely ingested by macrophages at the same time. Even though the assay described here results in suitable numbers of bacteria becoming associated with macrophages firmly enough to avoid being washed off by a strong jet of saline, some of the bacteria are already completely interiorized at the time of washing, while others are still in the process of being ingested. The rate of bacterial inactivation from T_0 on will depend, therefore, on the rate at which the partly ingested organisms are completely ingested, assuming, of course, that bactericidal mechanisms depend on complete ingestion. This problem becomes serious when the bactericidal activities of normal and activated macrophages are being compared, because activated macrophages possess an intrinsically enhanced capacity for ingesting bacteria at a faster rate. There is no way of knowing, therefore, whether increased bactericidal activity displayed by activated macrophages is caused by the possession of more potent bactericidal mechanisms, or whether it is simply the result of the same bactericidal mechanisms acting on more rapidly ingested bacteria. One way of overcoming this problem is to employ subagglutinating quantities of opsonic antibodies to ensure that bacteria are ingested by control and activated macrophages at similar rates and to similar extents. Assuring that this is achieved involves a lot of trial and error and painstaking microscopic examination of the cultures.

Acknowledgment

Supported by Grants AI-10351 from the National Institute of Allergy and Infectious Diseases, CA-21360 from the National Cancer Institute and by RR05705 from the Biomedical Research Support Grant Program, Division of Research Resources, National Institutes of Health.

REFERENCES

1. R. J. North. Cell-mediated immunity and the response to
    infection. *In* "Mechanisms of Cell-Mediated Immunity"
    (R. T. McCluskey and S. Cohen, eds.), pp. 185-220.
    Wiley, New York, 1973.
2. G. L. Spitalny. Suppression of macrophage bactericidal
    activity in ascites tumors. *J. Reticuloendothel. Soc.*
    28:223-235, 1980.
3. P. Cole and J. Brostoff. Intracellular killing of
    Listeria monocytogenes by activated macrophages (Mackaness
    system) is due to antibiotics. *Nature (London) 256*:515-
    517, 1975.
4. P. D'Arcy Hart. Critical approach to the technique of
    assessment of antibacterial effects of activated mouse
    peritoneal macrophages. *In* "Activation of Macrophages"
    (W. H. Wagner, H. Hahn, and R. Evans, eds.), pp. 131-317.
    American Elsevier, New York, 1974.

69

INGESTION AND DESTRUCTION OF *Candida albicans*

Robert I. Lehrer

I. GENERAL INTRODUCTION

Candida albicans, a commensal yeast that can cause superficial or disseminated infection in appropriately predisposed
hosts, is useful for probing the phagocytic functions of mononuclear phagocytes. We shall describe simple, but serviceable
methods for measuring uptake and phagocytic destruction of
this organism by mononuclear phagocytes. Although our own
studies have dealt either with human blood monocytes or rabbit
alveolar and peritoneal macrophages, the methods should have
general applicability (1, 2).

II.   PHAGOCYTIC ACTIVITY BY MONONUCLEAR PHAGOCYTES

A. *Introduction*

Method I applies the venerable dye-exclusion concept (3, 4) so that extracellular or surface-adherent heat-killed *C. albicans* cells can be distinguished clearly from fully ingested yeast cells.

B. *Reagents*

1. *Staining Solution*

To prepare 100 ml of staining solution, prepare and mix together the following ingredients.

(a) 40 ml of a 1% aqueous solution of trypan blue (C.I. 23850, K and K Labs, Plainview, New York, and many other suppliers).

(b) 20 ml of a 1% solution of eosin Y (C.I. 43580, MCB, Norwood, Ohio, and many other suppliers). Note, that if eosin Y is obtained as the free acid, it should be dissolved in 0.1 *N* NaOH. If the sodium salt is obtained, the solution can be prepared in distilled water.

(c) 10 ml of a 10X concentrated phosphate-buffered saline solution (GIBCO No. 310-4200, Grand Island, New York, for example).

Correct the pH to 7.4 (use 0.1 *N* HCl if 0.1 *N* NaOH was used to dissolve the eosin Y), dilute to 100 ml, Millipore filter, and place in a sterile bottle. The stain can be used for several years and is stable at room temperature. Check a drop microscopically before using it. It should be refiltered if a sediment has formed or if visible microbial contamination exists.

2. *Candida albicans*

Clinical isolates can be obtained from any hospital microbiology laboratory, from the American Type Culture collection, or (possibly) from the author. We maintain our stock cultures at room temperature on Sabouraud's agar slants (Difco No. 0109-01, Detroit, Michigan), passaging them at six-month intervals. Alternatively, a washed suspension of *C. albicans* in sterile distilled water will remain viable for several years. Working cultures are prepared by transferring a loopful (from slants) or a drop (from a *Candida* broth culture) to 50 ml of Sabouraud's 2% dextrose broth (BBL No. 10986, Becton Dickinson, Cockeysville, Maryland) contained in a sterile 100-ml container. The culture vessel, loosely capped, is incubated in room air without shaking for 3 - 5 days at 30°C to achieve a stationary phase culture. Under these conditions, the organism is completely in yeast phase. Most of its forms appear as single yeasts or attached doublets, and filamentous forms are absent. To prepare the yeasts for an experiment, centrifuge 5 - 10 ml of the culture (400 g for 10 min), remove the supernatant Sabouraud's broth, resuspend the yeast cells in 5 - 10 ml of distilled water and centrifuge again as before. After removing the clear supernatant, resuspend the yeast in 2 ml of distilled water.

To prepare heat-killed organisms, immerse the tube in a beaker of boiling water for 30 min, then wash the killed yeasts twice again with distilled water. This preparation will remain useful for several weeks if kept refrigerated and sterile. We generally store the suspensions at a concentration of 2×10^8 yeast cells/ml. Prior to use, the heat-killed organisms are centrifuged, washed once with Hanks' BSS (GIBCO No. 406, Grand Island, New York) or an equivalent medium, counted in an hemocytometer and resuspended in the medium to be used for the mononuclear phagocytes.

Our studies with rabbit macrophages (2) were primarily designed to examine intracellular killing (see below) rather than to define the minimal opsonic requirements for uptake. In our studies of phagocytosis, we used preopsonized yeast, prepared by resuspending 10^8 heat-killed *C. albicans* cells in 1 ml of fresh frozen (-70°C) human group AB serum containing a 1:20 dilution of conventionally raised specific rabbit antiserum to *C. albicans*. After incubation for 15 min at 37°C, the suspension was centrifuged, washed twice with Hanks' BSS, and suspended in Hanks' BSS at the desired concentration cells/ml.

3. Mononuclear Phagocytes

Human monocytes are obtained by Ficoll-Hypaque purification from peripheral blood (1). Rabbit alveolar and peritoneal macrophages are obtained from New Zealand White rabbits weighing 2 - 3 kg (2). We use untreated rabbits to provide "resident" macrophage populations. Other rabbits, injected 21 days earlier with 1 ml of complete Freund's adjuvant containing *Mycobacterium butyricum* (Difco No. 0638-60) via a marginal ear vein, provide "elicited" macrophages. Some rabbits receive, concurrently with their intravenous injection, an intraperitoneal injection of 20 ml of heavy paraffin oil (Fisher Chemical, Fair Lawn, New Jersey) containing 0.5 ml of complete Freund's adjuvant. Elicited macrophages have modestly enhanced ability to kill *C. albicans,* relative to "resident" macrophages (2).

To collect macrophages, injected and control rabbits are
anesthetized intravenously with 90 mg of sodium pentobarbitol
(Diabutal, Diamond Labs, Des Moines, Iowa) and killed by a
60-ml air embolism, both delivered through the marginal ear
vein. Alveolar and peritoneal macrophages are obtained promptly thereafter by pulmonary and/or peritoneal lavage with
300 - 500 ml of Dulbecco's phosphate-buffered saline (Grand
Island Biologicals, Grand Island, New York) containing 5 IU of
sodium heparin (Riker, Northridge, California), 100 μg/ml of
penicillin G and 100 μg/ml of streptomycin.

With these techniques we recover approximately (geometric
mean ± SEGM) $4.7 ± 0.1 × 10^7$ cells from the alveoli of unstimulated rabbits $(n = 22)$ and $2.8 ± 0.1 × 10^8$ cells from the
alveoli of Freund's adjuvant-stimulated rabbit $(n = 19)$. Resident alveolar cells consist of 94.8 ± 3.4% macrophages
(mean ±SD), 1.8 ± 1.6% granulocytes, and 3.2 ± 2.4% lymphocytes.
Alveolar cells elicited by Freund's adjuvant consist of
90.3 ± 5.6% macrophages, 5.0 ± 5.4% granulocytes, and
4.7 ± 3.6% lymphocytes.

Should it be desired to purify alveolar macrophages from
contaminated neutrophils (not required for the two methods described in this chapter, but useful for enzymatic or metabolic
studies), it can be done as follows: Suspend $\leq 1 × 10^8$ alveolar
lavage cells in 30 ml of a solution composed of 2 parts
phosphate - buffered saline + 1 part Ficoll-Hypaque (density$_{20}$
1.079 ± 0.002 gm/cc) and underlay this with 15 ml of Ficoll-
Hypaque (density 1.079) in a 50-ml plastic tube (Falcon No.
2070, Becton, Dickinson and Co., Oxnard, California). Centrifuge at 250 g for 45 min at 20°C in a swinging bucket rotor
(International PR-J centrifuge or equivalent). Granulocytes
will sediment through the lower Ficoll-Hypaque solution, whereas macrophages will accumulate at the interface. Recovery (approximately 80%) and viability (>95%) of macrophages are good.

Resident peritoneal cavities yield $8.9 ± 0.1 × 10^6$ cells/
rabbit $(n = 14)$, (88.4 ± 7.9% macrophages, 6.8 ± 8.2% granulocytes, 4.8 ± 2.9% lymphocytes) and stimulated peritoneal cavities provide $5.7 ± 1.6 × 10^7$ cells/rabbit $(n = 13)$, of which
71.9 ± 12.1% are macrophages, 23.1 ± 11.1% granulocytes, and
4.6 ± 4.5% lymphocytes. Macrophages are kept in suspension at
room temperature in polypropylene tubes (Falcon No. 2070, Becton, Dickinson and Co., Oxnard, California) containing Hanks'
balanced salt solution with 0.1% bovine serum albumin.

C. *Miscellaneous Reagents and Equipment*

(1) Hanks' balanced salt solution (HBSS, GIBCO, Grand
Island, New York)
(2) Bovine serum albumin, crystallized (Sigma, St. Louis,
Missouri)

(3) Tube rotator (BLL No. 60448, or equivalent)
(4) Laboratory differential counter (Clay Adams No. 4318, or equivalent)

D. Safety Considerations

Candida albicans, despite opportunistic proclivities in immunoincompetent hosts, does not pose significant safety problems in the laboratory. The organism does not form airborne or resistant spores and, consequently, does not menace nearby tissue culture operations. Laboratory workers are more likely to introduce *C. albicans* infection from their own resident flora than to acquire it. Reasonable laboratory technique suffices. This includes using cotton-plugged pipettes and rubber aspirating bulbs instead of pipetting by mouth; wiping up any spills with a germicide such as 70% alcohol, various commercial phenol-containing compounds, or Zephiran; and autoclaving wastes prior to their disposal.

E. Procedures

Rabbit macrophages are suspended at a concentration of 5×10^6 phagocytes/ml in Hanks' BSS containing 20% fetal calf serum and brought to 37°C in a water bath. Heat-killed *C. albicans,* freshly opsonized as described in Section II.B.2 are washed twice with distilled water to remove the serum and suspended in Hanks' BSS at 2.5×10^7 yeast cells/ml at 37°C. The washing can be done in a conventional centrifuge (400 g, 10 min) or can be completely rapidly with 30 sec centrifugations in an Eppendorf Model 3200 centrifuge (Brinkmann Instruments, Westbury, New York) using 1.5 ml polypropylene microfuge tubes (Kew Scientific, Columbus, Ohio).

For studies with human peripheral blood monocytes, 20% fresh frozen normal group AB serum replaces the fetal calf serum, and the heat-killed yeast are merely washed and not preopsonized. Rabbit serum is not used.

The assay is begun by mixing equal volumes, typically 0.5 ml each, of the phagocyte and yeast suspensions in a tube that is placed on an efficient rotator at 37°C. At intervals, e.g., 5, 15, and 30 min, a small drop of the mixture is transferred to a microscope slide, mixed with an equal amount of staining solution, placed beneath a coverslip and examined microscopically with the oil immersion lens.

F. Calculation of Data

Intracellular yeasts, unstained by the trypan-eosin mixture, are readily visible by virtue of their size (3 - 5 μm)
and relatively thick and refractive cell walls. Extracellular
yeasts are stained purple, thus allowing surface-adherent organisms (stained) to be unambiguously differentiated from fully
ingested yeasts. In addition, nonviable macrophages (stained)
are easily distinguished from viable ones. We examine 100 - 200
macrophages, and use a Laboratory hand counter designed for differential blood counts to tally the number of viable macrophages containing 0,1,2,3,4, etc., ingested yeast cells. From
these data, we calculate two indices: the percentage of macrophages that have ingested one or more yeast cells and the mean
number of yeasts ingested per macrophage. The latter is done
by summing the total number of ingested yeasts and dividing this
by the total number of viable macrophages counted.

G. Critical Comments

The assay takes advantage of the fact that ingested killed
yeast cells are protected from exposure to stains that are excluded from the viable surrounding phagocyte. The test has the
virtue of simplicity and, with minor modifications, could equally well be applied to cells on monolayers. We have found that
in 20 min at $37°C$, 68 ± 7% of elicited rabbit alveolar macrophages are phagocytic, containing 1.6 ± 0.2 yeast cells/macro-
phage. In contrast, 92.5 ± 3.3% of Freund's adjuvant elicited
peritoneal macrophages are phagocytic and these contain
2.9 ± 0.6 yeasts/macrophage. Resident alveolar and peritoneal
macrophages closely resemble elicited cells in performance (2).
It is likely that our opsonization procedure can be further
simplified without diminishing phagocytic uptake. As opsonic
requirements will vary according to the type (and state) of mononuclear phagocyte under study, they should be experimentally
determined. In general, phagocytosis of *C. albicans* is facilitated by heat-stabile and heat-labile components that are adequately provided by concentrations of normal serum equalling or
exceeding 10% v/v (5 - 7). Thus, specific immune serum may well
be superfluous, and fresh or fresh frozen $(-70°C)$ normal serum
sufficient to permit optimal rates of uptake.

III. CANDIDACIDAL ACTIVITY BY MONONUCLEAR PHAGOCYTES

A. *Introduction*

   This visual method is based on the fact that ingested *C. albicans* undergo characteristic changes in morphology or Giemsa-staining properties that correlate with their viability as determined by more laborious methods, such as colony counting. The method is rapid to perform and does not require strict sterile technique. If it is interpreted with an understanding of its basis and limitations, it can provide reliable, quantitative data.

B. *Reagents*

   1. *Viable Yeast-Phase C. albicans*

   It is essential to begin with *C. albicans* cultures of high (preferably >97%) viability, a condition generally met by following the procedures described in the first paragraph of Section II.B.2. The initial viability of the culture can be assessed in two ways. The simpler of these requires only reagents 1 - 5, and usually suffices. The reagents are as follows:

   (a) 3 - 5 Day-old yeast-phase *C. albicans* culture, as described in Section II.B.2.
   (b) Aqueous methylene blue 0.01%. This reagent is indefinitely stable at room temperature. We keep it in a plastic "squirt bottle."
   (c) Hemocytometer chamber, tally counter and microscope
   (d) Standard glass microscope slides, clean but not necessarily sterile
   (e) Hanks' BSS
   (f) Fetal calf serum or fresh frozen normal human serum (stored at -70°C)
   (g) Agarose (Sigma, St. Louis, Missouri), a 5% solution in distilled water, autoclaved (or remelted by boiling if previously prepared) and maintained fluid in a 40°C water bath
   (h) A mixture of reagents 5,6,7. The final mixture consists of Hanks' solution with 25% serum and 1% agarose and is kept at 40°C to prevent the gel from setting.

   2. *Viability Test I*

   Cell viability is most conveniently checked at the same time that the cell concentration is determined in an hemocyto-

meter. To do so, remove 50 µl of washed culture and add 1.95 ml
of aqueous methylene blue. Mix well, examine microscopically
under high dry magnification. Nonviable yeast cells are intensely blue, viable ones are devoid of any blue tinge. If there
is any appreciable percentage (i.e., >3%) of light-blue-tinged
organisms, remove another 50 µl of the washed culture, add 450
µl of HBSS, and incubate it for 30 min at 37°C. Then add 1.5 ml
of methylene blue, mix, transfer a drop to an hemocytometer and
again microscopically examine. If the light-blue-tinged organisms persist, they are nonviable (and probably extensively auto-
lysed). If they are no longer apparent, the slight bluish tinge
initially noted represented an inactive metabolic state (see
below).

3. *Viability Test II*

An elegant, but less rapid (4 hr), alternative method of
assessing the viability of the initial culture is the "slide
filamentation test." At 37°C in the presence of serum *C. albicans* (but not other *Candida* species) undergoes a characteristic
and rapid morphologic change. Rather than growing by budding,
the viable yeast cells produce one or more filamentous cylindrical processes, longer than they are wide, that resemble germ
tubes. By using this test to assess viability, one essentially
employs the equivalent of a colony-count procedure. In this
instance, however, it is not necessary to wait for multiple
divisions to occur so that a viable colony appears. Instead,
the first division is recognizable because of the altered morphology of the filamentous first-daughter cell.

To perform the test, add a drop of *Candida* suspension
$(1 - 3 \times 10^8$ yeast cells/ml) to 4 ml of the Hanks'/serum/aga-
rose mixture (reagent 8), mix the tube to distribute the
yeasts, and transfer several drops to a clean microscope slide,
where it will almost immediately gel. Transfer the slide culture to a humidified petri dish (one containing a damp gauze
pad or filter paper) and incubate for 4 hr at 37°C. Examine
microscopically with the high dry or oil immersion lens (press
down a small section of the agarose gel under a coverslip if
using oil immersion) and determine the percentage of cells bearing the pseudo-germ tubes. This provides a minimal estimate of
the percentage of viable yeasts in the starting inoculum and ordinarily agrees quite well with the simpler and more rapid
methylene blue screening test. Illustrations of these filamentous processes can be found in reference (2). Early filaments
are short cylindrical (rather than spherical or ovoid) processes and are readily recognized.

4. Monocytes or Macrophages

Human blood monocytes or rabbit alveolar or peritoneal macrophages are obtained as described in Section II.C. The monocyte-containing fraction obtained by Ficoll-Hypaque centrifugation of human blood is quite heterogeneous, containing 10 - 38% monocytes, 62 - 87% lymphocytes, and 0.5 - 2.5% granulocytes (neutrophils and basophils) (1).

As the present method is applicable to mixed cell populations, even mononuclear phagocyte preparations containing other phagocytic cell types (1, 8), it suffices to perform a hemocytometer chamber differential count. We mix 50 µl of leukocyte suspension with 0.96 ml of a white cell staining solution comprised of 0.05% methyl violet 2B in 0.5% acetic acid to dilute the cells for counting and to stain clearly their nuclei. Most rabbit macrophages are readily distinguished from other cell types by their large size, abundant cytoplasm, and roundish nucleus. Similarly, a folded or kidney-bean-shaped nucleus allows blood monocytes to be estimated with acceptable accuracy by an experienced observer. More definitive classification based on fixed slides stained for α-naphthyl butyrate esterase activity or with Giemsa can also be performed.

5. Serum

Fresh or fresh frozen $(-70°C)$ normal group AB human serum and rabbit antibody to *C. albicans* are obtained or raised by conventional techniques.

C. Miscellaneous Equipment and Supplies

(1) Incubator, 37°C, air or 5% CO_2

(2) Tube rotator, BBL-60448 or equivalent

(3) Cytocentrifuge (Cytospin, Shandon-Elliott Co., Sewickley, Pennsylvania) and perforated blotters to fit microscope slides

(4) Polystyrene tubes, Falcon No. 2054, sterile 12 × 75 mm with cap (Falcon, Oxnard, California)

(5) Microscope slides, staining dishes (Coplon jars or equivalents)

(6) Cytocentrifuge diluent (Hanks' BSS with 25% fetal calf serum or albumin)

(7) Absolute methanol

(8) Giemsa blood stain (MCS, No. GX85, Norwood, Ohio). Dilute by adding 10 ml of Giemsa stock solution to 10 ml of 0.1 M tris buffer, pH 7.4, and 80 ml of distilled water.

In my opinion, the stain works best when used within an hour of its preparation, and when used but for a single group of slides.

D. Procedure

(1) Monocytes or macrophages are prepared at 1×10^7 mononuclear phagocytes/ml, based on chamber differentials, in Hanks' BSS containing 10% normal human serum (human monocytes) or 10% fetal calf serum (rabbit macrophages) and kept at room temperature in plastic tubes (III.B.4).

(2) Viable *C. albicans* are suspended at 2×10^7 yeast cells/ml in serum-free Hanks' BSS. Although they are preopsonized for studies with rabbit macrophages (see Sections II.B.2 and II.G.2), preopsonization is not required when human monocytes are to be studied.

After exposure to the human + rabbit serum (Section II.B.2) (neither normal nor immune sera kill *C. albicans* or other *Candida* species), the opsonized organisms could be washed twice with glucose-free phosphate-buffered saline, and finally resuspended in Hanks' BSS just prior to their addition to the macrophages. As these yeasts are vigorous acid producers in media, such as Hanks' BSS, that contain glucose, they should be prepared and resuspended after all other components of the assay mixture have been combined and preincubated at 37°C.

(3) To test purified human monocytes, the final incubation mixture should contain, in a volume of 1 ml, 2.5×10^6 monocytes, 5×10^6 *C. albicans* cells and 25% group AB normal serum. In mixtures substantially contaminated by granulocytes, the number of *C. albicans* cells added should also be increased to provide two *C. albicans*/granulocyte.

Our procedure is to mix 0.5 ml of Hanks' BSS containing 45% AB serum with 0.25 ml of the monocyte suspension (Section III.D.1), and to bring these to 37°C by placing the tube for 15 min in a water bath. This period of temperature equilibration is used to count the yeasts (in methylene blue), to centrifuge them (while counting), and to resuspend them in warm (37°C) Hanks' BSS at 2×10^7 yeast cells/ml. We then add 0.25 ml of this yeast suspension to the 0.75 ml mixture of serum and monocytes, cap the tube, and place it on a tube rotator in a 37°C incubator.

To test rabbit macrophages, the final incubation mixture contains, in a volume of 1 ml, 2.5×10^6 macrophages, 7.5×10^6 preopsonized *C. albicans* and 10% fetal calf serum.

We accomplish this by mixing 0.5 ml of Hanks' BSS containing 15% fetal calf serum with 0.25 ml of the rabbit macrophage suspension (Section D.1), bringing these to 37°C by placing the tube for 15 min in a water bath. This period of temperature equilibration is used to count the yeasts (in methylene blue), to centrifuge them (while counting), and to resuspend them in warm (37°C) Hanks' BSS at 3×10^7 yeast cells/ml. We then add 0.25 ml of this yeast suspension to the 0.75 ml macrophage mixture, cap the tube, and place it on a tube rotator in a 37°C incubator.

At intervals during the incubation (15 min, 2.5 hr, 4 hr),
we prepare cytocentrifuge slides of the mixtures by adding
3 drops of incubation mixture + 3 drops of diluent (Section
III.C) to each chamber and centrifuging for 6 min at approximately 800 rpm. We immediately air dry the slides, and fix
them in methanol for 3 min, air dry again, and then stain with
Giemsa stain for 20 min. Overstained slides can sometimes be
toned by brief exposure (5 sec) to 50% methanol/water. Alternatively, they can be destained in 100% methanol, washed with
water, then restained with Giemsa using either a shorter staining time (8 - 10 min) or a decreased concentration of Giemsa.
Coverslips are not used on these slides.

Properly stained slides are quite beautiful. The mono-
cyte/macrophage nucleus is purplish red and the cytoplasm is
light blue. The yeast cell's cytoplasm is intense, homogeneous
dark blue, and the small (reddish-purple) yeast cell nucleus is
ordinarily obscured by the intensity of the cytoplasmic staining. Giemsa does not stain the cytoplasmic granules of human
neutrophils, their cytoplasm appearing pale orange. Eosinophil
granules are stained a distinctive vivid orange color. Rabbit
granulocytes (heterophils) have orange-stained granular cytoplasm, probably reflecting the affinity of the eosin component
of Giemsa stain (a mixture of methylene blue, methylene azure,
and eosin) for the abundant cationic proteins in the primary
heterophil granules.

The stained slides are examined under oil immersion (1000X
magnification), with good lighting and centering. We follow an
orderly search pattern across the field of cells (↓ → ↑ → ↓ →,
etc.), stopping at each new field to focus up and down with the
fine adjustment. We score all intracellular yeast cells (i.e.,
yeasts completely surrounded by the phagocyte's blue cytoplasm)
into three mutually exclusive classes, reflecting their shape
and staining characteristics. These are "filamentous forms,"
"unchanged yeasts," and "ghosts." "Filamentous forms" consist
of blue-staining yeast cells bearing one (and rarely, two) tu-
bular processes denoting their germination and growth within
the cell. "Unchanged yeasts" are spherical-to-ovoid yeast-phase
organisms that have maintained a homogeneous blue cytoplasmic
staining pattern, generally obscuring the small eccentrically
placed nucleus. "Ghosts" are yeast-phase (very rarely filamentous phase) organisms that have lost their cytoplasmic blue
staining properties. Instead, the cytoplasm stains pale gray
or pink. If not yet degraded, the nucleus of yeast "ghosts"
may be quite visible due to loss of the obscuring cytoplasmic
stain. The refractile cell wall of the yeast may be visible as
well, particularly if one floats a drop of immersion oil over a
thin film of water on the slide, and then uses the oil immersion
lens to examine the cells. I have no idea why this "trick,"

noted as a consequence of my usual impatience to examine the slides, works. Because the "ghosts" are quite faint, relative to the other two classes of intracellular yeasts, good microscope lighting and continual play with the fine adjustment are essential to avoid their being overlooked. The classification of yeasts into the three classes continues, until 200 yeasts within macrophages/monocytes have been counted and tallied on a manual differential counter. Illustrations (photomicrographs) of these yeast classes are published elsewhere (2, 9).

E. Calculation of Data

The candidacidal activity is expressed as a "candidacidal index," which is calculated as follows:

$$\frac{\text{number of intracellular yeasts that are "ghosts"}}{\text{total number of intracellular yeasts counted (all 3 classes)}} \times 100$$

In general, a substantially diminished candidacidal index is associated with an increased filamentation index. Or, otherwise stated, if fewer ingested yeasts are killed and degraded, then more will be viable and show evidence of intracellular growth.

F. Critical Comments

Two assumptions that underlie the "specific staining" assay require consideration. The first, that all intracellular *Candida* "ghosts" are the remnants of dead cells, is manifestly correct, and shortly will be explained. The second assumption, that all dead intracellular *C. albicans* have the appearance of "ghosts" is untrue, but a reasonable approximation of this circumstance holds under the circumstances we have described.

To explain, we must consider both the concept of microbial "death" and the nature of *Candida* "ghosts." Microbial death is usually defined as the irreversible loss of replicative ability, and is generally preceded by significant alterations in one or more critical areas requiring homeostasis (membrane integrity, transport, macromolecular synthesis, or assembly, etc.). Giemsa-stained, heat-killed *C. albicans* cells, unequivocally dead, are indistinguishable from similarly stained viable cells unless the heat-killed yeasts have also been treated with ribonuclease. When their RNA undergoes enzymatic hydrolysis, however, their cytoplasm loses its affinity for the basic components (methylene blue and methylene azure) of Giemsa, and stains pink or gray like a typical intracellular "ghost." Thus, "ghosts" are yeast cells that have been killed and substantially degraded by hydrolytic enzymes of the enveloping phagocyte. As the nucleus and especially the thick cell wall resist the phagocyte's degradation processes substantially longer than does the cytoplasmic RNA, the *Candida* remnant is easily visible by careful microscopy. Of course, in time, the nucleus and finally even the cell wall disappear, leaving only a featureless vacuole (at light level microscopy) to hint at the antecedent events. The assay therefore gives a reasonable approximation of killing because: (1) it appears to take approximately 60 - 90 min after an organism is killed before it is sufficiently degraded to manifest "ghost" staining; (2) phagocytosis occurs relatively rapidly when either rabbit macrophages or human monocytes are studied as outlined (virtually all organisms are ingested by 30 min, few extracellular ones remain); (3) killing of *C. albicans* (as measured by conventional colony-count procedures) is most effective during the initial 60 - 90 min of incubation; (4) the thick cell wall of *C. albicans* allows it to be identified with certainty for several hours after its intracellular death and partial degradation; and (5) by using stationary phase organisms, the viable survivors do not begin to sprout pseudogerm tubes for 2 - 3 hr, and these enlarging processes do not become large enough to rupture the phagocyte for at least 4 hr, allowing the assay to approach equilibrium.

The assay would not work if: (1) decolorization of the cytoplasm of nonviable organisms to Giemsa stain was irregular or incomplete (*C. parapsilosis* and certain other species) or (2) if degradation occurred so rapidly that "ghosts" faded completely from view too rapidly (*C. pseudotropicalis* and other yeasts) or if (3) the phagocytic block was in postmortem digestion of the yeast rather than in killing it. Possibility (3) should be excluded by verifying that heat-killed yeasts are converted to ghosts with high efficiency. Possibilities (1) and (2) suggest that the assay may be less suitable than conventional alternatives (colony counting, etc.) for nonalbicans *Candida*. When we applied the assay to normal human monocytes in mixed cell preparations containing many neutrophils, we found normal monocytes to contain 63.4 ± 10.2% "ghosts" (mean ± S.D., n = 91) after 2½ hr, whereas 10.5 ± 6.0% of the intracellular organisms had formed filaments, and 26.4 ± 9.2% had maintained their original shape and staining characteristics. In contrast, after 2.5 hr of incubation monocytes from three patients with myeloperoxidase deficiency contained approximately 5% ghosts, 55% filamentous forms, and 35% unaltered yeasts and monocytes from three boys with chronic granulomatous disease contained approximately 2.5% ghosts and over 90% filamentous forms.

Curiously, when normal monocytes were purified by Ficoll-Hypaque centrifugation only 24.7 ± 1.2% (mean S.E.M., n = 5) of ingested *C. albicans* were converted to ghosts in 2.5 hr, whereas when they were supplemented with normal neutrophils, the percentage of intramonocytic ghosts almost doubled

(47.4 × 3.7%). The nature of this evident neutrophil-monocyte interaction has not been clarified.

Our applications of this assay to rabbit macrophages yielded the results summarized in Table I. We have found the assay to be especially useful for characterizing the mechanisms used by mononuclear phagocytes to kill *C. albicans* (1, 2).

It is worth mentioning that the methylene blue dye-exclusion method used to check initial yeast cell viability (Section III.B.2) has a different basis than does the Giemsa staining method. Methylene blue, a redox dye, can exist in an oxidized (blue) or reduced (colorless, leuko-) form. The blue dye freely gains access to nonviable yeast cells, staining them blue by virtue of (1) the failure of their metabolism to reduce it to the colorless, leuko-form and (2) the stain's affinity for cytoplasmic RNA. Metabolically dormant cells may be stained pale blue, but this rapidly reverses after brief exposure to a fresh nutrient medium (see Section III.B.2) as their metabolic activity and homeostatic mechanisms become revitalized. Dead yeasts that have lost their RNA (through autolysis or enzymatic degradation) will not stain well with methylene blue, but the faint staining will persist after exposure to fresh medium.

It should also be realized that although the concentration of methylene blue employed in this assay (approximately 0.01%) does not kill *C. albicans*, it will inhibit its growth rate considerably. Other *Candida* species may be substantially more sensitive to the stain, and the method should not be blindly extrapolated to nonalbicans *Candida* species without considering this possibility. Aqueous methylene blue is also useful in a candidacidal method applicable to human neutrophils (5), but we now consider this dye-exclusion procedure to be less conve-

TABLE I. *Candidacidal Activity of Rabbit Macrophages*

| Cell type | State | Candidacidal index[a] | |
		2.5 hr	4 hr
Alveolar macrophage	Resident	16.4 ± 2.1 (19)[b]	28.1 ± 1.9 (19)
	Elicited	22.9 ± 2.2 (19)	32.9 ± 2.3 (22)
Peritoneal macrophage	Resident	10.8 ± 2.4 (8)	15.2 ± 1.3 (9)
	Elicited	24.0 ± 4.2 (8)	28.2 ± 3.1 (14)

[a]*The data are expressed as a candidacidal index (% of intracellular Candida that are "ghosts") after 2½ or 4 hr of incubation.*

[b]*Data shown as mean ± S.E.M., with (n) signifying the number of animals tested in each group. A full description of this study appears in ref. 2.*

nient than the "specific staining" method described herein. It
also substantially underestimates the candidacidal activity of
human monocytes, attributable largely to their rapid breakdown
of cytoplasmic RNA in *C. albicans* cells that they have killed.
As this property actually enhances the "specific staining" assay method, it is preferable to the dye-exclusion procedure
when mononuclear phagocytes are tested.

Acknowledgment

This study was supported in part by research grants
AI 16252 and AI 26005 from the U.S. Public Health Service.
This is Publication No. 3 of the Collaborative California Uni-
versities-Mycology Research Unit. I thank J. Patterson-
Delafield and L. G. Ferrari for their valuable contributions
to this work.

REFERENCES

1. R. I. Lehrer. The fungicidal mechanisms of human monocytes.
   I. Evidence for myeloperoxidase-linked and myeloperoxidase-
   independent candidacidal mechanisms. *J. Clin. Invest. 55*:
   338-346, 1975.
2. R. I. Lehrer, L. G. Ferrari, J. Patterson-Delafield, and
   T. Sorrell. Fungicidal activity of rabbit alveolar and
   peritoneal macrophages against *Candida albicans. Infect.
   Immun. 28*: 1001-1008.
3. E. Metschnikoff. Sur la lutte des cellules de l'organisme
   contre l'invasion des microbes. *Ann. Inst. Pasteur 1*: 321-
   336, 1887.
4. G. Knaysi. A microscopic method of distinguishing dead
   from living bacterial cells. *J. Bacteriol. 30*: 193-206,
   1935.
5. R. I. Lehrer and M. J. Cline. Interaction of *Candida albicans* with human leukocytes and serum. *J. Bacteriol. 98*:
   996-1004, 1969.
6. P. C. J. Leijh, M. T. van den Barselaar, and R. van Furth.
   Kinetics of phagocytosis and intracellular killing of *Candida albicans* by human granulocytes and monocytes. *Infect.
   Immun. 17*: 313-318, 1977.
7. J. S. Solomkin, E. L. Mills, G. S. Giebink, R. D. Nelson,
   R. L. Simmons, and P. G. Quie. Phagocytosis of *Candida albicans* by human leukocytes: opsonic requirements. *J. Infect. Dis. 137*: 30-37,1978.
8. R. I. Lehrer. Measurements of candidacidal activity of

specific leukocyte types in mixed cell populations. I.
Normal, myeloperoxidase-deficient, and chronic granulomatous
disease neutrophils. *Infect. Immun.* 2: 42-47, 1970.

9.   R. I. Lehrer. The fungicidal activity of human leukocytes.
In "Phagocytic Mechanisms in Health and Disease" (R. C.
Williams, Jr. and H. H. Fudenberg, eds.), pp. 151-166.
Intercontinental Medical Book Corporation, New York, 1972.

70

QUANTITATION OF DESTRUCTION OF TOXOPLASMA

Rima McLeod
Jack S. Remington

I. GENERAL INTRODUCTION

Persistence and multiplication of *Toxoplasma gondii* in mo-nonuclear phagocytes *in vitro* provide a model in which microbi-cidal or inhibitory capacity of infected cells can be evaluated. Methods used to quantitate destruction of Toxoplasma include visual observation of inhibition of multiplication or destruc-tion of *T. gondii* (1 - 12), measurement of nucleic acid syn-thesized by intracellular *T. gondii* (5), and quantification of the number of organisms released from cells by plaquing tech-niques (13, 14). These assays have been employed to assess the microbicidal capacity of human peripheral blood and spleen mo-nonuclear phagocytes (1, 3, 10 - 12), mouse (2, 4, 5), ham-ster (6, 7), and guinea pig peritoneal macrophages, and mouse (4) and guinea pig alveolar macrophages. They have also been used to study microbicidal mechanisms (1 - 3), to assess lym-phokine production and response of mononuclear phagocytes to lymphokines (1, 5 - 7, 10 - 12), and to assess cell-mediated

immunity in humans with diseases (1, 3) and in animals of varying ages (8). Mononuclear phagocytes that are not inhibitory
to *T. gondii* have been employed to assay the effect of antibiotics on this organism (9).

   Toxoplasma gondii is a class 2 pathogen, and the National
Institutes of Health guidelines for work with class 2 pathogens (15) should be followed. Nonimmune pregnant women and
immunosuppressed individuals should not work with this organism. Safety precautions for other healthy individuals include
avoidance of skin puncture with needles contaminated with the
trophozoite form of the parasite and avoidance of contact of
trophozoites with breaks in skin or conjunctival or mucosal
surfaces. Serum from each individual who works with this organism should be tested for antibody to Toxoplasma prior to
working with *T. gondii*. Individuals who are accidentally inoculated with *T. gondii* and who do not have antibody are generally treated with a combination of pyrimethamine and sulfa-
diazine (or trisulfapyrimidines) (16).

II. Propagation of *Toxoplasma gondii* and *In Vitro* Challenge

A. *Introduction*

   The RH strain of Toxoplasma (obtainable from many investigators) is maintained for *in vitro* experiments by serial intraperitoneal passage in mice or in tissue culture because
T. gondii remains viable and replicates only within cells.
Prior to *in vitro* experiments, tachyzoites of Toxoplasma are
filtered (17) or centrifuged (2) free of cells. Cultures of
mononuclear phagocytes are then challenged with these tachyzoites.

B. *Reagents*

   Almost any mammalian cell line, as well as chick embryo
fibroblasts and many types of media, may be used for propagation and *in vitro* challenge. Representative methods that are
currently utilized (1 - 12, 14, 18, 19) are described below.

   1. For Passage in Mice

   Sterile normal saline.

2. For Passage in Tissue Culture

Eagle's minimal essential medium containing Earle's salts (MEM) (Grand Island Biological [GIBCO], Grand Island, New York); fetal calf serum, without Toxoplasma antibody as measured by the Sabin-Feldman dye test, heat-inactivated for 30 min at 56°C (FCS) (GIBCO); aqueous penicillin G (Pen); streptomycin (Strep); amphotericin B (utilized by laboratories in which contamination of tissue cultures with fungi is a problem).

3. For in Vitro Challenge

Hanks' balanced salt solution (HBSS) (GIBCO); heparin (Organon, West Orange, New Jersey); Medium 199 with Hanks' salts (M199); FCS; Pen; Strep; glutamine (GIBCO); aqua regia (3 parts concentrated HCl to 1 part concentrated HNO_3).

C. Procedures

1. For Passage in Mice

Swiss Webster female mice weighing 18 - 20 gm are used. It is not necessary to perform serologic testing for antibody to Toxoplasma in laboratory mice in the United States since they have not been found to be infected with this organism. A mouse in which *T. gondii* has been passaged 3 days earlier is sacrificed by inhalation of CO_2. The external abdominal wall is cleaned with 70% ethanol and incised, and the peritoneum is exposed. One and one-half milliliters of sterile saline are injected into the peritoneal space with a 22-gauge needle. The mouse is gently shaken from side to side to move the saline within the peritoneal space. Approximately 1.5 ml of the ascitic fluid-saline solution are aspirated with a 5-ml syringe and 22-gauge needle, and the solution is mixed using the needle and syringe to inject and aspirate the suspension into a 5-ml container. The Toxoplasma in the suspension are enumerated using a Nebauer hemocytometer under 40X objective of a light microscope. For passage, 0.2 ml of a suspension containing 2×10^7 organisms/ml is injected intraperitoneally into each mouse. To keep the organism constantly available for use in the laboratory, this is performed daily; donor mice are infected 3 days earlier. Passage of Toxoplasma for use in experiments is as described above except that 0.2 ml of a suspension containing 2×10^8 organisms/ml is injected intraperitoneally into each mouse. On the second day after inoculation, this yields from each mouse approximately 2×10^7 trophozoites after filtration with a Corning filter or approximately 2×10^8 trophozoites after filtration with a Millipore filter (see below). These trophozoites are used for *in vitro* challenge.

2. For Passage in Tissue Culture

Human diploid foreskin fibroblasts are grown in MEM containing 10% FCS, 100 U/ml Pen, 100 µg/ml Strep, and 0.25 µg/ml amphotericin B. The cultures are incubated in 5% CO_2 in plastic or glass tissue culture flasks. Medium overlying the adherent cells is decanted and is replaced twice weekly, and the cultures are split 1 to 3 when confluent. For passage to maintain the organism, confluent monolayers are infected with approximately one *T. gondii* trophozoite of the RH strain per 100 fibroblasts (a 25-cm² flask contains approximately 2×10^6 fibroblasts) and maintained in MEM containing Pen, Strep, amphotericin B, and 3% FCS. After 48 hr, parasites newly released by spontaneous lysis are collected by decanting the media. For passage for an experiment, confluent cultures are infected with approximately two Toxoplasma per fibroblast, and supernatants for the experiment may be collected later. Nearly all the infected and uninfected cells remain attached to the plastic culture vessels.

3. For in Vitro Challenge

When Toxoplasma passaged in mice are used for experimental studies, mice inoculated 48 hr earlier are sacrificed, the external abdominal wall is cleaned with 70% ethanol and incised, the peritoneum is exposed, and the peritoneal cavity is filled with about 5 ml of heparinized HBSS (10 U/ml heparin). Mice are gently shaken and fluid is withdrawn into a 12-ml syringe through a 22-gauge needle. Fluid from each mouse is collected separately, and samples containing visible blood are discarded. All collected fluid is poured into a 50-cc luer-lock syringe and forced through a 27-gauge needle to disrupt cells containing *T. gondii*. The stream of fluid is directed against the side of a siliconized 40-ml pyrex conical centrifuge tube to avoid bubble formation. These Toxoplasma may be separated from cells by filtering through a sintered glass filter (17) or by passing through a Millipore filter (polycarbonate membrane filter, 3 µm pore diameter; Nucleopore, Pleasanton, California) or by centrifugation at 50 g for 5 min at 22°C followed by centrifugation of the supernatant at 50 g for 10 min to collect Toxoplasma (2). Prior to passage through the sintered glass filter, the preparation is filtered through a Pyrex funnel that is 60 mm in diameter and is lined with glass wool (Corning, Corning, New York). To adjust the pH of the glass wool, HBSS is passed through the glass wool until the effluent HBSS is orange-red (phenol indicator in HBSS is orange-red when the pH is approximately 7). To adjust the pH of the sintered glass filter [90 mm in diameter, 600 ml, medium coarse porosity, 15 - 25 µm; Corning

(17)], approximately 200 ml of HBSS are passed through the
filter into a 500-ml Pyrex flask with side arm attached to
suction until the effluent HBSS is orange-red. The effluent
HBSS is discarded, and the Toxoplasma preparation is then
passed through the sintered glass filter into the flask with
side arm attached to suction. An additional 250 ml of HBSS
are poured through the sintered glass filter. The filtered
Toxoplasma are then distributed to 250-ml centrifuge bottles
(Nalgene, Rochester, New York) and centrifuged at 600 g for
15 min at 4°C. The supernatant is discarded, the Toxoplasma
are resuspended in 10 ml of M199 containing Pen, Strep, and
10% FCS, and an aliquot is counted using 0.025% trypan blue in
normal saline.

When 1×10^6 mouse peritoneal macrophages or human mononuclear phagocytes are challenged with 2×10^6 Toxoplasma,
usually 20% to 60% of the mononuclear phagocytes are infected
30 min after the challenge is removed. One-half milliliter
of Toxoplasma suspension is added to each culture chamber, and
the Toxoplasma challenge is incubated with cell cultures in 5%
CO_2 for 1 hr at 37°C. Extracellular Toxoplasma are then removed by washing five times with 37°C HBSS, and cultures are
reincubated with M199 containing 100 U/ml Pen, 100 µg/ml Strep,
2 mM fresh glutamine, and 10% FCS (mouse macrophages) or 40%
autologous or AB human serum (human mononuclear phagocytes).
After use, the sintered glass filter is rinsed with deionized
water and 500 ml of aqua regia are poured through the filter
to clean it. It usually takes about 12 hr for the aqua regia
to pass through the filter. The filter is then backwashed with
approximately 24 liters of deionized water that has been distilled twice in glass containers. Suspensions of Toxoplasma
are maintained on ice throughout these procedures, except when
poured through the sintered glass filter and immediately prior
to challenge of mononuclear phagocytes. All glassware should
be sterile and suitable for use in tissue culture. Passage
and preparation of Toxoplasma are performed using sterile technique. Because Toxoplasma do not survive extracellularly for
a prolonged time, it is critical that no more than 1 hr elapse
between the time that Toxoplasma are obtained from the peritoneal fluid of mice and the time that monolayers are challenged.

III.   QUANTITATION OF DESTRUCTION OF TOXOPLASMA USING LIGHT OR
       PHASE MICROSCOPY

A. *Introduction*

Toxoplasma gondii multiply and synthesize nucleic acid
within phagocytic vacuoles of peritoneal macrophages from nonimmune mice, hamsters, and guinea pigs, and alveolar macrophages
from nonimmune mice and guinea pigs. Human peripheral blood
monocytes have the capacity to destroy the majority of *T. gondii*
that invade or are phagocytized by them. *Toxoplasma gondii* that
survive in human monocytes multiply and synthesize nucleic acid.
Multiplication or destruction of *T. gondii* within mononuclear
phagocytes may be observed by light microscopy in preparations
fixed with aminoacridine (used to better visualize phagocytic
vacuoles) and stained with Giemsa (1, 4, 6 - 8) or by phase microscopy in preparations fixed with glutaraldehyde (11, 12, 18).
Nucleic acid synthesis by intracellular Toxoplasma may be observed by autoradiography and light microscopy in preparations
incubated with radiolabeled nucleic acid precursors (10, 11).

B. *Reagents*

   1. *For All Methods of Evaluation*

M199; FCS; autologous human serum; mononuclear phagocytes;
37°C HBSS; ethidium bromide (Calbiochem-Behring, La Jolla,
California); acridine orange (Calbiochem-Behring).

   2. *For Light Microscopy (with and without Autoradiography)*

Aminoacridine fixative (0.4% aminoacridine hydrochloride
[Sigma Chemical, St. Louis, Missouri] in 50% ethanol, fixed for
at least 1 hr at 4°C before washing and staining); Giemsa stain
(original azure blend 7.415 gm/liter in methyl alcohol; Harleco,
Gibbstown, New Jersey).

   3. *For Autoradiography*

Uridine (Calbiochem-Behring); [^{3}H]uridine (28 Ci/mmol; New
England Nuclear, Boston, Massachusetts); [5,6-^{3}H]uracil (48
Ci/mmol; Amersham Searle, Arlington Heights, Illinois); anhy-
drous calcium sulfate (Drierite, Xenia, Ohio); NTB2 emulsion
(Kodak, Rochester, New York); black slide box (Scientific
Products, Sunnyvale, California); D19 developer (Kodak); 1%
glacial acetic acid (acid rinse is 2 ml of glacial acetic acid,
brought to 200 ml with deionized water); fixer (16.88 ml of

fixer [Edwall Quick Fix; Edwall Scientific Products, Chicago,
Illinois] plus 2.55 ml of hardener, brought to 200 ml with deionized water); citric acid (0.1 M solution, i.e., 21.014 gm
of citric acid per liter of distilled water); dibasic sodium
phosphate (0.2 M solution, i.e., 28.4 gm of Na_2HPO_4 per liter
of distilled water; use sterile distilled water, but sterile
glassware is not necessary); buffer, pH 5.75 [prepared from
the two preceding solutions (85 ml of 0.1 M citric acid solution and 150 ml of 0.2 M dibasic sodium phosphate solution)
and 765 ml of distilled water; the concentrated solution can
be refrigerated and distilled water can be added just before
use but, before using, the pH should be checked to be certain
it is 5.75 ± 0.5]; methanol.

4. For Phase Microscopy

Glutaraldehyde (2.5% in sodium cacodylate buffer, pH 7.4)
(18).

C. Procedures

1. For All Methods of Evaluation

Cultures of mononuclear phagocytes are prepared in chambers
of Labtek slides (4 chamber; Labtek Products, Naperville, Illinois) or on 15-mm glass coverslips (Bellco Glass, Vineland, New
Jersey) and placed in wells of 24-well culture trays (FB-16-24-
7C; Linbro Chemical, Los Angeles, California). The coverslips
are first cleaned by soaking in 1 M of KOH overnight, rinsing
thoroughly with deionized water, and then rinsing in boiling
twice-distilled deionized water. They are then sterilized by
dry heat. Medium containing 40% human serum (employed to culture human mononuclear phagocytes) may dissolve adhesive material on Labtek slides and, therefore, coverslips are used for
these cultures. Cultures are maintained at 37°C in an atmosphere containing 5% CO_2. The time at which the challenge is
removed is defined as zero time.

2. For Light Microscopy (without Autoradiography)

One-half hour after the challenge is removed and at later
times, usually at 12 hr and at 18 to 24 hr, medium containing
serum is washed from the slides with HBSS, the slides are fixed
in aminoacridine for 1 hr and stained with Giemsa stain (1 part
Giemsa stain, 7.415 gm/liter, to 9 parts water), and then coverslips are permounted on these preparations. If cells have been
cultured on round coverslips in Linbro trays, the coverslips
are removed from the Linbro trays, mounted with permount face-up

on slides, and stained, and then an additional coverslip is
permounted on top of this stained preparation.

3. For Light Microscopy (with Autoradiography)

If [^{3}H]uridine is used as the radioactive precursor, cell
cultures are incubated for 3 hr with cold uridine (0.01 M)
prior to Toxoplasma challenge. Either [^{3}H]uridine (5 µCi per
culture chamber) or uracil (10 µCi per culture chamber) is
added for 1 hr prior to fixation of slides. Extracellular
radiolabel is washed from slides by rinsing them thoroughly
with HBSS. Slides are fixed in aminoacridine as described
above. Emulsion is applied in a darkroom, and slides are
placed within a lead shield for 1 week at 15°C. Slides are
developed in a darkroom by placing them in developer for 2 min,
acid rinse for 2 sec, and fixer for 2 min, and then rinsing
them in cool running tap water for 6 to 8 min. The slides are
then Giemsa stained as follows (20): The slides are dehydrated
and hydrated by placing radioautographs in each of the following
solutions for 6 min: 50% methanol plus 50% pH 5.75 buffer (for
staining boat, use 90 ml of methanol and 90 ml of pH 5.75 buffer); then 95% methanol plus 5% pH 5.75 buffer (use 171 ml of
methanol and 9 ml of pH 5.75 buffer); then pH 5.75 buffer.
The slides are dried. Stain is prepared with 18 ml of Giemsa
stain and 5.4 ml of methanol, brought to 200 ml with pH 5.75
buffer. Slides are stained for 15 min, rinsed in pH 5.75 buffer for 1 min, and dried, and coverslips are mounted with permount.

4. For Phase Microscopy

Culture and challenge of cells are the same as described
above with the exception that cells are cultured for 24 hr
before infection with Toxoplasma to allow for adequate spreading. The glutaraldehyde-fixed specimens are examined by microscopy with a 63X planapo phase oil emersion objective or 100X
phase oil emersion objective.

D. Calculation of Data

1. For Light Microscopy (without Autoradiography)

Percentage infected cells, mean number of Toxoplasma per
vacuole, and cells per field are counted using a 40X objective.
To determine percentage infected cells and mean number of Toxoplasma per vacuole, at least 500 to 1000 total cells should be
counted if infection rates are <20%, and at least 200 cells
should be counted if infection rates are >20%. Ten fields ob-

served with 40X objective are counted to determine cells per
high-power field. All areas of the slide should be inspected
to determine that the 200 to 1000 cells in ten fields counted
are representative of the entire experiment. Equivalence of
cell numbers in different cultures may also be assessed by
quantitating amount of DNA or cell nuclei[21] in the cultures.

2. For Light Microscopy (with Autoradiography)

Slides are evaluated in the same manner as described above.
In addition, in slides in which uridine is used as the radiolabeled precursor, the number of grains overlying Toxoplasma
are also counted. Toxoplasma with five or more overlying
grains are considered viable. In experiments in which radiolabeled uracil is utilized as the precursor, the Toxoplasma
take up this substance so avidly that evaluating mean number
of Toxoplasma per vacuole is not possible since organisms are
obscured by radiolabel (Fig. 1).

3. For Phase Microscopy

The percentage infected cells and mean number of Toxoplasma
per vacuole are quantitated as described above.

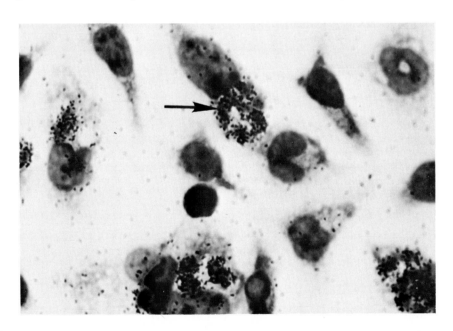

Fig. 1. Light microscopy (with autoradiography) showing
Toxoplasma in a culture labeled with 10 μCi/ml [5,6-³H]uracil.
Arrow indicates grains over the organisms.

E.   Critical Comments

These methods are reproducible and sensitive for assessment of microbicidal capacity of mononuclear phagocytes. Peritoneal mononuclear phagocytes from mice, hamsters, and guinea
pigs that do not have infection with *T. gondii* permit multiplication of this organism. For example, there are approximately
8 to 16 Toxoplasma per vacuole by 24 hr and lysis or detachment
of cells soon afterwards, there is uptake of radiolabeled
nucleic acid precursors by intracellular organisms, and there
is <50% reduction in percentage infected macrophages between
30 min and 18 to 24 hr after challenge. If microbicidal capacity is enhanced, multiplication and nucleic acid synthesis by
intracellular *T. gondii* are impaired and the percentage infected macrophages at 18 to 24 hr after challenge is reduced
substantially when compared to the percentage infected macrophages noted at 30 min. In almost all instances, >80% of human
monocytes and ≥50% of monocyte-derived macrophages from individuals with and without antibody to Toxoplasma destroy the
organism in the first 6 hr after challenge. Toxoplasma that
remain within human monocytes and macrophages after 6 hr multiply; at 18 to 24 hr, there are from 2 to 8 Toxoplasma per
vacuole and synthesis of nucleic acid by these organisms is reflected in their uptake of radiolabeled nucleic acid precursor.
If reduction in percentage infected monocytes is being assessed,
viability of the challenge inoculum of Toxoplasma must be
demonstrated by simultaneous challenge of cells without microbicidal ability (e.g., normal mouse peritoneal macrophages).
Viability of Toxoplasma has also been confirmed by acridine
orange staining (2, 22). Acridine orange (Allied Chemical,
Morristown, New Jersey) in a final concentration of 5 µg/ml is
incubated with the parasites for 10 min at 37°C. Viable Toxoplasma show bright orange-red punctate lysosomal fluorescence
against a homogeneous dark green cytoplasm when examined by
fluorescence microscopy with a photomicroscope (exciter filter
BG 12, barrier filter 53). Observer bias is a potential difficulty in using these methods.

IV.   QUANTITATION OF NUCLEIC ACID SYNTHESIS BY INTRACELLULAR
      T. gondii

A.   Introduction

This method involves measurement of incorporation of
[^{3}H]uracil into nucleic acids of the obligate intracellular
parasite *T. gondii*. The method is based on an observation by

Pfefferkorn and Pfefferkorn (19) that [³H]uracil is incorporated in substantially greater amounts by *T. gondii* than by certain mammalian cell types. Differential uptake of [³H]uracil by Toxoplasma in infected and uninfected cultures allows for evaluation of the ability of macrophages or monocytes to inhibit or kill this organism. This method has been employed with mouse peritoneal macrophages and human monocytes and monocyte-derived macrophages (1, 5).

B. Reagents

[5,6-³H]Uracil (specific activity 48 Ci/mmol; Amersham Searle); sodium dodecyl sulfate; uracil (Sigma); 0.3 N trichloroacetic acid; ethanol; omniflor (New England Nuclear); toluene (4 liters of toluene should contain 16.7 gm of omniflor).

C. Procedures

Culture of mononuclear phagocytes and preparation of lymphocyte supernatants are as previously described (5, 10), and Toxoplasma challenge is as described above. Mononuclear phagocytes are cultured directly on the plastic surfaces of wells in the Linbro trays. Radiolabeling and extraction procedures are performed at the desired intervals following infection with Toxoplasma (for growth curves, optimal times are every 6 hr for 24 hr). Monolayers of infected and uninfected cells are pulsed with 10 µCi of [³H]uracil. Incorporation of [³H]uracil into acid precipitable material is measured by a filtration procedure: Monolayers are dissolved in 1% sodium dodecyl sulfate containing 100 µg/ml of uracil employed as a carrier, adjusted to a final concentration of 0.3 N trichloroacetic acid, and are stored for at least 1 hr at 4°C. The resulting precipitates are kept on ice and are collected on glass filters (type a e, 24 mm; Gelman Instrument, Ann Arbor, Michigan). The material retained by the filters is washed with cold 0.3 N trichloroacetic acid, rinsed with 95% ethanol, dried for 1 hr in an oven at 60°C, placed in scintillation vials containing toluene and omniflor (5 ml/vial), and counted in a scintillation counter.

D. Calculation of Data

These studies are usually performed with at least three sets of infected and uninfected cultures. Data are expressed as counts per minute (cpm) or difference in cpm between infected and uninfected cultures (Δcpm). Statistical evaluation of the

differences between test and control results is by the Student's
t test, other than for comparison of Δcpm of groups. For comparison of Δcpm of test and control groups, the size of the difference, corrected for background, is determined using the normal significance test.

E. Critical Comments

This method obviates the potential observer bias in the
visual methods described above and is a simple and rapid technique. The visual methods and this method permit assessment
of monocyte or macrophage function without need for antibiotics
in the media and without concern about multiplication of extracellular organisms (as in systems that assess effect of phagocytic cells on bacteria). It is critical, however, that monolayers being studied are of comparable density. Cultures of
uninfected mouse peritoneal macrophages and human peripheral
blood mononuclear phagocytes incorporate approximately 200 to
500 cpm [^{3}H]uracil. Cultures of mouse peritoneal and human
peripheral blood mononuclear phagocytes infected with Toxoplasma incorporate approximately 5000 to 30,000 cpm [^{3}H]uracil.

V. QUANTITATIVE PLAQUING OF TOXOPLASMA IN CULTURES OF FIBRO-
BLASTS

A. Introduction

Plaque techniques that employ agar overlay (13) and liquid
overlay (14) have been used to determine quantitatively the
number of Toxoplasma in a suspension capable of infecting fibroblasts. Although reports of this method have not specifically described its usefulness for assessment of the microbicidal
capacity of mononuclear phagocytes, it is reasonable to assume
that it could be used to determine the number of T. gondii in
supernatants of cultures of mononuclear phagocytes. The procedure using liquid overlay is simpler than and as reliable as
the method using an agar overlay (14) and, therefore, it will
be described here.

B. Reagents

Eagle's MEM; FCS; Pen; Strep; amphotericin B.

C. Procedures

Human diploid fibroblast cells are grown to confluency in 25 cm^2 plastic tissue culture flasks in MEM containing Pen, Strep, amphotericin B, and 10% FCS (14, 19). Medium is discarded and replaced with fresh medium containing Pen, Strep, amphotericin B, and 3% FCS. Extracellular *T. gondii*, which could be obtained from supernatants of cultures of mononuclear phagocytes, are diluted in Eagle's MEM containing Hanks' salts, antibiotics, and 3% FCS. Dilutions of supernatant containing toxoplasma in volumes varying from 25 to 500 μl are added to flasks of confluent fibroblasts, and the flasks are then incubated for 4 days at 37°C. The infectious parasites produce irregularly shaped plaques that are 1 to 2 mm in diameter. Under these conditions, microscopically visible secondary plaques are not observed unless the culture is disturbed early in the incubation period. The plaques are counted, without aid of staining, using oblique illumination on a dark background (14, 19).

D. Calculation of Data

The data are recorded as plaque-forming units (PFU). PFU of supernatants of cultures of mouse peritoneal and human peripheral blood mononuclear phagocytes could be obtained at 6-hr intervals after challenge to detect viable Toxoplasma released from the mononuclear phagocytic cells.

E. Critical Comments

This method is reproducible (14) and could be used to measure the number of Toxoplasma released from mononuclear phagocytes but would also reflect the ability of the organisms to infect and replicate within fibroblasts.

Acknowledgment

This work was supported by Grant AI 04717 from the National Institutes of Health and Biomedical Research Support Grant SO7RR05476-17, Michael Reese Medical Center Institutional Award.

REFERENCES

1. R. McLeod, K. G. Bensch, S. M. Smith, and J. S. Remington.
    Effects of human peripheral blood monocytes, monocyte-
    derived macrophages, and spleen mononuclear phagocytes on
    Toxoplasma gondii. *Cell. Immunol.* *54*: 330-350, 1980.
2. H. W. Murray and Z. A. Cohn. Macrophage oxygen-dependent
    antimicrobial activity. I. Susceptibility of *Toxoplasma
    gondii* to oxygen intermediates. *J. Exp. Med.* *150*: 938-
    949, 1979.
3. C. B. Wilson, V. Tsai, and J. S. Remington. Failure to
    trigger the oxidative metabolic burst by normal macro-
    phages: A possible mechanism for survival of intracellu-
    lar pathogens. *J. Exp. Med.* *151*: 328-346, 1980.
4. F. W. Ryning and J. S. Remington. Effect of alveolar
    macrophages on *Toxoplasma gondii.* *Infect. Immun.* *18*:
    746-753, 1977.
5. R. McLeod and J. S. Remington. A method to evaluate the
    capacity of monocytes and macrophages to inhibit multipli-
    cation of an intracellular pathogen. *J. Immunol. Methods*
    27: 19-29, 1979.
6. R. L. Hoff and J. K. Frenkel. Cell-mediated immunity
    against Besnoitia and Toxoplasma in specifically and cross-
    immunized hamsters and in cultures. *J. Exp. Med.* *139*:
    560-580, 1974.
7. R. E. Lindberg and J. K. Frenkel. Cellular immunity to
    Toxoplasma and Besnoitia in hamsters: Specificity and the
    effects of cortisol. *Infect. Immun.* *15*: 855-862, 1977.
8. I. D. Gardner and J. S. Remington. Aging and the immune
    response. II. Lymphocyte responsiveness and macrophage ac-
    tivation in *Toxoplasma gondii*-infected mice. *J. Immunol.*
    120: 944-949, 1978.
9. P. L. Grossman and J. S. Remington. The effect of tri-
    methoprim and sulfamethoxazole on *Toxoplasma gondii in
    vitro* and *in vivo.* *Am. J. Trop. Med. Hyg.* *28*: 445-455,
    1979.
10. S. E. Anderson, Jr., and J. S. Remington. Effect of nor-
    mal and activated human macrophages on *Toxoplasma gondii.*
    J. Exp. Med. *139*: 1154-1174, 1974.
11. S. E. Anderson, S. C. Bautista, and J. S. Remington. Induc-
    tion of resistance to *Toxoplasma gondii* in human macro-
    phages by soluble lymphocyte products. *J. Immunol.* *117*:
    381-387, 1976.
12. J. S. Borges and W. D. Johnson, Jr. Inhibition of multi-
    plication of *Toxoplasma gondii* by human monocytes exposed
    to T-lymphocyte products. *J. Exp. Med.* *141*: 483-496,
    1975.
13. V. L. Foley and J. S. Remington. Plaquing of *Toxoplasma*

gondii in secondary cultures of chick embryo fibroblasts. *J. Bacteriol. 98*: 1-3, 1969.

14. E. R. Pfefferkorn and L. C. Pfefferkorn. *Toxoplasma gondii*: Isolation and preliminary characterization of temperature-sensitive mutants. *Exp. Parasitol. 39*: 365-376, 1976.

15. "Classification of Etiologic Agents on the Basis of Hazard," 4th edition, U.S. Department of Health, Education, and Welfare, Public Health Service, Center for Disease Control, Office of Biosafety, Atlanta, Georgia, 1979.

16. R. McLeod and J. S. Remington. Toxoplasmosis. *In* "Harrison's Principles of Internal Medicine" (K. J. Isselbacher, R. Adams, E. Braunwald, R. Petersdorf, and J. D. Wilson, eds.), pp. 879-885. McGraw-Hill, New York, 1980.

17. J. S. Remington, M. M. Bloomfield, E. Russel, Jr., and W. S. Robinson. The RNA of *Toxoplasma gondii*. *Proc. Soc. Exp. Biol. Med. 133*: 623-626, 1970.

18. T. C. Jones, L. Len, and J. G. Hirsch. Assessment *in vitro* of immunity against *Toxoplasma gondii*. *J. Exp. Med. 141*: 466-482, 1975.

19. E. R. Pfefferkorn and L. C. Pfefferkorn. Specific labeling of intracellular *Toxoplasma gondii* with uracil. *J. Protozool. 24*: 449-453, 1977.

20. V. J. Pasanen and L. B. Epstein. An appraisal of an autoradiographic technique for enumeration of antibody containing cells in response to Salmonella somatic polysaccharide. *Int. Arch. Allergy 32*: 149-163, 1967.

21. K. Burton. Study of conditions and mechanisms of diphenylamine reaction for colorimetric estimation of deoxyribonucleic acid. *Biochem. J. 62*: 315-323, 1956.

22. D. R. Parks, V. M. Bryan, V. T. Oi, and L. A. Herzenberg. Antigen-specific identification and cloning of hybridomas with a fluorescence-activated cell sorter. *Proc. Nat. Acad. Sci. USA 76*: 1962-1966, 1979.

71

DESTRUCTION OF RICKETTSIAE

Carol A. Nacy
Stanley C. Oaks

I. INTRODUCTION

The rickettsiae are obligate intracellular bacteria that
infect a variety of cells *in vitro*, including macrophages
(1 - 3). The process by which rickettsiae enter cells is unknown, but may involve "induced phagocytosis" in a manner similar to that described for Chlamydia (4). Both host cell and
rickettsia must be metabolically active for penetration to occur, and the rickettsiae are initially bound by a host-derived
phagocytic vacuole. Within 15 min the phagosome is destroyed,
and the rickettsiae are free in the cytosol of the cell.
Rickettsia tsutsugamushi, the etiologic agent of scrub typhus,
replicates preferentially in the cytoplasm of the perinuclear
region of the macrophage (1). As with all rickettsiae in the
spotted fever group, *R. akari*, the etiologic agent of rickettsial pox, replicates in both the cytoplasm and the nucleus (5).
The rate of replication of rickettsiae varies with the host
cell. In cultured peritoneal macrophages of mice, *R. tsutsuga-*

METHODS FOR STUDYING
MONONUCLEAR PHAGOCYTES

mushi doubling time is approximately 18 - 20 hr. *Rickettsia akari,* on the other hand, replicates more rapidly, and has a doubling time of 12 - 15 hr. Both rickettsiae migrate out of infected cells a short time after they begin replication: Secondary infections of cultured cells occur immediately with *R. akari,* and after 2 days with *R. tsutsugamushi* (1).

Several studies suggest that immunologically activated macrophages are effector cells of antirickettsial immunity *in vivo* and *in vitro* (6 - 9). The role of macrophages in immunity to rickettsial infections was further emphasized in studies with *R. akari.* Certain strains of mice fail to develop activated tumoricidal macrophages after treatment *in vivo* with BCG or *C. parvum,* or *in vitro* with lymphokines (13): Macrophages from these same mouse strains failed to develop rickettsiacidal activity after treatment with macrophage activating agents, and mice were highly susceptible to the lethal effects of *R. akari* infection (10). Analysis of macrophage activation for rickettsiacidal activity indicates two separate and distinct mechanisms by which the activated macrophage remains free of intracellular rickettsiae (9):

(1) When macrophages are pulsed with lymphokines 4 hr prior to rickettsial infection, substantially fewer treated cells contain intracellular rickettsiae immediately after the rickettsial adsorption period. The rickettsiae lose their infectivity for macrophages: 35% fewer viable rickettsiae can be recovered from macrophage lysates in treated cultures compared to control macrophage lysates. This loss of rickettsial infectivity is not due to soluble products released from the macrophage (unpublished observations).

(2) Intracellular killing of rickettsiae occurs in lymphokine-pretreated macrophage cultures with additional incubation of 24 hr. This intracellular killing can be dissociated from the immediate effect of lymphokine activation by infecting macrophages first, and adding lymphokines only after infection. A 75 - 85% reduction in percentage macrophages infected with rickettsiae or viable rickettsiae recovered from macrophage lysates, occurs in macrophage cultures treated with lymphokines after infection.

The rickettsiae have several unique characteristics that make them useful for studying immunologic activation of murine macrophages: (1) they are obligate intracellular parasites: they do not replicate in the extracellular environment and, in fact, have a very short lifespan (less than 1 hr) outside of cells; (2) they have a long generation time: differences in numbers of intracellular rickettsiae in activated and untreated macrophage cultures reflects killing without complication of rapid multiplication in a few infected cells; and (3) rickettsiae are killed by immunologically activated macrophages only: cells in various states of "stimulation" due to sterile eliciting agents support the growth of rickettsiae as do resident macrophages.

Although the rickettsiacidal assay is somewhat more diffi-cult to establish in the laboratory, it is one of very few as-says available to study microbicidal activities of activated macrophages.

II. REAGENTS

A. Rickettsial Stocks

(1) Rickettsia akari, Kaplan strain (American Type Culture Collection (ATCC), Rockville, Maryland) propagated in irra-diated L-929 cells. Rickettsia akari is now classified as a class 2 agent and may be used in "laboratories whose staff have levels of competency equal to or greater than one would expect in a college department of microbiology. Requests for agents in class 2 are placed on institutional letterhead (11)."

(2) Rickettsia tsutsugamushi, strain Gilliam (ATCC) propa-gated in irradiated L-929 cells. Rickettsia tsutsugamushi is classified as class 3 microorganism and may be used in "labora-tories whose staff have levels of competency equal to or greater than one would expect in a college department of microbiology and who have had special training in handling dangerous agents, and are supervised by competent scientists.... Requests for agents in class 3 are signed by the chairman of the department or the heat of the laboratory or research institute where the work will be carried out. Conditions for containment include:

(1) a controlled access facility--separated from the general traffic pattern of the rest of the building;

(2) negative air pressure--at the site of work in a prepa-ration cubicle or under a hood. Air should be decontaminated by high efficiency filter before recirculation;

(3) animal experiments--are conducted with a level of pre-caution equivalent to conditions required for laboratory experi-ments;

(4) personnel at risk are immunized against agents for which immune prophylaxis is available (1).

(NOTE: There is no prophylactic immunization for scrub typhus.)

B. *Cell lines: L-929 Cells (No. CCL-1, ATCC).*

C. *Culture Media, Solutions*

   L-cell growth medium: Medium 199 supplemented with 2 mM
L-glutamine and 10% heat-inactivated fetal bovine serum (FBS)
   Macrophage harvest and rickettsiacidal assay medium: RPMI
1640 supplemented with 2 mM L-glutamine and 10% heat-inactivated
FBS
   Trypsin-EDTA solution: 0.05% trypsin, 0.02% disodium salt
of EDTA (Flow Laboratories, Rockville, Maryland)
   Earl's or Hank's balanced salt solution (M. A. Bioproducts,
Walkersville, Maryland)
   Snyder I diluent (12): Sucrose, 75.0 ; KH_2PO_4, 0.52 ;
Na_2HPO_4, 1.22 ; Glutamic acid, 0.72 . Dissolve sucrose in
150 ml of distilled water. Add buffer salts in order, then
glutamic acid. Add distilled water to 1000 ml. Adjust pH to
7.4 with 10 N NaOH, then dispense in 50 ml quantities and auto-
clave for 20 min at 10 lb pressure. Store at 4C.
   Neutral red staining solution, 1/300 (GIBCO, Grand Island,
New York)
   Trypan blue, 0.4% (GIBCO)
   *Agarose, Seakem brand (M. A. Bioproducts)
   Brain Heart Infusion broth (BHI) (Difco Laboratories,
Detroit, Michigan)
   70% Alcohol in a squirt bottle
   Distilled water

D. *Plasticware*

   150-cm^2 tissue culture flasks (No. 3150, Costar, Cambridge,
Massachusetts)
   50-ml sterile polypropylene centrifuge tubes (No. 2070,
Falcon Plastics, Oxnard, California)
   12 × 75 mm sterile polypropylene* tubes with caps (No. 2063,
Costar)
   30-cc polypropylene disposable syringes
   1-, 5-, and 10-cc sterile cotton-plugged serological pipettes (Costar)

E. *Glassware*

   500-ml bottles, screw-capped, sterilized (MA Bioproducts)
   600-ml beakers, covered with 2 layers of gauze
   1 dram sterile glass screw-capped vials (Lawshe Instrument
Company, Inc., Bethesda, Maryland

50- and 250-cc sterile cotton-plugged graduated cylinders
Pasteur pipettes
Two small funnels
Two 250-ml Ehrlenmeyer flasks

F. *Equipment*

CO_2 incubator, humidified, solid stainless steel shelves
Refrigerated centrifuge
Binocular microscope
Inverted tissue culture microscope
Vortex mixer
Autoclave (fast and slow exhaust)
Water baths (3): 37°C, 46° - 48°, and 56°C
Balance
Pipette-aid (Bellco, Vineland, New Jersey)
Vertical laminar flow hood for use with biological agents
Rh typing box (Fisher Scientific Company, Silver Spring, Maryland
Homogenizer with stainless steel, aerosol-proof cup (Sorvall, Newtown, Connecticut)
Gamma radiation source
Cytocentrifuge (Cytospin, Shandon Southern Instruments, Sewelicky, Pennsylvania)

G. *Mice*

*Use only inbred mouse strains; mice must be healthy. Avoid using mouse strains with characterized *in vivo* and *in vitro* macrophage defects (13).

H. *Stains*

1. Diff-Quick (Harleco, Gibbstown, New Jersey) can be used for differentials on peritoneal cells.
2. Giemsa stain (Reagent Chemicals, Saugerties, New York) can be used for detection of *R. tsutsugamushi* in macrophages. Prepare stain according to package directions; flood slides with stain for 25 min and wash with tap water.
3. Gimenez stain must be used for detection of *R. akari* in macrophages:

    (a) Reagents
        (1) Carbol basic fuchsin stock: 100 ml 10% basic
            fuchsin in 95% ethanol (10 gm basic fuchsin in
            100 ml 95% ethanol)

250 ml 4% aqueous phenol (10 ml phenol in 240 ml distilled water)
650 ml distilled water
Incubate stock solution at 37°C for 48 hr. Refrigerate.
(2) Dilution buffer for carbol basic fuchsin:
3.5 ml 0.2 M NaH$_2$PO$_4$, pH 4.2 - 4.6 (2.76 gm/100 ml
d/H$_2$O)
15.5 ml 0.2 M Na$_2$HPO$_4$, pH 9.1 - 9.2 (2.84 gm/100 ml
d/H$_2$O)
19.0 ml distilled H$_2$O (should be pH 7.45)
(b) Preparation of working strains
(1) Carbol basic fuchsin: 4 ml stock carbol basic
fuchsin
10 ml buffer, pH 7.45
Filter immediately (use Whatman No. 1 filter in conical funnel: filter stain into 250 ml flask) and
again before every stain. Remains unstable for 48
hr, if kept at 4°C.
(2) malachite green counter stain: 0.8% aqueous malachite green (0.8 gm/100 ml d/H$_2$O)
Filter before use. Refrigerate.
(c) Staining procedure for macrophage cytocentrifuge smears
(1) Air dry cytocentrifuge smears
(2) Heat fix smears
(3) Stain with working carbol basic fuchsin 3.5 min.
(4) Wash thoroughly with tap water
(5) Stain with filtered malachite green for 3.5 min
(6) Wash thoroughly with tap water
(7) Air dry
(8) Observe cell smears under oil immersion; cell cytoplasm and nucleus will be green, and the rickettsiae will stain red.

* Indicates brand or type of material that is critical for
success of procedure.

III. PROCEDURE

A. *Culture of Rickettsiae in Irradiated L-929 Cells*

Rickettsiae obtained from ATCC have been propagated in yolk
sacs of eggs; it is necessary to grow rickettsiae in cultured
cells for use in the rickettsiacidal assay, as ingested yolk sac
obscures the intracellular organisms when macrophages are microscopically observed.

1. Growth and Subculture of L-929 Cells

(a) Place trypsin-EDTA and growth medium into 37°C water bath 30 min prior to use.

(b) Select a 150-cm^2 flask of L-929 cells to be subcultured. Remove medium by pouring into gauze-covered beaker (gauze prevents medium from splashing back into flask).

(c) Wash cells by pipetting 4 ml of warmed trypsin-EDTA into flask (not directly onto monolayer). Rock flask to distribute solution and immediately pour into gauze-covered beaker.

(d) Pipette 8 ml of warmed trypsin-EDTA solution into the flask; replace cap and allow to stand on level surface for 5 - 8 min. Alternatively, flasks may be incubated at 34° - 37°C for several minutes to speed up trypsinization.

(e) Tap side of flask against palm of hand to loosen cells that have not already detached. Triturate the cell suspension with a 10-ml pipette and transfer to a sterile 50-ml plastic centrifuge tube containing 10 ml of growth medium and 3 ml FBS (to inactivate the trypsin).

(f) Centrifuge cell suspensions at 800 g for 10 min. Decant supernatant fluid and resuspend cells in 10 ml growth medium. Triturate well to ensure an even distribution of single cells.

(g) Using 1-ml pipette, transfer 0.5 ml of cell suspension to a 12 × 75 mm test tube containing 1 ml of trypan blue solution (1/3 dilution of cell suspension). Triturate well using a Pasteur pipette and then carefully load both chambers of a clean hemocytometer.

(h) Count the number of viable cells (those that do not take up blue stain) in each of the four corner squares of each of the two chambers (each corner square contains 16 smaller divisions). Using this total, calculate the number of viable cells per ml of the cell suspension:

Number of cells/ml = total number cells for 8 squares/8 × dilution factor × 10^4

Example: cells/ml = 408/8 × 3   10^4
= 1.53 × 10^6 cells/ml

Total number of cells = number of cells/ml × total number of ml.

(i) Transfer 5 × 10^6 cells into each 150-cm^2 flask containing 50 ml growth medium. Tighten caps, shake each flask gently to ensure an even distribution of cells, and immediately place in a humidified incubator at 37°C and 5% CO_2. Loosen all flask caps 1/2 turn to allow free exchange of gases; tighten caps after 18 - 24 hr. Cells are ready for use after 3 - 5 days of incubation.

2. Preparation of Irradiated Cell Monolayers

(a) Select several flasks (number depends on number of cells required) containing moderately heavy (20 - 30 × 10^6 cells/flask) monolayers of L-929 cells.

(b) Follow steps (a) - (e) of Section III.A.1 above, treating each flask in the same manner. Cells from three flasks may be combined into a single 50-ml centrifuge tube.

(c) Place tubes containing cell suspension into a gamma radiation source. Irradiate cells with a 3000 rad total dose.

(d) Follow steps (f) - (h) of Section III.A.1. On step (g), however, a second 1/3 dilution of cells is necessary to attain the appropriate number of cells in each square of the hemocytometer (i.e., transfer 0.5 ml from the initial 1/3 dilution into a second 12 × 75 mm tube containing 1 ml of trypan blue solution). Fill the hemocytometer, count the cells, and calculate the number of cells per milliliter of suspension as noted in steps (g) - (h) of Section III.A.1.

(e) Determine the number of milliliter of this suspension required to obtain 18 - 20 × 10^6 cells. Pipette this volume into 150-cm^2 flasks, each containing 50 ml of growth medium. Tighten caps, shake gently to ensure an even distribution of cells, and immediately place in a humidified incubator at 34° - 37°C with 5% CO_2. Loosen all caps 1/2 turn to allow free exchange of gases; tighten caps after 18 - 24 hr. Flasks will be ready for use after overnight incubation.

3. Growth of Rickettsiae in Cell Culture

(a) Prepare monolayers of irradiated L-929 cells in 150-cm^2 flasks the day before this procedure. Examine monolayers microscopically to ensure that cells are healthy, monolayers are confluent, and there is no gross contamination.

(b) Prepare dilution blank by pipetting 9 ml of cold BHI broth into a sterile screwcapped tube, and place in ice bath. Rapidly thaw (at 37°C) a vial containing the appropriate rickettsial suspension, and immediately pipette 1 ml of this suspension into the dilution blank. Mix thoroughly on a vortex mixer.

(c) Immediately pour growth medium from flasks with irradiated monolayers into a gauze-covered beaker. Pipette 1 ml of the diluted rickettsial suspension into each flask. Tilt the flasks back and forth to distribute inoculum, and place on a level surface at room temperature (23° - 27°C) to allow rickettsiae to adsorb to the cells. Tilt the flasks every 10 min to redistribute inoculum and prevent monolayers from drying out.

(d) After 1 hr, wash infected monolayers by adding 25 - 30 ml warmed Earl's or Hank's balanced salt solution to each flask;

distribute solution over monolayer and pour into gauze-covered
beaker. Repeat the process again, and then add 50 ml of L-cell
growth medium.

(e) Incubate flasks (tightly capped) at 34°C for 6 - 9 days,
checking daily for any indication of bacterial or fungal contamination (turbidity, cell death, or pH change). After 3 - 5
days, cells should begin to show signs of infection. Rickettsial cytopathogenic effect (CPE) is granulation of the cytoplasm, cell rounding, and release of some of the cells from the
monolayer. Cells should be harvested when 10 - 20% of the cells
have been released from the surface.

(f) To harvest rickettsiae, pour medium from infected flasks
into sterile 50-ml centrifuge tubes, rinse infected monolayers
with 3 ml warmed trypsin-EDTA, and then pour this fluid into the
centrifuge tubes. Add 5 ml of the trypsin-EDTA to each flask
and allow to stand on a level surface for 5 - 8 min. Tighten
caps and tap the side of the flask against palm of hand to release the rest of the cells. Pour the infected cell suspension
into the centrifuge tubes. Care should be taken to ensure that
each tube has approximately the same volume (for balancing centrifuge cups during centrifugation).

(g) Centrifuge tubes at 800 g for 10 min and carefully decant supernatant fluid into gauze-covered beaker. Resuspend
pellets in a small volume (1.0 - 1.5 ml of fluid per original
flask) of cold Snyder I diluent. Pipette infected cell suspensions into sterile homogenizer cup. Immediately attach cup to
homogenizer, and blend at maximum speed (15 - 16,000 rpm) for
30 sec, with bottom half of cup immersed in ice bath. Repeat
twice with 10 - 15 sec intervals in between to allow contents
to settle. Disconnect cup from the homogenizer.

(h) Immediately pipette contents into sterile plastic centrifuge tube. Pipette 0.5 ml aliquots into labeled sterile
1-dram glass vials. Cap each vial tightly and place into an
ethanol/Dry Ice bath. Transfer to a -70°C freezer as soon as
possible after the contents of the vials are frozen.

B. *Quantitation of Viable Rickettsiae in Rickettsial Seed*
    Suspensions

The plaque assay technique (14) provides a convenient, sensitive, and reproduceable means for enumeration of rickettsiae
in a sample. Titers achieved with this method are very similar
to those calculated from LD_{50} determinations in mice. This
technique is also useful for determining the number of viable
rickettsiae in macrophage lysates:

1. Preparing monolayers of irradiated L-929 cells in 60-mm
dishes the day prior to the assay.

(a) Irradiate L-929 cells by following steps (a) through
(d) in Section III.A.2.

(b) Determine the total volume of growth medium needed by
multiplying the number of dishes required times 5 ml/dish.
Then determine total number of cells required by multiplying
the number of dishes times 2.5 × 10^6 cells/dish. Divide the
number of cells per milliliter (determined in step A.2(d)) into
the total number of cells required to obtain the volume of cell
suspension to add to the growth medium. Subtract this volume
from the total volume of growth medium required and transfer
this amount of growth medium into sterile 500-ml screw-capped
bottle, using a sterile, cotton-plugged graduated cylinder.
Add volume of cell suspension calculated to growth medium.
This results in a cell suspension containing 5 × 10^5 cells/ml.

(c) Pipette 5 ml into each dish, tilting dish <u>slightly</u> to
ensure that the liquid covers the entire area of the dish.
Do this <u>very</u> gently, since any excessive movement will cause
the cells to collect in the middle of the dish, rendering monolayers unfit for use in plaquing. An even distribution of
cells is essential due to the low cell density per dish.

(d) Allow dishes to stand <u>undisturbed</u> for 30 min to facilitate cell attachment and to ensure an even distribution of cells
over the entire surface; this is a critical step.

(e) After 30 min, <u>carefully</u> transfer dishes to incubator
tray (use a solid tray to reduce contamination) and cover
dishes with a piece of plastic-baked absorbent paper (also to
reduce contamination). Tape the edges of the paper to the tray
with autoclave tape; regular masking tape does not work, as the
high humidity in the incubator causes the tape to loosen. Carefully place the incubator tray into the incubator.

(f) The dishes will be ready for use after overnight incubation.

2. Plaque assay for viable rickettsiae

(a) Before beginning the assay, microscopically examine the
monolayers in several of the dishes to ensure that the cells are
healthy, the monolayers are confluent, and to check for gross
contamination. Return the dishes to the incubator.

(b) Prepare six dilution blanks, each containing 1.8 ml of
cold BHI broth; use 12 × 75 mm polypropylene tubes with caps.
Place tubes in refrigerator until needed.

(c) Weigh out agarose according to Table I. Place powder
in a sterile 500-ml screw-capped bottle and add the indicated
volume of distilled water. Place the bottle, loosely capped,
in a pan of water and autoclave at 15 lb pressure (121°C) for
15 min (water in the pan prevents bottle from cracking around
bottom edge).

(d) Again, from Table I, determine the volume of medium required. Measure this volume in a sterile graduated cylinder

TABLE I.   Preparation of Agarose Feeder and Staining Over-
lays

No. of dishes[a]	Agarose (gm)	Distilled water (ml)	Growth medium (ml)	Neutral red (ml)
0.5% Agarose feeder overlay				
20	0.56	11	101	--
30	0.84	17	152	--
40	1.13	22	203	--
50	1.41	28	254	--
60	1.69	34	304	--
0.5% Agarose neutral red staining overlay				
20	0.56	11	98	3.3
30	0.84	17	147	4.9
40	1.13	22	196	6.5
50	1.41	28	245	8.1
60	1.69	34	294	9.8

[a]Recipe makes enough overlay to fill indicated number of
dishes with 5 - 10% excess.

and transfer to a second sterile 500-ml screw-capped bottle.
Place the bottle, tightly capped, in a water bath set at
46° - 48°C.

(e) Remove dishes containing monolayers from the incubator,
pour supernatants into a beaker covered with gauze, and label
dishes with dilutions to be used. Generally, dilutions 10^{-3}
to 10^{-6} will ensure plates with a countable number of plaques.

(f) Rapidly thaw the rickettsial inoculum and pipette 0.2
ml into the first 1.8-ml BHI dilution blank. Continue serial
tenfold dilutions through the sixth tube, mixing each dilution
well with a vortex mixer.

(g) Pipette 0.1 ml of each dilution to be plaqued onto
dishes labeled with the appropriate dilution, beginning with
the highest dilution (10^{-6}). Pipette the inoculum into the
center of the monolayer, and touch the tip of the pipette very
gently to the surface. Disperse inoculum evenly over the monolayers by tilting the dishes several times in each of two different directions.

(h) Allow the rickettsiae to adsorb to cells for 1 hr.
Tilt dishes every 8 - 10 min; this is a critical step. Failure
to observe these time constraints can result in large areas of
dead cells due to drying of monolayer.

(i) While the rickettsiae are adsorbing, prepare the agarose
overlay by pouring the warmed medium into the bottle containing

the hot autoclaved agarose, and mix gently by swirling. Pour
this mixture back into the original bottle and place into the
46° - 48°C water bath to cool. Transfer of hot overlay back
into the cooler bottle eliminates breakage that can occur when
placing bottles into water bath.

(j) After the adsorption period, pipette 5 ml of cooled
46°C overlay into each dish, directing fluid against inside
edge of the dish to prevent cell damage. Tip the dishes
slightly to disperse the overlay over the entire monolayer,
and allow dishes to stand on a level surface for 10 - 15 min
so that the overlay solidifies. It is important that the overlay not be too warm when it is applied. To check the temperature, hold bottle of overlay against your cheek for 5 - 10 sec.
It should be warm, but not enough to cause discomfort. Even
though the overlay will gel, it is still quite soft (concentration of agarose is only 0.5%). For this reason, handle dishes
very gently.

(k) Arrange dishes on a clean UV-irradiated tray, cover
with absorbent paper, seal with autoclave tape, and return to
the incubator. It is critical that neither the tray nor the
incubator be jolted from now to the end of the assay, as shift-
ing of the monolayers may occur.

(l) If you are assaying R. tsutsugamushi, a feeder overlay
must be applied on day 8 to prevent dishes from drying out:
These plates will be incubated for 16 days. The feeder overlay
is identical to the initial overlay: it should be applied
carefully to the center of the dishes. Assay of R. akari does
not require the feeder overlay, as these plates are only incubated 9 days.

(m) On day 8 (R. akari) or day 15 (R. tsutsugamushi), prepare a neutral red staining overlay according to Table I, and
instructions in steps (c), (d), and (i) of this section. Neutral red solution (volume shown in Table I) must be added to
the warmed medium just prior to mixing the medium with hot
agarose. Note also that the volume of the medium is adjusted
slightly to compensate for the volume of neutral red solution
added. Addition of neutral red to the medium earlier than indicated above can result in difficulty in reading plaques.

(n) After the staining overlay has cooled to 46° - 48°C,
pipette 5 ml into the center of each dish, allow agarose to
gel for a few minutes, and return plates to the incubator after
covering them with absorbent paper. Light affects the stain,
with loss of plaque/monolayer contrast, hence do not allow the
plates to be exposed to light for more than a few minutes after
the overlay has been applied.

(o) After overnight incubation, the plaques may be counted
using transmitted light such as that obtained from an Rh-typing
box. Neutral red stains living cells a light orange-red color.
The unstained areas (dead cells) will appear as plaques. As

you count, mark each plaque with a marking pen. Use a hand
tally counter to record the number of plaques. Count and record the plaques on all dishes with 200 or fewer plaques. Calculate the rickettsial titer in plaque-forming units per milliliter as shown in Section IV of this chapter.

C. *Mouse Peritoneal Macrophages*

Activated macrophages can be induced in the peritoneum of
mice by intraperitoneal inoculation of viable *M. bovis* strain
BCG (Phipps substrain, Trudeau Institute, Saranac Lake, New
York; 10^6 CFU) or formalinized *C. parvum* (70 mg/kg). Macrophages are harvested 8 - 12 days after inoculation of these
agents. Alternatively, resident or exudate macrophages can be
activated *in vitro* by exposure to lymphokines induced by either
antigen or mitogen stimulation of spleen cells (see Chapter 75).

Total peritoneal cells × % macrophages = total peritoneal
macrophages.

The peritoneal cells are obtained and counted (see Chapter 7).

D. *Preparation of Cells*

(1) Centrifuge pooled peritoneal fluids at 400 *g* for 10
min at 4°C, and discard supernatant.
(2) Adjust cell pellet to 1 × 10^6 macrophages/ml with assay
medium and dispense into 12 × 75 mm polypropylene capped tubes
in 0.5 ml aliquots.
(3) If macrophages are activated *in vitro*, add 0.1 ml lymphokines to each appropriate tube.
(4) All macrophage cultures are incubated 2 hr; lymphokine-
activated macrophages must be incubated a minimum of 4 hr
(6 - 8 hr is optimum).

E. *Infection of Macrophage Cultures*

(1) Thaw tissue culture-grown rickettsiae rapidly (37°C
water bath) and dilute immediately to approximately 5 PFU/
macrophage in cold BHI or assay medium.
(2) Add 0.1 ml rickettsial suspension to each appropriate
tube. Remember to include (i) one sample of macrophages only
(monitors aseptic technique), and (ii) greater than two samples
of normal macrophages infected with rickettsiae (control) for
each time point.

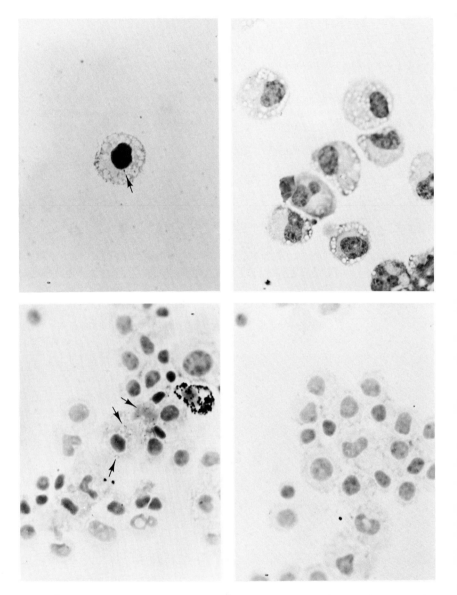

Fig. 1. Stained cytocentrifuge preparations of macrophage cultures infected with R. tsutsugamushi or R. akari. (A) Macrophage infected with R. tsutsugamushi (arrow indicates rickettsia) and stained with giemsa. (B) Lymphokine-activated macrophages stained with giemsa. (C) Macrophages infected with R. akari (arrows indicate rickettsiae) and stained by the Gimenez method. (D) Activated macrophages stained with the Gimenez method.

(3) Incubate cells for 1 hr at room temperature, shaking tubes every 10 min.

(4) To remove inoculum, centrifuge tubes at 500 g for 10 min, aspirate supernatant, and replace with fresh assay medium (0.5 ml).

(5) Sample test and control macrophages for cell counts and cytocentrifugation and staining immediately after step 4 above (1-hr sample).

(6) Incubate remaining samples for 24 hr at 34° - 37°C with 5% CO_2 in moist air; remove samples for cell counts and staining at 24 hr.

(7) Determine kiling of rickettsiae by formula in Section IV.

(8) Alternate mechanisms of determining rickettsial killing by macrophage cultures include: (i) LD_{50} determination of viable rickettsiae in macrophage lysates in susceptible C3H/He mice, or (ii) plaque titration of viable rickettsiae in macrophage lysates using methods outlined in Section III.B.1 and III.B.2.

(a) Macrophages can be lysed without loss of rickettsial titer by blending for three 30-sec intervals with microadapter attachment to Sorvall homogenizer. Use aerosol-proof stainless steel cups; optimum volume for the stainless steel cups is 5 ml of washed cell suspension.

IV. CALCULATION OF DATA

Quantitation of viable rickettsial seed suspensions: Results of a typical plaque assay using *R. tsutsugamushi* is shown in the following tabulation.

Dilution	Plaque counts/dish	Average plaques
10^{-3}	TNTC[1]	--
10^{-4}	140, 167, 163, 147, 181	159.6
10^{-5}	16, 13, 21, 18, 15	16.6
10^{-6}	1, 2, 2, 0, 1	1.2

(1) Select the dilution whose average plaque count is 30 or greater. Calculate titer by the following formula:

PFU/ml = average No. of plaques × dilution factor × 10 (to compensate for 0.1 ml inoculum).

[1] *TNTC equals plaques too numerous to count.*

(2) Using the above figures:

PFU/ml $= 159.6 \times 10^4 \times 10 = 1.596 \times 10^7$ PFU/ml, or 1.6×10^7 PFU/ml

Rickettsial killing by activated macrophages is determined by the following formula:

$$100 \times \frac{\% \text{ infected control macrophages} - \% \text{ infected control macrophages}}{\% \text{ infected control macrophages}}$$

Analysis of intracellular killing by activated macrophages in a typical experiment:

At 1 hr: 37% of control macrophages contain intracellular rickettsiae
23% of lymphokine treated macrophages contain intracellular rickettsiae

$$100 \times \frac{37-23}{37} = \underline{38\% \text{ rickettsiacidal activity by activated macrophages.}}$$

At 24 hr: 39% of control macrophages contain intracellular rickettsiae
5% lymphokine-treated macrophages contain intracellular rickettsiae

$$100 \times \frac{39-5}{39} \quad \underline{91\% \text{ rickettsiacidal activity by activated macrophages}}$$

Measurement of macrophage activation is the difference in percentage macrophages infected in activated macrophage cultures compared to control cultures. Therefore, an appropriate number of control cultures must be examined to generate statistically valid 95% confidence limits. Duplicate smears of two samples (100 cells observed/smear) is the minimum: Usually from control samples and two each of test samples are used for each time of sampling.

V.   CRITICAL COMMENTS

A.   *Growth and Quantitation of Rickettsiae in L929 Cells*

The procedures for growth and quantitation of rickettsiae in seed suspensions are the most difficult part of the rickettsiacidal assay. Once the rickettsial stocks are obtained, however, they will last several years with storage at $-70°C$. Ten flasks of irradiated L-cells produce enough rickettsiae for approximately 30 rickettsiacidal assays.

Do not refreeze rickettsial seed suspension after use: Freezing and thawing drastically reduce rickettsial titer.

All work with rickettsiae must be done in the ABSENCE OF
ANTIBIOTICS. Strict adherence to aseptic technique is essential.

B. Rickettsiacidal Assay

Since antibiotics cannot be used for the rickettsiacidal
assay, this technique is somewhat more difficult to establish
in the laboratory than others for macrophage activation. With
the recent dissociation of microbicidal and tumoricidal activities of activated macrophages, however, the rickettsiacidal assay may prove a powerful tool for analysis of lymphokines inducing microbicidal activity in macrophages and studying mechanisms of intracellular killing (13).

The Gimenez stain for R. akari has not been remarkably consistent in our hands. Efforts to locate other staining protocols effective for R. akari may be useful. We can obtain consistent results only if the working carbol fuchsin is made
immediately prior to staining cell smears.

Most information on intracellular killing of rickettsiae
by macrophages has been obtained with R. tsutsugamushi. This
is the organism of choice for macrophage studies IF one has a
P3 containment facility (see above); R. tsutsugamushi has a
slower generation time, does not produce secondary infections
as rapidly, and stains consistently with giemsa.

Data obtained by microscopic analysis are identical to results obtained by plaque assay for viable rickettsiae (9);
choice of the method for analysis is then left to individual
preference. If plaque assay or LD_{50} determinations are used
for quantitation of destruction of rickettsiae, cultures must
be washed at least two times and adjusted to equal cell numbers
(macrophages and lymphocytes) prior to blending. Results can
be calculated by percentage reduction in viable rickettsiae:
titer of treated macrophage culture/titer of control macrophage
cultures.

Lymphokines have no direct effect on rickettsiae and do not
need to be washed out of pretreated macrophage cultures during
infection.

Lymphokines added after infection induce macrophage activation as long as lymphokines remain in the culture at least 4 hr.
In this instance, one observes only intracellular killing.

REFERENCES

1. C. A. Nacy and J. V. Osterman. Host defenses in experi-
    mental scrub typhus: Role of normal and activated macro-
    phages. *Infect. Immun. 26*: 744-750, 1979.
2. D. J. Hinrichs and T. R. Jerrells. *In vitro* evaluation
    of immunity to *Coxiella burnetii*. *J. Immunol. 117*: 996-
    1003, 1976.
3. M. R. Gambril and C. L. Wisseman, Jr. Mechanisms of im-
    munity in typhus infections. II. Multiplication of typhus
    rickettsiae in human macrophage cell cultures in the non-
    immune system: Influence of virulence of rickettsial
    strain and of chloramphenicol. *Infect. Immun. 8*: 519-527,
    1973.
4. G. I. Byrne and J. W. Moulder. Parasite-specified phago-
    cytosis of *Chlamydia psittaci* and *Chlamydia trachomatis*
    by L and HeLa cells. *Infect. Immun. 19*: 598-606, 1978.
5. W. C. Buhles, Jr., D. L. Huxsoll, and B. L. Elisberg.
    Isolation of *Rickettsia rickettsii* in primary bone marrow
    cell and circulating monocyte cultures derived from ex-
    perimentally infected guinea pigs. *Infect. Immun. 7*:
    1003-1005, 1973.
6. P. J. Catanzaro, A. Shirai, P. K. Hildebrandt, and J. V.
    Osterman. Host defenses in experimental scrub typhus:
    Histopathological correlates. *Infect. Immun. 13:* 861-
    875, 1976.
7. P. J. Catanzaro, A. Shirai, L. D. Agniel, Jr., and J. V.
    Osterman. Host defenses in experimental scrub typhus:
    Role of spleen and peritoneal exudate lymphocytes in cel-
    lular immunity. *Infect. Immun. 18*: 118, 1977.
8. C. A. Nacy, M. S. Meltzer, P. K. Russell, and J. V. Oster-
    man. Immunity to *Rickettsia tsutsugamushi* infection in-
    duced by nonspecific macrophage activating agents. *Fed.
    Proc. 38*: 1978, 1979.
9. C. A. Nacy and M. S. Meltzer. Macrophages in resistance
    to rickettsial infection: Macrophage activation *in vitro*
    for killing of *Rickettsia tsutsugamushi*. *J. Immunol. 123*:
    2544-2549, 1979.
10. M. S. Meltzer and C. A. Nacy. Macrophages in resistance
    to rickettsial infections: Susceptibility to lethal ef-
    fects of *Rickettsia akari* infection in mouse strains with
    defective macrophage function. *Cell. Immunol. 54*: 487,
    1980.
11. Classification of etiologic agents on the basis of hazard.
    U.S. Public Health Service, Center for Disease Control,
    Office of Biosafety, Atlanta, GA. 4th ed., 1974.
12. E. B. Jackson and J. E. Smadel. Immunization against scrub
    typhus. II. Preparation of lyophilized living vaccine. *Am.*

J. Hyg. 53: 326–331, 1951.

13. D. Boraschi and M. S. Meltzer. Macrophage activation for
     tumor cytotoxicity: Genetic variation in macrophage tu-
     moricidal capacity among mouse strains. *Cell. Immunol.*
     45: 188–194, 1979.

14. S. C. Oaks, Jr., J. V. Osterman, and F. M. Hetrick.
     Plaque assay and cloning of scrub typhus rickettsiae in
     irradiated L-929 cells. *J. Clin. Microbiol. 6:* 76–80,
     1977.

72

DESTRUCTION OF LEISHMANIA[*]

Carol A. Nacy
Michael G. Pappas

I. INTRODUCTION

The *Leishmania* are protozoan parasites that exist in two
discrete forms: the motile promastigote is found in the in-
sect vector, and this form converts to a nonmotile amastigote
form in vertebrate hosts. *Leishmania* amastigotes are obligate
intracellular parasites of macrophages *in vivo*, where they reside and multiply within phagolysosomes (1). Several reports
demonstrate that immunologically activated macrophages kill the
intracellular parasite (2 - 4). Studies on intracellular kill-

[*]*In conducting the research described in this report, the
investigators adhered to the "Guide for Laboratory Animal Facilities and Care" as promulgated by the Committee of the
Guide for Laboratory Animal Facilities and Care of the Institute of Laboratory Animal Resources, National Academy of
Sciences, National Research Council.*

METHODS FOR STUDYING
MONONUCLEAR PHAGOCYTES
745

ing, however, have been hampered by poor multiplication of
Leishmania in vitro in monolayer cultures of macrophages obtained from guinea pigs (5), mice (2, 4), and humans (1).
Prolonged cultivation of the infected macrophage cultures resulted in spontaneous cure of infection. Recent examination
of culture conditions necessary for multiplication of *Leishmania tropica in vitro* suggests that adherence of macrophages
may alter the physiology of the cell, inducing an environment
hostile for survival and/or multiplication of the parasite.
Mouse peritoneal macrophages maintained in suspension and infected with *L. tropica in vitro* supported continuous multiplication of the parasite, with tenfold increases in numbers of
amastigotes over 96 hr of culture (6). Replication of *Leishmania* in suspension cultures continued through 9 days: spontaneous cure of infected macrophages was not observed. Addition of lymphokines to the infected cultures, however, induced macrophage-mediated killing of the parasite reminiscent
of macrophage killing of rickettsiae (7, and Chapter 71). Two
distinct interactions of activated macrophages and *L. tropica*
could be distinguished and analyzed separately:

(1) Macrophage cultures treated with lymphokines before
infection induced an immediate loss of infectivity of *Leishmania* for the activated macrophage population. One hour after
addition of *Leishmania,* 25 - 35% fewer macrophages contained
intracellular parasites in cultures pretreated with lymphokines than in control cultures. Although *Leishmania* enter
macrophages by phagocytosis, this decrease in percentage infected cells was <u>not</u> secondary to alterations in phagocytic
ability of activated macrophages, since nonspecific phagocytosis
of latex beads remained the same in treated and untreated cultures. Efforts to isolate soluble factors released from activated macrophages that could affect viability of *Leishmania*
have, as yet, been unsuccessful.

(2) Macrophage cultures infected with *Leishmania* and
treated with lymphokines after infection acquire the capacity
to kill the intracellular parasite: Within 72 hr, 80 - 95%
fewer macrophages contain *Leishmania* than control cultures, and
the mean number of amastigotes in residual infected macrophages
of lymphokine-treated cultures is a fraction of those in infected control macrophages.

A number of similarities exist in the activation of macrophages for killing of *Leishmania* and for killing of rickettsiae.
These two organisms exist in different cellular compartments
(rickettsia multiply free in the cytosol of the cell, while
Leishmania replicate inside phagolysosomes), but have in common
the obligate nature of their intracellular parasitism. Like
the rickettsiae (7, 8, 9), the *Leishmania*

(1) are killed by immunologically activated (*in vivo* or

in vitro) macrophages only: macrophages induced by sterile inflammatory agents do not kill *Leishmania* unless further exposed
to lymphokines *in vitro*;
        (2) macrophages from mouse strains with characterized de-
fects in development of macrophage activation for tumor cytotoxicity are also defective in one or both microbicidal activities for killing of *Leishmania*; and
        (3) lymphokine signals for activation of macrophages to
kill *L. tropica* elute in three peaks from Sephadex G-200 fractionation of lymphocyte supernatants: the peaks are approximately 135,000, 45,000, and 10,000 MW.

        As with all assays of macrophage activation, there are
advantages and disadvantages to using *Leishmania* as the target
for macrophage-mediated killing. Included among the advantages
are (1) the parasite replicates only intracellularly in macrophages at 37°C (10), (2) the parasite is a large organism compared to rickettsiae and other bacteria, and can be visualized
easily by light microscopy under oil immersion, (3) unlike
facultative intracellular bacteria, only immunologically activated macrophages kill replicating *Leishmania*, and (4) amastigotes can easily be propagated for *in vitro* use by infecting
footpads of BALB/c mice and harvesting amastigotes 2 - 4 wks
later. There are, however, several disadvantages that should
be mentioned: (1) Although amastigotes do not replicate outside of cells, they also do not die extracellularly, as do the
rickettsiae. The number of macrophages containing intracellular *Leishmania* remains stable from 1 - 8 hr after introduction
of the parasite; by 24 hr, however, there is an increase in
the percentage macrophages containing amastigotes. This increase in percentage macrophages infected at 24 hr can be reduced by altering the number of amastigotes present in the
original inoculum. Nevertheless, it is clear that removal of
the amastigote inoculum by low-speed centrifugation is not completely effective. (2) Reliable and simple techniques for assaying viability of *L. tropica* in macrophage populations are
not currently available.
        Despite cautions of the preceding paragraph, *Leishmania*
may prove to be a powerful tool in dissecting the microbicidal
properties of various macrophage populations.

II. REAGENTS

A. *Culture Media and Solutions*

    (1) Macrophage harvest medium: RPMI 1640 supplemented
with 2 mM L-glutamine, 10% heat-inactivated fetal bovine
serum (FBS), 50 µg/ml Garamycin (M. A. Bioproducts, Walkersville, Maryland), 10 u/ml sodium heparin (Panheprin, Abbott
Laboratories, King of Prussia, Pennsylvania).
    (2) Microbicidal assay medium: RPMI 1640 supplemented
with 2 mM L-glutamine, 10% heat-inactivated FBS, 50 µg/ml
Garamycin (M. A. Bioproducts)
    (3) PBG (phosphate-buffered glucose solution): NaH_2PO_4,
1.62 gm; KH_2PO_4, 0.49 gm; and dextrose, 5.40 gm. Dissolve
buffer salts and dextrose in 200 ml distilled H_2O and adjust
pH to 7.2 with 10 N NaOH. Filter sterilize and store at 4°C.
    (4) Normal saline: 0.85% NaCl in distilled H_2O, sterile
    (5) Sodium azide solution: Dissolve 0.1 gm NaN in 100 ml
normal saline.
    (6) Gluteraldehyde solution (0.2%): dilute gluteralde-
hyde stock solution (25%) 1:125 in PBG. CAUTION: contact
with gluteraldehyde can cause both blindness and lung and tissue damage. Wear rubber gloves and prepare working solution
in biological safety hood.
    (7) Diff-Quick differential stain (Scientific Products,
Columbia, Maryland)
    (8) Ether, anesthesia grade
    (9) Iodine disinfectant solution (Wescodyne or Betadiene)
    (10) Crushed ice
    (11) 70% Alcohol
    (12) Distilled H_2O

B. *Equipment*

    (1) Refrigerated centrifuge
    (2) Binocular microscope
    (3) Vortex mixer
    (4) Balance
    (5) Pipette-aid (Bellco, Vineland, New Jersey)
    (6) Vertical laminar flow hood for use with biological
agents
    (7) Cytocentrifuge (Shandon Southern Instruments, Sewelicky,
Pennsylvania)
    (8) Water baths: 37°C, 56°C
    (9) pH Meter
    (10) CO_2 Incubator with humidity control
    (11) Autoclave

C. Plasticware

(1) 15-ml sterile conical centrifuge tubes (No. 2095, Falcon Plastics, Oxnard, California)

(2) 50 ml sterile polypropylene centrifuge tubes (No. 2070, Falcon Plastics)

*(3) 12 × 75 mm sterile polypropylene snap-cap tubes (No. 2063, Falcon Plastics)

(4) 35 × 10 mm sterile disposable petri dishes (No. 3001, Falcon Plastics)

(5) 1, 10, 30 cc polypropylene disposable syringes

(6) 1, 5, 10 cc sterile cotton-plugged serological pipettes (Costar, Cambridge, Massachusetts)

D. Glassware

(1) Sterile Pasteur pipettes, cotton-plugged and unplugged

(2) Three 100-ml beakers, one 50-ml beaker, sterile

(3) Tissue homogenizer (Dounce or Tindall), sterile

(4) 12 × 75 mm culture tubes

E. Mice

*Use only inbred mouse strains; mice must be healthy. Avoid using mouse strains with characterized *in vivo* and *in vitro* macrophage defects (11).

F. Leishmania

Leishmania tropica NIH strain 173, obtained from Dr. D. J. Wyler, is used routinely in our laboratory. This organism was isolated from a patient with Oriental sore in Iran, and given to NIH by A. Ebrahimzadeh, Shapur University School of Medicine, Ahwaz, Iran. Several other strains of *L. tropica* have been used successfully in this assay. *Leishmania tropica* can be purchased from the American Type Culture Collection (Rockville, Maryland) or obtained from Walter Reed Army Institute of Research.

*Indicates brand or type of material that is critical for success of procedure.

III. PROCEDURE

A. *Propagation of L. tropica Amastigotes in Footpads of Mice*

(1) Anesthetize BALB/c mice with ether. Other inbred
strains of mice can be used for propagating amastigotes; however, most commonly used strains resolve *Leishmania* footpad
lesions after approximately 4 - 5 weeks. Numbers of amastigotes obtained from footpad lesions of these mouse strains are
considerably lower than those obtained from BALB/c footpads
infected at the same time.
(2) Inject 50 λ of a 10^6/ml amastigote preparation
(5 × 10^4 amastigotes) into each footpad of mouse. Use a tuberculin syringe with 27-gauge needle.
(3) Leishmanial lesions, indicated by swelling of footpad,
are evident 10 - 14 days after injection.
(4) Footpad lesions should be used for amastigote harvest
on weeks 2 - 4 after inoculation; lesions older than 4 weeks
may have secondary bacterial infections.
(5) Recovery of amastigotes ranges between 1 - 3 × 10^7
amastigotes per footpad.
(6) To harvest amastigotes, euthanize infected mouse with
ether and immerse entire body and limbs in 100-ml beaker containing 20 ml iodine (Betadiene or Wescodyne) and 80 ml distilled H_2O. Allow mouse to soak for 15 min, and repeat procedure in second beaker containing the iodine solution.
(7) Immerse mouse in 100-ml beaker containing 70% alcohol
for 15 min.
(8) Grasping toes of infected foot with forceps, cut foot
off at ankle with small scissors and place infected foot in
sterile petri dish.
Leishmania tropica can be obtained from the American type
culture collection (ATCC, Rockville, Maryland).
(9) In laminar flow biological safety hood, place one foot
(footpad up) on #50 wire mesh sieve placed over 50-ml beaker;
flood footpad with several ml assay medium to wash away 70%
alcohol. Discard wash medium.
(10) Split swollen footpad longitudinally with sterile scalpel and turn footpad down; mash footpad into wire mesh with
10-cc rubber-tipped syringe plunger. This step requires a
modest amount of strength, as foot should be reduced to bones
and skin at the end of procedure. Occasionally wash footpad
with a few milliliters of medium and allow medium to drain into beaker. If large numbers of amastigotes are needed, remove
and repeat procedure with second foot. Combine amastigote-rich
medium from both footpads; remove foot debris and rinse mesh
with 3 - 4 ml medium and add to amastigote suspension.

(11) Pour amastigote suspension into 50-ml tissue homogenizer and grind 10 times; for safety, wrap tissue homogenizer in several layers of 4 × 4 gauze pads.

(12) Transfer suspension to sterile conical screw-capped tube and centrifuge for 10 min at 400 g (removes large cell debris and intact cells from the suspension). Pour amastigote-rich supernatant into second sterile tube; the suspension will appear cloudy.

(13) Infected tissue and disposable equipment should be autoclaved; nondisposable equipment and glassware should be soaked in 70% of alcohol for 1/2 hr and transferred to soapy water for an additional 1/2 hr. Equipment should be washed thoroughly, rinsed in distilled water, and sterilized.

B. Quantitation of Amastigotes Obtained from Footpad Lesion

Prepare and quantify gluteraldehyde-fixed chicken red blood cells as follows:

(1) Chicken red blood cells should be 5 - 21 days old before treatment with gluteraldehyde and should be stored in 50% Alsever's solution at 4C.

(2) Wash 1 ml suspension of chicken red blood cells four times in 10 - 15 ml normal saline for 5 min at 500 g. Aspirate buffy coat (white blood cells) from top of red cell pellet after each wash and discard. Pack cells for 10 min at 500 g and discard supernatant.

(3) Suspend erythrocytes to 20% in PBG (see reagents).

(4) With constant stirring (a magnetic stirrer may be used), add an equal volume of 0.2% gluteraldehyde solution to the 20% suspension of red cells (final concentration of erythrocytes is 10%).

(5) Incubate suspension for 15 min in 37°C water bath with occasional mixing. Remove from waterbath and wash red cells five times in normal saline for 10 min at 500 g.

(6) Resuspend chicken red cells to 10% in 0.1% NaN_3 solution: This is STOCK RED CELL suspension. Determine red cells per milliliter in STOCK suspension by counting in hemocytometer. Adjust concentration of portion of erythrocytes to 3×10^6/ml with 0.1% NaN_3 solution: This is WORKING RED CELL SUSPENSION. Refrigerate STOCK and WORKING suspensions at 4°C until use.

Quantify Leishmania amastigotes as follows:

(1) Using lambda pipette gun or pipette aid, mix 100λ amastigote suspension with 100λ of WORKING SUSPENSION gluteraldehyde-fixed chicken red blood cells in 12 × 75 mm culture tube. Mix thoroughly. (It is essential that the chicken red cells be

vigorously suspended just prior to addition to amastigotes.)

(2) Spread 200λ of amastigote/chicken red blood cell suspension on a glass microscope slide and allow to air dry. Drying can be hastened by cold air from laboratory dryer; other methods have not been shown to result in reasonable slide preparations, although logical reasons for this remain obscure.

(3) Amastigotes stain nicely with the simple Diff-Quick modified Wright's stain: (i) fix slide 30 sec in fixative solution, (ii) stain slide 30 sec in Diff-Quick solution I; and (iii) counter-stain slide 45 sec in Diff-Quick solution II.

(4) Wash slide thoroughly with tap water and air dry or dry by pressing between two leaves of bibulous paper.

(5) Observe amastigote/chicken erythrocyte preparation under oil immersion: amastigotes are 1 - 2 μm long, tear-drop shaped, with dark-staining nucleus and kinetoplast; chicken erythrocytes are considerably larger, with a prominent nucleus.

(6) Count chicken red cells and associated amastigotes in each field; a minimum of 100 chicken red cells should be counted. Number of amastigotes per milliliter is calculated by the ratio:

$$\frac{\text{number of amastigoes}}{\text{number red cells}} \times 3.0 \times 10^6$$

C. Mouse Peritoneal Macrophages

Activated macrophages can be induced in the peritoneum of mice by intraperitoneal inoculation of viable *M. bovis* strain BCG (Phipps substrain, Trudeau Institute, Saranac Lake, New York, 10^6CFU) or formalinized *C. parvum* (70 mg/kg). Macrophages are harvested 8 - 12 days after inoculation of these agents. Alternatively, resident or exudate macrophages can be activated *in vitro* by exposure to lymphokines induced by either antigen or mitogen stimulation of spleen cells (see chapter 75). Peritoneal cells and macrophages are obtained, pooled and counted (see chapter 7).

Centrifuge pooled peritoneal fluids at 400 *g* for 10 min at 4°C, and discard supernatant. Resuspended cell pellet to 1 × 10^6 macrophages/ml with assay medium and dispense into 12 × 75 mm polypropylene capped tubes in 0.5 ml aliquots. If macrophages are treated with lymphokines prior to infection, add 0.1 ml lymphokines to each appropriate tube; add 0.1 ml medium to corresponding control tubes. All macrophage cultures are incubated 2 hr including macrophages activated *in vivo*. Macrophages treated with lymphokine before infection must be incubated a minimum of 4 hr (6 - 8 hr is optimum).

D. Infection of Macrophage Cultures

(1) Adjust amastigote suspension to approximately
1.5 - 1.8 × 10^6 amastigotes/ml in assay medium. Mix well.

(2) Add 0.1 ml of amastigote suspension to all tubes.
Shake samples to ensure thorough mixing and incubate all
samples for 1 hr at 37°C, shaking tubes every 15 min.

(3) Centrifuge infected macrophage samples at 100 g for
5 min and aspirate supernatant; take care not to disturb cell
pellet.

(4) Add 0.5 ml fresh assay medium to each tube and mix.

(5) Remove several cultures of control and activated infected macrophage populations for 1 hr sample; cytocentrifuge
samples and stain cell smears with Diff-Quick. Observe stained
smears for percentage infected macrophages and numbers of intracellular *Leishmania* per infected macrophage.

(6) For macrophage populations treated with lymphokines
after infection, or samples treated with lymphokines both before and after infection, add 0.1 ml lymphokines to each tube;
add 0.1 ml assay medium to controls. Mix (no further manipulations after step 5 are necessary for macrophage populations
activated *in vivo*: proceed to step 7).

(7) Incubate macrophages for 72 hr at 37°C with 5% CO_2 in
moist air. Repeat step 5 with cultures incubated 72 hr.

IV. CALCULATION OF DATA

Microbicidal activity by activated macrophages (killing of
L. tropica) is determined by the following formula:

$$100 \times \frac{\% \text{ infected control macrophages} - \% \text{ infected treated macrophages}}{\% \text{ infected control macrophages}}$$

Analysis of microbicidal activity in a typical experiment with
lymphokine-activated C3H/HeN mouse macrophages might generate
data similar to

<u>1 hr</u>: 30% control macrophages contain intracellular
Leishmania; 22% treated macrophages contain intracellular
Leishmania.

$$100 \times \frac{30 - 22}{30} = 27\% \text{ microbicidal activity}$$

<u>72 hr</u>: 55% control macrophages contain intracellular

Leishmania; 2% treated macrophages contain intracellular
Leishmania.

$$100 \times \frac{55 - 2}{55} = 96\% \text{ microbicidal activity}$$

Measurement of macrophage activation is the difference in percentage macrophages infected in activated macrophage cultures
compared to control cultures. Therefore, an appropriate number of cultures must be examined to generate statistically
valid 95% confidence limits. Duplicate smears of two samples
(200 cells observed/smear) is the minimum; usually four control
samples and two each of test samples are used for each time of
sampling.

V. CRITICAL COMMENTS

    Propagation of amastigotes of *L. tropica* (and other species
causing cutaneous leishmaniasis) in footpads of BALB/c mice is
a convenient and reliable way of maintaining a stock of amastigotes for *in vitro* use. A recent report by K. P. Chang (12)
suggests that macrophage cell lines may also be useful as a
source of large quantities of amastigotes. This *in vitro* propagation is not currently in use in our laboratory, and so we
cannot offer comparisons between amastigotes derived from *in
vivo* or *in vitro* cultivation. However, it might be pointed out
that Dr. Chang's methods could be useful for (1) those with
limited animal facilities or (2) those interested in *L. donovani*, which causes systemic infection, and for which there is
no convenient source in mice of large numbers of amastigotes
in vivo.
    Repeated attempts to find a consistent, reliable method of
quantifying amastigotes in suspension suggest that estimation
with known concentrations of chicken red blood cells is the
easiest and most reproduceable technique. However, the accuracy of this technique is clearly dependent upon proper mixing
of both red blood cell and amastigote suspensions prior to combining appropriate quantities and proper mixing of the combined amastigote-red blood cell suspension before application
to slide. Accuracy is helped by independent observation by two
investigators, and observation of 200 - 400 chicken red cells.
    Macrophages can be elicited into the peritoneal cavity of
a mouse with sterile inflammatory agents such as casein, latex
beads, and phosphate-buffered saline; these macrophage populations support the growth of *L. tropica* equally as well as resident cells, with percentage macrophages infected and number of

amastigotes per infected cell increasing similarly over 72 hr.
Inflammatory macrophages, however, in contrast to macrophage
activation for tumor cytotoxicity (13), respond less well to
lymphokines for intracellular killing of *Leishmania* than resident peritoneal macrophages. Nevertheless, the 2 - 5-fold increase in cell yield following elicitation is very useful when
examining macrophage responses in individual mice. When using
inflammatory macrophages, pretreat cells with lymphokines for
6 - 8 hr, and use the lowest dilution of lymphokines possible
(1/6 final dilution).

Macrophages from certain strains of mice, i.e., BALB/c,
are notably inconsistent in their response to activating
stimuli *in vivo* or *in vitro* for tumor cytotoxicity (11). We
have also observed inconsistent results with lymphokine activation for intracellular killing of *Leishmania*: Occasionally
macrophages from BALB/c mice respond to lymphokines for cytostatic rather than cytocidal activity. In this case, the percentage of infected macrophages remains the same in control
and lymphokine-treated cultures, but the mean number of
Leishmania per infected macrophage and amastigote distribution
in macrophages at 72 hr changes dramatically in control cultures and remains the same in treated cultures, compared to
the 1 hr samples.

Removal of leishmanial inoculum by low-speed centrifugation
and aspiration is partially effective in reducing the 24-hr increase in percentage of infected macrophages which were observed in our original studies. Approximately 70% of the inoculum can be accounted for by intracellular amastigotes and
amastigotes present in supernatants removed by aspiration.
Repeated washing did not improve this figure and increased the
risk of cell loss during the procedure. By reducing the multiplicity of infection (MOI) to 1:1 amastigote/macrophage, we
could further minimize the interaction of macrophages and remaining extracellular *Leishmania*. The recommended MOI in the
procedure for infection of macrophages is approximately 0.5:1
amastigotes/macrophage; in our hands, this reliably produces
25 - 30% infected macrophages at 1 hr and 30 - 35% infected
macrophages at 72 hr in control macrophage populations. The
metabolic condition of amastigotes that enter macrophages 6 - 8
hr after the usual infection period is currently unknown.

Lymphokines have no direct effects on *Leishmania* amastigotes. Therefore, it is not necessary to wash lymphokine-
pretreated macrophage cultures prior to infection.

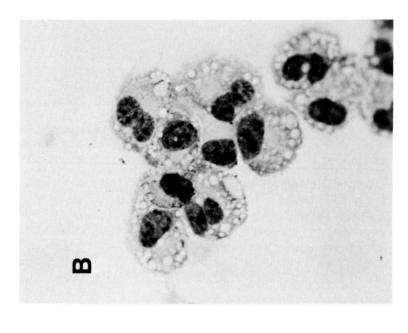

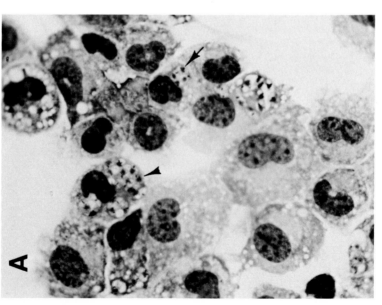

Fig. 1. Macrophage cultures were infected with Leishmania, washed, and incubated in medium (A) or 1/6 dilution lymphokines (B) for 72 hr. Arrows indicate presence of intracellular leishmania.

REFERENCES

1. J. D. Berman, D. W. Dwyer, and D. J. Wyler. Growth of *Leishmania* in human macrophages *in vitro Infect. Immun.* *26*: 375, 1979.
2. J. Mauel, Y. Buchmuller, and R. Behin. Studies on the mechanisms of macrophage activation I. Destruction of intracellular *Leishmania enriettii* in macrophages activated by cocultivation with stimulated lymphocytes. *J. Exp. Med. 148*: 393, 1978.
3. Y. Buchmuller and J. Mauel. Studies on the mechanisms of macrophage activation II. Parasite destruction in macrophages activated by supernatants from concanavalin A-stimulated lymphocytes. *J. Exp. Med. 150*: 359, 1979.
4. E. Handman and A. W. Burgess. Stimulation by granulocyte-macrophage colony-stimulating factor of *Leishmania tropica* killing by macrophages. *J. Immunol. 122*: 1134, 1979.
5. R. Behin, J. Mauel, B. Noerjasin, and D. S. Rowe. Mechanisms of protective immunity in experimental cutaneous leishmaniasis of the guinea pig II. Selective destruction of different *Leishmania* species in activated guinea-pig and mouse macrophages. *Clin. Exp. Immunol. 20*: 351, 1975.
6. C. A. Nacy and C. L. Diggs. Intracellular replication of *Leishmania tropica* in suspension cultures of mouse peritoneal macrophages. (Submitted for publication.)
7. C. A. Nacy and M. S. Meltzer. Macrophages in resistance to rickettsial infection: Macrophage activation *in vitro* for killing of *Rickettsia tsutsugamushi*. *J. Immunol. 123*: 2544, 1979.
8. C. A. Nacy, G. Radlick, and M. S. Meltzer. Activated macrophages in natural resistance to *Rickettsia akari. In* "Genetic Control of Natural Resistance to Infection and Malignancy, Perspectives in Immunology" (E. Skamene, ed.). Academic Press, New York, 1981.
9. C. A. Nacy, E. J. Leonard, and M. S. Meltzer. Macrophages in resistance to rickettsial infection: Characterization of lymphokines that induce intracellular killing in macrophages. *J. Immunol. 126*: 204, 1981.
10. H. J. Akiyama and J. C. Taylor. Effect of macrophage engulfment and temperature on the transformation process of *Leishmania donovani*. *Am. J. Trop. Med. Hyg. 19*: 747, 1970.
11. D. Boraschi and M. S. Meltzer. Macrophage activation for tumor cytotoxicity: genetic variation in macrophage tumoricidal capacity among mouse strains. *Cell. Immunol. 45*: 188-194, 1979.

12. K. P. Chang. Human cutaneous *leishmania* in a mouse macro-
     phage line: Propagation and isolation of intracellular
     parasites. *Science 209*: 1240, 1980.
13. L. P. Ruco and M. S. Meltzer. Macrophage activation for
     tumor cytotoxicity: Increased lymphokine responsiveness
     of peritoneal macrophages during acute inflammation. *J.
     Immunol. 120*: 1054, 1978.

73

DESTRUCTION OF VIRUSES

Stephen S. Morse
Page S. Morahan

I. GENERAL INTRODUCTION

Destruction of viruses by mononuclear phagocytes can be defined in several ways. Phagocytes may adsorb virus and then
either actively destroy the virus intracellularly or be nonper-
missive for virus replication (intrinsic antiviral activity)
(1 - 3). Mononuclear phagocytes can also reduce virus production in other infected cells (extrinsic antiviral activity)
(1, 4), possibly by unusual mechanisms, in addition to such
classical mechanisms as macrophage-mediated cytotoxicity for
virus-infected cells (5), production of antiviral substances
such as interferon, toxic metabolites, or growth-limiting
products (6, 7), and antibody-dependent cellular cytotoxicity,
ADCC (8).

This chapter will describe two assays for macrophage antiviral activity. The first is a procedure to determine macrophage intrinsic antiviral activity. The second assesses extrinsic antiviral activity by measuring the ability of the

759

macrophage to reduce virus growth in infected susceptible host cells in mixed culture. The procedures described are applicable to any mononuclear phagocyte, although mouse peritoneal cells have been investigated most extensively and will be referred to in this chapter. It is assumed that the reader has a basic understanding of virologic assay techniques (9). The virus used in these protocols is herpes simplex virus (HSV), but other viruses may be substituted as desired. Required biocontainment precautions will be discussed in the concluding section.

II. DETERMINATION OF INTRINSIC ANTIVIRAL ACTIVITY

A. *Introduction*

Most viruses can adsorb to mononuclear phagocytes (10, 11). Several outcomes are possible. With a few viruses (poxviruses in nonimmune hosts, lactate dehydrogenase-elevating virus, and several others), the virus may grow in the mononuclear phagocyte and eventually be spread wherever the infected phagocyte wanders (1, 11). More frequently perhaps, the virus is adsorbed and penetrates into the cytoplasm, but is then unable to replicate in the macrophage, and is eventually destroyed. This phenomenon, which we have termed intrinsic antiviral activity, has been described with many viruses, including herpes simplex virus (3, 12). The effect can be measured easily by monitoring virus growth in monolayers of phagocytes, as is done in the following procedure.

B. *Reagents*

(1) Eagle's Minimum Essential Medium with Earle's balanced salts (EMEM) supplemented with 10% (v/v) heat-inactivated fetal bovine serum (FBS), 2 mM L-glutamine, and antibiotics (e.g, 50 μg Gentamicin per milliliter). All the components are commercially available. Prepare sterile and store at 4°C.

(2) Herpes simplex virus (HSV). Available from American Type Culture Collection (ATCC), Rockville, Maryland. We use Type 2 (HSV-2), but HSV Type 1 or other viruses can be substituted. CAUTION: BIOHAZARD. For preparation of virus stocks consult standard references (9).

(3) Virus diluent, GLB: Hanks' balanced salt solution with 0.5% (w/v) gelatin (Difco, Detroit, Michigan) and 0.25% (w/v) lactalbumin hydrolysate (Difco).

(4) Materials for plaque assay of virus (see Section IV).

(5) Tissue culture plates, 35 mm (6 well) (Costar Division

of Data Packaging Corp., Cambridge, Massachusetts or Linbro
Chemical Co., New Haven, Connecticut). The assay can be scaled
down (to one-quarter) by using 24-well plates (16-mm wells).

(6) Hanks' balanced salt solution (HBSS). Store at $4°C$.

(7) Mononuclear phagocyte preparation. See the appropriate
chapter in Section I of this volume.

All reagents should be sterile. The cells should be kept
in a CO_2 incubator (at 5% CO_2 in air). Glassware required includes sterile cotton-plugged 1-ml and 10-ml pipettes and
sterile capped tubes (12 × 75 or 13 × 10mm glass, polypropylene,
or polystyrene).

C. Procedure

(1) Obtain mononuclear phagocytes and resuspend in culture
medium [Section II.B.(1)]. A convenient concentration is
6 - 9 × 10^6 peritoneal cells (approximately 3 × 10^6 macrophages) per milliliter. Different types of mouse peritoneal
macrophages, human monocytes, and macrophage cell lines have
been studied (1).

(2) With a sterile 10-ml pipette, pipette approximately
2 - 3 × 10^7 peritoneal cells (or about 1 × 10^7 macrophages) per
well. Use minimum of two wells per group; one plate per time
point plus an additional plate for virus uptake at 1 hr. (4
plates minimum). Leave 2 wells, or an additional plate, without cells; these wells will be used later for virus thermal inactivation controls. If the supply of macrophages is sufficient,
pipette macrophages into 1-2 additional wells which will be left
uninfected to serve as morphologic controls for evaluation of
virus cytopathic effect in step (8). Shake gently to evenly
disperse cells and incubate ($37°C$) 2 hr for cell attachment.

(3) Wash with HBSS [Section II.B.(6)] three times to remove
nonadherent cells. This is done by vigorously pipetting sterile
HBSS (approximately 5 ml/well) into each well and then removing
the wash liquid by dumping or aspirating the plates. Repeat
two more times, leaving HBSS in the wells the last time.

(4) Prepare dilution of virus in GLB [Section II.B.(2) and
(3)]. In general, a suitable dilution will be ≥ 1 virus plaque-
forming unit (PFU) per cell. Thus, the final dilution should
contain about 2.5 × 10^7 PFU/ml if 0.4 ml of virus will be adsorbed to 1 × 10^7 macrophages. Keep virus on ice until added
to cells. Save aliquot for virus titration (store at $-70°C$).

(5) Drain wells (by dumping or aspirating off liquid) and
add 0.4 ml of the virus dilution to each well (including thermal inactivation control wells) with a sterile 1 ml pipette.
Gently rock plate to spread the liquid over the cells and incubate plates for 1 hr at $37°C$. Shake the plates gently every
15 min to ensure even distribution of virus.

(6) At end of hour, add 3.6 ml EMEM to each well containing cells and pipette off fluid. Save (-70°C) for later determination of the amount of virus adsorbed. Add 13 ml EMEM to the wells reserved for the thermal inactivation controls and take a 0.5 - 1 ml sample from each of these control wells.

(7) Wash wells (except thermal inactivation controls) three times with HBSS, as in step (3). (This is essential in order to remove nonadsorbed virus. If not washed, such initially nonadsorbed virus can attach to cells and give a false impression of virus growth.) Drain wells and add 5 ml EMEM to each well containing macrophages. Place the 1 hr plate in a freezer (-70°C) for later determination of initial virus uptake. Incubate remaining plates at 37°C. The thermal inactivation controls should also be concurrently incubated.

(8) At 24 hr after infection, look for microscopic signs of cytopathic effect (cell damage), and place one plate in -70°C freezer (the freezing and later thawing will disrupt the cells sufficiently to release cell-associated virus). This is the 24-hr sample. Also freeze aliquot of thermal inactivation control to be titrated later with the other samples. Repeat this procedure at 48 and 72 hr.

(9) When ready to perform the virus assay (Section IV), remove plates and control samples from freezer and thaw (at room temperature or 37°C). Collect fluids from each well as soon as thawed and keep on ice until the virus dilutions are placed on the assay cells.

D. Calculation of Results

Virus titers are calculated from the plaque counts and the dilutions as explained in Section IV.D. On a semi-log scale, plot virus thermal inactivation control and macrophage virus titers for each time point. Calculate amount of virus adsorbed at 1 hr by subtracting unadsorbed virus (virus titer, calculated in PFU/well, of supernatant fluid in step (6)) from input virus (calculated from titer of aliquot from step (4)). [To calculate input virus in step (5), PFU/well = 0.4 × PFU/ml. Step (6) represents a tenfold dilution; therefore, for actual titer of unadsorbed virus in PFU/well, multiply titer (calculated as shown in Section IV.D) by ten.]

Demonstration of virus growth in the macrophage requires that virus titer of the macrophage wells be above amount initially adsorbed and significantly above thermal inactivation controls at one or more time points. Impression of virus growth is strengthened if virus titer in infected macrophage wells after 24 hr increases over time. With HSV, virus growth, if any, is characteristically modest (often $\leq 0.5 - 1 \log_{10}$ over amount adsorbed) and statistical analysis (e.g., by t-test) may be required to demonstrate significance.

Virus titer of macrophages lower than corresponding thermal inactivation controls suggest virus clearance from the macrophage or prolonged eclipse phase of virus in the macrophage. Slope of curve can be used to determine rate of clearance.

Alternative assays are discussed in the next section (Critical Comments).

E. *Critical Comments*

The intrinsic antiviral assay involves measurement of virus growth in mononuclear phagocytes. With HSV, many macrophages are refractory to infection, including resident peritoneal macrophages (12), and less than 10^2 PFU/ml of virus is observed. Thioglycollate-elicited macrophages are reported to be permissive for virus growth (13). The multiplicity of infection (number of virus PFU per cell in initial infection) may be critical to detection of growth, and a higher MOI (1 - 5 PFU/cell) may be necessary to ensure infection of every cell. Confluency of the phagocyte monolayer may also be important. The figures given should allow about 80% confluency. If a virus that does not exhibit cell-to-cell spread is used, a slightly heavier monolayer may be desirable. The length of time which the mononuclear phagocytes have been kept in culture may also be important. With HSV, macrophages cultured *in vitro* for seven days appear to gain permissiveness for virus replication (13, 14). In all cases a thermal inactivation control must be used; even so, it may be difficult at times to distinguish between true virus growth and decreased thermal inactivation due to protective effect of cell association. In the procedure described total virus yield (intracellular and extracellular) was determined, but each can be separately determined by removing supernatant medium at each time point and lysing cells with distilled water as described in the following paragraph.

Destruction of virus may be determined in several other ways. It may be of interest in some cases to determine virus clearance per se within the macrophage. This can be done by taking earlier time points (e.g., 2, 4, 8, 12, and 24 hr). Step (8) is slightly modified. The supernatant fluid should be removed (and saved for titration of extracellular virus) and the plate for that time point washed three times with HBSS. Distilled water (5 ml) is then added and the plates are frozen-thawed as described. The remainder of the procedure is as described. Virus titers in supernatant fluid and in cell lysate are then separately determined [Section IV].

Virus clearance can also be determined by following the fate of viral antigens (by immunofluorescence or immunoperoxidase techniques) or of other virus components or products (e.g.,

nucleic acid by hybridization). Replication of HSV in infected
cells is preceded (early after infection) by increased cellular
uptake of thymidine which can therefore be used to monitor virus infection. In our hands, both virus yield and thymidine uptake in *Corynebacterium parvum*-elicited macrophages are generally low, indicating the relative nonpermissiveness of these cells
for HSV replication.

An alternative method is to determine the presence of potentially infectious virus (rather than virus growth) by infectious
center assay. Infected macrophages in step (7) are overlaid
with susceptible indicator cells (for HSV, 2×10^6 Vero cells
per well) which are allowed to form an even monolayer. Semisolid overlay medium [Section II.B.(4)] is added to the wells.
The cells are incubated for 48 - 72 hr and then fixed and
stained for virus plaques [Section IV]. The number of plaques
gives the number of infectious centers, that is, the number of
macrophages containing infectious or potentially infectious virus. This assay is reasonably sensitive and can serve as a
method for following clearance or persistence of virus in the
macrophage.

III. ASSAY FOR EXTRINSIC ANTIVIRAL ACTIVITY

A. *Introduction*

Extrinsic antiviral activity, the ability of certain mononuclear phagocytes to reduce virus growth in infected susceptible host cells on mixed culture, is another means by which
macrophages may assist in host defense against viruses. It has
been described with several viruses, including herpes simplex
virus (1, 4), vesicular stomatitis virus (4), vaccinia virus
(1), and encephalomyocarditis virus (15). Although the exact
mechanisms are not known, the activity can be distinguished
from other macrophage activities such as cytotoxicity (16).
The specific mechanisms involved appear to vary with different
viruses and host cells. Interferon is probably not involved in
extrinsic activity against HSV (16), but appears to be important in the activity against encephalomyocarditis virus (15).

B. *Reagents*

Those listed here are in addition to those required in Section II.B with the exception of item (5) of Section II.B.

(1) EMEM with 2% FBS [prepared as described in Section II.B.(1), but with 2% FBS v/v].

(2) Vero cells (African green monkey kidney cell line). Available from ATCC, Rockville, Maryland or Microbiological Associates, Walkersville, Maryland. These are grown in EMEM with 10% FBS [Section II.B.(1)] and kept at 37°C in 5% CO_2.

(3) Tissue culture plates, 16 mm (24 well), sterile. Available from Costar, Cambridge, Massachusetts or Linbro Chemical Co., New Haven, Connecticut.

(4) Overlay medium for virus plaque assay: EMEM with 2% FBS [Section II.B.(1)] and 1% (w/v) methylcellulose (4000 cp; Fisher Scientific Co., Fair Lawn, New Jersey). Store at 4°C. (To prepare, suspend methylcellulose, 2% (w/v), in distilled water, mix, and autoclave. When cool, shake vigorously to dissolve methylcellulose, aseptically add proper amount of 10X EMEM, FBS, antibiotics and sterile distilled water to final volume (for final methylcellulose concentration of 1%), adjust pH with sterile sodium bicarbonate, and stir at room temperature for 1 hr to mix. Do not be alarmed by initial appearance, which should improve with stirring. Final product should be fairly viscous.)

C. Procedures for Yield Reduction and Plaque Reduction Assays of Extrinsic Antiviral Activity

All steps are done under sterile conditions and with biohazard precautions.

1. Before Assay

(a) If necessary, treat animals with macrophage-eliciting agents. With mice, we find good activity with peritoneal macrophages elicited by Brewer's thioglycollate broth (preferably aged at least 2 weeks) (available from Difco; make up as directed by manufacturer and inject 1 ml/mouse intraperitoneally on day 5 before harvest) or Corynebacterium parvum vaccine (Burroughs Wellcome, Research Triangle Park, North Carolina; 70 mg/kg intraperitoneally on day -7), as well as with peritoneal macrophages from mice infected intraperitoneally with virus (4). Controls should include resident macrophages (from untreated animals). If a virus is used to elicit macrophages, animals treated with virus diluent should also be used as controls.

(b) On the day before assay, prepare the monolayer of host (Vero) cells in plates. Seed the Vero cell suspension (in EMEM with 10% FBS) [Section II.B.(1)] at $2 - 2.5 \times 10^5$ cells per 16 mm well (1 ml/well), gently shake plates until cells are evenly dispersed, and incubate at 37°C. The Vero cells should

be evenly suspended before pipetting onto plates. At least
two plates will be required.

2. On Day of Assay

(a) Harvest macrophages, wash, and resuspend in EMEM with
2% FBS [Section III.B.(1)] at approximately $6 \times 10^6 - 1 \times 10^7$/ml.
Keep cells on ice until ready to dispense.

(b) Prepare dilution of stock HSV. The dilution should contain approximately 500 PFU/ml in virus diluent (GLB). Keep on
ice until ready to use.

(c) Drain or aspirate liquid from wells of Vero cells to be
infected. Duplicate plates will be infected and set up with
phagocytes. For each plate, at least 3 - 4 wells per treatment
group of macrophages should be infected, plus the same number
of wells with virus but without macrophages as virus controls.
Leave uninfected at least 2 wells per group as macrophage nonspecific cytotoxicity controls, plus 2 - 3 additional wells per
plate as cell controls. Removing the liquid can be done with a
sterile 10-ml pipette or aspirator or by inverting the plates
(carefully, to avoid contamination) over absorbent material.

(d) To each well to be infected, add 0.1 ml of the virus
dilution. This should represent approximately 50 PFU/well.
Rock plate gently to distribute virus over the cell monolayer
and incubate at 37°C for 1 hr, gently shaking the plate every
15 min to ensure even distribution of the virus.

(e) At end of hour, you may wash each well once to remove
unadsorbed virus. [Washing at this point is optional. Do as
described in Section II.C.(3). This is really only necessary
if a MOI $\geq$ 0.1 is used.]

(f) To the duplicate plates, add 3×10^6 peritoneal cells
(representing approximately $1 - 1.5 \times 10^6$ macrophages or monocytes) per well (except the cell and virus control wells,
which do not receive macrophages). Shake plates gently to
evenly distribute macrophages. The groups used might typically
include for each plate (depending on sources of mononuclear
phagocytes, etc.):

Resident macrophages + infected Vero cells (3 - 4 wells per
   plate)
Elicited macrophages + infected Vero cells (3 - 4 wells per
   plate for each group)
Infected Vero cells alone (virus controls; 3 - 4 wells per
   plate)
Resident macrophages + uninfected Vero cells (cytotoxicity
   controls; 2 wells per plate)
Elicited macrophages + uninfected Vero cells (cytotoxicity
   controls; 2 wells per plate for each group of macrophages)
Uninfected Vero cells alone (cell controls; 2 wells per
   plate)

The number of macrophages added in the assay corresponds to a final macrophage - host cell ratio of about 2:1.

(g) Incubate plates 2 hr at 37°C to allow macrophage adherence.

(h) Remove nonadherent cells by washing three times with HBSS (as described above)

(i) Drain or pipette off liquid from plates. To one plate (or set of plates) add 1 ml EMEM with 2% FBS [Section III.B.(1)] per well. The duplicate plate will receive overlay medium [Section II.B.(4)]. Return to incubator and incubate 72 hr (37°C, 5% CO_2).

(j) The plate which received EMEM with 2% FBS will be used for a YIELD REDUCTION ASSAY; the plate with overlay medium is used for a PLAQUE REDUCTION ASSAY. After 72 hr postinfection, remove plates from incubator and collect supernatant culture medium from each well of the YIELD ASSAY PLATE with sterile 1-ml pipettes. Pipette into sterile glass vials or capped tubes and store at -70°C for subsequent virus titration by plaque assay (Section IV).

(k) For plaque reduction assay, the plate which received overlay medium is fixed and stained as for plaque assay [Section IV.C.(5) and subsequent steps] at 72 hr postinfection.

D. Calculation of Results

In the extrinsic antiviral assay, plaque reduction is determined by comparing the macrophage wells (for each group of macrophages) with virus controls. Plaque reduction may be expressed as percentage reduction in plaque number or size compared with virus controls.

In the yield reduction assay, virus yield is most easily expressed as log_{10} titer (PFU/ml) and activity is then expressed as log_{10} reduction of virus titer relative to virus controls.

E. Critical Comments

Extrinsic antiviral activity is assayed by either plaque reduction or virus yield inhibition. Both can be done concurrently, as described here, and are generally well correlated although they measure somewhat different aspects of virus growth. In general, the virus yield assay may be somewhat more sensitive, and can be used alone if desired.

Typical results (for C. parvum or thioglycollate-elicited macrophages) are 2 - 3 log_{10} reduction in yield and ≥90% plaque reduction. Resident macrophages typically have little activity; if considerable activity (1 log_{10} yield reduction or 90% plaque

reduction) is observed, the possibility of nonspecific infection
of the macrophage donors should be considered. This assay may
therefore serve as an additional test of activated macrophage
function.

For determination of antiviral activity against a new virus,
some of the conditions may need to be optimized. The input MOI
is critical. We have found that a very low MOI gives best results in both yield and plaque reduction assays. Activity is
reduced or abrogated at MOI more than five to ten times higher
than that used here. The time of addition of effector cells,
while not critical, can have an effect. Activity is reduced if
addition of effector cells is delayed much beyond 12 hr.
Choice of host cell is also important, although the assay works
equally well with mouse embryo fibroblasts (4). We have used a
xenogeneic system in order to minimize effects of interferon
and possible lymphocyte cytotoxicity. It is wise to ensure that
adequate controls are used, including the cytotoxicity controls
described. In practice, we generally do not observe nonspecific
cytotoxicity at the macrophage - host cell ratio used. The assay should be repeated with fresh macrophages if cytotoxicity is
observed.

IV. TITRATION OF VIRUS BY PLAQUE ASSAY

A. *Introduction*

Growth or presence of most viruses is determined by plaque
assay (9). Plaque assay is based on the observation that many
viruses cause cell death after infecting susceptible cells; if
enough cells in an area are damaged, a clear area, or plaque,
is visible in the cell monolayer. It is assumed (and has been
proved for many viruses) that the number of plaques formed is
proportional to the number of infectious virus particles originally present. The amount of virus is calculated as plaque-
forming units (PFU) from the number of plaques counted.

B. *Reagents*

All reagents are sterile. Biohazard precautions should be
observed. Most of the reagents required have been listed in
other sections. These include Section II.B.(1) (EMEM with 10%
FBS) for growing the monolayers, Section II.B.(3) (virus diluent), Section III.B.(2) (Vero cells), Section III.B.(3)
(16 mm, 24 well plates), and Section III.B.(4) (overlay medium).

Additional items required include the following nonsterile reagents:

(1) Fixative: Aqueous formaldehyde, 4% (made by diluting commercial concentrated formalin 1:10 with water). Store at r-om temperature.

(2) Crystal violet stain: Dissolve 3 gm crystal violet (Fisher Scientific Co., Fair Lawn, New Jersey) in 132 ml 95% ethanol and add distilled water to 600 ml. Filter (Whatman No. 1 or equivalent) into bottles and store at room temperature.

C. Procedure

(1) Prepare Vero cell monolayers in 24 well plates as in Section III.C.1.(b); this should be done 24 hr before starting assay. (Required number of plates will depend on number of samples.)

(2) Prepare serial tenfold dilutions of virus in GLB. To do this, first aseptically dispense 1.8 ml GLB diluent into sterile culture tubes (12 × 75 or 13 × 100 mm), one tube per dilution. Keep virus samples and tubes in ice. (In general, for the extrinsic antiviral yield assay, dilutions from 10^{-1} through 10^{-5} will be required. For the intrinsic antiviral assay, undiluted through 10^{-3} dilution can be used, 10^{-1} through 10^{-5} for controls). With a sterile 1-ml pipette, add 0.2 ml of the virus sample to the first dilution tube (be careful not to place the pipette tip in the diluent), and discard pipette. Using a second sterile pipette, pipette the liquid up and down several times to mix and withdraw 0.3 ml of the dilution. Add 0.2 ml to the next dilution tube. Discard pipette and use new pipette to mix. Continue in this fashion until all required dilutions have been done. The original sample is the undiluted; the first dilution is termed 10^{-1}; and so on.

(3) Drain or aspirate liquid from the Vero cell plates [Section III.C.2.(c)]. To each well, add 0.1 ml of sample (undiluted sample or a dilution, as required); this is best done in duplicate. Gently rock plate to distribute virus over cell monolayer. Incubate 1 hr at 37°C, gently shaking plates every 15 min.

(4) After 1 hr, add 1 ml overlay medium [Section III.B.(4)] to each well. Incubate (37°C, 5% CO_2) 72 hr.

(5) At end of incubation, add formaldehyde fixative [Section IV.B.(1)] to each well (approximately 1.5 ml, enough to almost fill the well). Fix at room temperature for 30 min.

(6) Drain plates. Wash wells three times under gentle stream of tap water to remove remaining methylcellulose. (Drain wash water into sink.)

(7) Add sufficient crystal violet stain [Section IV.B.(2)] to each well to cover cells. Stain at room temperature for 15 min.

(8) Drain stain into sink and wash again as in step (6). Invert plates over absorbent material and allow to dry.

(9) Virus plaques will be seen as clear areas in a blue cell sheet (may be best seen under dissecting microscope). Count plaques and calculate virus titer from dilution.

D. *Calculation of Results*

The virus titer is calculated from the plaque counts and the dilution. For each sample, use those dilutions with the greatest number of countable plaques (roughly 10 - 50 plaques). The titers of these wells can be averaged together to give a mean titer. The titer in plaque-forming units per ml is given by the formula

Titer (PFU/ml) = Plaques counted × (1/dilution) × volume correction

Since the amount of sample used in each well was 0.1 ml, it is necessary to multiply by 10 to give PFU/ml. The last (volume correction) term is therefore 10. For example, if two wells of a 10^{-3} dilution have 20 and 22 plaques each, the titer in PFU/ml will be

$$[(20 + 22/2] \times 10^3 \times 10 = 21 \times 10^4 = 2.1 \times 10^5 \text{ PFU/ml}$$

It is convenient in many cases to express the titer in units of $\log_{10}$, in which case the answer would be 5.3 $\log_{10}$ (rounded to one decimal place).

E. *Critical Comments*

Plaque assay is a standard enumeration method for many viruses and the procedure given here is easily adapted to other viruses. The Vero cell line works well with many viruses. In addition, other cell lines are available for different viruses (9). For viruses that plaque poorly, other techniques (such as hemagglutination inhibition, hemadsorption, or immunofluorescence) are available (9).

Herpes simplex virus plaques well on Vero cell monolayers. A few considerations should be mentioned. The cells should be in a confluent monolayer, but should not be allowed to overgrow. Seeding the cells as directed about 24 hr before beginning titrations should give good results. The overlay medium incorporates 2% heat-inactivated fetal bovine serum (FBS). Most batches of FBS, and some other sera, are satisfactory for

plaque assays; new batches should always be tested with a standard virus preparation. In performing the titrations, care
should be taken to avoid contamination and drying out of cells
(see Section V.A). The 3-day incubation recommended is a guide.
After formalin fixation, all traces of methylcellulose should
be washed out before staining. Fixation and staining times are
approximate, and may be increased if desired.

Accuracy and reproducibility of the plaque assay depends on
many factors, including cell type, age and density of cells,
culture medium used, virus strain, and operator proficiency.
For this procedure, with HSV, variation within samples should
be less than 0.3 $\log_{10}$. Dilution and pipetting errors are the
commonest source of error. Automatic pipettes (Pipetman or
Eppendorf-type) can be used in place of regular 1-ml pipettes
if desired. A "Vortex" mixer can be used (with HSV dilutions
in capped tubes) to mix samples if desired.

V. CONCLUDING REMARKS

A. Technical Precautions

All the procedures described here require multiple washings
of plates. Careful technique should be used to prevent contamination of the cells. During adsorption steps, drying of the
cells in the drained wells can occur if care is not taken to
prevent it. This is especially true when work is done under
a vertical laminar flow ("biocontainment") hood. Drying can be
prevented by working quickly and uncovering only that part of
the plate actually being worked on at the moment.

Virus samples and dilutions should always be kept on ice
when not actually in contact with cells. HSV may be refrigerated at $4°C$ for short-term storage (less than 24 hr). For long-
term storage, freeze at $-70°C$ or below (never at $-20°C$).

B. Biohazard Precautions

Although herpes simplex virus is widespread in nature, it
is a human pathogen and should be handled with care. Biohazard
precautions should therefore be carefully observed (9). The
Vero cell line is transformed and may also be potentially
hazardous. The following precautions apply generally to work
with any virus.

Mouth pipetting should be prohibited. We have found an
electric pipette pump ("Pipet-Aid," Drummond Scientific, Bro-
mall, Pennsylvania) very useful for washing and emptying

wells, adding cells, etc.

Whenever possible, all work should be done in a vertical laminar flow ("biocontainment") hood. Disposable gloves and a laboratory coat reserved for virus work should be used whenever working with virus. If work is done with respiratory viruses, a surgical mask should also be worn. All contaminated liquids and recyclable materials (pipettes, tubes, etc.) should be placed immediately after use into covered buckets or pans containing disinfectant (such as 0.6% sodium hypochlorite), and these vessels should be autoclaved daily before the contents are processed. Disposable items (such as gloves) should also go into autoclavable bags or containers that are autoclaved before being discarded. General hygiene (e.g., washing hands after all work) should be observed. Eating, drinking, or smoking in the laboratory should be prohibited. While work is being performed, laboratory doors should be kept closed and unauthorized personnel should be excluded. Special care should be taken to prevent exposing infants, debilitated elderly persons, pregnant women, and patients receiving immunosuppressive treatment or cancer chemotherapy. With these precautions, the assays can be done without serious danger to personnel or visitors.

C. *Comparison of Activities*

The antiviral assays detailed in this chapter measure two specific antiviral functions of macrophages. Both have been associated with *in vivo* resistance to virus infection (1), although intrinsic activity has been separated from genetic resistance to HSV (13); both activities may be important *in vivo*. It should be noted that intrinsic and extrinsic antiviral activity are not necessarily correlated, and that the mechanisms involved in each of these activities also vary with the virus and host cell used. It is therefore essential that all components (source of mononuclear phagocytes, virus, and host cells) be specified. Other factors that may affect the assays include time in culture (see Section II.E) and age of mononuclear phagocyte donors. We routinely use mice at age 8 - 10 weeks. Peritoneal macrophages of older mice have comparable activity, while cells from suckling mice may have less activity (3). Although we generally use BALB/c mice, other strains can be used.

In addition to the antiviral activities described, other activities of mononuclear phagocytes may also affect the outcome of virus infection. One can measure direct cytotoxicity for virus-infected cells as recently reported (5, 17). However, that activity appears to be detectable only at relatively high macrophage - target cell ratios (50:1 or greater), and when a high virus MOI (>1) is used. This activity may be complementary to the macrophage antiviral assays we have described.

It is also important to rule out NK cell involvement in the antiviral activity assays. In our systems, cytotoxicity is very low (16), suggesting that NK cells are probably not involved. This may need to be established when a new system is used. If virus is used as the eliciting stimulus for macrophages, possible ADCC activity or other effects of antibody may also need to be considered (8). The interrelationships of all these activities, and their role *in vivo*, require further elucidation.

Acknowledgment

Supported by Grants CA 24686 from the National Cancer Institute, DHHS and IN-105C from the American Cancer Society. SSM was a recipient of Postdoctoral Fellowship CA06332 from the National Cancer Institute, DHHS. We acknowledge the contributions of Dr. Lowell A. Glasgow to the original assay system.

REFERENCES

1. P. S. Morahan and S. S. Morse. Macrophage - virus interactions. *In* "Virus-Lymphocyte Interactions: Implications for Disease" (M. R. Proffitt, ed.), pp. 17-35. Elsevier North Holland, New York, 1979.
2. S. C. Mogensen. Role of macrophages in natural resistance to virus infections. *Microbiol. Rev. 43*: 1-26, 1979.
3. R. T. Johnson. The pathogenesis of herpes virus encephalitis. II. A cellular basis for the development of resistance with age. *J. Exp. Med. 120*: 359-374, 1964.
4. P. S. Morahan, S. S. Morse, and M. B. McGeorge. Macrophage extrinsic antiviral activity during herpes simplex virus infection. *J. Gen. Virol. 46*: 291-300, 1980.
5. S. K. Chapes and W. A. F. Tompkins. Cytotoxic macrophages induced in hamsters by vaccinia virus: Selective cytotoxicity for virus-infected targets by macrophages collected late after immunization. *J. Immunol. 123*: 358-364, 1979.
6. L. A. Glasgow. Transfer of interferon-producing macrophages: New approach to viral chemotherapy. *Science 170*: 854-856, 1970.
7. J. T. Kung, S. B. Brooks, J. P. Jakway, L. L. Leonard, and D. W. Talmage. Suppression of *in vitro* cytotoxic response by macrophages due to induced arginase. *J. Exp. Med. 146*: 665-672, 1977.
8. S. Kohl, D. L. Cahall, D. L. Walters, and V. E. Schaffner. Murine antibody-dependent cellular cytotoxicity to herpes simplex virus-infected target cells. *J. Immunol. 123*:

25-30, 1979.

9. E. H. Lennette and N. J. Schmidt, eds. "Diagnostic Procedures for Viral, Rickettsial and Chlamydial Infections," 5th edition. American Public Health Association, Washington, D.C., 1979.

10. S. C. Silverstein. The role of mononuclear phagocytes in viral immunity. *In* "Mononuclear Phagocytes in Immunity, Infection and Pathology" (R. Van Furth, ed.), pp. 557-573. Blackwell Scientific Publishers, Oxford, 1975.

11. C. A. Mims. Aspects of the pathogenesis of viral disease. *Bacteriol. Rev. 28*: 30-62, 1964.

12. J. G. Stevens and M. L. Cook. Restriction of herpes simplex virus by macrophages. An analysis of the cell-virus interaction. *J. Exp. Med. 133*: 19-38, 1971.

13. C. Lopez and G. Dudas. Replication of herpes simplex virus type 1 in macrophages from resistant and susceptible mice. *Infect. Immun. 23*: 432-437, 1979.

14. C. A. Daniels, E. S. Kleinerman, and R. Snyderman. Abortive and productive infections of human mononuclear phagocytes by type I herpes simplex virus. *Am. J. Pathol. 91*: 119-136, 1978.

15. A. M. Pusateri, L. C. Ewalt, and D. L. Lodmell. Nonspecific inhibition of encephalomyocarditis virus replication by a Type II interferon released from unstimulated cells of *Mycobacterium tuberculosis*-sensitized mice. *J. Immunol. 124*: 1277-1283, 1980.

16. S. S. Morse and P. S. Morahan. Macrophage extrinsic antiviral activity *in vitro*. *Fed. Proc. 38*: 1158, 1979.
   S. S. Morse and P. S. Morahan. Activated macrophages mediate interferon-independent inhibition of herpes simplex virus. *Cellular Immunol. 58*: 72-84, 1981.

17. E. J. Stott, M. Probert, and L. H. Thomas. Cytotoxicity of alveolar macrophages for virus infected cell. *Nature 255*: 710-712, 1975.

74

CYTOSTASIS OF TUMOR
AND NONTUMOR CELLS

Alan M. Kaplan

I. INTRODUCTION

In vitro inhibition of tumor growth (cytostasis) and tumor
cytolysis (cytotoxicity) have been shown to be mediated by T
cells, K cells, natural killer cells, and macrophages (MØ)
[reviewed in (1)]. Cytostasis mediated by activated macrophages (AMØ) has been demonstrated by reduced cell counts of
target cells, reduced target cell clonability, inhibition of
mitosis, and by the reduced ability of target cells to incorporate [^{3}H]- or [^{125}]-labeled nucleosides into DNA (2-6).
Macrophage-mediated cytostasis, unlike cytotoxicity, is exhibited against both neoplastic and normal target cells (2,7)
as well as proliferating normal lymphocytes (7,8,9). While
soluble factors have been implicated in MØ-mediated cytostasis,
most reports have suggested that cell-to-cell contact is a prerequisite for cytostasis to occur (10).
The implication that interaction of AMØ with target cells
results in inhibition of proliferation is of great potential

consequence, not only in tumor immunology but in cell biology
in general. With respect to MØ, recent data suggest that
growth regulatory properties extend to immunologically unrelated systems such as wound healing (11). Unfortunately, tumor cell growth as measured either by actual cell counts or
isotope incorporation is subject to a series of culture conditions including vessel shape, specific activity of the radiolabeled nucleoside, degree of activation of the effector cells,
release of a series of effector cell products including arginase (12,13) and thymidine (14-17), and cytolytic effects
generated during the culture (1). These problems which, for
the most part, are ignored have prompted Gyongyossay *et al.* (1),
in a recent article discussing the methodological problems inherent in cell-mediated cytostasis, to raise the question as to
whether or not cell-mediated cytostasis as a distinct *in vitro*
phenomenon exists.

II. REAGENTS

      Target cells (Lewis lung carcinoma, mouse embryo fibro-
blasts, methylcholanthrene fibrosarcomas, B-16 melanoma, etc.)
      Trypsin: EDTA (10X) (GIBCO 610-5405, GIBCO, Grand Island,
New York)
      Eagle's minimum essential medium (EMEM) with Earle's
balanced salt solution, 2X essential amino acids, vitamins,
100 U penicillin/ml, 100 μg streptomycin/ml and 20% heat-inactivated fetal bovine serum
      Tissue culture flasks
      Trypan blue
      96-Well microtest plates (Linbro Scientific, Inc., Hamden,
Connecticut)
      Sterile 4 x 4 in. gauze pads
      Hanks' balanced salt solution (HBSS)
      Brewer's thioglycollate (Difco Laboratories, Detroit,
Michigan)
      Protease peptone (Difco Laboratories, Detroit, Michigan)
      Pyran copolymer (lot XA124-177, Hercules, Inc., Wilming-
ton, Delaware)
      Corynebacterium parvum (Burroughs-Wellcome, Research
Triangle, North Carolina)
      Glycogen (type II from Oyster, Sigma G-8751, Sigma Chemi-
cal Co., St. Louis, Missouri)
      Mycybacterium bovis, strain BCG (Phipps substrain TMC
No. 1029 (Trudeau Inst., Saranac Lake, New York)
      Purified protein derivative (PPD, Connaught Laboratories,
Toronto, Canada) [125]Iododexoyuridine (IUdR, >2000 Ci/mmol,
NEX-072, New England Nuclear, Boston, Massachusetts)

5-Fluorodeoxyuridine (FUdR, Hoffman-La Roche, Nutley,
New Jersey)
Methanol
Clear lacquer varnish

III. PROCEDURES

A. *Target Cell Preparation*

Target cells (Lewis lung carcinoma, mouse embryo fibroblasts, methylcholanthrene fibrosarcomas or B-16 melanoma)
are trypsinized from tissue culture after growth for two to
three days. The cells are usually approximately 90% confluent
at the time of use. Cells are trypsinized from 75 cm^2 culture
flasks by pouring off the culture supernatant, washing twice
with 5 ml of sterile saline and adding 2.5 ml of 0.25% trypsin-
EDTA solution. After incubation at 37°C for 5 to 10 min, the
flasks are tapped several times on the bench top to dislodge
the cells, and 2.5 ml of complete EMEM is added. The cells
are removed from the flasks by repeated pipetting to break up
clumps, centrifuged at 200 g, resuspended in complete EMEM,
and viability determined by trypan blue dye exclusion. Target
cells are diluted to 5 × 10^4 cells/ml in complete EMEM, 0.2 ml
(10^4 cells) added to the wells of a 96-well microtest plate,
and the plates incubated at 37°C for 24 hr. Prior to adding
effector cells, the medium is dumped from the wells and the
plate drained on sterile gauze pads. The wells are washed
twice with complete EMEM by gently pipetting 0.2 ml medium
down the side of each well, and dumping the medium as before.

B. *Peritoneal Cell Preparation*

Peritoneal exudate cells (PEC) are obtained from normal
or treated mice by washing the peritoneal cavity twice with
4 ml of Hanks' balanced salt solution (HBSS) without serum.
The PEC are pooled in 50 ml sterile plastic centrifuge tubes
and collected by centrifugation at 200 g, washed twice with
HBSS, and resuspended in complete EMEM. (We do not routinely
use heparin in the wash fluid but 10 U preservative-free hep-
arin/ml reduces clotting.) To obtain "elicited" or "activated"
macrophages, mice may be inoculated ip with any of a number of
sterile inflammatory agents or immunomodulators. Some typical
substances, doses and schedules are given below with respect
to time of inoculation prior to harvest

Saline, sterile pyrogen free, 1.0 ml ip, day −2.
Brewer's thioglycollate, 10%, 1.0 ml ip, day −3 to −5.
Protease peptone, 10%, 1.0 ml ip, day −3 to −5.
Glycogen, 2.5%, 1.0 ml ip, day −3 to −5.
Pyran copolymer, 25 mg/kg in 0.2 ml ip, day −7.
Killed *C. parvum*, 17.5 − 70 mg/kg in 0.2 ml ip, day −7.
Mycobacterium bovis, strain BCG (Phipps substrain, TMC
No. 1029, 5×10^6 colony-forming units (CFU), id day −30 to
−90, 5×10^6 CFU ip, day −3 to −7.
Mycobacterium bovis, BCG, 5×10^6 CFU id on day −30 to
−90, PPD, 50 μg ip, day −1 to −3.

The washed PEC in complete EMEM are added to the microtest
wells to provide ratios of 20:1 (10^6/ml or 2×10^5/0.2 ml/well),
10:1, 5:1, and 1:1. After 2-hr incubation at 37°C, the nonadherent cells can be removed by washing two to three times as
described above. In general, we have found that there is
little or no difference in the results obtained when total
cells or the adherent cell population are used. Alternatively,
any of a number of procedures can be utilized to purify MØ
prior to their addition to the microtest plates including purification by adherence to collagen-coated plates and removal by
collagenase (18), purification by adherence to FCS-treated
plates and removal by EDTA (19), and purification by adherence
to parafilm and removal at 4°C (20).

C. Incorporation of ^{125}IUdR

At various times after cocultivation of peritoneal macrophages (PM) and target cells (usually 24 and/or 48 hr), the
medium is dumped and the plates washed three times as described
above. The isotope ^{125}IUdR is added at 0.5 μCi/ml in 0.2 ml in
complete EMEM containing 5×10^{-5} M FUdR and the plates are incubated at 37°C for 2 hr in 5% CO_2. After incubation, the medium with ^{125}IUdR is dumped and the plates are washed three
times as described above. The plates are fixed with methanol
for 10 min, allowed to air dry, then sprayed with clear lacquer
varnish and allowed to air dry. The plates are cut with a band
saw to separate the individual wells and the individual wells
are placed in carrier tubes and counted in a gamma scintillation spectrometer. The assay is carried out in quadruplicate
and controls include target cells alone, effector cells alone,
target cells with resident PM, and target cells with the appropriate diluent for any agent being tested for induction of
cytostatic macrophages.

IV. CALCULATION OF DATA

The data can most simply be expressed as counts per minute of [125]IUdR incorporated at a given effector:target cell ratio. Alternatively,

$$\% \text{ Inhibition} = [1 - \frac{\text{cpm target cells + effector cells}}{\text{cpm target cells + control cells}}] \times 100,$$

where control cells are obtained from mice treated with the diluent used for the agent tested for its capacity to induce cytostatic macrophages. This formula assumes that incorporation into effector and control macrophages is negligible and must be modified if this is found not to be the case.

V. CRITICAL COMMENTS

The cytostasis assay as outlined is, for the most part, a straightforward, highly reproducible assay within a given experiment. [^{3}H]-Thymidine or [125]IUdR incorporation as a technique for assessing the relative amount of DNA synthesis has obvious advantages over counting cells in a hemocytometer or an automated counter. The technique is extremely rapid compared to visual means, and allows large numbers of samples to be processed in an objective manner.

Several alternatives exist for various steps in the cytostasis assay. Peritoneal exudate MØ can be purified by adherence directly onto the microtest plates before adding the target tumor cells. Cells can be harvested with sodium dodecysulfate after incubation with [125]IUdR and washing and extracted with 10% cold trichloroacetic acid (TCA) to precipitate acid insoluble DNA-bound [125]I (21). While as much as 25% of the counts of ^{125}I associated with the tumor cells can be non-TCA precipitable, the results of a given assay are quite similar regardless of whether whole cells or TCA precipitable DNA is counted (4). Lastly, [^{3}H]-thymidine can be used instead of [125]IUdR to measure DNA synthesis. The use of [125]IUdR is substantially simpler and less expensive in that preparation for liquid scintillation counting is avoided. Similarly, the plate assay that we have described while overestimating the cpm [125]IUdR provides a fast and accurate assessment of relative DNA synthesis among different groups.

Target susceptibility to MØ-mediated cytostasis is varied and includes cells of varied species, both lymphoid and non-lymphoid tumors and cells grown in both monolayer and suspension including L-929 (4), EMT-6 mouse adenosarcoma (4), transitional cell bladder tumor 4934 (4), Lewis lung carcinoma

(3,7), mouse embryo fibroblasts (3,7), lymphocytes (7,9), SL2 lymphoma cells (17), methylcholanthrene and dimethylbenzan-threne-induced fibrosarcomas (5), polyoma virus-induced tumors (5), rat fibroblasts (2), human melanomas, MEL-1 and RPMI 7932 (2), Burkitt's lymphoma, RAJI (2), human osteogenic sarcoma (2) and human WI-38 lung fibroblasts (3,7). The relative cyto-static activity of various macrophage populations (normal, eli-cited, activated) differ somewhat from publication to publica-tion perhaps due to the varying background flora from mouse colony to mouse colony. In general, lymphocyte blastogenesis is not severely inhibited by normal macrophages, only weakly inhibited at high normal macrophage-to-lymphocyte ratios and enhanced at low normal macrophage-to-lymphocyte ratios (9,22, 23). Activated mouse macrophages (pyran and *C. parvum*) inhibit PHA, con A, and LPS-induced lymphocyte blastogenesis (9,23), while elicited (protease peptone) but not normal rat macro-phages also inhibit lymphocyte blastogenesis (22). The cyto-static effect of elicited rat peritoneal macrophages for both lymphocytes and tumor cells and the cytocidal activity of eli-cited rat peritoneal macrophages for tumor cells is in contrast to the mouse system where elicited macrophages are not cyto-cidal. In the mouse model normal peritoneal macrophages are generally not cytostatic or only weakly cytostatic to tumor and normal target cells while activated macrophages tend to be strongly cytostatic (7,24,25).

A major problem in the cytostasis assay is in intrepreting the data and avoiding the numerous artefacts that either di-rectly or indirectly alter cell growth and, while causing the appearance of cytostasis in the *in vitro* environment, are un-likely to be relevant *in vivo*. This is particularly problem-atic when a single technique is used to assess cell prolifera-tion since several laboratories have demonstrated that cell-free supernatants of macrophages inhibit thymidine or [125]IUdR uptake by cells without blocking cell proliferation (14-17).

The factor that is inhibiting thymidine or [125]IUdR incor-poration is synthesized by macrophages, has been identified as thymidine, and acts as a cold inhibitor of labeled nucleo-side incorporation (15-17). Under normal experimental condi-tions washing the cultures before pulsing with thymidine or IUdR removes the competitive inhibitor and prevents the appar-ent cytostatic effect (17) except in the EL4 system that is uniquely sensitive to thymidine blockade resulting in inhibi-tion of DNA synthesis and cell growth (16).

Another problem frequently overlooked in evaluating cyto-stasis experiments is the potential cytotoxicity of the effec-tor cells. Activated macrophages that are cytotoxic for tumor cells also appear to be extremely cytostatic, however, if the target cells are dying in culture, the resulting decrease in cell number and/or isotope incorporation would be wrongfully interpreted as cytostasis. Cytostasis can be detected earlier after the initiation of cultures (approximately 2 to 6 hr) than cytotoxicity, but it is not known whether or not cytostasis is a prerequisite for cytotoxicity, shares a common mechanism with cytotoxicity, or is irrelevant to cytotoxicity. Perhaps the ideal target cell for cytostasis assays would be a tumor cell that is resistant to the cytotoxic effects of macrophages or any other effector cell in question; however, it is not clear that such a tumor target cell exists. Interestingly, normal cells in culture and lymphocytes are generally susceptible to activated macrophage-mediated cytostasis while being resistant to the cytotoxic effects of macrophages and, therefore, may make good targets for a cytostasis assay. However, the relevance of the cytostatic activity of activated macrophages or any other effector cell for normal targets is of questionable *in vivo* significance.

Acknowledgment

Supported in part by American Cancer Society Grant #IM183 and NIH Grant #CA28308.

REFERENCES

1. M. I. C. Gyöngyössy, A. Liabeuf, and P. Goldstein. Cell-mediated cytostasis: A critical analysis of methodological problems. *Cell. Immunol.* 45:1-14, 1979.
2. R. Keller. Susceptibility of normal and transformed cell lines to cytostatic and cytotoxic effects exerted by macrophages. *J. Natl. Cancer Inst.* 56:369-374, 1976.
3. A. M. Kaplan, P. M. Walker, and P. S. Morahan. Tumor cell cytotoxicity versus cytostasis of pyran activated macrophages. *In* "Modulation of Host Immune Resistance" (M. Chirigos, ed.), pp. 277-286. Fogarty International Center Proceedings, U. S. Government Printing Office, Washington, D.C., No. 28, 1977.
4. J. L. Krahenbuhl, L. H. Lambert, and J. S. Remington. The effects of activated macrophages on tumor target cells: Escape from cytostasis. *Cell. Immunol.* 25:279-293, 1976.
5. R. Keller. Cytostatic elimination of syngeneic rat tumor cells *in vitro* by nonspecifically activated macrophages. *J. Exp. Med.* 138:625-644, 1973.
6. J. L. Krahenbuhl and J. S. Remington. Inhibition of target cell mitosis as a measure of the cytostatic effects of activated macrophages on tumor target cells. *Cancer Res.* 37:3912-3916, 1977.

7. A. M. Kaplan, L. G. Baird, and P. S. Morahan. Macrophage regulation of tumor cell growth and mitogen-induced blastogenesis. *In* "Control of Neoplasia by Modulation of the Immune System" (M. A. Chirigos, ed.), pp. 461-474. Raven Press, New York, 1977.

8. L. G. Baird and A. M. Kaplan. Macrophage regulation of mitogen-induced blastogenesis. I. Demonstration of inhibitory cells in the spleens and peritoneal exudates of mice. *Cell. Immunol. 28:*22-35, 1977.

9. L. G. Baird and A. M. Kaplan. Macrophage regulation of mitogen-induced blastogenesis. II. Mechanism of inhibition. *Cell. Immunol. 28:*36-50, 1977.

10. J. L. Krahenbuhl and L. H. Lambert. Cytokinetic studies of the effects of activated macrophages as tumor target cells. *J. Natl. Cancer Inst. 54:*1433-1437, 1975.

11. S. J. Leibovich. Production of macrophage-dependent fibroblast-stimulating activity (M-FSA) by murine macrophages. *Exp. Cell. Res. 113:*47-56, 1978.

12. J. T. Kung, S. B. Brooks, J. P. Jakway, L. L. Leonard, and D. W. Talmage. Suppression of *in vitro* cytotoxic response by macrophages due to induced arginase. *J. Exp. Med. 146:*665-672, 1977.

13. G. A. Currie and C. Basham. Differential arginine dependence and the selective cytotoxic effects of activated macrophages for malignant cells *in vitro. Br. J. Cancer 38:*653-659, 1978.

14. H. G. Opitz, D. Niethammer, H. Lemke, H. D. Flad, and R. Huget. Inhibition of [^{3}H]-thymidine incorporation of lymphocytes by a soluble factor from macrophages. *Cell. Immunol. 16:*378-388, 1975.

15. H. G. Opitz, D. Niethammer, R. C. Jackson, H. Lemke, R. Huget, and H. D. Flad. Biochemical characterization of a factor released by macrophages. *Cell. Immunol. 18:*70-75, 1975.

16. M. J. Stadecker, J. Calderon, M. L. Karnovsky, and E. R. Unanue. Synthesis and release of thymidine by macrophages. *J. Immunol. 119:*1738-1743, 1977.

17. R. Evans and C. G. Booth. Inhibition of ^{125}IUdR incorporation by supernatants from macrophage and lymphocyte culture: A cautionary note. *Cell. Immunol. 26:*120-126, 1976.

18. G. A. Miller and J. D. Feldman. Genetic role of rat macrophage cytotoxicity against tumor. *Int. J. Cancer 18:*168-175, 1976.

19. K. Kumagai, K. Itoh, S. Hinuma, and M. Tada. Pretreatment of plastic petri dishes with fetal calf serum. A simple method for macrophage isolation. *J. Immunol. Methods 29:*17-25, 1979

20. D. E. Tracey. The requirement for macrophages in the
     augmentation of natural killer cell activity by BCG.
     J. Immunol. *123*:840-845, 1979.
21. A. M. Kaplan, J. Brown, J. M. Collins, P. S. Morahan,
     and M. J. Snodgrass. Mechanism of macrophage-mediated
     tumor cell cytotoxicity. *J. Immunol.* *121*:1781-1789,
     1978.
22. R. Keller. Major changes in lymphocyte proliferation
     evoked by activated macrophages. *Cell. Immunol.* *17*:542-
     551, 1975.
23. E. J. Wing and J. S. Remington. Studies on the regula-
     tion of lymphocyte reactivity by normal and activated
     macrophages. *Cell. Immunol.* *30*:108-121, 1977.
24. J. L. Krahenbuhl, L. M. Lambert, and J. S. Remington.
     Effects of *Corynebacterium parvum* treatment and *Toxo-
     plasma gondii* infection on macrophage-mediated cytostasis
     of tumor target cells. *Immunology* *31*:837-846, 1976.
25. G. R. Pasternack, R. T. Johnson, and H. S. Shin. Tumor
     cell cytostasis by macrophages and antibody *in vitro*. I.
     Resolution into contact-dependent and contact-independent
     steps. *J. Immunol.* *120*:1560-1566, 1978.

75

CYTOLYSIS OF TUMOR CELLS
BY RELEASE OF [^{3}H-] THYMIDINE

Monte S. Meltzer

I. INTRODUCTION

Mouse peritoneal macrophages activated during chronic localized infection with *Mycobacterium bovis* strain BCG develop
nonspecific cytotoxic activity against a wide variety of tumor
target cells *in vitro* (1, 2). While exact mechanism(s) of
cytotoxicity are poorly understood, macrophage cytotoxic activity is effected through two major pathways: tumor cytostasis or inhibition of growth and actual cytolysis (3). Either
effect can be measured to quantify macrophage-tumor cell interactions. Cytostatic effects of activated macrophages, however,
are difficult to evaluate. Cells in culture (activated and
normal macrophages, fibroblasts, and even tumor cells) may be
cytostatic to other cells through poorly understood mechanisms
collectively termed "contact inhibition of cell growth" (4).
At the outset then, tumor cytolysis seems a more interpretable
endpoint for quantitation of macrophage cytotoxic activity. It
should be emphasized, however, that measurement of cytolysis as

METHODS FOR STUDYING
MONONUCLEAR PHAGOCYTES

785

a cytotoxicity endpoint would consistently underestimate the extent of macrophage - tumor cell interaction.

The major problem in measurement of tumor cytolysis is that unlike the relatively rapid effects of antibody and complement, of sensitized lymphocytes, or even antibody and macrophages, tumor cytotoxicity by activated macrophages generally requires at least 18 - 24 hr to become evident. Cinemicroscopic analysis of activated macrophage - tumor cell cultures revealed target cell death as early as 2 hr, but maximal toxicity was not seen until 20 - 30 hr (3). This long period of effector - target cell interaction before cytolysis can limit the choices for a radioisotopic cytotoxicity assay. Commonly used cytoplasmic labels such as ^{51}Cr may have a high "spontaneous release" of label over 20 - 30 hr (approximately 2%/hr). Nuclear labels such as $[^{125}I]$uridine on the other hand may themselves inhibit normal target cell proliferation. Alterations in cell growth cycles induced by radiolabel may then profoundly affect macrophage - tumor cell interaction. The macrophage cytotoxicity assay with $[^3H]$ or $[^{14}C]$thymidine-prelabeled tumor target cells avoids both problems: Spontaneous release of label (label released by tumor cells alone or cultured with normal macrophages) is consistently less than 10 - 15% of the total incorporated counts over 72 hr; growth rates of labeled and unlabeled target cells were identical by cinemicroscopic analysis (3, 5).

II. PROCEDURE

A. *Activation of Mouse Peritoneal Macrophages*

(1) Clean and healthy animals are essential for accurate and reproducible assays of mononuclear phagocyte function. This point cannot be overemphasized. Mice obtained from many commercial sources have chronic inapparent infections. Sendai virus, LDH-virus, minute virus of mice, and mouse hepatitis virus are common contaminants.

(2) Certain strains of mice with characterized genetic defects in macrophage cytotoxic activity should be avoided: (i) strains with the defective Lps gene (C3H/HeJ, C57BL/10ScN); (ii) strains derived from the A strain (A/J, A/HeJ, AL/N); and (iii) the P/J strain (6).

(3) Macrophage activation for tumor cytotoxicity by *in vivo* treatments in *Mycobacterium bovis,* strain BCG-infection, is one of the most consistent stimulants of activation *in vivo*. Activated macrophages can be recovered 7 - 35 days after a single intraperitoneal injection of 1×10^6 colony-forming units of viable BCG (Phipps substrain, TMC No. 1029, Trudeau Mycobacte-

rial Collection, Saranac Lake, New York). Other chronic activation stimuli include: (i) killed *Corynebacterium parvum*
(Burroughs-Wellcome, Triangle Park, North Carolina) 70 mg/kg:
harvest 7 - 21 days; and (ii) pyran copolymer (Hercules XA 124-
177, Hercules Chemical Corp., Wilmington, Delaware 25 mg/kg:
harvest 7 - 21 days.

Activated tumoricidal macrophages can also be harvested
from peritoneal cavities of mice treated intraperitoneally
24 - 48 hr previously with (i) 100 µg PPD (Connaught Medical
Laboratories) in mice immunized intradermally with BCG 3 - 6
weeks previously; (ii) 50 µg purified PHA (Burroughs-Wellcome,
Research Triangle Park, North Carolina or (iii) 100 µg con A
(Miles-Yeda, Rehovot, Israel) (7, 8).

(4) Macrophage activation for tumor cytotoxicity by *in
vitro* treatment with lymphokines. Lymphokines are prepared as
follows: Spleens are removed and pressed through 50 mesh
stainless steel sieves into 100-mm plastic petri dishes held
on ice. The resultant splenic fragments in RPMI 1640 with
buffer are passed through 19- and then 23-gauge needles.
Single-cell suspensions are placed in polypropylene tubes on
ice with 3:1 (v/v) erythrocyte lysing buffer (0.16 M NH$_4$Cl,
0.01 M KHCO$_3$, $10^{-4}M$ Na$_2$EDTA, pH 7.4) for 1/2 min. Lysed spleen
cell suspensions are centrifuged at 300 g for 10 min at 4°C
and resuspended to 5 - 10 × 10^6 leukocytes/ml in RPMI 1640 with
25 mM HEPES buffer, 50 µg/ml gentamicin and 1 - 3% heat-
inactivated (56°C for 30 min) fetal bovine serum. Spleen cell
suspensions are then cultured in 20 ml of medium/75 cm^2 plastic
flask with 50 g/ml PPD (spleens from BCG-immune mice) or
3 - 5 µg/ml con A (spleens from normal or BCG-immune mice) for
48 hr. Sephadex G-10 (Pharmacia Fine Chemicals, Piscataway,
New Jersey) 10 mg/ml is added to supernatants of con A-stimulated spleen cells to remove the lectin. Supernatants can be
stored at 4°C for 1 - 3 months or at -20°C for up to 6 months
without loss of activity. Lymphokine activity for macrophage
activation can usually be detected through a 1/30 dilution of
active supernatant. As an alternative procedure, spleen cells
can be suspended to 50 - 100 × 10^6 cells/ml and cultured for
4 hr with antigen or lectin in 50 ml polypropylene centrifuge
tubes (volume should not exceed 20 ml). After incubation,
cells are washed free of stimulant and cultured at 5 - 10 × 10^6
cells/ml in 20 ml/75 cm^2 flask for 48 hr.

Macrophages from sterile irritant-induced peritoneal exudates are more responsive to lymphokine activation than resident
peritoneal cells. We have found 0.02 M phosphate-buffered
saline, pH 7.4, to be the most innocuous irritant. Agents such
as mineral oil, casein, starch, or thioglycollate may remain
within the macrophage and be continuously released into the
medium through exocytosis. Peritoneal exudate cells are har-

vested 18 - 36 hr after intraperitoneal injection of 1.0 ml PBS (9).

B. Preparation of [^3H]Thymidine-Prelabeled Target Cells

(1) Almost any adherent mouse fibrosarcoma can be used as the tumor target cell. The C3H/HeN fibrosarcoma, L-929, is readily available through several commercial sources. Tumor cells are grown in Dulbecco's modified Eagle's medium with 4.5 gm/liter glucose and 2.0 gm/liter $NaHCO_3$ supplemented with 50 µg/ml gentamicin and 10% v/v heat-inactivated fetal bovine serum.

(2) Tumor cell cultures in log growth (about 40 - 60% confluent) are labeled with 0.2 µc/ml [^3H]thymidine (specific activity 2 mCi/mmol) or [^{14}C]thymidine (specific activity 50 mCi/mmol) for 16-24 hr in medium. [^{14}C]Thymidine is less toxic to target cells than an equal activity of [^3H]thymidine.

(3) Radiolabeled tumor cell cultures are washed free of unincorporated label about 4-6 hr before use and cultured in medium. This interval decreases label in cytoplasmic pools and, in turn, decreases spontaneous release of label during assay. For harvest of target cells, monolayers are washed with Dulbecco's modified PBS without Ca^{2+} or Mg^{2+}. Add 1.0 ml 0.25% trypsin in EDTA (GIBCO, Grand Island, New York) to each 75-cm^2 flask for about 1-2 min (trypsin solution must be warmed to 37°C) and observe digestion under inverted microscope. When monolayer shows first signs of disruption, strike flask against bench surface to remove cells mechanically from the plastic. Add 10 ml medium with 10% fetal bovine serum and pipette cell suspension several times to separate clumps. Cell suspensions are washed twice in medium and resuspended to 0.4 × 10^5 cells/ ml. Target cells should have no more than 10,000 cpm/4 × 10^4 cells. ^{3}HTdR-Incorporation above this level may be toxic.

C. Tumor Cytotoxicity by Activated Macrophages

(1) All cell and medium manipulations in this assay are easily and accurately done with a Biopette (Becton, Dickinson and Company) automatic pipette (adjustable to 1.0 ml in 0.1-ml intervals). Add 4 - 8 × 10^5 macrophages (not total peritoneal cells)/0.5 ml medium to 16-mm plastic culture wells (Linbro or Costar Plastics, Hartford, Connecticut and Cambridge, Massachusetts. Incubate multiwell plates 37°C in 5% CO_2 in moist air for 1 - 3 hr.

(2) Adherent macrophage monolayers are prepared by washing peritoneal cell cultures with 0.7 ml warm medium delivered directly onto the monolayer through the Biopette tip. Medium in

the well can be aspirated through a 19-gauge needle attached
to a cut tuberculin syringe connected to a trapped vacuum line
by rubber tubing. The wash-aspirate cycle should be repeated
three times.

(3) Adherent peritoneal cells from mice treated with *in
vivo* activation agents are cytotoxic without further treatment
in vitro. However, the level of cytotoxicity decays with time
in culture (about 3%/hr). By 24 - 36 hr in culture, *in vivo*-
activated macrophages have completely and irreversibly lost cytotoxic activity.

(4) Adherent peritoneal exudate cells from PBS-treated mice,
about 90% macrophages, can be activated by lymphokines for tumor
cytotoxicity. Macrophages are cultured in dilutions of lymphokines for 4 - 12 hr (optimal activation occurs at about 8 hr).
Lymphokine-treated cells are washed twice with warm medium and
then cultured with ^{3}HTdR-prelabeled tumor cells (6 - 8 × 10^5
macrophages in 16-mm wells with 4 × 10^4 target cells.

(5) The level of cytotoxic activity by lymphokine-activated
macrophages can be synergistically increased by 0.1 - 10 ng/ml
phenol-extracted bacterial endotoxin added during the lymphokine treatment and removed before addition of target cells (10).
It should also be noted that cytotoxic activity of lymphokine-
activated macrophages decays with time in culture. The rate of
decay is similar to that of *in vivo* activated cells (9 - 10).

(6) ^{3}HTdR-Labeled tumor cells are added to adherent peritoneal cell monolayers in 1.0 ml medium. Labeled tumor cells
are added to wells without macrophages to determine "spontaneous
release" (release by tumor cells alone). Total incorporated
counts are estimated from 1:1 mixtures of labeled target cells
and 0.5 - 1.0% sodium dodecyl sulfate detergent (SDS) in water.
After 48 hr in culture, 0.5 ml of each macrophage-tumor cell
culture supernatant and of the SDS digest is removed with a
Biopette and placed into 5 - 10 ml Biofluor liquid scintillation
cocktail (New England Nuclear Corp., Boston, Massachussets).
Results are expressed as a percentage of total incorporated
counts from the SDS digest. Each point should be done in duplicate or triplicate.

III. CALCULATION OF DATA

Typical results at 48 hr	Radioactivity (% of total)
SDS total counts	10,000 cpm (100%)
Spontaneous release	1000 cpm (10%)
Normal resident or exudate macrophages	1000 cpm (10%)
Lymphokine-activated macrophages	4000 cpm (40%)
Lymphokine-activated macrophages and LPS	6000 cpm (60%)
BCG-activated macrophages	5000 cpm (50%)

IV.   COMMENTS

(1) Estimation of target cell death be release of nuclear label into culture supernatants involves at laeast two mechanisms: Target cells must first die; cell death is then followed by autolysis and release of nuclear label. The delay in label release after cell death is dependent upon the rate of cytolysis. Examination of macrophage-induced tumor cytolysis by [3H] thymidine release and by cinemicroscopic analysis under identical conditions resulted in superimposable cytotoxicity curves: Both assays measured the same event (cell death) but [3H] thymidine release was delayed after actual cell death by a factor of 2. [3H]Thymidine in supernatants harvested at 48 hr reflected cell death at 24 hr. This relationship was true for all points between 0 - 72 hr (5).

REFERENCES

1. J. B. Hibbs, Jr. The macrophage as a tumoricidal effector cell: A review of *in vitro* and *in vivo* studies on the mechanism of the activated macrophage nonspecific cytotoxic reaction. *In* "The Macrophage in Neoplasis" (M. A. Fink, ed.). Academic Press, New York, 1976.
2. R. P. Cleveland, M. S. Meltzer, and B. Zbar. Tumor cytotoxicity *in vitro* by macrophages from mice infected with *Mycobacterium bovis*, strain BCG. *J. Natl. Cancer Inst.* *52*: 1887-1895, 1974.
3. M. S. Meltzer, R. W. Tucker, and A. C. Breuer. Interaction of BCG-activated macrophages with neoplastic and non-neoplastic cell lines *in vitro*: Cinemicrographic analysis. *Cell Immunol. 17*: 30-42, 1975.
4. M. S. Meltzer, M. M. Stevenson, R. W. Tucker, and E. J. Leonard. Peritoneal macrophages from BCG-infected mice: Tumor cytotoxicity and chemotactic responses *in vitro*. *In* "The Macrophage in Neoplasia" (M. A. Funk, ed.). Academic Press, New York, 1976.
5. M. S. Meltzer, L. P. Ruco, and E. J. Leonard. Macrophage activation for tumor cytotoxicity: Mechanisms of macrophage activation by lymphokines. *In* "Macrophages and Lymphocytes: Nature, Functions and Interactions" (M. Escobar and H. Friedman, eds.). Plenum, New York, 1979.
6. D. Boraschi and M. S. Meltzer. Macrophage activation for tumor cytotoxicity: Genetic variation in macrophage tumoricidal capacity among mouse strains. *Cell. Immunol. 45*: 18-194, 1979.

7. L. P. Ruco and M. S. Meltzer. Macrophage activation for tumor cytotoxicity: Induction of tumoricidal macrophages by PPD in BCG-immune mice. *Cell. Immunol. 32*: 203-215, 1977.

8. L. P. Ruco and M. S. Meltzer. Macrophage activation for tumor cytotoxicity: Induction of tumoricidal macrophages by supernatants of PPD-stimulated Bacillus Calmette Guerin-immune spleen cell cultures. *J. Immunol. 119*: 889-896, 1977.

9. L. P. Ruco and M. S. Meltzer. Macrophage activation for tumor cytotoxicity: Increased lymphokine responsiveness of peritoneal macrophages during acute inflammation. *J. Immunol. 120*: 1054-1062, 1978.

10. L. P. Ruco and M. S. Meltzer. Macrophage activation for tumor cytotoxicity: Development of macrophage cytotoxic activity requires completion of a sequence of short-lived intermediary reactions. *J. Immunol. 121*: 2035-2042, 1978.

76

QUANTIFICATION OF CYTOLYSIS OF NEOPLASTIC CELLS
BY RELEASE OF CHROMIUM-51

Stephen W. Russell

I. INTRODUCTION

Release of ^{51}Cr from prelabeled target cells is a convenient and objective means of measuring damage to target cell
membranes. Lysis (or membrane changes that herald lysis) is
characterized by increased plasma membrane permeability and,
thus, an increased rate of leakage of this cytoplasmically
localized radioisotope. Such increased release can be quantified in a gamma spectrometer, with the standard deviation between samples assayed in triplicate being <2% of the total release (freeze - thaw) value. No scintillant is required,
thereby reducing costs over isotope release assays that require beta counting (It should be emphasized, however, that
the sensitivity of the ^{51}Cr release assay can be increased significantly if radioactivity is quantified in a liquid scintillation spectrometer.). The main disadvantage is a relatively
high level of spontaneous, background release that decreases
the usefulness of this technique if assays of >24 hr duration

are attempted. Spontaneous release increases markedly if
target cells are mishandled during the labeling procedure.

II. REAGENTS

Note: All reagents should be tested to ensure that they
are free of contaminating endotoxin. This is of extraordinary importance in assays of mouse macrophage-mediated tumor
cell killing (1). Although nonspecificity can be a problem
(2), the most sensitive and reliable assay for endotoxin now
generally available is the *Limulus* amebocyte lysate test. The
assay is available in kit form (e.g., Associates of Cape Cod,
Inc., Woods Hole, Massachusetts).
    (1) Minimum essential tissue culture medium (Eagle's), or
any other standard medium, buffered to pH 7.2 with 15 mm
HEPES.
    (2) Fetal bovine serum, heated 30 min at 56°C and filtered
to remove sediment. This reagent often is contaminated with
endotoxin, unless special precautions are taken in its collection. A source that guarantees their product to be free of
detectable endotoxin is Sterile Systems, Inc., Logan, Utah.
    (3) ^{51}Cr, as $Na_2{}^{51}CrO_4$ in sterile, isotonic saline (Amer-
sham Corp., CJS-11).
    (4) 16-mm or 6-mm Diameter, flat-bottomed wells in 24- or
96-place plastic plates, respectively (available from a number
of manufacturers, e.g., Costar or Linbro).

III. PROCEDURE

A. *Preparation of Macrophage Monolayers*

The objective here is to obtain a confluent monolayer of
mononuclear phagocytes. This is important because low population density can depress or even prevent the expression of
killing by cytolytic macrophages in this assay (3, 4). Because different mononuclear phagocyte populations behave differently, it is impossible to generalize as to the number that
should be added per well to ensure that a confluent monolayer
is produced. The figures given below should be viewed, therefore, as suggestions and each investigator should derive a
value for his or her own system and conditions. In all cases,
it is helpful to perform a differential analysis on the starting suspension so that cells can be seeded on the basis of num-

ber of mononuclear phagocytes per well, rather than total cell number.

1. 16-mm Diameter Wells

Adjust the mononuclear phagocyte concentration to $1 - 2 \times 10^6$/ml. Add 0.5 ml to each well. Just before placing the plate into the incubator, shake it several times at right angles to ensure uniform distribution of cells after they have settled (movements caused by walking tend to create a vortex, resulting in uneven distribution of the macrophages). After 1 hr (or longer, if necessary), wash monolayers by jetting medium onto them from a Pasteur pipette (or similar device) until nonadherent cells have been removed. Three washes will usually suffice.

2. 6-mm Diameter Wells

Seed between $1.5 - 2.5 \times 10^5$ mononuclear phagocytes per well in 0.2 ml (equivalent to $7.5 - 12.5 \times 10^5$/ml). Allow cells to settle and adhere for 1-2 hr. Wash the resultant monolayers, either by repeatedly jetting medium onto them from a Pasteur pipette, or by repeatedly throwing the medium out of the wells (by inverting the plate and sharply shaking downward several times), after which a drop of medium is rapidly added to each well to prevent drying. The drops of medium are vigorously shaken in the wells, after which they are vigorously expelled. The number of washes needed will be governed by the extent to which cell types other than mononuclear phagocytes contaminate monolayers. In our hands, three washes usually have proved adequate.

B. Preparation and Labeling of Target Cells

If nonspecific, direct killing is being measured, try to choose a target cell that is antigenically unrelated to the system being investigated. By so doing, killing that is attributable to antibody-dependent, macrophage-mediated cytotoxicity and/or T lymphocyte-mediated cytotoxicity can be avoided, if it is a potential problem. The target cell of choice is the P815 mastocytoma cell. This particular cell is characterized by a high degree of ^{51}Cr retention and is susceptible to killing during the relatively short (16 hr) time that target cells are exposed to macrophages in this assay.

The target cells should be certified free of contamination by mycoplasma and be in an exponential phase of growth. All forms of mechanical injury, such as vortexing, vigorous pipetting, violent shaking, high-speed centrifugation, etc., should be avoided during the labeling procedure or background release will be markedly increased. If adherent cells are used, they should not be exposed to trypsin (during removal from flasks) for any longer than necessary or, again, increased ^{51}Cr leakage will result.

Centrifuge (200 g, 5 min) the cells. Resuspend in approximately 0.5 ml of medium containing 10% FBS. Add approximately 250 μCi of ^{51}Cr. Bring the final volume to 1 ml with medium + 10% FBS. The batch of chromium used should ideally be no more than one month old, as the decay products of ^{51}Cr are toxic to cells. The incubation should be conducted in a conical, 50-ml, polypropylene centrifuge tube. A lead container should be placed in a 37°C water bath for this purpose. With gentle shaking at 10 - 15 min intervals, the incubation should be continued for 1 hr. Terminate the uptake of ^{51}Cr by diluting the cells (and ^{51}Cr-containing medium) to 50 ml with warm (37°C) medium containing 10% FBS, in the same tube that was used for the incubation. Cap and mix gently by inverting the tube several times. Pellet the cells (200 g, 10 min) and remove all of the supernatant medium. Add a few drops of fresh medium, flick the bottom of the tube several times to resuspend the cells (as gently as possible) and dilute up to 10 ml using 37°C medium containing 10% FBS. Return the cells to the water bath and incubate them by gently inverting the tube every 15 min for an additional hour. During this period dead and injured cells will leak their ^{51}Cr. This step is important in reducing the background level of ^{51}Cr release. After the hour has elapsed, pellet the cells as before, being certain to remove all supernatant medium (it is important to allow the sides of the emptied tube to drain, after which the residiuum of ^{51}Cr-contaminated medium can be removed). After a few drops of fresh medium have been added, the tube should be flicked to resuspend the cells, after which they can be diluted to a convenient volume (usually 5 ml) for counting. After a final adjustment in concentration is made, the labeled target cells are ready to use. If clumping has occurred, the larger of these can be eliminated by allowing them to settle out. If clumps are dispersed by vigorous pipetting, background release probably will be increased.

C. Conduct of the Assay

With the target cells fully prepared for use, add whatever experimental reagents are needed to the assay wells, being sure to leave enough room in the well for the target cells. In the 16-mm diameter wells targets are conveniently added in 0.5 ml, bringing the total volume in each well to 1.5 ml. For 6 mm-diameter wells, we usually add targets in 0.1 ml, bringing the total volume to 0.2 ml. A useful number of targets per well is

10^5 or 10^4 for 16- and 6-mm diameter wells, respectively. Targets should be added using an automatic pipette that has a high degree of accuracy. Reproducibility well-to-well can be compromised at this step if care is not taken to ensure that a reproducible number of cells is dispensed into each well. With the large wells, after seeding care must be taken to shake the plate just prior to putting it into the incubator, thereby ensuring that the target cells will settle evenly onto the monolayer.

After 16 hr, supernate from each well should be removed for quantification of radioactivity that has been released into the medium. To harvest each 16-mm diameter well, the plate is tipped at about a 30° angle. One ml of medium is drawn up into an automatic pipette, expelled back into the well to mix the contents, and again withdrawn. It is then transferred to a 12 × 75 mm tube, the number of which corresponds with that of the well. The procedure is repeated, using the same pipette tip for each of the three wells that constitute the replicates for a given sample. After harvesting has been completed, cork the tubes and centrifuge them (750 g, 10 min, 4°C) to sediment the cells. While this step is being performed, prepare a second set of tubes with the same series of numbers. After centrifugation has been completed, transfer 0.5 ml of the cell-free supernate (using the automatic pipette) from each centrifuged tube into the correspondingly numbered tube in the new set. Cork and quantify the radioactivity in a gamma counter. If the Costar 24-place plate is used, it will fit into a centrifuge carrier that is designed to hold the 96-place, microtiter plate (e.g., the carrier made by Dynatech Laboratories, Alexandria, Virginia). After mixing the supernatant medium in each well as described, use of such a carrier will eliminate the need for centrifugation in tubes, as the suspended cells can be sedimented in the wells. For the smaller, 6-mm diameter wells, it is possible to avoid mixing and centrifugation altogether. The upper 0.1 ml of supernatant medium is simply aspirated for counting using a microliter pipette, being careful not to introduce the tip of the pipette any deeper into the well than is necessary.

Controls for spontaneous release should consist of target cells incubated for 16 hr, either alone or on monolayers of thioglycollate-elicited, peritoneal macrophages. The presence of the noncytotoxic macrophages usually enhances retention of label by the targets, compared to cells cultured alone. Maximum release of the label is determined by adding target cells to each of three tubes containing distilled water. The volume of target cells and distilled water should be appropriate for the well size being used, e.g., 0.1 ml of targets and 0.1 ml of distilled water for the 6 mm diameter wells. Freeze – thaw tubes are held overnight at -20°C, and then thawed and frozen

twice more (ethanol/dry ice bath) during the next morning.
After the third round of freezing and thawing, the tubes are
mixed by vortexing (very important) and then centrifuged
(750 g, 10 min, 4°C) to remove cell debris. A sample of cell-
free supernate is then removed from each tube for counting.

IV. CALCULATION OF DATA

Two types of values must be reported for each assay:
background release and percent-specific ^{51}Cr release.

A. *Background Release*

This is reported as the percentage of the total releasable
counts that is released spontaneously from the target cells
per hour. The calculation for a 16-hr assay is

$$\% \text{ Release/hr} = \frac{\text{Total spontaneous release}}{16 \times \text{freeze - thaw release}} \times 100$$

B. *Percent-Specific ^{51}Cr Release*

The calculation is

$$\frac{\% \text{ Specific}}{^{51}\text{Cr release}} = \frac{\text{Exp. release - total spont. release}}{\text{Freeze - thaw release - total spont. release}} \times 100$$

This value should be reported as the arithmetic mean ±1
standard deviation.

V. CRITICAL COMMENTS

The ^{51}Cr release method of quantifying mononuclear
phagocyte-mediated cytolysis has as its main advantages the
relatively short duration of the assay and its reproducibility
well-to-well. Chief among its disadvantages is the relative
high background release. With care the level can be reduced
to acceptable limits, however. For example, one can expect a
rate of 1 - 1.5%/hr with the P815 target, resulting in release

of from 16 - 24% of the total label in 16 hr. Another disadvantage is that not all target cells retain ^{51}Cr well, resulting in unacceptably high levels of background release with
some cells, no matter how careful one is during the labeling
procedure. Conversely, not all target cells release ^{51}Cr well
after they are injured, and some may resist injury during the
relatively short exposure to macrophages that is a characteristic of this assay. Thus, one should consider this a relatively specialized method that works best when used with a target such as the P815 mastocytoma cell. This limitation is not
as great a detraction as it may first appear to be, however,
as in correlative experiments we have found that macrophages
that killed P815 cells were capable of killing many other kinds
of tumor cells when they were examined using the longer cytotoxicity assays, e.g., [^{3}H]-thymidine release, even though
killing of these same target cells was not detectable using the
^{51}Cr release assay.

Acknowledgment

     The author thanks Ms. Brenda Brown for typing the manu-
script. Supported by the United States Public Health Service
research grant CA 31199 and Research Career Development Award
CA 00497.

REFERENCES

1. J. B. Weinberg, H. A. Chapman, Jr., and J. B. Hibbs, Jr.
    Characterization of the effects of endotoxin on macrophage
    tumor cell killing. *J. Immunol.* *121*: 72-80, 1978.
2. R. J. Elin and S. M. Wolff. Nonspecificity of the *Limulus*
    amebocyte lysate test: Positive reactions with polynucleo-
    tides and proteins. *J. Infect. Dis.* *128*: 349-352, 1973.
3. W. F. Doe and P. M. Henson. Macrophage stimulation by bac-
    terial lipopolysaccharides. I. Cytolytic effect on tumor
    cells. *J. Exp. Med.* *148*: 544-556, 1978.
4. S. W. Russell and A. T. McIntosh. Macrophages isolated
    from regressing Moloney sarcomas are more cytotoxic than
    those recovered from progressing sarcomas. *Nature 268*:
    69-71, 1977.

77

ASSESSMENT OF CYTOLYSIS OF TUMOR CELLS
BY RELEASE OF $[^{125}I]$IODODEOXYURIDINE

Ronald B. Herberman

I. INTRODUCTION

^{125}I-Iododeoxyuridine (^{125}IUdR) is a useful compound for
labeling a wide variety of tumor cells and other cells.
^{125}IUdR is incorporated into target cell nuclear DNA in place
of sterically similar thymidine. There is very little or no
spontaneous release of radioisotope from living cells and reutilization is minimal. Therefore, release of this isotope
from cells into the supernatant is a direct and quantitative
reflection of the proportion of cells being killed and losing
their structural integrity (1). ^{125}IUdR release assays have
been successfully used for measurement of humoral and cell-
mediated cytotoxicity of a variety of adherent and suspension
animal and human tumor cell lines (1 - 8). Results with this
label have compared favorably with those obtained with other
isotopes (9). Although ^{125}IUdR has not been as widely used as
[^{3}H]thymidine or ^{51}Cr for assays of cytolysis by macrophages,
the studies that have been performed with ^{125}IUdR have had

801

satisfactory results with a variety of different cells (e.g., 10 - 13). Target cells labeled with this radioisotope should also be useful in exploring the *in vivo* role of macrophages in resistance to tumor growth, as has been done recently with natural killer cells (14, 15).

Assays that measure the release of ^{125}IUdR or [^{3}H]thymidine over an incubation period of 48 - 72 hr are sufficiently sensitive to detect cytolytic activity by normal rodent or human macrophages or monocytes (e.g., 16, 17) as well as the higher reactivity of *in vivo* or *in vitro* activated macrophages.

II. REAGENTS

(1) Sterile plastic tissue culture flask, 75 cm^2 (3024, Falcon Plastics, Oxnard, California)
(2) Sterile 50-ml graduated conical plastic centrifuge tubes (Falcon Plastics, Oxnard, California)
(3) Plastic perti dishes, 10 cm (Falcon, Oxnard, California)
(4) Sterile plastic pipettes
(5) Microtest plates, 6.4-mm flat-bottomed wells (3596, Costar, Cambridge, Massachusetts)
(6) Biopette (1 ml Biopette, Schwarz/Mann, Orangeburg, New York 10962)
(7) RIA Microharvest Tips (Cooke Engineering, Rockville, Maryland)
(8) Counting tubes for gamma counting or vials for scintillation counting

Other equipment includes:
Standard microscope with hemocytometer
Coulter counter (Model Z, Coulter Electronics, Hialeah, Florida)
Incubator with 5% CO_2 humidified atmosphere (37°C)
Mash II automatic harvester (Microbiological Assoc., Bethesda, Maryland) for suspension target cells
Gamma counter (Beckman Biogamma, Irvine, California 92664)
Beta scintillation counter (Isocap 300, Searle Analytic, Inc., Des Plaines, Illinois 60018)

Solutions and Chemicals

Incubation media. A variety of incubation media can be utilized for this test. The tissue culture media in which the cells are normally carried are satisfactory for the assay. Our assays are all done in RPMI 1640 medium with 10% fetal bovine serum (Biofluids, Rockville, Maryland). Hanks' balanced salt

solution (BSS) or phosphate-buffered saline (PBS) is utilized
to wash the cells.

Trypsin.   0.25% crude trypsin-EDTA, GIBCO, Grand Island,
New York was used as needed to detach cells for labeling.

Antibiotics.   For the assay, the media utilized are supplemented with 50 µg/ml gentamicin (Schering Corp., Kenilworth,
New Jersey).

[125]Iododeoxyuridine.   [125]IUdR (New England Nuclear, Boston,
Massachusetts or Amersham Searle, Arlington Heights, Illinois).
Stock solutions of 50 µCi/ml are prepared on arrival by dilution
with RPMI 1640 medium. The stock solution is stored at $4°C$.

Fluorodeoxyuridine (FUdR) 10^{-4} molar stock solutions were
prepared. This chemical has been obtained from Hoffmann La-
Roche, Nutley, New Jersey as well as from the NIH Chemotherapy
Branch. FUdR stock solution is kept at $4°C$ but the FUdR concentrated solution ($10^{-2}M$) is held frozen at $-70°C$.

If liquid scintillation counter is used: Aquasol beta
scintillation fluid (New England Nuclear, Boston, Massachusetts
02118). Because water is present in the samples to be counted,
a scintillation fluid that will tolerate water is necessary.

C. Effector Cells

For studies of natural cytolytic activity of macrophages,
peritoneal macrophages from normal mice or rats or peripheral
blood monocytes from normal human donors may be used. For
studies of cytolysis by activated macrophages, *in vivo* or *in
vitro* stimulated macrophages are used.

1. Normal Mouse Macrophages

Peritoneal macrophages from most strains of mice [main exception, C3H/HeJ (16)] have substantial levels of natural cytolytic activity. Peritoneal cells are collected immediately
from intraperitoneal injection of 10 ml of RPMI 1640 medium containing heparin (40 U/ml, GIBCO, Grand Island, New York). The
resident peritoneal cells are washed twice with PBS and resuspended in culture medium with 10% FBS. Adherent cells can be
obtained by either of the following methods:

(a) Ten to 15 ml of cell suspensions are seeded in tissue
culture flasks and incubated for 45 min at $37°C$. Nonadherent
and loosely adherent cells are removed by vigorous agitation
and the flasks are then thoroughly washed five times with 20 ml
of culture medium. Adherent cells are then recovered from the
flasks by scraping with a rubber policeman, washed with 50 ml
of PBS, and resuspended in culture medium with 10% FBS.

(b) According to the method of Ackerman and Douglas (18),

microexudate-coated tissue culture flasks can be used to obtain
adherent cells.

Adherent cells prepared by the two methods showed no difference in cytotoxic activity or yield (25 - 30%). However, the
cells from the microexudate flasks had higher viability (99%
versus 65 - 75% after scraping with rubber policeman). By
either method, 97 - 99% of the adherent cells were macrophages,
capable of ingesting latex particles.

2. Activated Mouse Macrophages

(a) *In vivo* activated macrophages: Macrophages can be harvested from the peritoneal cavity of mice pretreated with various stimulants. Two suitable procedures are the following:

(i) Bacille Calmette-Guerin (BCG), $1 - 3 \times 10^7$ viable organisms intraperitoneally, 7 - 14 days before harvest.

(ii) *Corynebacterium parvum* (Burroughs Wellcome, Research
Triangle Park, North Carolina), 2.1 mg intraperitoneally, 7 - 11
days before harvest. Adherent peritoneal cells are harvested as
described above.

(b) *In vitro* activated macrophages: Adherent peritoneal
cells from normal mice are harvested as described above. These
cells, at $5 \times 10^4/0.1$ ml are seeded into each well of microplates and incubated for 45 min at $37°C$. After washing, 0.1 ml
of culture medium with 10% FBS is added to each well. To
evaluate the *in vitro* activation of macrophages by lymphokines,
0.1 ml of a lymphokine-containing supernatant is added to the
wells. The lymphokine supernatants may be left in throughout
the 48-hr assay, since they did not affect the percentage cytolysis of target cells in the absence of effector cells.

Lymphokine supernatants, suitable for activation of macrophages, may be prepared by stimulation of lymphoid cells with
mitogens or antigens *in vivo* or *in vitro*. One method that we
have used for producing active supernatants has been to immunize
C3H/HeN mice with BCG, by intradermal inoculation of $2 - 3 \times 10^6$
viable organisms (Phipps strain, Trudeau Institute, Saranac Lake,
New York). After 3 - 6 weeks, the spleen cells from these mice
$(5 \times 10^6/ml)$ are incubated for 4 hr at $37°C$ with 100 μg/ml purified protein derivative (PPD), washed twice by centrifugation at
150 g for 10 min, suspended at $5 \times 10^6/ml$ and incubated at $37°C$
in a humidified 5% CO_2 incubator for 48 hr. The culture supernatants can be stored at $-70°C$ until use.

3. Normal Human Monocytes

Heparinized (40 U/ml, GIBCO, Grand Island, New York) peripheral venous blood (50 - 300 ml) are obtained from normal adult

donors and diluted 1:4 with PBS. Alternatively, leukocytes are
obtained by leukophoresis or plateletpheresis. Mononuclear
cells are separated by centrifugation at 400 g for 30 min on
Ficoll-Hypaque (LSM, Litton Bionetics, Kensington, Maryland),
washed twice with FBS, and then resuspended at 1×10^6/ml in
culture medium with 10% FBS. Adherent cells are then obtained
by either of the two procedures described in Section II.C.1.
The yields and viabilities of monocytes harvested by the microexudate method (mean of 5.9% of mononuclear cells and viability
> 90%) have generally been higher than those obtained by
scraping (mean yield of 5.3% and viability of 70%). By either
procedure, > 90% of the adherent cells were monocytes, as assessed by morphology, nonspecific esterase staining (19) or latex phagocytosis.

4. *In vitro Activated Human Monocytes*

Monocytes are prepared as described above and added to the
wells, followed by a lymphokine-containing supernatant, to give
a total volume of 0.2 ml. Target cells are then prepared and
about 60 min later added to the wells in a volume of 0.1 ml.
As with the mouse macrophages, the presence of lymphokine-
containing supernatants throughout the 48-72 hr assay did not
affect the percent release in the medium controls.
Supernatants of lymphocytes cultured with phytohemagglutinin
(PHA), PPD (for skin test positive donors) or *C. parvum* have all
been quite effective in increasing the levels of macrophage-
mediated cytolysis (20).
The procedure for preparing lymphokine-containing supernatants with PHA or PPD is as follows: Peripheral blood mononuclear cells, depleted or firmly adherent monocytes but still
containing 2 - 4% monocytes, are cultured at $2 - 5 \times 10^6$/ml in
plastic tubes (2070 Falcon) in 7 - 10 ml culture medium in the
presence of 10 µg/ml PHA (HA17, Wellcome Research Laboratories,
Beckenham, England) or 20 g/ml PPD (Connaught Medical Research
Laboratories, Toronto, Canada). After 20 hr at 37°C in a humidified 5% CO_2 incubator, the cells are washed three times with
50 ml culture medium and after resuspension in the original
volume, incubated for 24 (PHA) or 48 (PPD) hr. The culture
fluids can either be tested immediately or stored at -70°C until
used.

D. *Target Cells*

A wide variety of transformed target cells are sensitive to
cytolysis by macrophages and are suitable for this assay. Adherent target cells have been predominantly used but recent
studies indicate that some suspension lymphoma cell lines are

particularly sensitive to macrophage-mediated cytolysis (21).
Since reactivity by macrophages is not species-restricted,
there is no requirement to use target cells from the same species as the effector cells. Of the various adherent cell lines
tested in our laboratory, the mouse line, TU5, and the human
line, G11, have been most susceptible to lysis (17). Nontrans-
formed fibroblasts have shown little or no susceptibility (16,
22). Our standard target cell line, TU5, has been useful for
studies with both mouse macrophages and human monocytes (16, 17).
TU5, or more completely designated mKSA-TU5, is a BALB/c mouse
kidney line transformed by SV40 (23). The cell line is maintained in Minimal Essential Medium plus 10% FBS in tissue culture flasks.

III. PROCEDURE

A. *Labeling of Target Cells*

1. *Adherent Monolayers*

Cells from confluent monolayers are harvested by exposure
for 5 min at 37°C to 5 ml of trypsin-EDTA, diluted with at
least 5 ml of RPMI medium plus 10% FBS to inhibit further action
by the trypsin and counted. One - two million cells in 5 - 10
ml are added to another flask, which is then incubated for 2 - 4
hr to allow the cells to adhere and form a subconfluent monolayer. Then ^{125}IUdR, 2.5 μCi (optimal amount varies among cell
lines and higher amounts are needed to label certain lines),
plus 10^{-5} M FUdR are added and the flask is incubated at 37°C
for 4 hr (overnight labeling time may be utilized, to result in
higher radioactivity per cell, but this larger exposure may be
toxic to some cell lines). It is desirable to achieve labeling
at an average of 0.5 - 1 count per minute (cpm) per target cell.
The rate of DNA synthesis, the amount of ^{125}IUdR added, and the
length of the labeling period are all significant factors that
influence the level of radioactivity of the target cells (1).
After labeling, the supernate in the flask is poured off
and the monolayer gently washed twice with Hanks' BSS to remove
excess isotope. Cells are then detached with trypsin-EDTA as
described above, washed once with culture medium, and diluted
to the appropriate concentration.

2. *Suspension Cells*

The same general procedure is used as for adherent target
cells, with labeling done either in tissue culture flasks or in

tubes. Washing of cells and other steps requiring separation of supernatant from cells must be done by centrifugation rather than the pouring off of supernatants from monolayers. The suspension cell lines, particularly lymphomas, are often more sensitive to toxicity from the ^{125}IUdR and lower amounts of isotope (0.5 - 2 µCi) and short labeling times (2 - 4 hr) usually give optimal labeling and low spontaneous release during the assay.

B. Assay Procedure

Target cells (10^4/well) are added to the test plates, followed by a range of concentrations of macrophages (effector: target cell ratios usually from 40:1 to 1:1) to give a final volume of 0.3 ml RPMI 1640 medium plus 10% FBS. Before plating, an aliquot of target cells should be counted to assure that adequate labeling has occurred. Aliquots of the target cells are also placed in counting tubes, to be counted at the end of the assay along with the test samples, to give the total incorporation into the cells. Replicates of at least four for each group should be prepared. The plates are incubated at 37°C in a humidified incubator with 5% CO_2 in air for a period of 48 - 72 hr.

C. Harvesting of Assay and Counting of Radioactivity

1. Adherent Target Cells

At the end of the incubation, 0.1 ml of the supernatant can be removed with a 0.1 ml Biopette or with the RIA tips. With each cell line, some pilot studies need to be done to determine whether any of the target cells become detached spontaneously or during incubation with macrophages and thus are counted in the supernatant along with released isotope. This is done simply by centrifuging the culture fluid and separately counting the pellet and centrifuged supernatant. If appreciable radioactivity is found in the pellets, the plates need to be centrifuged before removal of the supernatants.

2. Suspension Target Cells

For suspension targets, the simplest harvesting procedure is by the automatic harvesting apparatus (7). The labeled cells are retained on the filter paper, and the released isotope in the supernatant can be discarded or collected in counting tubes. The supernatants from adherent target cells can also be harvested by this procedure.

3. Measurement of Radioactivity

^{125}I emits both gamma and beta rays and therefore can be
counted in either a gamma counter or in a liquid scintillation
counter with comparable results. For gamma counting, the cpm
can be determined directly from each sample. For beta counting,
10 ml of scintillation fluid is mixed with each sample and,
prior to counting, incubated at room temperature overnight to
allow equilibration and to decrease chemoluminescence.

IV. CALCULATION OF RESULTS

One can determine the cpm in the supernatant, the cpm remaining in the cells, and the total cpm incorporated [measure-
ment of any two of these values allows calculation of the
third, since cpm in total volume of supernatant (cpm in 0.1 ml
aliquot × 3) plus cpm remaining in target cells = total cpm incorporated into cells]. The percentage cytotoxicity for each
group is calculated as

$$\frac{\text{cpm supernatant}}{\text{total cpm incorporated}} \times 100$$

Net lysis in test group is determined by subtracting the percentage spontaneous release of tumor cell incubated in the absence of effectors (medium control) from the percentage cytotoxicity of the test group. It is highly desirable to work out
conditions with the target cells and labeling procedure to have
the medium control be less than 30% over a 48- to 72-hr incubation period.

V. CRITICAL COMMENTS

A. Potential Advantages of ^{125}IUdR as a Label

^{125}IUdR is an excellent marker for measuring target cell
lysis. As with any nuclear label, the release of the isotope
into the supernatant is strong evidence of cell lysis. However, it is necessary to rule out the possibility that some of
the radioactivity in the supernatant is due to detached but
still viable cells. Assays with this or other radioisotopes
that only measure cpm remaining in the monolayer cells may actually measure a combination of cytolysis plus loss of adherence.

Some cytoplasmic labels, e.g., ^{51}Cr and [^{3}H]proline, appear to
be released to some extent from cells without overt cell lysis
and therefore may give high spontaneous release values and possibly optimistic indications of the levels of cytotoxic activity. Reutilization of ^{125}IUdR is minimal (1, 5) in contrast to
some reutilization with [^{3}H]thymidine. ^{125}IUdR also produces
cytostasis of most target cells: this can be both an advantage
and a disadvantage. On the one hand, the inhibition of proliferation will keep the effector:target cell ratios relatively
constant over the period of the assay and prevent the labeled
cells from being diluted out and cold target-inhibited by proliferating unlabeled cells. However, it is possible that the
cytostatic effects of the compound may alter the susceptibility
of the target cells to lysis by macrophages. There is no clear
evidence that this potential problem significantly affects the
results, since direct comparative studies with other labels
have generally given parallel results.

B. *Potential Disadvantages of ^{125}IUdR as a Label*

The main disadvantage of this isotope is that synthesis of
DNA and hence replicating cells are necessary for incorporation.
Thus, cells with metabolic but little or no replicative activity
incorporated low amounts of ^{125}IUdR into the nucleus, which may
be insufficient for accurate quantitation of results. In general, only established tissue culture cell lines are suitable for
this isotope. ^{125}IUdR also has some inherent toxicity that must
be assessed for each target cell (1, 6).
Another potential problem is that ^{125}IUdR or other nuclear
labels are usually not released immediately after cell death.
Loss of integrity of the nucleus must occur prior to release of
radioactivity. In some systems, it has been useful to treat
target cells with trypsin at the end of the assay, to facilitate
release of the label from damaged cells (5, 7, 8). However,
with assays of 48 - 72 hr, this additional step is usually not
required.
The methods used to calculate results in assays of this
nature can have an appreciable effect on the values reported.
Calculation of data by a cytotoxic index will often indicate
substantially higher levels of cytotoxicity than those seen
with the percentage cytotoxicity calculation (5). Even among
the procedures used for calculation of percentage cytotoxicity,
substantial variation can be produced, depending on the denomi-
nator used in the formula. Use of the total cpm incorporated
is rather conservative but appears to give a more stable and
reliable value than that obtained by attempts at maximally
lysing the targets cells with detergents or freezing and thawing. Some cell lines are very resistant to disruption by such

physical treatments and may give spuriously low values. A common practice is to subtract the spontaneous release values from the total cpm in the cells or from the maximal release. This procedure is of some concern, since it tends to magnify the levels of cytotoxicity when the spontaneous release becomes high. The problems with subtraction of the spontaneous release may be further compounded when the spontaneous release is actually a group containing normal macrophages in place of activated macrophages. This procedure masks the degree of natural macrophage-mediated cytotoxicity that can occur against the target cell, and in assays lasting 48 - 72 hr, this is usually appreciable (16, 17, 24).

REFERENCES

1. B. P. Le Mevel, R. K. Oldham, S. A. Wells, and R. B. Herberman. An evaluation of ^{125}I-iododeoxyuridine as a cellular label for *in vitro* assays: Kinetics of incorporation and toxicity. *J. Nat. Cancer Inst. 51*: 1511-1558, 1973.
2. B. P. Le Mevel and S. A. Wells. Development of a microassay for the quantitation of cytotoxic antitumor antibody. Use of ^{125}I-iododeoxyuridine as a tumor cell label. *J. Nat. Cancer Inst. 50*: 803-806, 1973.
3. A. M. Cohen, J. F. Burdick, and A. S. Ketcham. Cell-mediated cytotoxicity: An assay using ^{125}I-idodeoxyuridine-labeled target cells. *J. Immunol. 107*: 895-898, 1971.
4. R. K. Oldham, D. Siwarski, J. L. McCoy, E. J. Plata, and R. B. Herberman. Evaluation of a cell-mediated cytotoxicity assay utilizing ^{125}I-iododeoxyuridine-labeled tissue-culture target cells. *Nat. Cancer Inst. Monogr. 37*: 49-58, 1973.
5. R. K. Oldham and R. B. Herberman. Evaluation of cell-mediated cytotoxic reactivity against tumor associated antigens, utilizing ^{125}I-iododeoxyuridine labeled target cells. *J. Immunol. 111*: 1862-1871, 1973.
6. R. C. Seeger, S. A. Rayner, and J. J. T. Owen. An analysis of variables affecting the measurement of tumor immunity *in vitro* with ^{125}I-iododeoxyuridine-labeled target cells. Studies of immunity to primary Moloney sarcomas. *Int. J. Cancer 13*: 697-713, 1974.
7. C. C. Ting, G. S. Bushar, D. Rodrigues, and R. B. Herberman. Cell-mediated immunity to Friend virus-induced leukemia. I. Modification of [125]IUdR release cytotoxicity assay for use with suspension target cells. *J. Immunol. 115*:

1351, 1356, 1975.

8. R. K. Oldham and R. B. Herberman. Determination of cell-mediated cytotoxicity by the ^{125}I-iododeoxyuridine-labeled microcytotoxicity assay. *In* "*In Vitro* Methods in Cell-Mediated and Tumor Immunity" (B. R. Bloom and J. R. David, eds.), pp. 461-470. Academic Press, New York, 1976.

9. G. Fossati, H. Holden, and R. B. Herberman. Evaluation of the cell-mediated immune response to murine sarcoma virus by ^{125}I-iododeoxyuridine assay and comparison with ^{51}Cr and microcytotoxicity assays. *Cancer Res. 35*: 2600-2608, 1975.

10. I. J. Fidler. Activation *in vitro* of mouse macrophages by syngeneic, allogeneic, or xenogeneic lymphocyte supernatants. *J. Nat. Cancer Inst. 55*: 1159-1164, 1975.

11. I. J. Fidler, J. H. Darnell, and M. B. Budmen. *In vitro* activation of mouse macrophages by rat lymphocyte mediators. *J. Immunol. 117*: 666-673, 1976.

12. M.-L. Lohmann-Matthes, W. Domzig, and H. Taskov. Antibody-dependent cellular cytotoxicity (ADCC) against tumor cells. I. Cultivated bone-marrow macrophages kill tumor targets. *Eur. J. Immunol. 9*: 261-267, 1979.

13. A. Raz, W. E. Fogler, and I. J. Fidler. The effects of experimental conditions on the expression of *in vitro*-mediated tumor cytotoxicity mediated by murine macrophages. *Cancer Immunol. Immunotherapy 7*: 157-163, 1979.

14. C. Riccardi, P. Puccetti, A. Santoni, and R. B. Herberman. Rapid *in vivo* assay of mouse NK cell activity. *J. Nat. Cancer Inst. 63*: 1041-1045, 1979.

15. C. Riccardi, A. Santoni, T. Barlozzari, P. Puccetti, and R. B. Herberman. *In vivo* natural reactivity of mice against tumor cells. *Int. J. Cancer 25*: 475-486, 1980.

16. A. Tagliabue, A. Mantovani, M. Kilgallen, R. B. Herberman, and J. L. McCoy. Natural cytotoxicity of mouse monocytes and macrophages. *J. Immunol. 122*: 2363-2370, 1979.

17. A. Mantovani, T. R. Jerrells, J. H. Dean, and R. B. Herberman. Cytolytic and cytostatic activity on tumor cells of circulating human monocytes. *Int. J. Cancer 23*: 18-27, 1979.

18. S. K. Ackerman and S. D. Douglas. Purification of human monocytes on microexudate-coated surfaces. *J. Immunol. 120*: 1372-1378, 1978.

19. R. Koski, D. G. Poplack, and R. M. Blaese. A nonspecific esterase stain for the identification of monocytes and macrophages. *In* "*In Vitro* Methods in Cell-Mediated and Tumor Immunity" (B. Bloom and J. R. David, eds.), pp. 359-362. Academic Press, New York, 1976.

20. A. Mantovani, J. H. Dean, T. R. Jerrell, and R. B. Herberman. Augmentation of tumoricidal activity of human monocytes and macrophages by lymphokines. *Int. J. Cancer 25*: 691-699, 1980.

21. T. Taniyama and H. T. Holden. Cytotoxic activity of
     macrophages isolated from primary murine sarcoma virus
     (MSV)-induced tumors. *Int. J. Cancer 24*: 151-160, 1979.
22. A. Mantovani, A. Tagliabue, J. H. Dean, T. R. Jerrells,
     and R. B. Herberman. Cytolytic activity of circulating
     human monocytes on transformed and untransformed human
     fibroblasts. *Int. J. Cancer 23*: 29-31, 1979.
23. S. Kit, T. Kurimura, and D. R. Dubbs. Transplantable
     mouse tumor cell line induced by injection of SV40 trans-
     formed mouse kidney cells. *Int. J. Cancer 4*: 384-392,
     1969.
24. R. Keller. Regulatory capacities of mononuclear phago-
     cytes with particular reference to natural immunity
     against tumors. *In* "Natural Cell-Mediated Immunity
     against Tumors" (R. B. Herberman, ed.). Academic Press,
     New York, 1980.

78

ANTIBODY-DEPENDENT CELLULAR CYTOTOXICITY (ADCC)
OF ERYTHROID AND TUMOR CELLS

Hillel S. Koren
Dina G. Fischer

I. INTRODUCTION

The phenomenon of antibody-dependent cellular cytotoxicity
(ADCC) has attracted much attention since its original description by Möller (1) and by Perlmann and Holm (2). Their investigations established that a variety of different target cells,
including fowl erythrocytes and mammalian tissue culture cells,
could be destroyed through the interaction of specific antibody
absorbed to the target cells with normal lymphoid or monocytic
cells. Although the exact mechanism of ADCC is still not completely understood, there is a general agreement that the
specificity of this immunologic reaction is determined by antibody bound to membrane-associated antigens and that the effector cells bear receptors for the Fc fragment of the immunoglobulin (Ig) molecule. The range of effector cells mediating
ADCC has been shown to include: K lymphocytes, T cells, polymorphonuclear leukocytes, platelets, monocytes/macrophages
[for review see (3-4)] and macrophage-like cell lines (5).

METHODS FOR STUDYING
MONONUCLEAR PHAGOCYTES

813

The major goal of this chapter is to describe and discuss a short-term ^{51}Cr-release ADCC assay using purified mononuclear phagocytes as effector cells against hapten-modified antibody-coated target cells (6). This technique can be readily adapted to various ADCC systems employing effector cells from different tissues and species or cell lines, antibodies (allo- or xenogeneic) and target cells (erythroid and lymphoid). The use of hapten-modified target cells facilitates a standardization of the ADCC assay and enables one to compare the cytotoxic activities of an effector cell population against different target cells (e.g., erythroid versus lymphoid) modified with the same hapten and coated with the same antiserum.

II. REAGENTS

A. Materials and Methods

1. Effector Mononuclear Phagocytes
Macrophages obtained from peritoneal cells of thioglycollate-induced (stimulated) and BCG-immunized (activated) mice; monocytes derived from human peripheral blood leukocytes (PBL) and the U937 macrophage-like cell line (other macrophage-like cell lines with ADCC activity could be used as well).

2. Target Cells
Chicken red blood cells (CRC), obtained by venous puncture of adult chickens using Alsever's solution (diluted 1:2 with the blood). CRC can be stored at 4°C up to one week.

Cultured murine and human cell lines can be used as tumor targets. We have found the human HSB cell line (7) to be most suitable as a target for both murine and human effector cells.

3. Preparation of Anti-TNP Serum
BDF$_1$ and C57BL/6 mice are injected in the footpads with trinitrophenyl (TNP)-modified *Mycobacterium tuberculosis* strain H37Ra incorporated in incomplete Freund's adjuvant. After 2 weeks the mice are boosted with 100 μg of TNP-modified *M. tuberculosis,* intraperitoneally, and bled 2-3 weeks later. Sera can also be obtained from mice immunized with TNP-modified keyhole limpet hemocyanin (TNP-KLH). All sera are heat-inactivated at 56°C for 30 min. New sera should be titered in the ADCC assay and the optimal dilution determined. It should be mentioned that mouse anti-TNP serum can be used effectively with human and murine effector cells though other anti-TNP sera raised in other species (e.g., rabbit) may be more suitable with human effector cells.

4. Media
Phosphate-buffered saline (PBS), E-MEM supplemented with 10% heat inactivated fetal calf serum (FCS), 2 mM L-glutamine, 1 mM sodium pyruvate, nonessential amino acids (1x concentration), and 50 µg/ml gentamicin. This medium will be termed EMEM-10%.

5. Chemicals
2,3,6-Trinitrobenzyl sulfonic acid (TNBS) and Triton X-100 (Sigma Chemical Company).

6. Plastics
Flat- and round-bottom microtiter plates (e.g., Linbro, 76-003-05), 50-ml conical tubes and pipettes.

7. Stains
Wright stain: (Harelco Dif. Quick, Arthur Thomas Incorp., Philadelphia, Pennsylvania).

Nonspecific esterase stain: Used to determine the purity of the monocyte preparation, as described by Tucker *et al.* (8). (See Chapter 40.)

Peroxidase stain: Helpful in identifying especially the small monocytes that are morphologically indistinguishable from lymphocytes. The procedure for this stain has been described by Kaplow (9). (See Chapter 39.)

8. *Radiolabel:* Na$_2{}^{51}$CrO$_4$ - Specific activity 250-500 mCi/mg (New England Nuclear, Boston, Massachusetts, Catalog No. NEZ-030).

III. PROCEDURES

A. Preparation of Purified Murine Macrophage Monolayers

Peritoneal cells are obtained by lavage of the peritoneal cavity with 10 ml EMEM containing 10 U heparin/ml. The cells are washed once (250 g for 10 min), resuspended in EMEM-10%, counted in a hemocytometer and the cellular composition determined by preparing smears on a cytocentrifuge followed by staining with Wright's stain. Cell suspensions are adjusted based on viable macrophages and depending on the desired effector-target (E:T) ratio. One hundred µl of these suspensions are delivered into 96-well microtiter plates (flat bottom), which are then incubated for 2 hr at 37°C in a humidified 5% CO$_2$ incubator followed by three vigorous washings with PBS containing 10% FCS. The wells are then replenished with 100 µl of EMEM-10%.

B. *Preparation of Purified Peripheral Blood Monocytes*

To obtain purified monocytes, mononuclear cells obtained
from the interface of a Ficoll-Hypaque gradient (10) are subjected to the newly developed technique of reversible adherence to serum-coated surfaces as described in detail in a
separate chapter (11) and elsewhere (12). The recovered monocytes are highly purified (97-99% by nonspecific esterase and
peroxidase stains) and can be used as effector cells for ADCC.
They are resuspended in MEM-10% and adjusted according to the
desired E:T ratio. Since this effector cell population is
already purified, further adherence steps are not necessary.
Therefore, 100 µl aliquots of the monocyte suspension are delivered into 96-well microtiter plates (round bottom) to which
target cells and antibodies can be added immediately.

C. *The Use of the U937 Cell Line as Effector Cells*

The ADCC activity and other properties of this human mono-
cyte-like cell line have been previously described (13,14).
This cell line grows under standard tissue culture conditions
and is therefore readily available as a source of effector
cells as described in Section II. B. However, it should be
mentioned that unstimulated U937 cells can kill only erythroid
targets, whereas killing of antibody-coated tumor cells requires prior stimulation of the cell line with lymphokines (14).

D. *Preparation of Target Cells*

1. ^{51}Cr *Labeling*

Sixty-100 × 10^6 CRC are washed once in PBS and resuspended
in 0.2 ml of PBS, to which 200 µCi of $Na_2{}^{51}CrO_4$ are added.
The cells are then incubated for 1 hr in a 37°C water bath,
and washed twice in PBS (without serum). Five to 10 × 10^6 HSB
tumor cells from a logarithmically growing culture (optimally
the cell suspension is diluted on the day prior to the assay)
are washed once and resuspended in 0.2 ml of EMEM-10%, to
which 200 µCi of $Na_2{}^{51}CrO_4$ are added and incubated for 1 hr in
a 37°C water bath. The cells are then washed twice in PBS
(without serum).

2. *Hapten Modification of Target Cells*

The ^{51}Cr-labeled and washed cells are resuspended in 5 ml
(using 50-ml conical tubes) of 10 m*M* TNBS (pH 7.2) and incubated for 10 min in a 37°C water bath. The reaction is stopped
by adding a large excess of cold EMEM-10% followed by two additional washes with the same medium. The TNP-modified cells

are then counted in a hemocytometer and adjusted to 3×10^4 cells/50 μl or 1×10^4 cells/50 μl for CRC-TNP and HSB-TNP targets, respectively.

E. Assay Procedure

The TNP-modified targets are added in 50 μl aliquots wells already containing the 100 μl of purified mononuclear phagocyte effector cells. Fifty μl of an appropriate diluted hyperimmune anti-TNP serum are then added to the appropriate wells. The plates are spun to 50 g for 3 min (using special plate carriers and a suitable head) to enhance contact between the effectors and targets. Plates containing CRC-TNP targets are incubated for 2 hr at 37°C and those with HSB-TNP targets are incubated for 3 hr at 37°C. Assays are terminated by spinning the trays at 500 g for 5 min and harvesting 100 μl of the supernatant from each well. Samples are counted in a welltype gamma counter.

F. Controls

To determine the spontaneous release of the ^{51}Cr-labeled targets, they are incubated with 150 μl of EMEM-10% in the absence of macrophages. To determine the antibody dependency ("specificity") of the cytolytic reaction, targets are added to wells containing macrophages and medium in the absence of anti-TNP serum. If a new batch of antiserum is tested, an additional control containing targets and serum only is added. To determine the maximum releasable CPM from the target, 150 μl of 1% Triton X-100 is added to wells containing 50 μl targets.

IV. CALCULATIONS

Specific lysis (SL) is calculated by the formula:

$$\%SL = \frac{E_{ADCC} - C}{MR - C} \times 100$$

where E_{ADCC} = released cpm in experimental wells; C = cpm released in control wells containing targets and medium alone or target and effector in the absence of anti-TNP; MR = maximal releasable cpm of wells containing target cells incubated with 1% Triton X-100, which usually exceeds 90% of the total incorporated radioactivity. Experiments should be set up in triplicates or quadruplicates and all data presented as percentage specific lysis ± S.E. (see Table I).

TABLE I. *ADCC by Thioglycollate and BCG Macrophages*[a]

Macrophage population	Anti-TNP[c]	% Specific Lysis ± S.E.[b] E:T Ratio				Slope[d]	Slope ratio
		5:1	2.5:1	1.2:1	0.6:1		
Thioglycollate	–	1.1±0.2					
Thioglycollate	+	7.8±1.0	3.1±0.4	2.3±0.4	1.9±0.3	1.3	
BCG	–	1.0±0.9					8.1
BCG	+	32.1±1.3	25.9±1.6	11.2±1.3	4.7±0.3	11.1	

[a]Data from (18).
[b]Specific lysis was determined in a 2-hr assay with 3×10^4 CRC-TNP per well. The spontaneous release = 0.6%.
[c]Anti-TNP serum was used at a final dilution of 1:1000.
[d]For calculating slopes the three lowest E:T values were employed.

V. CRITICAL COMMENTS

Contamination by neutrophils (previously shown to function as ADCC effector cells (3-4)) of up to 10% (mainly in the BCG population) was occasionally detected. Therefore, it is advantageous to let the plates incubate for an additional period of 18 hr at 37°C followed by additional washings. Monolayers of macrophages of 99% purity are thus obtained.

Since TNBS binds readily to proteins, it is essential to wash the ^{51}Cr-labeled target cells free of serum-containing medium prior to the modification step. It is equally important to stop the reaction after 10 min with cold EMEM-10%. Longer modification time results in target cell damage leading to high spontaneous release.

One has to be aware of the fact that when antibody-coated erythroid targets are used with effector macrophages, significant immune phagocytosis occurs as well. It is therefore important to test to what extent phagocytosis affects ADCC. Inhibition of phagocytosis by iodoacetate (16) or 2-deoxy-D-glucose (17), for example, can be employed.

Acknowledgments

The authors thank Ms. Linda Nash for her excellent secretarial assistance. This work was supported by a grant from the National Institutes of Health CA 23354. HSK is a recipient of a Research Career Development Award CA 00581.

REFERENCES

1. E. Möller. Contact-induced cytotoxicity by lymphoid cells containing foreign isoantigens. *Science 147*:873. 1965.
2. P. Perlmann and G. Holm. Cytotoxic effects of lymphoid cells *in vitro*. *Adv. Immunol. 11*:117, 1969.
3. P. Perlmann. Cellular immunity: Antibody-dependent cytotoxicity (K-cell activity). *In* "Clinical Immunobiology," Vol. 3. (F. H. Bach and R. A. Good, eds.), p. 107. Academic Press, New York, 1976.
4. H. S. Shin, R. J. Johnson, G. R. Pasterneck, and J. S. Economu. Mechanism of tumor immunity: The role of antibody and nonimmune effectors. *In* "Progress in Allergy," Vol. 25. (P. Kallos, G. Waksman, and A. De Weck, eds.), p. 163. Karger, Basel, 1978.

5. V. Defendi. Macrophage cell lines and their use in
    immunobiology. *In* "Immunobiology of the Macrophage"
    (D. S. Nelson, ed.), p. 275. Academic Press, New York,
    1976.
6. B. S. Handwerger and H. S. Koren. The nature of the
    effector cell in antibody-dependent, cell-mediated cyto-
    lysis (ADCC): The cytotoxic activity of murine tumor
    cells and peritoneal macrophages. *Clin. Immunol. Pathol.*
    *5:*272, 1976.
7. I. R. Royston, W. Smith, D. N. Buell, E. S. Huang, and
    J. S. Pagano. Autologous human B and T lymphoblastoid
    cell lines. *Nature 251:*745, 1974.
8. S. B. Tucker, R. B. Pierre, and R. E. Jordon. Rapid
    identification of monocytes in a mixed mononuclear cell
    preparation. *J. Immunol. Methods 14:*267, 1977.
9. L. S. Kaplow. Simplified myeloperoxidase stain using
    benzidine dihydrochloride. *Blood 26:*215, 1965.
10. A. Boyum. Separation of lymphocytes from blood and bone
    marrow. *Scand. J. Clin. Lab. Invest. 97* (Suppl. *21):*77,
    1968.
11. D. G. Fischer and H. S. Koren. Antibody-Dependent Cellu-
    lar Cytotoxicity (ADCC) of Erythroid and Tumor Cells.
    In "Methods for Studying Mononuclear Phagocytes," this
    volume (D. O. Adams, P. Edelson, and H. S. Koren, eds.),
    Academic Press, New York, 1981.
12. D. G. Fischer, W. H. Hubbard, and H. S. Koren. Tumor
    cell killing by freshly isolated peripheral blood mono-
    cytes. *Cell. Immunol., 58:*426, 1981.
13. C. Sundstrom and K. Nilsson. Establishment and charac-
    terization of a human histiocytic lymphoma cell line
    (U-937). *Int. J. Cancer 17:*565, 1976.
14. H. S. Koren, S. J. Anderson, and J. W. Larrick. *In vitro*
    activation of a human macrophage-like cell line.
    *Nature 279:*328, 1979.
15. D. Finney. *In* "Statistical Methods in Biological Assays."
    Hafner, New York, 1964.
16. W. S. Walker and A. Demus. Antibody-dependent cytolysis
    of chicken erythrocytes by an *in vitro* established line
    of mouse peritoneal macrophages. *J. Immunol. 114:*765,
    1975.
17. J. Michl, D. J. Ohlbaum, and S. C. Silverstein.
    2-Deoxyglucose selectively inhibits Fc and complement-
    mediated phagocytosis in mouse peritoneal macrophages.
    *J. Exp. Med. 114:*1465, 1976.
18. H. S. Koren, S. J. Anderson, and D. O. Adams. The effect
    of cytolytic activation on macrophage function in ADCC.
    *Cell Immunol. 57:*51, 1981.

79

OVERVIEW: THE MACROPHAGE IN CELL BIOLOGY

David Vaux
Siamon Gordon

I. INTRODUCTION

Because of its varied function and remarkable adaptability, the macrophage is not only of interest to the immunologist and pathologist, concerned with its special role in host defense and injury, but also to the cell biologist, who can use macrophages to study many processes common to all cells. Since macrophages can be obtained in good yield and purity and since they maintain many of their differentiated properties in culture, a great deal has been learned in the past two decades about their physiology, especially with regard to endocytosis, lysosomal function, and the synthesis and secretion of various biologically active molecules.

In this chapter, we discuss selected aspects of macrophage cell biology to illustrate the versatility of the cell and the ingenuity of some of its investigators. We have chosen to present the spectrum of research with the aid of several summary tables, to conserve space and for ease of reference.

METHODS FOR STUDYING
MONONUCLEAR PHAGOCYTES

821

Earlier reviews provide useful information and several topics
are dealt with in greater detail elsewhere in this volume
(1 - 4).

II.   SOURCES AND HETEROGENEITY

   Mononuclear phagocytes can be obtained from various sources
for experimental purposes (Table I). It is important to recognize that cells from different species and from different sites
in the body differ in development and state of activation.
Heterogeneity of this kind makes it possible to compare the
structure and function of closely related types of cell. Although cell lines provide a more homogeneous cell population,
their origin and stage of differentiation are usually ill-
defined and the cells could change their properties after long
periods in culture. Primary cells may also show properties
reflecting their adaptation to conditions *in vitro* rather than
those within the animal.

III. GROWTH AND DIFFERENTIATION

   Like other hemopoietic cells, precursors for macrophages
originate in bone marrow in the adult animal and undergo
several divisions during differentiation. Cells enter the
blood stream as monocytes and are then widely distributed in
peripheral tissues, especially the liver (Kupffer cells), lung
(alveolar macrophages), spleen, and serosal cavities. Some of
the methods used to study the origin and growth of macrophages
are listed in Table II. Development of differentiated mouse
macrophages in culture depends on a specific growth factor,
colony-stimulating factor(s) (CSF), which is produced by mononuclear phagocytes under certain conditions or by other cells
such as mouse fibroblasts (26). Methods have been developed
for clonal analysis of cell growth in soft agar and for mass
culture in liquid systems (see Chapter 2).
   Mouse bone marrow contains only a small proportion of
colony-forming precursors (CFU-C), approximately 1 per 1000.
Cell culture with CSF initially favors production of polymorphonuclear leukocytes that die rapidly, and, subsequently,
after 2 - 7 days, of a relatively homogeneous population of
adherent macrophages. Such bone marrow cultured macrophages
(BMCM) continue to proliferate for some weeks if the CSF is
renewed.

TABLE I. Sources of Mononuclear Phagocytes

Site	Species	Method	Comments	Reference
Serous cavities	Mouse	(a) Sterile peritoneal washout	A "resident" population, not exposed to inflammatory agents	5
		(b) Sterile peritoneal washout after inflammatory agent (Proteose peptone thioglycollate broth) given intraperitoneally	Higher yields, but cells are "stimulated," an intermediate activation state	6
		(c) As above after infection by an intracellular pathogen, e.g., BCG	Activated macrophages display nonspecifically enhanced activity against microorganisms and cells, especially after further stimulation, e.g., by PMA	7, 8
Lung	Rabbit Rat Human	(a) Bronchial lavage, often after BCG iv		9
		(b) Resected lung tissue extracted with salt solutions without trypsin and purified by adherence	Major source of human macrophages	10
Blood	Any	Density centrifugation of peripheral blood gives band of mononuclear cells further purified by adherence	Source of defined stage of development, e.g., monocyte. Note species differences in centrifugation protocol	11

823

Parenchy-matous organs	Any	Single-cell suspensions by enzyme digestion puri-fied by adherence	Source of tissue macrophages	12
Bone marrow	Mouse Rat Human	Sterile washout of bone marrow cultured with source of CSF	Good yields of proliferating cells. Differentiation series present in culture. Population initially hetero-geneous	13
Cell lines	Mouse	In vitro or in vivo passage of transformed cell lines carrying macrophage markers	High yields of homogeneous population, but macrophage status may be uncertain. Viral antigens present	14

TABLE II. Macrophage Precursors and Growth

Method of study	Purpose	Reference
In Vivo		
Parabiosis	Hematogenous origin	15
Adoptive transfer into	of tissue macro-	16
syngeneic, irradiated	phages. Bone marrow	17
recipient using chromo-	origin of stem cell	
somal marker; colony	precursor for tissue	
formation in spleen by	macrophages and other	
limiting dilution	hemopoietic cells	
	(CFU-S).	
In Vitro		
Cloning in suspension	Assay CFU-C and pro-	18
in a semisolid medium,	liferative capacity	19
in liquid culture or	of precursors in	20
after adherence, all	bone marrow and of	
in presence of CSF	tissue and exudate	
	macrophages.	
Mass liquid culture of	DNA synthesis and	13
bone marrow, in pres-	proliferation in	21
ence of CSF	macrophages gener-	
	ated in culture.	
Mass liquid cultures	DNA synthesis and	22, 23
of macrophages	proliferation.	
Culture of bone marrow	Cycling of CFU-C in	24, 25
with a bone marrow	vitro, without dif-	
derived feeder system,	ferentiation.	
under special condi-		
tions, without exo-		
genous CSF		

Although tissue macrophages are typically in the resting (G_0) phase of the cell cycle, up to 20% of macrophages obtained from inflammatory exudates, e.g., after stimulation with thioglycollate broth, give rise to colonies in agar in the presence of CSF, after a lag period of up to 4 weeks (20). In general, the speed and extent of macrophage proliferation diminish as the cells mature from precursor to end cell.

CSF has been purified considerably, partially characterized as a glycoprotein approximately 70,000 MW and is composed of two identical subunits (27). The effect of CSF is mostly

TABLE III.   Studies with Primary Cultures of Proliferating Macrophages

Purpose of study	Reference
1. *Differentiation* Precursor-product relationships, relation to other hemopoietic cells and acquisition of markers, e.g., adherence, esterases, lysozyme, Fc receptors, antigens, and plasminogen activator secretion.	*29, 30, 31, 13, 32*
2. *Heterogeneity of mononuclear phagocytes* Variation in expression of markers (e.g., differentiation antigens) within and among clones	
3. *Growth control* Stimulation by colony-stimulating factor(s), serum, and other growth factors, e.g., transferrin, selenium. Inhibitors, e.g., glucocorticoids, lactoferrin, and prostaglandins.	*33, 34, 35, 36*
4. *Properties of proliferating cell* Response of target to CSF varies, BMCM > inflammatory > resident. CSF receptors specifically found on mononuclear phagocytes.	*28*
5. *Associated phenotype* Plasminogen activator secretion. Cytostatic activity; microbicidal activity.	*37, 38, 39*
6. *Transformation by tumor viruses* murine; avian	*40, 41, 42*
7. *Cell hybridization*	

restricted to target cells of the same species, and a specific receptor for CSF has been identified on cells of the mononuclear phagocyte system (28).

Dexter and his colleages have developed a specialized culture system, not completely defined, to maintain some precursor cells in a cycling state in culture, without differentiation. CSF is not added and adherent cells, often laden with lipid, perform a poorly understood accessory function (25). Such accessory cells can be obtained from mouse bone marrow by cultivation at a lower temperature, 33°C, or by using horse serum supplemented with glucocorticoids.

As shown in Table III, these culture systems have been used to define the stages of macrophage differentiation and the acquisition of cell-specific markers in relation to other hemopoietic cells. A question that has not been resolved concerns the nature of the heterogeneity observed among different mononuclear phagocytes. Variation in expression of various markers can be ascribed to differences in the stage of development and growth or in the degree of cell activation by various inflammatory, immunologic, and endocytic stimuli. The role of unusual factors in the local environment, e.g., in the lung, has not been defined. Although no evidence for independent subsets of mononuclear phagocytes has yet been obtained, analysis of markers such as monoclonal antigens within and among independent clones of macrophages derived from bone marrow or tissue sources will provide a powerful test for their existence.

An unusual feature of proliferation and its control in the MPS is the ability of immature precursors to form colonies in semisolid medium, a trait often associated with malignancy in the case of other cells. Maturation of mononuclear phagocytes results in loss of this property. Unlike the growth of malignant cells, growth of macrophage precursors is tightly controlled and dependent on the continuous presence of CSF. Other molecules have been reported, which regulate growth when CSF is not limiting.

Very little is known about the properties that determine the response of a macrophage to CSF or about the complex phenotype associated with proliferation. BMCM are exquisitely sensitive to CSF compared with resident macrophages. Production and secretion of plasminogen activator are coordinated with cell proliferation and CSF is able to enhance both activities in close sequence (37). Microbicidal and cytocidal activities, other characteristic effector functions of activated macrophages, may be induced at the same time.

Two limitations to the present use of bone marrow cultures should be noted. The preadherent precursors of macrophages are poorly characterized and present in small numbers in the heterogeneous cell populations found early in culture. Moreover, differentiation *in vitro* may differ from that *in vivo*, with the role of CSF or surface adherence unlike that of hematologic and local influences in the body.

IV. STRUCTURE AND FUNCTION OF MACROPHAGE MEMBRANES

The membranes of the macrophage, both surface and intracellular, are of central interest because so many of the specialized functions of macrophages are membrane mediated. These include all types of endocytosis, associated delivery of vesicles to the lysosomal compartment by a specific intracellular membrane fusion, and possible retrieval and redeployment of any receptors involved. Exocytosis is another important membrane-dependent event and intracellular membranes are important in the complex oxidative killing systems delivering high-energy

TABLE IV. *Plasma Membrane Components of the Macrophage*

Class	Example	Characteristics	Reference
"Receptor"	Fc receptor	Receptor molecules specific for the Fc portion of some subclasses of immunoglobulin G. Trypsin-resistant and trypsin-sensitive receptors have been described. Mediate phagocytosis of antibody-coated particles and antigen-antibody complexes	1, 2, 44, 45
	C3b receptor	Receptor for cleaved third component of complement cascade, mediates phagocytosis of IgM-coated particles in the presence of complement. Trypsin sensitive.	2
	"Denatured surface receptor"	Immunologically nonspecific "receptors" recognizing chemically modified biological particulates and nonphysiological stimuli, e.g., oil red O droplets or latex microspheres.	46, 47
	Mannosyl/ fucosyl terminal receptor	Pinocytosis-mediating receptor-binding mannose or fucose terminated glycoproteins (including various lysosomal glycosidases). Requires Ca^{2+} for binding. Trypsin sensitive. May function as retrieval pathway for lysosomal glycoproteins and may also be involved in clearance of antigen IgM antibody complexes.	48, 49, 50, 51
	α_2-Macroglobulin receptor	Mediates clearance of protease complexes.	52
	Lymphokine receptor	Reported to be blocked by fucose in guinea pig macrophages.	53
	CSF receptor	Restricted to phagocytic cells and their precursors	28

Table IV (Cont'd.)

Class	Example	Characteristics	Reference
Enzymes	ATPase	Macrophages are rich in a divalent cation-dependent ATPase activity of unknown function.	54
	5'Nucleo-tidase	Plasma membrane marker [although also present on some intracellular membranes in polymorphs (87)] which is internalized during phagocytosis. Function unknown, but present in much higher activity on resident peritoneal macrophages than thioglycollate elicited macrophages.	55
	Alkaline phospho-diester-ase I	Macrophages carry a membrane-associated activity, which liberates 5'nucleoside monophosphates from polyribonucleotides with free 3'-OH. Most activity on plasma membrane, but significant intracellular activity representing either a second site of localization or internalization of plasma membrane. Reduced half-life for this activity in activated cells suggests the latter, showing endogenous pinocytic rate as an important determinant of the enzyme turnover.	56
	Protein kinase	Plasma membrane associated activity capable of transferring γ-phosphate of ATP to specific membrane components or exogenous acceptor has been described in guinea pig peritoneal macrophages. Such selective phosphorylation may be fundamental in control of	57

Table IV (Cont'd.)

Class	Example	Characteristics	Reference
		membrane functions.	
	Specific adherence components	*Macrophages are highly adhesive to glass and culture plastic, spreading widely over the surface and exhibiting membrane ruffling. Mouse peritoneal macrophages express a trypsin-resistant surface iodinatable 195,000 Mr component that appears with development of adhesive phenotype in culture. Human monocytes express surface receptors for fibronectin.*	*58, 58a*
Antigens	*MHC*	*Antigens coded by the major histocompatibility complex are present on the macrophage.*	*59*
	Ia	*The presence and possible functional significance of Ia and DRw antigens on the macrophage membrane remain controversial*	*60, 61*
	Mac I	*Monoclonal antibodies are now being used to probe the macrophage membrane, no function has been assigned to the antigens*	*62, 63*
	F4.80	*recognized by these antibodies, but their almost complete restriction to cells of the mononuclear phagocyte series suggests the possibility of interesting specialized functions.*	
Lipids		*The phospholipid composition of the macrophage plasma membrane may be modified by culturing cells in serum-free medium containing fatty acid-*	*64*

Table IV (Cont'd.)

Class	Example	Characteristics	Reference
		bovine serum albumin. Analysis reveals increase in ratio of saturated/unsaturated fatty acid and reduction in both phagocytic and pinocytic activity.	

oxygen metabolites to the lumen of the phagosome without causing damage to the cell.

This breadth of membrane activity is both an important reason for using macrophages to study problems in membrane biology and the biggest drawback that hinders such work. In addition to the common elements such as plasma membrane, nuclear membrane, rough and smooth endoplasmic reticulum, Golgi and mitochondrial membrane, macrophages contain large populations of lysosomes, secretory vesicles, phagosomes, and pinosomes. This has meant that it is very difficult to isolate individual types of membrane for biochemical characterization. It is partly for this reason that the modification of the technique of Wetzel and Korn (43) for flotation of latex-filled phagolysosomes on discontinuous sucrose density gradients dominate several areas of membrane research.

The composition of the various membrane compartments of the macrophage remains largely unknown, although a wide variety of plasma membrane components has been described (Table IV) and some differences have been noted between plasma membrane and phagolysosomal membrane. It is to be expected that the composition of the plasma membrane will be further complicated by changes due to differentiation and activation of the cell. The composition of intracellular membranes may be substantially different again, and the plasma membrane interiorized in endocytosis could represent an intermediate state. Studies in the fibroblast have revealed plasma membrane specializations involved in endocytosis, which take the form of areas of high receptor density in the membrane with a web of filaments beneath (65). It may be that lateral differentiations in the plasma membrane are widespread, and experiments aimed at demonstrating selective internalization of plasma membrane components during endocytosis could be the first to show this (see Selective internalization, Table VI).

It is a characteristic of the mature macrophage to be highly adherent to tissue culture plastic and glassware.

Fibroblast adherence appears to be dependent on fibronectin
(cell adherence substance, LETS) on the cell surface. Recently,
it has been established that macrophages synthesize fibronectin
(66) and express receptors for fibronectin on the cell surface
(58a). Other components of the plasma membrane have been implicated in the adhesion process in macrophages (see Table IV).

Among the components described on the plasma membrane of
the macrophages are a variety of receptors for specific ligands
mediating their endocytic uptake into the cell. The best
studied of these is the Fc receptor, but there are also receptors for the cleaved third component of the complement cascade
and "nonspecific receptors" for such artificial polymers as
latex or cross-linked cell surfaces (e.g., after glutaraldehyde
fixation), which the macrophage shares with other cell types,
such as fibroblasts. There is also a receptor for synthetic
chemotactic peptides (see Chapter 85).

Mature macrophages express receptors capable of binding the
Fc portion of certain classes of immunoglobulin G. Although
present on a variety of cell types (including B lymphocytes,
stimulated T lymphocytes, PMN, and mononuclear phagocytes), Fc
receptors appear to mediate immune phagocytosis only in "professional" phagocytes, the macrophage, and PMN. The Fc receptor is an important marker because it is possessed by all macrophages and its expression is stable in long-term culture.
The Fc receptor has been intensively studied, and the results
are prototypical of those that may eventually be achieved for
other components. Table V sets out these studies, and reveals
the wide range of cell biological fields that can be examined
using the macrophage Fc receptor.

Macrophages also express a receptor for mannose/fucose terminal moieties, which mediates binding and internalization of
glycoproteins, glycoconjugates, and lysosomal glycosidases.
This receptor, probably involved in retrieval of secreted lysosomal enzymes, is of considerable interest since it appears to
recycle from the cell surface to the interior and back again.
The rapid influx of macrophage plasma membrane and the constant
volume of intracellular membrane compartments in resting and
endocytosing cells have been interpreted for some time as a
bulk recycling of membrane, despite labeling studies assigning
long half-lives to many plasma membrane components. The fundamental question remains whether the bulk of the plasma membrane
recycles, tracing the path revealed by the mannosyl/fucosyl receptor, or is degraded after internalization, leaving only
certain components to escape and recycle. If the latter is
true, then it implies the existence of hitherto unknown mechanisms for singling out receptors that are to recycle from the
rest of the membrane. Either way, further study in this area
should provide new insights into the dynamics of plasma membrane movement within the cell.

TABLE V. *The Fc Receptor as a Tool in Cell Biology*

Use	Characteristic	Reference
Cell Marker	(a) Depletion of Fc receptor (FcR) positive cells by density centrifugation after rosetting with antibody-coated sheep red blood cells. Important technique for evaluating role of FcR bearing cells in in vitro immunological systems.	67
	(b) Drug targeting to FcR bearing cells, for example, depletion of FcR positive cells with antibody-coated sheep red blood cells preloaded with tubercidin or by uptake of immune complexes of the toxic chain of ricin.	68
	(c) Selection of macrophage variants in cell lines, mutagenesis followed by selective toxicity as in (b).	69
Differentiation Marker	(a) FcR is an easily demonstrated macrophage marker in heterokaryons and hybrids.	70
	(b) Appearance of FcR bearing cells can be used to follow the differentiation of in vitro cultures of bone marrow cells.	29
Membrane marker	(a) Plating macrophages onto immobilized immune complexes clears the free cell surface of the appropriate FcR, allowing examination of receptor mobility in the plane of the plasma membrane.	71, 72
	(b) Monoclonal antibodies against the FcR give plasma membrane marker and enable measurements of receptor at different stages of differentiation and activation.	73
FcR structure	(a) FcR can be precipitated from macrophages and analyzed by polyacrylamide gel electrophoresis or density gradient centrifugation.	74, 75, 76
	(b) Development of monoclonal	73

Table V (Cont'd.)

Use	Characteristic	Reference
	antibodies against FcR have enabled more rapid isolation of FcR for structural characterization.	
	(c) The FcR is thought to be heterogeneous, with trypsin-sensitive and trypsin-resistant types exhibiting different subclass binding specificity.	77
Role of FcR in phagocytosis	(a) FcR and C3b receptors mediate phagocytosis of antibody-coated particles via a distinctive mechanism. Receptor mobility and continued sequential ligand-receptor interaction are important during internalization.	2
	(b) 2 Deoxy-glucose blocks ingestion of particles via the FcR and C3b receptor without affecting the nonspecific ingestion of latex particles. This observation may lead to a further dissociation of the sequence of events during internalization.	78
	(c) FcR facilitates the uptake of certain viral-antibody complexes with resultant enhancement rather than neutralization of virus growth in macrophage cell lines or monocytes.	79
Immunological function	(a) FcR mediates immune phagocytosis, endocytic clearance of circulating immune complexes as well as extracellular antibody dependent lysis of appropriate target cells.	80
	(b) Binding of immune complexes to the FcR can elicit increased superoxide and H_2O_2 activity; this system may be used to examine the genesis of the metabolic burst associated with phagocytosis as well as the mechanisms of oxidative killing.	81

TABLE VI. Analysis of Endocytosis

Phenomenon	Experimental techniques	Comments	Reference
Receptor mobility	(a) Capping of membrane glyco-proteins by lectin, e.g., concanavalin A.		82
	(b) Loss of appropriate FcR on free plasma membrane surface when macrophages are plated on immobilized immune complexes.		71
	(c) Macrophage x nonmacrophage heterokaryons exhibit FcR and ATPase on all plasma membrane soon after formation		70
Membrane flow	(a) In pinocytosis, small pino-cytic vesicles may be visualized by loading with horse radish peroxidase, detected with dia-minobenzidine, and quantified by stereology.	Kinetic, cytochemical, and biochemi-cal criteria allow differentiation between phagosome and secondary ly-sosome. Technique reveals destina-tion for contents of most pinocytic vesicles is the lysosomal compart-ment, and rate of membrane flux high.	83
	(b) In phagocytosis, uptake may be estimated by counting in the cells, by extraction of par-ticle material from cells or by using labeled particle for rate of uptake.	Distinction between binding and up-take can be difficult.	46, 47, 84

835

Table VI (Cont'd.)

Selective internalization	(a) Involvement of whole plasma membrane in internalization at endocytosis may be examined by looking for changes in specific activity of membrane functions after extensive endocytosis.	V_{max} and K_m of adenosine and lysine plasma membrane transport sites unaffected by large ingestion of latex beads, exclusion from phagosome probably involves microtubules. Macrophage 5' nucleotidase is internalized during phagocytosis of latex beads.	85, 86, 55
	(b) Labeling of plasma membrane, followed by extraction of phagosome membrane and comparing labeling pattern with plasma membrane	In L cells all surface iodinatable components of plasma membrane can be isolated from phagosomes. In PMN, selective exclusion and inclusion of plasma membrane components into phagosomes have been claimed.	87
	(c) Labeling of phagosome membrane from within, compared with plasma membrane label	All surface iodinatable components appear to be accessible to labeling by iodination catalyzed by lacto-peroxidase immobilized on latex beads, after phagosome formation.	88
Fate of internalized membrane	(a) Marking plasma membrane, and tracing label after internalization	Enzyme marker (5' nucleotidase) or surface iodination reveals that most internalized components enter a lysosomal compartment and are degraded with a half life of a few hours.	89, 90
	(b) Stereological measurement of surface area of intracellular membrane compartments during endocytosis	Measurements of area of lysosomal compartment during HRP-marked pinocytosis reveals constant value despite plasma membrane internalization	83

Table VI (Cont'd.)

Phenomenon	Experimental techniques	Comments	Reference
		within 30 min. Unlikely de novo synthesis could account for re-placement at this rate.	
	(c) Iodination of phagosomes from within intact cells followed by autoradiograph time course shows subsequent path for these mem-brane components	Despite low levels of labeling, auto-radiography at the light or electron microscope level supports redeploy-ment of phagosomal membrane compo-nents back to the plasma membrane.	88
	(d) Use of probes for specific membrane species, for example, labeled ligand to known receptor or monoclonal antibody against a membrane constituent, to trace dynamics of expression of these components within the various membrane compartments of the cell.	Continuous substantial reexpression of proteolytically removed surface component in conditions of no pro-tein synthesis reveal either a large intracellular pool or a recycling system. Comparison of uptake rate with surface density of receptor (i.e., binding capacity) may confirm existence of recycling. Monoclonal antibodies have yet to be exploited in this area.	50
Involvement of the ly-sosomal compart-ment	(a) In vivo, clearance role of macrophages suggest lysosomal degradation of phagosome con-tents as the usual conclusion to phagocytosis.	Sensitive assays for lysosomal hydro-lases, based on appropriate umbel-liferyl derivatives and fluorescent detection, reveal very rapid asso-ciation of lysosomes with the pha-gosome fraction.	91
	Lysosomal hydrolases may be as-sayed for in fractions of discon-tinuous sucrose gradients used to isolate latex phagosomes.	Single and double label studies of turnover of membrane proteins re-veals short half lives for each com-	

837

Table VI (Cont'd.)

Pulse chase studies using surface radioiodination can be used to estimate half lives for many membrane components.	ponent in some cells, and a heterogeneous distribution of half-lives in other cell types. Only the former result is consistent with bulk delivery of membrane proteins to lysosomes, since iodinated components internalized on latex show short homogeneous half lives.
(b) Essential for any degradation of phagosomal contents is phagolysosomal fusion. Phagolysosomal fusion may be examined by preloading the lysosomes with a marker such as acridine orange or colloidal thorium (Thorotrast) and monitoring its subsequent transfer to the phagosomes. Presence of lysosomal hydrolases in phagosomes is diagnostic of phagolysosomal fusion. In vitro, fusion of two vesicle populations may be monitored by preloading each separately with one of a pair of synergistic fluorochromes.	It is relatively easy to distinguish transfer of lysosomal marker such as the fluorescent acridine orange into phagosomes if the test particles are larger than lysosomes, for example, yeasts, latex beads or antibody-coated erythrocytes. Pinolysosomal fusion is harder to demonstrate since both vesicle populations are similar in size. However, appearance of HRP after DAB staining reveals pinosomes with a rim of staining, whereas after fusion with lysosomes staining was diffuse and throughout the vesicle. Synthetic fluorochromes have been developed, which only emit at a particular wavelength when both components are adjacent in the same membrane, so fusion may be monitored by recording emission at this wavelength. Techniques like this may enable a

References: 88, 89, 90; 92, 93; 94

Table VI (Cont'd.)

Phenomenon	Experimental techniques	Comments	Reference
	(c) Inhibition of phagolysosomal fusion may be fundamental to the survival of many intracellular parasites.	separation of fusion event from its cellular control.	
	Experimental inhibitors of phagolysosomal fusion are of two types, lysosomotropic polyanionic compounds such as poly-D-glutamic acid and the semisynthetic chlorite oxidized amylose, and plasma membrane active compounds like concanavalin A.	It is possible that both types of inhibitor function in basically the same way, by multivalent attachment to membrane components (in the pinosome for concanavalin A, and in the lysosome for the polyanions) compromising normal membrane fluidity by this extensive cross-linking. Recent demonstrations of the inhibition of phagolysosomal fusion by ammonia suggest that the mechanism may be more subtle than this.	95, 96, 97
Role of receptors	*(a) In pinocytosis, receptor-ligand interaction required for internalization (N.B. Fluid phase pinocytosis does not involve receptors.)*	Receptor – ligand interaction confers specificity and ability to concentrate ligand from the extracellular medium.	2
	(b) In phagocytosis, segmental response of membrane to phagocytic stimulus can be demon-	In nonactivated macrophages binding via C3b receptor does not lead to	2

Table VI (Cont'd.)

strated using two separate test particles ingested via different receptors.	internalization, surrounding membrane can ingest particles via Fc receptors without affecting C3b-bound markers.	
(c) Internalized particles/molecules are normally delivered to the lysosomes.		
For peptide hormone receptors, degradation of both the ligand and the receptor probably results and may account for down regulation.	Possible difference between receptors for uptake, which appear to recycle, and receptors for triggering metabolic changes, which may be "one-shot."	98, 99
For particles internalized by "immune" phagocytosis, total lysosomal degradation occurs, with additional possibility of activity of oxidative killing pathway.	Macrophages achieve intracellular (and extracellular) killing by means of high-energy oxygen metabolites (e.g., Superoxide, H_2O_2) and this pathway is activated by phagocytosis.	100, 81
Recently, comparison of surface binding with uptake rate in the presence of cycloheximide have suggested for a variety of receptors (LDL receptors in fibroblasts, mannose-fucose receptors in macrophages, mannose-6-phosphate receptors in fibroblasts) that lysosomal degradation is not inevitable.	Evidence is now compelling that a variety of receptors in several cell types engage in continuous recycling from plasma membrane to intracellular membrane compartment and back again. Since ligand, if present, must be removed and probably degraded, it seems likely that a traverse of the lysosomal compartment is part of the recycling route; the survival of the receptor is then an intriguing problem.	101, 50

Table VI (Cont'd.)

Phenomenon	Experimental technique	Comments	Reference
	(d) Measurement of surface binding of mannose receptor using 125I-Mannose-BSA, a "neoglycoprotein." Time course of recovery at 37°C after clearance of surface receptor at 4°C suggests ligand-independent recycling of receptors to the plasma membrane of alveolar macrophages.	Essential to these studies is the temperature-dependence of receptor-mediated endocytosis, so that measurements at 4°C record only surface binding.	50
	(e) In fibroblasts, similar behavior is found for the LDL receptor, movement of which may be visualized using ferritin-LDL, revealing association of LDL receptor with specialized regions of membrane, having a novel cytoskeletal underlay of clathrin.	It is not yet known whether macrophage receptors are concentrated into specialized coated pits prior to internalization or role of clathrin in macrophages.	65
	(f) Redeployment of mannose receptors to the plasma membrane can be inhibited with chloroquine and ammonium ions that are known to dissipate lysosomal pH gradients.	These inhibitors have no effect on surface binding, or internalization at 37°C of ligand prebound at 4°C, but reduce 37°C recovery of surface receptors after trypsin clearance at 4°C.

Conditions within the lysosomes may influence survival and redeployment of receptors. | 102 |

Table VI (Cont'd.)

Membrane signal transduction	(a) Electron microscopy reveals assembly of complex web of cytoskeleton adjacent to site of surface binding of particle destined for phagocytosis.	There must be some signal for the activation of the intracellular contractile system as a result of binding to receptors present on the outer face of the plasma membrane.	103
	(b) Use of voltage-sensitive chemical probes or direct recording of potential using intracellular microelectrodes reveals hyperpolarization.	Lipophilic cation triphenylmethyl phosphonium ion distributes across membranes according to the potential across them and has been used to show hyperpolarization responses to endocytic stimuli in human PMN. This has been confirmed by intracellular microelectrode recording in rat macrophages phagocytosing latex beads.	104, 105, 106
	(c) Measurement of changes in phospholipid turnover with endocytic activity in macrophages.	Phagocytosis of immune stimulants (e.g., C. parvum) leads to increased phosphatidylinositol turnover in mouse resident peritoneal cells.	107
Involvement of the contractile system	(a) Biochemical characterization of lysate of macrophages by SDS-PAGE and in vitro reassembly of components.	Mononuclear phagocytes contain actin, myosin, an actin-binding protein and a cofactor required for activation of actomyosin ATPase, which may be a myosin light chain kinase. Actin-, myosin-, and actin-binding protein together gel at room temperature and exhibit Mg^{2+}-sensitive contraction.	108, 109

Table VI (Cont'd.)

Phenomenon	Experimental techniques	Comments	Reference
	(b) Examination of control of contraction in gels formed in tubes, looking for messenger-linking surface-binding of phagocytic target with adjacent actomyosin contraction.	Recently, a new component has been isolated from macrophages. Named gelsolin, it has the ability to confer Ca^{2+}-dependent directionality of contraction on the gel matrix.	110
	(c) Electron microscopic morphology of phagocytosing cells.	The pseudopodia that engulf phagocytic targets contain networks of interdigitating filaments, some of which bind exogenous heavy meromyosin.	103
	(d) Immunocytochemical localization of contractile system components within phagocytosing cells.	Immunofluorescence localization of myosin and actin-binding protein shows highest concentrations within pseudopodia engaged in phagocytic engulfment.	111
Role of ionic calcium	(a) Biochemical search for macrophage cytosolic equivalents of muscle Ca^{2+}-dependent contraction triggers.	Macrophages do not contain tropinin or tropomyosin, which connect changes in (Ca^{2+}) to changes in contraction in muscle systems.	110
	(b) Addition of troponin and tropomyosin to macrophage actomyosin	Macrophage actomyosin ATPase activity remains Ca^{2+}-independent suggesting that control of the contractile system in macrophages is fundamentally different from that in muscle. However, see (b) of previous section.	110

Table VI (Cont'd.)

	(c) Ultrastructural cytochemical localization of divalent cations (e.g., by pyroantimonate complexes) during phagocytosis.	*None of these techniques have yet been applied to macrophages, but it seems possible that they will prove important in elucidating role of Ca^{2+} in macrophage endocytosis.*	*112, 113, 114*
	(d) X-Ray microprobe localization of Ca^{2+} in conjunction with electron microscope.		
	(e) Microinjection of Ca^{2+}-sensitive photoprotein into phagocytosing cells.		
Energy requirements of phagocytosis	*(a) Phagocytosis: Examination of temperature dependence of internalization of test particles*	*Binding to macrophage surface occurs down to 4°C, but internalization can only result above a critical temperature of 18 – 21°C.*	*2*
	(b) Temperature dependence of HRP-marked solute-phase pinocytosis.	*No critical temperature found: Pinocytic rate is linearly related to temperature from 2 – 38°C.*	
	(c) Effects of metabolic inhibitors.	*Phagocytosis is reduced by inhibitors of glycolysis (NaF, iodoacetic acid) but not inhibitors of oxidative metabolism (CN^-). Conclusion from these and other results suggested phagocytosis to be an ATP-dependent energy requiring process.*	

Table VI (Cont'd.)

Phenomenon	Experimental techniques	Comments	Reference
	(d) Dissection of metabolic inhibitor effects with a competitive glucose analog, 2-deoxyglucose	Like glycolytic inhibitors, 2-deoxyglucose causes large falls in cellular (ATP), but does not affect uptake of inert particles (however it does reduce phagocytosis via Fc and C3b receptors). Glycoprotein synthesis may also be affected.	78
	(e) Estimates of ATP turnover during phagocytosis by measuring incorporation of $[^{32}P]P_i$ into ATP	Reduction of specific activity of ATP labeled in macrophages undertaking phagocytosis compared to controls suggests existence of another high-energy phosphate reservoir apart from ATP. Creatine phosphate is present in three- to fivefold molar excess over ATP and its turnover is substantially increased during phagocytosis. It is possible that creatine phosphate replenishes the ATP pool such that it does not appear to change in size during phagocytosis.	115

845

The mononuclear phagocytes are highly active endocytic cells and have been extensively used in the elucidation of the mechanisms involved in this process. The wide area covered by this research is outlined in Table VI. Although many of the techniques mentioned have not been exploited to the limit, there is one in particular which seems likely to contribute very much more in the future. The complexity of macrophage membranes has made isolation or marking of individual components difficult. This problem can be overcome by utilizing the high specificity of an antigen-antibody reaction by raising antisera. However, antisera have the disadvantage of polyspecificity, small yields, and lack of reproducibility between batches. The recent advent of the spleen cell-myeloma fusion technique (116) for production of clonal hybrid lines producing large quantities of pure monospecific antibody has profound implications in this field.

Early studies of macrophages using monoclonal antibodies have centered mainly on recognition and immunoprecipitation of specific plasma membrane components such as the Fc receptor or putative differentiation markers. Clearly, this will revolutionize the characterization of specific components of the plasma membrane, but it is far from the limit of exploitation of the technique. The production of monoclonal antibodies in other fields has involved use of indirect radioimmunoassay to detect active supernatants containing antibodies binding to cell surface determinants. However, it is possible to employ a functional assay so that selection is based on an antibody interfering with some cellular process, rather than simply the presence of a determinant on a complex cell surface. A selection protocol of this sort, based on inhibition of rosetting of antibody-coated erythrocytes on macrophages, has been used to select a monoclonal antibody against the mouse macrophage Fc receptor (73). A second substantial area in which monoclonal antibodies have yet to be used is in the examination of intracellular components. This is somewhat more difficult as the indirect radioimmunoassay on whole cells is no longer adequate for screening of fusion supernatants for activity against intracellular components. In order to use a radioimmunoassay, then the intracellular components of interest must be isolated in considerable quantity, the latex phagolysosome is a good candidate here. Another approach is to use a functional inhibition assay in a cell-free system, for example, to select for an antibody recognizing a determinant on a molecule involved in intracellular membrane fusion, inhibition of an *in vitro* assay measuring fusion of two vesicle populations (by fluorescence enhancement, double labeling, single label transfer, see role of lysosomal compartment, Table VI) could be employed as a supernatant screen.

One drawback of making antibodies against intracellular

components is the difficulty of getting them into intact cells to test their effects. Microinjection has been extensively used to introduce fluorescent antibodies into intact live cells (117), this gives a good way of examining antigen distribution in a small number of cells, but to observe biochemical effects it is necessary to introduce antibody into a large number of cells. An as yet little-utilized technique here is the virally induced fusion of antibody-preloaded red cells with the cells of interest (118); there is now evidence to suggest delivery of functionally intact antibody into the cytoplasm of the target cells (119).

A number of obligate intracellular parasites that penetrate macrophages appear to do so via a specific surface receptor. The fact that the cells continue to express such an apparently disadvantageous receptor suggests that it has some normal physiological role and binding of the microorganism is the result of an adaptive modification by the microorganism or parasite. For example, *Toxoplasma* and *Chlamydia* enter the cell by an apparently normal endocytic process, prevent phagolysosomal fusion and replicate within the phagosome until the cell is lysed (20). Recent evidence suggests that survival of *Toxoplasma gondii* inside cells may be due to a failure to trigger the burst of oxidative metabolism normally associated with immune phagocytosis (121). Since it is clear that intracellular parasites are using isolated elements of the normal endocytic pathway to gain entry and to survive within macrophages, these microorganisms may prove very important in the dissection of the endocytic process and the analysis of its component parts.

The consequences of endocytosis are far-ranging and the exact sequence of events is uncertain. Electrical changes are briefly discussed in Table VI. The reader is referred to Chapter 51 for a brief discussion of the oxidative metabolic burst.

V. SOMATIC CELL GENETICS

Since the macrophage phenotype remains stable in culture, this cell is suitable for analysis by cell fusion and related techniques. Some examples of studies of this kind are listed in Table VII. The study of human inborn errors has lagged, in part because of the difficulty of obtaining adequate yields of proliferating human macrophages, e.g., from bone marrow, in part because of the paucity of defined genetic disorders with exclusive involvement of cells of the mononuclear phagocyte system.

TABLE VII. Somatic Cell Genetics of the Macrophage

Category	Use	Reference
1. Heterokaryons	Expression of plasma membrane receptors (fluidity, masking) and control of DNA synthesis in G_0 cell.	
2. Enucleation	Role of nucleus in expression of plasma membrane receptors.	122
3. Cell hybridization	Isolation of intraspecific hybrids (macrophage × non-macrophage), which extinguish or express a macrophage specific phenotype (lysozyme, Fc receptors with variant function).	37
	Rescue of rat alveolar macrophage receptors for glycoconjugates by fusion with receptor negative mouse macrophage cell line.	
	Mapping of mouse chromosome loci by segregation analysis	123
4. Cell lines	Variant expression of macrophage phenotype; Membrane antigens, adenylcyclase.	124
5. Inborn errors of metabolism	Complement deficiencies (C_4); chronic granulomatous disease, Chediak - Higashi syndrome and beige mutation, and myeloperoxidase deficiency.	125, 126
6. Resistance to virus infections	Genetic control of host susceptibility is expressed by the macrophage.	127, 128

Heterokaryon studies with mouse macrophages have been used to study the fate of plasma membrane markers such as ATPase and Fc receptors after Sendai-virus induced fusion with mouse melanoma cells. Membrane reorganization is complex and involves a rapid intermixing of markers, probably due to difffusion within the plane of the membrane, and concurrent masking of macrophage Fc receptors by surface proteins under control of the melanoma nucleus. The ability of such heterokaryons to continue to synthesize macrophage specific receptors has not been demonstrated, because of the difficulty in distinguishing new and old receptor molecules at the level of the single cell.

Macrophage heterokaryons have also proved suitable to study cytoplasmic reorganization, especially the role of microtubules, and the reactivation of DNA synthesis in the G_0 macrophage nucleus, a process controlled by the melanoma cell nucleus.

VI.   MACROPHAGE HYBRIDIZATION

Permanent cell lines of macrophage hybrids have been used to map the mouse genome and to study expression of a macrophage-specific phenotype. Intra- and interspecies hybrids have been produced by using primary macrophages or macrophage-like lines with suitable drug markers. Primary macrophages offer the advantage that the parental cells cannot proliferate indefinitely so that only half-selection systems are required to eliminate the other unfused parent line. An important problem is caused by the presence of other cells like fibroblasts when primary populations are used for fusion. Thus, hybrids obtained by fusing peritoneal cells with human SV40-transformed cell lines express a mouse fibroblast and not a macrophage phenotype and are likely to originate from contaminant cells (129).

Thioguanine-resistant variants of mouse macrophage lines, J774 and P388D$_1$, have been prepared for use with selection in HAT medium. Ouabain resistance provides another suitable method to isolate mouse macrophage X human fibroblas hybrids. These markers involve metabolic products found in all cell types. Macrophage specific markers, e.g., lysozyme secretion and Fc receptors, provide simple nondestructive screening systems to identify hybrids that express a macrophage phenotype. The use of surface markers with FACS and cell panning methods permit some enrichment of macrophagelike hybrids, but lack efficiency. Improved methods of positive and negative selection are needed to isolate rare hybrids.

Little is known about stability of the karyotype of macrophage hybrids. Intraspecies hybrids with primary diploid cells may be less stable than those with macrophage cell lines and a pattern of reverse segregation of mouse chromosomes in interspecies hybrids with human cells could occur (130).

Early experiments in which mouse peritoneal macrophages were fused with mouse L cell fibroblasts or melanoma cells yielded hybrids in which the macrophage-specific traits were often extinguished. More recently we have isolated hybrids of this type which continue to secrete lysozyme and to express Fc receptors and cell-specific antigens. Such hybrids, however, show a variant phenotype in that Fc receptors result in binding of antibody-coated red cells, but fail to internalize these particles. The defect in ingestion is selective since the hybrids take up latex and immune complexes. These variants should provide useful insights into normal cellular function.

The lack of subset heterogeneity in mononuclear phagocytes makes it difficult to distinguish the parental origin in macrophage X macrophagelike hybrids. Species differences can be useful in this regard. The absence of a receptor for glycoconjugates on the mouse macrophage line J774 has recently made it possible to rescue this marker by hybridization with rat alveolar macrophages.

Although several examples are known in which a genetically determined deficiency in the host, such as complement biosynthesis or susceptibility to virus infection, is expressed by macrophages in culture, the cellular mechanisms remain to be characterized. The macrophage cell lines now available also lend themselves to mutagenesis and selection of variants with an interesting phenotype. It is, however, important to recognize that such variants are often complex and may express a variety of defects in addition to the one under investigation.

REFERENCES

1. R. van Furth, ed. "Mononuclear Phagocytes in Immunity, Infection and Pathology." Blackwell Scientific Publications, England, 1975.
2. S. C. Silverstein, R. M. Steinman, and Z. A. Cohn. Endocytosis. *Ann. Rev. Biochem. 46*: 669-722, 1977.
3. S. Gordon and Z. A. Cohn. The macrophage. *Int. Rev. Cytol. 36*: 171-214, 1973.
4. S. Gordon. Regulation of enzyme secretion by mononuclear phagocytes: Studies with macrophage plasminogen activator and lysozyme. *Fed. Proc. 37*: 2754-2758, 1978.
5. Z. A. Cohn and B. Benson. The differentiation of mononuclear phagocytes: Morphology, cytochemistry, and biochemistry. *J. Exp. Med. 121*: 153-170, 1965.
6. Z. A. Cohn. The activation of mononuclear phagocytes: Fact, fancy, and future. *J. Immunol. 121*: 813-816, 1978.
7. S. Gordon and Z. A. Cohn. Bacille Calmette-Guérin infection in the mouse. Regulation of macrophage plasminogen activator by T lymphocytes and specific antigen. *J. Exp. Med. 147*: 1175-1188, 1978.

8. C. F. Nathan and R. K. Root. Hydrogen peroxide release from mouse peritoneal macrophages: Dependence on sequential activation and triggering. *J. Exp. Med. 146*: 1648-1662, 1977.
9. Q. N. Myrvik, E. S. Leake, and S. Oshima. A study of macrophages and epithelioid-like cells from granulomatous (BCG-induced) lungs of rabbits. *J. Immunol. 89*: 745, 1962.
10. R. Mason, F. Brodsky, J. Austyn, and S. Gordon. Submitted.
11. A. Boyum. Separation of leukocytes from blood and bone marrow. *Scand. J. Clin. Lab. Invest. 21* (Suppl. 97): 1, 1968.
12. R. Seljelid. Properties of Kupffer cells. *In* "Mononuclear Phagocytes; Functional Aspects" (R. van Furth, ed.), pp. 157-199. Martinus Nijhoff, Boston, The Hague, London, 1980.
13. H-S. Lin and S. Gordon. Secretion of plasminogen activator by bone marrow-derived mononuclear phagocytes and its enhancement by colony-stimulating factor. *J. Exp. Med. 150*: 231-245, 1979.
14. P. Ralph. Functions of macrophage cell lines. *In* "Mononuclear Phagocytes, Functional Aspects" (R. van Furth, ed.), pp. 439-456. Martinus Nijhoff, Boston, The Hague, London, 1980.
15. A. Volkman and J. L. Gowans. The origin of macrophages from bone marrow in the rat. *Br. J. Exp. Pathol. 46*: 62, 1965.
16. J. E. Till and E. A. McCulloch. A direct measurement of the radiation sensitivity of normal mouse bone marrow cells. *Radiat. Res. 14*: 213, 1961.
17. M. Virolainen. Hematopoietic origin of macrophages as studied by chromosome markers in mice. *J. Exp. Med. 127*: 943, 1968.
18. T. R. Bradley and D. Metcalf. The growth of mouse bone marrow cells *in vitro*. *J. Exp. Biol. 44*: 287, 1966.
19. D. H. Pluznik and L. Sachs. The cloning of normal 'mast' cells in tissue culture. *J. Cell. Physiol. 66*: 319, 1965.
20. C. C. Stewart, H. Lin, and C. Adles. Proliferation and colony-forming ability of peritoneal exudate cells in liquid culture. *J. Exp. Med. 141*: 1114-1132, 1975.
21. M. A. Sumner, T. R. Bradley, G. S. Hodgson, M. J. Cline, P. A. Fry, and L. Sutherland. The growth of bone marrow cells in liquid culture. *Br. J. Haematol. 23*: 221, 1972.
22. M. Virolainen and V. Defendi. Dependence of macrophage growth *in vitro* upon interaction with other cell types. *Wistar Inst. Symp. Monogr. 7*: 67, 1967.
23. J. Mauel and V. Defendi. Regulation of DNA synthesis in

mouse macrophages. Studies on mechanisms of action of the macrophage growth factor. *Exp. Cell Res. 65*: 377-385, 1971.

24. T. M. Dexter, T. D. Allen, L. G. Lajtha, R. Schofield, and B. I. Lord. Stimulation of differentiation and proliferation of hemopoietic cells *in vitro*. *J. Cell Physiol. 82*: 461-474, 1973.

25. J. S. Greenberger, P. B. Davisson, and P. J. Gans. Murine sarcoma viruses block corticosteroid-induced differentiation of bone marrow preadipocytes associated with long-term *in vitro* hemopoiesis. *Virology 95*: 317-333, 1979.

26. B. Clarkson, P. A. Marks, and J. E. Till, eds.). "Differentiation of Normal and Neoplastic Hematopoietic Cells." Cold Spring Harbor Conferences on Cell Proliferation No. 5, 1978.

27. E. R. Stanley and P. M. Heard. Factors regulating macrophage production and growth. Purification and some properties of the colony stimulating factor from medium conditioned by mouse L cells. *J. Biol. Chem. 252*: 4305, 1977.

28. L. J. Guilbert and E. R. Stanley. Specific interaction of murine colony-stimulating factor with mononuclear phagocytic cells. *J. Cell Biol. 85*: 153-159, 1980.

29. M. J. Cline and M. A. Sumner. Bone marrow macrophage precursors. I. Some functional characteristics of the early cells of the mouse macrophage series. *Blood 40*: 62, 1972.

30. T. J. L. M. Goud, C. Schotte, and R. van Furth. Identification and characterization of the monoblast in mononuclear phagocyte colonies grown *in vitro*. *J. Exp. Med. 142*: 1180-1199, 1975.

31. L. Sachs. Control of normal cell differentiation and the phenotypic reversion of malignancy in myeloid leukaemia. *Nature 274*: 535-539, 1978.

32. E. M. Rabellino, G. D. Ross, H. T. K. Trang, N. Williams, and D. Metcalf. Membrane receptors of mouse leukocytes. II. Sequential expression of membrane receptors and phagocytic capacity during leukocyte differentiation. *J. Exp. Med. 147*: 434-445, 1978.

33. L. J. Guilbert and N. N. Iscove. Partial replacement of serum by selenite, transferrin, albumin, and lecithin in haemopoietic cell cultures. *Nature 263*: 594, 1976.

34. Z. Werb. Biochemical actions of glucocorticoids on macrophages in culture. Specific inhibition of elastase, collagenase, and plasminogen activator secretion and effects on other metabolic functions. *J. Exp. Med. 147*: 1695-1712, 1978.

35. J. I. Kurland, L. M. Pelus, P. Ralph, R. S. Bockman, and M. A. S. Moore. Induction of prostaglandin E synthesis in normal and neoplastic macrophages. Role for colony-

stimulating factor(s) distinct from effects on myeloid progenitor cell proliferation. *Proc. Natl. Acad. Sci. USA 76*: 2326-2330, 1979.

36. H. E. Broxmeyer, A. Smithyman, R. R. Eger, P. A. Meyers, and M. de Sousa. Identification of lactoferrin as the granulocyte-derived inhibitor of colony-stimulating activity production. *J. Exp. Med. 148*: 1052-1067, 1978.

37. S. Gordon. Unpublished results.

38. M-L. Lohmann-Matthes, W. Domzig, and J. Roder. Promonocytes have the functional characteristics of natural killer cells. *J. Immunol. 123*: 1883-1886, 1979.

39. E. Handman and A. W. Burgess. Stimulation by granulocyte-macrophage colony stimulating factor of *Leishmania tropica* killing by macrophages. *J. Immunol. 122*: 1134-1137, 1979.

40. N. G. Testa, T. M. Dexter, D. Scott, and N. M. Teich. Malignant myelomonocytic cells after *in vitro* infection of marrow cells with Friend leukaemia virus. *Br. J. Cancer 41*: 33-39, 1980.

41. T. Graf, H. Beug, and M. J. Hayman. Target cell specificity of defective avian leukemia viruses: Hematopoietic target cells for a given virus type can be infected but not transformed by strains of a different type. *Proc. Nat. Acad. Sci. USA 77*: 389-393, 1980.

42. L. Gazzolo, C. Moscovici, and M. G. Moscovici. Response of hemopoietic cells to avian acute leukemia viruses: Effects on the differentiation of the target cells. *Cell 16*: 627-638, 1979.

43. M. G. Wetzel and E. D. Korn. Phagocytosis of latex beads by *Acanthamoeba castellanii*: III. Isolation of the phagocytic vesicles and their membranes. *J. Cell Biol. 43*: 90-104, 1969.

44. J. C. Unkeless. The presence of two Fc receptors on mouse macrophages: Evidence from a variant cell line and differential trypsin sensitivity. *J. Exp. Med. 145*: 931-947, 1977.

45. W. S. Walker. Separate Fc receptors for immunoglobulins IgG_{2a} and IgG_{2b} on an established cell line of mouse macrophages. *J. Immunol. 116*: 911-914, 1976.

46. T. P. Stossel, R. J. Mason, J. Hartwig, and M. Vaughan. Quantitative studies of phagocytosis by polymorphonuclear leukocytes: Use of paraffin oil emulsions to measure the initial rate of phagocytosis. *J. Clin. Invest. 51*: 615, 1972.

47. M. Ito, P. Ralph, and M. A. S. Moore. *In vitro* stimulation of phagocytosis in a macrophage cell line measured by a convenient radiolabeled latex bead assay. *Cell. Immunol. 46*, 48-56, 1979.

48. P. Stahl, P. H. Schlesinger, J. S. Rodman, and T. Doebber.

Recognition of lysosomal glycosidases *in vivo* inhibited by modified glycoproteins. *Nature 264*: 86-88, 1976.

49. P. D. Stahl, J. S. Rodman, M. J. Miller, and P. H. Schlesinger. Evidence for receptor-mediated binding of glycoproteins, glycoconjugates, and lysosomal glycosidases by alveolar macrophages. *Proc. Nat. Acad. Sci. USA 75*: 1399-1403, 1978.

50. P. Stahl, P. H. Schlesinger, E. Sigardson, J. S. Rodman, and T. C. Lee. Receptor-mediated pinocytosis of mannose glycoconjugates by macrophages: Characterization and evidence for receptor recycling. *Cell 19*: 207-215, 1980.

51. J. F. Day, R. W. Thornburg, S. R. Thorpe, and J. W. Baynes. Carbohydrate-mediated clearance of antibody-antigen complexes from the circulation. *J. Biol. Chem. 255*: 2360-2365, 1980.

52. J. Kaplan. Evidence for reutilization of surface receptors for α macroglobulin-protease complexes in rabbit alveolar macrophages. *Cell 19*: 197-205, 1980.

53. H. G. Remold. Requirement for α-L-fucose on the macrophage membrane receptor for MIF. *J. Exp. Med. 138*: 1065-1076, 1973.

54. S. Gordon and Z. A. Cohn. Macrophage-melanocyte heterokaryons: Preparation and properties. *J. Exp. Med. 131*: 981-1003, 1970.

55. Z. Werb and Z. A. Cohn. Plasma membrane synthesis in the macrophage following phagocytosis of polystyrene latex particles. *J. Biol. Chem. 247*: 2439-2446, 1972.

56. P. J. Edelson and C. Erbs. Plasma membrane localization and metabolism of alkaline phosphodiesterase I in mouse peritoneal macrophages. *J. Exp. Med. 147*: 77-86, 1978.

57. E. Remold-O'Donnell. Protein kinase activity associated with the surface of guinea pig macrophages. *J. Exp. Med. 148*: 1099-1104, 1978.

58. E. Pearlstein, S. R. Dienstman, and V. Defendi. Identification of macrophage external membrane proteins and their possible role in cell adhesion. *J. Cell Biol. 79*: 263-267, 1978.

58a. M. P. Bevilacqua, D. Amrani, M. W. Mosesson, and C. Bianco. Receptors for cold-insoluble globulin (plasma fibronectin) on human monocytes. *J. Exp. Med. 153*: 42-60, 1981.

59. S. Gordon, C. S. Ripps, and Z. A. Cohn. The preparation and properties of macrophage-L cell hybrids. *J. Exp. Med. 134*: 1187-1200, 1971.

60. D. I. Beller and E. R. Unanue. IA antigens and antigen-presenting function of thymic macrophages. *J. Immunol. 124*: 1433-1440, 1980.

61. D. I. Beller, J.-M. Kiely, and E. R. Unanue. Regulation of macrophage populations. 1. Preferential induction of Ia-rich peritoneal exudates by immunological stimuli.

J. *Immunol*. *124*: 1426-1432, 1980.

62. T. Springer, G. Galfré, D. S. Secher, and C. Milstein. Mac I: A macrophage differentiation antigen identified by monoclonal antibody. *Eur. J. Immunol*. *9*: 301-306, 1979.

63. J. Austyn and S. Gordon. Submitted.

64. E. M. Mahoney, A. L. Hamill, W. A. Scott, and Z. A. Cohn. Response of endocytosis to fatty acyl composition of macrophage phospholipids. *Proc. Nat. Acad. Sci. USA 74*: 4895-4899, 1977.

65. R. G. W. Anderson, E. Vasile, R. J. Mello, M. S. Brown, and J. L. Goldstein. Immunocytochemical localization of coated pits and vesicles in human fibroblasts: Relation to low density lipoprotein receptor distribution. *Cell 15*: 919-933, 1978.

66. K. Alitalo, T. Hovi, and A. Vahieri. Fibronectin is produced by human macrophages. *J. Exp. Med*. *151*: 602-613, 1980.

67. S. V. Hunt. Separation of lymphocyte subpopulations. *In* "Handbook of Experimental Immunology," 3rd ed. (D. M. Weir, ed.), Chapter 24. Blackwell, England, 1978.

68. K. Refnes and A. C. Munthe-Kaas. Introduction of B-chain inactivated ricin into mouse macrophages and rat Kupffer cells via their Fc receptors. *J. Exp. Med*. *143*: 1464-1474, 1976.

69. R. J. Muschel, N. Rosen, and B. R. Bloom. Isolation of variants in phagocytosis of a macrophage-like continuous cell line. *J. Exp. Med*. *145*: 175-186, 1977.

70. S. Gordon and Z. A. Cohn. Macrophage-melanocyte hetero-karyons: Preparation and properties. *J. Exp. Med*. *131*: 981-1003, 1970.

71. J. Michl, M. M. Pieczonka, J. C. Unkeless and S. C. Silverstein. Effects of immobilized immune complexes on Fc and complement receptor function in resident and thio-glycollate elicited mouse peritoneal macrophages. *J. Exp. Med*. *150*: 607-621, 1979.

72. C. G. Ragsdale and W. P. Arend. Loss of Fc receptor activity after culture of human monocytes on surface bound immune complexes: Mediation by cyclic nucleotides. *J. Exp. Med*. *151*: 32-44, 1980.

73. J. C. Unkeless. Characterization of a monoclonal antibody directed against mouse macrophage and lymphocyte Fc receptors. *J. Exp. Med*. *150*: 580-596, 1979.

74. C. L. Anderson and H. M. Grey. Solubilization and partial characterization of cell membrane Fc receptors. *J. Immunol*. *118*: 819-825, 1977.

75. A. Bourgois, E. R. Abney, and R. M. E. Parkhouse. Structure of mouse Fc receptor. *Eur. J. Immunol*. 7: 691-

695, 1977.

76. C. Cunningham-Rundles, F. P. Siegal, and R. A. Good. Isolation and characterization of a human mononuclear cell Fc receptor. *Immunochemistry 15*: 365-370, 1978.

77. H. M. Grey, C. L. Anderson, C. H. Heusser, B. K. Borthistle, K. B. von Eschen, and J. M. Chiller. *In* "Origins of Lymphocyte Diversity." Proceedings of 41st Cold Spring Harbor Symposium. "Structural and Functional Heterogeneity of Fc Receptors," pp. 315-321. Published by Cold Spring Harbor Laboratory, 1976.

78. J. Michl and S. C. Silverstein. Role of macrophage receptors in the ingestion phase of phagocytosis. Birth Defects: Original article *Series 14*: 99-117, 1978.

79. J. S. M. Peiris and J. S. Porterfield. Antibody-mediated enhancement of Flavivirus replication in macrophage-like cell lines. *Nature 282*: 509-511, 1979.

80. H. S. Koren, B. S. Handwerger, and J. R. Wunderlich. Identification of macrophage-like characteristics in a cultured murine tumor line. *J. Immunol. 114*: 894-897, 1975.

81. R. B. Johnston, Jr. Oxygen metabolism and the microbicidal activity of macrophages. *Fed. Proc. 37*: 2759-2764, 1978.

82. D. A. Williams, L. A. Boxer, J. A. Oliver, and R. L. Bachner. Cytoskeletal regulation of concanavalin A in pulmonary alveolar macrophages. *Nature 267*: 255-257, 1977.

83. R. M. Steinman, S. E. Brodie, and Z. A. Cohn. Membrane flow during pinocytosis: A stereological analysis. *J. Cell Biol. 68*: 665-687, 1976.

84. M. S. Al-Ibrahim, R. Chandra, R. Kishore, F. T. Valentine, and Lawrence H. Sherwood. A micromethod for evaluating the phagocytic activity of human macrophages by ingestion of radiolabeled polystyrene particles. *J. Immunol. Methods 10*: 207-218, 1976.

85. M. F. Tsan and R. D. Berlin. Effect of phagocytosis on membrane transport of nonelectrolytes. *J. Exp. Med. 134*: 1016-1035, 1971.

86. T. E. Ukena and R. D. Berlin. Effect of colchicine and vinblastine on the topographical separation of membrane functions. *J. Exp. Med. 136*: 1-7, 1972.

87. M. Willinger and F. R. Frankel. Rate of surface protein of rabbit polymorphonuclear leukocytes during phagocytosis. I. Identification of surface proteins. II. Internalization of proteins. *J. Cell Biol. 82*: 32-44, 45-56, 1979.

88. W. A. Muller, R. A. Steinman, and Z. A. Cohn. The membrane proteins of the vacuolar system. I. Analysis by a novel method of intralysosomal iodination. II. Bidirec-

tional flow between secondary lysosomes and plasma membrane. *J. Cell Biol.* *86*: 292-303; 304-314, 1980.

89. A. Hubbard and Z. A. Cohn. Externally disposed plasma membrane proteins. II. Metabolic fate of iodinated polypeptides of mouse L cells. *J. Cell Biol.* *64*: 461-479, 1975.

90. G. Kaplan, J. C. Unkeless, and Z. A. Cohn. Insertion and turnover of macrophage plasma membrane proteins. *Proc. Nat. Acad. Sci. USA 76,* 3824-3828, 1979.

91. D. H. Leaback. "An Introduction to the Fluorimetric Estimation of Enzyme Activities," 2nd ed. Koch-Light Laboratories, Colnbrook, United Kingdom, 1975.

92. P. D'Arcy Hart and M. R. Young. Interference with normal phagosome-lysosome fusion in macrophages, using ingested yeast and suramin. *Nature 256*: 47-49, 1975.

93. P. J. Oates and O. Touster. *In vitro* fusion of Acanthamoeba phagolysosomes. *J. Cell Biol. 68*: 319-338, 1976.

94. P. M. Keller, S. Person, and W. Snipes. A fluorescence enhancement assay of cell fusion. *J. Cell Sci. 28*: 167-177, 1977.

95. M. J. Geisow, G. H. Beaven, P. D'Arcy Hart, and M. R. Young. Site of action of a polyanion inhibitor of phagosome-lysosome fusion in cultured macrophages. *Exp. Cell Res. 126*: 159-165, 1980.

96. P. J. Edelson and Z. A. Cohn. Effects of concanavalin A on mouse peritoneal macrophages. I. Stimulation of endocytic activity and inhibition of phagolysosome formation. *J. Exp. Med. 140*: 1365-1386, 1974.

97. A. H. Gordon, P. D'Arcy Hart, and M. R. Young. Ammonia inhibits phagosome-lysosome fusion in macrophages. *Nature 286*: 79-80, 1980.

98. M. S. Brown and J. L. Goldstein. Receptor-mediated endocytosis: Insights from the lipoprotein receptor system. *Proc. Nat. Acad. Sci. USA 76*: 3330-3337, 1979.

99. J. L. Goldstein, R. G. W. Anderson, and M. S. Brown. Coated pits, coated vesicles, and receptor-mediated endocytosis. *Nature 279*: 679-685, 1979.

100. C. F. Nathan, L. H. Brukner, S. C. Silverstein, and Z. A. Cohn. Extracellular cytolysis by activated macrophages and granulocytes. 1. Pharmacologic triggering of effector cells and the release of hydrogen peroxide. *J. Exp. Med. 149*: 84-99, 1975.

101. A. Kaplan, D. Fischer, D. Achord, and W. Sly. Phosphohexosyl recognition is a general characteristic of pinocytosis of lysosomal glycosidases by human fibroblasts. *J. Clin. Invest. 60*: 1088-1093, 1977.

102. C. Tietze, P. Schlesinger, and P. Stahl. Chloroquine and ammonium ion inhibit receptor-mediated endocytosis of mannoseglycoconjugates by màcrophages: Apparent inhibition

of receptor recycling. *Biochem. Biophys. Res. Commun.* *93*: 1-8, 1980.

103. A. C. Allison, P. Davies, and S. De Petris. Role of contractile microfilaments in macrophage movement and endocytosis. *Nature N. Biol. 232*: 153-155, 1971.

104. H. M. Korchak and G. Weissmann. Changes in membrane potential of human granulocytes antecede the metabolic responses to surface stimulation. *Proc. Nat. Acad. Sci. USA 75*: 3818-3822, 1978.

105. E. K. Gallin and J. I. Gallin. Interaction of chemotactic factors with human macrophages. Induction of transmembrane potential changes. *J. Cell Biol. 75*: 277-289, 1977.

106. J. Kouri, M. Noa, B. Diaz, and E. Niubo. Hyperpolarization of rat peritoneal macrophages phagocytosing latex particles. *Nature 283*: 868-869, 1980.

107. H. M. Odmundsdottir and D. M. Weir. Stimulation of phosphatidylinositol turnover in the macrophage plasma membrane: A possible mechanism for signal transmission. *Immunology 37*: 689-696, 1979.

108. T. P. Stossel and J. H. Hartwig. Interactions of actin, myosin, and a new actin-binding protein of rabbit pulmonary macrophages. II. Role in cytoplasmic movement and phagocytosis. *J. Cell Biol. 68*: 602-619, 1976.

109. J. A. Trotter and R. S. Adelstein. Macrophage Myosin: Regulation of actin-activated ATPase activity by phosphorylation of the 20,000 dalton light chain. *J. Biol. Chem. 254*: 8781-8785, 1979.

110. O. I. Stendahl and T. P. Stossel. Actin-binding protein amplifies actinomysin contraction, and gelsolin confers calcium control on the direction of contraction. *Biochem. Biophys. Res. Commun. 92*: 675-681, 1980.

111. O. I. Stendahl, J. H. Hartwig, E. A. Brotschi, and T. P. Stossel. Distribution of actin-binding protein and myosin in macrophages during spreading and phagocytosis. *J. Cell Biol. 84*: 215-224, 1980.

112. S. T. Hoffstein. Ultrastructural demonstration of calcium loss from local regions of the plasma membrane of surface-stimulated human granulocytes. *J. Immunol. 123*: 1395-1402, 1979.

113. H. Plattner and S. Fuchs. X-Ray microanalysis of calcium-binding sites in *Paramecium*, with special reference to exocytosis. *Histochemistry 45*: 23-47, 1975.

114. R. Llinas, J. R. Blinks, and C. Nicholson. Calcium transient in presynaptic terminal of squid giant synapse: Detection with aequorin. *Science 176*: 1127-1129, 1972.

115. J. D. Loike, V. F. Kozler, and S. C. Silverstein. Increased ATP and creatine phosphate turnover in phagocytosing mouse peritoneal macrophages. *J. Biol. Chem. 254*:

9558-9564, 1979.

116. G. Kohler and C. Milstein. Derivation of specific antibody-producing tissue culture and tumour lines by cell fusion. *Eur. J. Immunol. 6*: 511-519, 1976.

117. D. Lansing Taylor and Y.-L. Wang. Fluorescently labeled molecules as probes of the structure and function of living cells. *Nature 284*: 405-410, 1980.

118. M. Yamaizumi, M. Furusawa, T. Uchida, T. Nishimura, and Y. Okada. Characterization of the Ghost fusion method: A method for introducing exogeneous substances into cultured cells. *Cell Structr. Funct. 3*: 293-304, 1978.

119. M. Yamaizumi, T. Uchida, E. Mekada, and Y. Okada. Antibodies introduced into living cells by red cell ghosts are functionally stable in the cytoplasm of the cells. *Cell 18*: 1008-1014, 1979.

120. B. R. Bloom. Games parasites play: How parasites evade immune surveillance. *Nature 279*: 21-26, 1979.

121. C. B. Wilson, V. Tsai, and J. S. Remington. Failure to trigger the oxidative metabolic burst by normal macrophages: Possible mechanism for survival of intracellular parasites. *J. Exp. Med. 151*: 328-346, 1980.

122. G. Poste and P. Reeve. Formation of hybrid cells and heterokaryons by fusion of enucleated and nucleated cells. *Nature N. Biol. 229*: 123-125, 1971.

123. C. Kozak, E. Nichols, and F. H. Ruddle. Gene linkage analysis in the mouse by somatic cell hybridization. Assignment of adenine phosphoribosyl-transferase to chromosome 8 and α-galactosidase to the X chromosome. *Somatic Cell Genet. 1*: 371-382, 1975.

124. B. R. Bloom, B. Diamond, R. Muschel, N. Rosen, J. Schneck, G. Damiani, O. Rosen, and M. Scharff. Genetic approaches to the mechanism of macrophage functions. *Fed. Proc. 37*: 2765-2771, 1978.

125. H. R. Colten. Biosynthesis of complement. *Adv. Immunol. 22*: 67-118, 1976.

126. S. J. Klebanoff and R. A. Clark. "The Neutrophil: Function and Clinical Disorders." North-Holland, Amsterdam, New York, Oxford, 1978.

127. F. B. Bang and A. Warwick. Mouse macrophages as host cells for the mouse hepatitis virus and the genetic basis of their susceptibility. *Proc. Nat. Acad. Sci. USA 46*: 1065, 1960.

128. O. Haller, H. Arnheiter, and J. Lindenmann. Natural, genetically determined resistance toward influenza virus in hemopoietic mouse chimeras. Role of mononuclear phagocytes. *J. Exp. Med. 150*: 117, 1979.

129. C. M. Croce and H. Koprowski. Somatic cell hybrids between mouse peritoneal macrophages and SV40 transformed human cells. I. Positive control of the transformed

phenotype by the human chromosome 7 carrying the SV40 genome. *J. Exp. Med.* *140*: 1221-1229, 1974.

130. J. D. Minna and H. G. Coon. Human x mouse hybrid cells segregating mouse chromosomes and isozymes. *Nature 252*: 401-404, 1974.

80

BIOSYNTHETIC RADIOLABELING OF CELLULAR AND
SECRETED PROTEINS OF MONONUCLEAR PHAGOCYTES

Zena Werb
Jennie R. Chin

I. GENERAL INTRODUCTION

   A complete description of the phenotype of mononuclear
phagocytes involves defining all the biochemical and functional properties of the cells. One approach is to examine the
pattern of total transcribable mRNA present in a macrophage
at any given point in its history. This can be achieved
either by translating isolated mRNA in cell-free systems, a
process unsuitable for examination of many samples, or by
studying the translation of mRNA into proteins using the
machinery of a live cell. If radiolabeled amino acids are
present during translation in live cells, the resulting biosynthesized proteins can be analyzed by polyacrylamide gel
electrophoresis to give detailed "fingerprints" of specific
macrophage phenotypes (1,2). These procedures offer high
resolution and specificity, require small numbers of cells
(as few as 1×10^5), and are applicable to a wide variety of
mononuclear phagocytes from man, mouse, rat, rabbit, and

861

guinea pig. In conjuction with other methods, such as specific immunoprecipitation of labeled proteins, it is possible
to examine in detail changes in the properties of macrophages
that may not be seen with a single assay such as receptor
binding or quantitation of a secreted proteolytic enzyme. In
addition, these methods can be used to detect contamination
by other cell populations by searching for biosynthesized
proteins specific for those cells.

II. [^{35}S]-METHIONINE LABELING AND SAMPLE PREPARATION OF
     SECRETED AND CELLULAR PROTEINS OF MACROPHAGES

A. *Introduction*

    Resident or elicited macrophages are harvested from the
peritoneal cavity or lungs by lavage with phosphate-buffered
saline containing 100 U/ml heparin (see Section II of this
volume). When rabbit alveolar macrophages are to be studied,
it is essential to isolate and plate them as quickly and
gently as possible to prevent clumping. Mouse cells are less
apt to undergo this aggregation.

B. *Reagents*

    All tissue culture media are obtained from Grand Island
Biological Co., Grand Island, New York, and stored at 4°C
except where noted. Culture plasticware is available from
standard suppliers (Flow Laboratories, M. A. Bioproducts,
GIBCO, Costar).

    (1) Heat-inactivated fetal calf serum. Thaw to room
temperature and heat in a 56°C water bath for 30 to 60 min.
    (2) Lactalbumin hydrolysate (extra-soluble, tissue cul-
ture grade) (LH). Sterilize a 10% stock solution in water
by filtration through a 0.22-μm filter. Store at -20°C.
    (3) Culture medium. Dulbecco's modified Eagle's medium
(DME) is supplemented with heat-inactivated fetal calf serum
to a final concentration of 10% (DME-10%) or with LH (DME-LH)
to 0.2%. Add penicillin-streptomycin solution to a final concentration of 50 U/ml penicillin and 50 μg/ml streptomycin.
RPMI-1640 or minimal essential medium can be substituted for
DME.
    Methionine-free medium can be purchased as a custom order
from GIBCO; or minimal essential medium and RPMI can be mixed
from "select-amine" kits available from GIBCO.

(4)   [^{35}S]-methionine.   Amersham, >1000 Ci/mmole.   Store
at -80°C until needed.   Labeling medium is made up fresh at
25 µCi/ml in methionine-free medium.

(5)   *Micrococcus lysodeikticus.*   Sigma.   Wash dried cells
once with saline and make up at 2 mg/ml with saline.   The
suspension is stored at 4°C and should be made up fresh every
2 weeks; prolonged storage may result in hydrolysis of the
cell suspension.

(6)   Trichloroacetic acid (45% w/v).   This is used for
precipitation of labeled proteins.

(7)   2X Sample buffer.   Section III. B.

(8)   Sample tubes.   Screwcapped cryotubes, 2- and 5-ml
sizes, manufactured by Nunc or Cooke, are available from
GIBCO.   Microfuge tubes (1.5 ml polypropylene) are available
from Beckman and other suppliers.

C. Procedures

(1).   Plate the macrophages in DME-10% at 5×10^5 to 10^6
cells per well in 12-well Linbro plates (2.4-cm diameter) or
24-well Costar plates (16-mm diameter).   Allow cells to adhere 2-24 hr at 37°C in 5% CO_2 in humidified air.   If the
cells are to be treated with drugs, proceed to the next step;
otherwise, go to step 4 for direct labeling.

(2).   Wash the cells at least three times with DME-LH to
remove serum and nonadherent cells.   Phosphate-buffered saline
or Hanks' balanced salt solution can also be used for preliminary washes.

(3).   Pretreat the macrophages with 0.5-1.0 ml of DME-LH
or DME-10% containing the drug for the desired time period.
Stock solutions of drugs are usually prepared 100X concentrated in methionine-free DME; ethanol content, if any, should
be 0.05% or less to maintain cell viability.

(4).   Wash the macrophages three times with methionine-
free DME and label with 0.5-1.0 ml methionine-free DME containing 25 µCi [^{35}S]-methionine per ml; usually any drug used
during pretreatment is also added.   Macrophages are generally
labeled for 2-4 hr, although periods as short as 10 min are
feasible for special purposes.   Up to 300 µCi [^{35}S]-methionine
per ml may be needed for very short labeling times.

(5).   At the end of the labeling period, collect the
conditioned medium in 1.5-ml microfuge tubes with Pasteur
pipettes.   Wash the cells 3-4 times with saline and lyse (in
the plate) with 0.2 to 0.5 ml of 1X sample buffer or 0.1%
sodium dodecyl sulfate (SDS) followed by an equal volume of
2X sample buffer.   Freeze plates at -80°C in ziplock plastic

bags. Just before electrophoresis, check for complete lysis
by microscopy and transfer the lysates to microfuge tubes or
cryotubes for boiling (step 11).

(6). Spin the collected medium 2.5 min in a Beckman
Microfuge B (approx. 8730 g) to remove any loose cells and
debris. This step is of utmost importance for analysis of
macrophage secretion products; otherwise, minor cellular contaminants will appear in the fluorographs along with proteins
from the medium. Presence of actin (42,000 daltons) in conditioned medium is a marker for contamination by cell debris.

(7). With a Pasteur pipette carefully transfer all but
the bottom 10 µl of medium to another microfuge tube; no
pellet will be visible.

(8). To each sample, add 150 µg (75 µl) *M. lysodeikticus*
cell suspension (kept stirring on a magnetic stirrer) as a
carrier. This carrier was chosen because it does not enter
the gel during electrophoresis, as would protein carriers such
as bovine serum albumin, and, consequently, there is less
chance of interference with the electrophoretic run.
Precipitate proteins with ice-cold trichloroacetic acid
(150 µl of 45% w/v) to a final concentration of 5-7%. Cap and
shake tubes and let stand in an ice bath for at least 20 min.

(9). Centrifuge, wash, and vortex the *M. lysodeikticus*-
containing pellet 1-2 times with 1 ml 5% trichloroacetic acid,
or imlacetone. Remove as much supernatant as possible with a
Pasteur pipette and discard the supernatant as radioactive
waste.

(10). Vortex the pellet in 100 µl of 1X sample buffer, if
necessary adjust to alkaline pH with 1-5 µl 1 N NaOH (yellow,
acidic sample becomes blue when basic). *Caution:* Excessively
high concentrations of NaOH (pH greater than 10) when boiled
will result in hydrolysis of the protein sample, *M. Lysodeikticus,* and stacker gel. Freeze the samples at -80°C until
the day of electrophoresis.

(11). Place tightly capped sample tubes into a boiling
water bath for 3 min. Microfuge tubes have a tendency to pop
open during boiling unless a weight is placed on their lids.
An alternative is to use screwtop cryotubes.

(12). Determine incorporation by putting 5-µl aliquots
into counting vials containing scintillant (work in the fume
hood), rinsing out the pipette tip with the scintillant. This
precaution is necessary because the glycerol and SDS-contain-
ing sample tends to adhere to the walls of the tip, resulting
in incorrect counts.

III.   SDS-POLYACRYLAMIDE GRADIENT GEL ELECTROPHORESIS AND
FLUOROGRAPHY OF LABELED MACROPHAGE PROTEINS

A. *Introduction*

Samples are electrophoresed on 7-18% polyacrylamide - 0.1%
SDS gradient slab gels, using the Tris-glycine-SDS buffer system of Laemmli (3). The resolving power of gradient gels is
far superior to that of uniform percentage gels, which tend to
yield fuzzier bands, especially with proteins in the conditioned medium. For some types of analysis it may be helpful to
add 2 M urea to gels and sample buffer.

Low plating efficiencies and short labeling periods will
obviously result in lower incorporation. Two fluorographic
methods are presented to increase the efficiency of detection
of bands up to tenfold for ^{35}S and ^{14}C and to allow visualization of ^{3}H-labeled proteins.

B. *Reagents*

All electrophoresis stock solutions are made from electrophoretic grade reagents from Bio-Rad. Many designs of electrophoresis apparatus can be used. A suitable design is available from Bio-Rad.

(1)   30% Acrylamide-N',N'-methylenebisacrylamide.
Dissolve 29.2 gm acrylamide and 0.8 gm bisacrylamide in triple
distilled water, adjust the volume to 100 ml, and filter
through a No. 1 Whatman filter paper. Store at 4°C in a brown
bottle. Avoid contact with skin; acrylamide in solution is a
neurotoxin.
(2)   4X Lower gel buffer.   1.5 M Tris-HCl, pH 8.8, with
0.4% SDS. Store at 4°C.
(3)   4X Upper gel buffer.   0.5% M Tris-HCl, pH 6.8, with
0.4% SDS. Store at 4°C.
(4)   10% Ammonium persulfate.   Make up fresh in water.
(5) N,N,N',N'-Tetramethylethylenediamine (TEMED).   Store
at 4°C. Prolonged gelling time may be due to weak or old
TEMED.
(6)   10X Electrode buffer.   0.25 M Tris, 1.9 M glycine,
and 1% SDS. Store at room temperature. Dilute with water
before use.
(7)   2X Sample buffer.   1% β-mercaptoethanol, 0.1% bromophenol blue, 0.0625 M Tris-HCl, pH 6.8, 50% glycerol, and 2%
SDS. Store at room temperature. For 1X sample buffer, dilute
with water.

(8) ^{14}C-Methylated protein markers.   Amersham. Contains myosin, phosphorylase B, bovine serum albumin, ovalbumin, carbonic anhydrase, and lysozyme (0.833 µCi/ml each).
(9) EN-HANCE.   New England Nuclear.   Store at 4°C.
(10) Kodak X-Omat AR X-ray film.

C. Procedures

(1). Gradient slab gels are prepared a day in advance of electrophoresis. The volumes needed depend on the design of the electrophoresis apparatus; best results are obtained with gels that are 0.75-mm thick and 10-20 cm long. For each slab gel containing 0.375 M Tris-HCl, pH 8.8, and 0.1% SDS, prepare one volume each of 7% and 18% acrylamide gel solution according to the following recipe: Mix gently in a beaker on ice: 0.25 vol lower gel buffer, 0.75 vol acrylamide - water (dilute stock acrylamide with appropriate volume of water to give a final concentration of 7% or 18%), 0.00145 vol 10% ammonium persulfate, and 0.0005 vol TEMED. A few grains of bromophenol blue are added to the 7% solution to aid in visualization of gradient formation and water overlaying.
(2). Pour the gradient gel with a linear gradient maker at a rate of 1 ml/min. Gently overlay the surface with water from a 22-gauge, beveled 2-in. needle and syringe. Let polymerize undisturbed for 20-30 min. Prolonged polymerization time is indicative of old TEMED and fresher catalyst should be used. Wash the surface twice with fresh water. The gel may be left at room temperature overnight. For longer storage (2-3 days) use 1X lower gel buffer to overlay the gel.
(3). Pour off the water and gently blot the surface with bibulous paper before adding the stacking gel solution. For a 3% stacker gel containing 0.125 M Tris-HCl, pH 6.8, and 0.1% SDS, mix gently in a beaker: 0.25 vol upper gel buffer, 0.1 vol acrylamide, 0.64 vol water, 0.01 vol 10% ammonium persulfate, and 0.0005 vol TEMED. Quickly pipette the solution onto the gradient gel and insert the sample-well comb, without forming any air pockets. Sample wells 1.8-2.8 cm long and 0.45-0.9 cm wide (10- or 20-well combs) are usually used. Let polymerize. Wash the wells twice with 1X electrode buffer.
(4). Apply samples to the wells with either equivalent counts or proportionate volumes. The former will show changes in incorporation by particular bands, whereas the latter will show overall changes in the whole secretory pattern. Reserve one well for ^{14}C-labeled protein markers (diluted 1 to 40 with 1X sample buffer and boiled 3 min.).
If different volumes are applied, a more "even" run is achieved by equalizing the volumes in each well with half-strength sample buffer before overlaying with electrode buffer.

(5). Electrophorese at 20 mA per gel. A typical run time for 10 × 14 × 0.75 mm gels is 3 hr.

(6). Fix the gels in 50% trichloroacetic acid for 1 hr or overnight. A staining step is usually eliminated because there is not enough protein to be detected visually. Any staining would be extracted by preparation for fluorography.

(7). One of two procedures can be used to fluorograph gels. Bonner and Laskey's method (4) involves replacement of water in the gel with dimethyl sulfoxide (DMSO), impregnation with the fluor, 2,5-diphenyloxazole (PPO), followed by precipitation with water. To summarize briefly:

a. Working in a fume hood and wearing gloves, immerse the fixed gel in 20 vol of DMSO for 30 min. Repeat with fresh DMSO.

b. Soak the gel for 3 hr in 22.2% (w/v) PPO in DMSO. Discard this solution after one use.

c. Precipitate the PPO by submerging the gel in water for 1 hr.

d. Dry the gel under vacuum on a standard slab gel drying apparatus.

The second procedure eliminates steps 1 and 2 and consists of soaking the gel for 1 hr in a commercial fluorographic solution, EN³HANCE, followed by precipitation with water for 1 hr.

(8). Preflash Kodak X-Omat AR X-ray film before exposure to the gel. According to Laskey and Mills (5), the absorbance of the fluorographic image is not linear with the amount of radioactivity or with exposure time. Preexposure of the film to a flash of light from a flash unit corrects for this nonlinearity and increases the efficiency of detection. Place the film against the gel and seal them inside the film envelope with photographic tape. If necessary, wrap the envelope with lead foil to prevent exposure from any stray radioactive sources. Secure between two boards with clamps and expose at −80°C.

IV. CALCULATION OF DATA

A. *Introduction*

Fluorographs can be scanned in a gel densitometer (Joyce-Loebl, Canalco, etc.) to determine molecular weights and relative incorporation by individual bands.

B. Procedures

(1). With a sharp pencil draw a line approximately 1-2 mm above the origin and below the front of the lane to be scanned. (Placing millimeter graph paper behind the film is very helpful.) This step produces a sharp peak and shows the exact beginning and end of the scan.

(2). Peak areas can be readily calculated by those densitometers equipped with integrators. An alternative method is to make several xerographic copies of the scan and to resolve and extend each peak down to the baseline. Each one is then cut out exactly and weighed on a Mettler balance. Knowing the individual peak weights, the total weight of all the peaks, and the number of counts in the applied sample, it is possible to calculate the percentage of the total incorporation and the absolute number of counts in a single band. For example:

Weight of all peaks = 1500 mg
Peak X = 100 mg = 6.7% of total weight
Counts in applied sample = 15,000 cpm
Therefore, counts in Peak X = 6.7% (15,000) = 1000 cpm

(3). Individual bands, once localized, can be cut out of the original gel, solubilized, and counted in a scintillation spectrometer for additional quantitation.

(4). Molecular weights can be determined by comparison of the R_f values of each band with those of the standards (6).

V.   CRITICAL COMMENTS

A. Expected Incorporation

Incorporation of [^{35}S]-methionine into cell-associated and secreted proteins varies with cell number and labeling time, as well as time in culture (see Section V. B. 2). Protein patterns from 10^6 macrophages can be detected in as little as 15 min of labeling; however, it should be noted that the exposure time will be longer than that for cells labeled 2-4 hr. If fewer cells are available, e.g., 10^5, the incorporation time can be increased to 4 hr and fluorographs can be readily examined after only 10 days of exposure at -80°C.

The total incorporation into the secreted proteins of macrophages varies from 1.5 to 20% of the total incorporated label. Typical labeling of 5×10^5 thioglycollate-elicited macrophages in a 2-hr labeling period under the conditions described here is approximately 2.3×10^4 cpm in the secreted proteins and about 1×10^6 cpm in the cell-associated proteins.

For similar numbers of resident macrophages, approximately 1×10^4 cpm are seen in the secreted proteins and about 1.2×10^5 cpm in the cell-associated proteins.

B. Reproducibility of Incorporation

The reproducibility of incorporation depends on the age and specific activity of [^{35}S]-methionine and the time in culture of the macrophages.

(1). Because the half-life of ^{35}S is only 87.5 days, the concentration of the isotope is recalculated with each use to maintain a constant concentration from experiment to experiment. It should also be noted that storage of radioisotope for 3 weeks at 20°C results in 50% loss of radiochemical purity. By 6 weeks, over 75% of [^{35}S]-methionine has decomposed to [^{35}S]-methionine sulfoxide. Therefore, Amersham recommends storage at or below -80°C.

[^{35}S]-methionine is commercially available with specific activity of 1000 Ci/mmol or 500 Ci/mmol. To get maximum incorporation, label with the former.

(2). Preliminary experiments have shown that incorporation by macrophages varies with time in culture (unpublished results). For example, $NaIO_4$-elicited mouse peritoneal macrophages were cultured in DME-10% for either 2 hr or 2 days (medium was changed once) before labeling. Cells in the 2-day culture incorporated approximately 30% less label in their secreted proteins than those in the 2-hr culture. With macrophages elicited by other means, incorporation was higher in the older cultures.

A comparison of fluorographs showed loss or change in a number of bands. Although this phenomenon needs to be investigated further, it is preferable to label macrophages that have been explanted into culture for less than 72 hr and to be consistent with culture time.

C. Sensitivity

Metabolic labeling with [^{35}S]-methionine is a very sensitive analytic technique for the study of both secreted and cellular proteins from macrophages. The high energy of ^{35}S combined with its short half-life and its high specific activity relative to ^{14}C- and ^{3}H-labeled amino acids allows greater incorporation. In addition, fluorography increases the efficiency of detection tenfold over conventional autoradiography. Bonner and Laskey (4) were able to detect 0.06 nCi/band after 24-hr exposure at -70°C. Exposure time will, of course, depend on the total number of bands present, as well as the number of counts applied. For example, 25,000 cpm distributed among 30 bands of secreted proteins were visible after 4 days of exposure at -70°C.

D. *Differences in Synthesis and Secretion Patterns in Mononuclear Phagocytes from Different Sources*

The procedures outlined here are powerful tools in tracing the history of mononuclear phagocytes. We have found that the gel patterns of both cell-associated and secreted proteins of macrophages from various inbred mouse strains, including the recombinant resistant strains, exhibited significant differences that cannot be attributed to differences in the *H-2* haplotype of the mice. The most striking distinctions observed were between resident and inflammatory macrophages, and several subclasses of inflammatory macrophages (e.g., thioglycollate-, endotoxin-, and pyran copolymer-elicited) can be differentiated by using [^{35}S]-methionine, [^{3}H]-mannose as labels. There are similarities between species: rat, rabbit, human, and mouse macrophages share some major secreted proteins but also differ significantly in others. Similarly, proliferating tumor-derived mouse macrophages share some major proteins with macrophages from normal mice. However, in this case, major differences are possibly due to the biosynthesis and secretion of viral proteins by these cells. These labeling procedures can also be used to examine modulation of macrophage function. For example, new proteins are biosynthesized in response to treatment of mouse macrophages with glucocorticoids, prostaglandins, and antibody-coated erythrocytes.

Another important use of this technique is to help evaluate the contamination of macrophages or other cell populations by other cells. For example, the presence of radiolabeled plasma proteins such as albumin and fibrinogen in the gel patterns of secreted proteins from Kupffer cell populations is indicative of hepatocyte contamination. Similarly, fibroblast-specific proteins can be used to evaluate fibroblast contamination in inflammatory macrophage monolayers, and similar evaluations can be made for thymocytes and B cells.

E. *Modifications*

The procedures outlined in Sections II and III involve the use of [^{35}S]-methionine as the biosynthetic label of choice. However, other isotopes, such as [^{3}H]-mannose, [^{3}H]-glucosamine, other amino acids, and even ^{32}P, can be used in this way (7-11). Indeed, the most dramatic differences between resident and inflammatory macrophages appear to be specific to the secreted glycoproteins. Carbohydrate labels are particularly useful in this regard.

Specific labeled proteins can be immunoprecipitated directly with immune serum or indirectly with specific immunoglobulins followed by protein A or a second antibody (12). These techniques have been applied to the investigation of macrophage α_2-macroglobulin (13), fibronectin (13), complement components (9,10,14), and β-glucuronidase (11).

Additional details about the biosynthesis and processing of macrophage proteins can be obtained by peptide mapping of specific proteins as described by Cleveland *et al.* (15) and Johnson *et al.* (16). These techniques have been applied to studies of lysosomal enzymes and complement proteins (9,11).

Acknowledgment

This work was supported by the U. S. Department of Energy.

REFERENCES

1. Z. Werb and J. Chin. The secretion phenotypes of resident and inflammatory mouse macrophages. Manuscript in preparation.
2. Z. Werb. The effects of toxic chemicals on the immune system: The interaction of macrophages with glucocorticoids as a model system. *In* "Proceedings of the 10th Conference on Environmental Toxicology," Dayton, Ohio, 13-15 November 1979, pp. 154-171, 1980.
3. U. K. Laemmli. Cleavage of structural proteins during the assembly of the head of bacteriophage T4. *Nature (London)* 227:680-685, 1970.
4. W. M. Bonner and R. A. Laskey. A film detection method for tritium-labeled proteins and nucleic acids in polyacrylamide gels. *Eur. J. Biochem.* 46:83-88, 1974.
5. R. A. Laskey and A. D. Mills. Quantitative film detection of ^{3}H and ^{14}C in polyacrylamide gels by fluorography. *Eur. J. Biochem.* 56:335-341, 1975.
6. K. Weber and M. Osborn. The reliability of molecular weight determinations by dodecyl sulfate-polyacrylamide gel electrophoresis. *J. Biol. Chem.* 244:4406-4412, 1969.
7. D. K. Struck, P. B. Siuta, M. D. Lane, and W. J. Lennarz. Effect of tunicamycin on the secretion of serum proteins by primary cultures of rat and chick hepatocytes. *J. Biol. Chem.* 253:5332-5337, 1978.

8. A. Tartakoff, P. Vassalli, and M. Detraz. Comparative studies of intracellular transport of secretory proteins. *J. Cell Biol.* 79:694-707, 1978.

9. J. E. Pennington, W. J. Matthews. Jr., J. T. Marino, Jr., and H. R. Colten. Cyclophosphamide and cortisone acetate inhibit complement biosynthesis by guinea pig broncho-alveolar macrophages. *J. Immunol.* 123:1318-1321, 1979.

10. C. Bentley, D. Bitter-Suermann, U. Hadding, and V. Brade. *In vitro* synthesis of factor B of the alternative path-way of complement activation by mouse peritoneal macro-phages. *Eur. J. Immunol.* 6:393-398, 1976.

11. M. D. Skudlarek and R. T. Swank. Biosynthesis of two lysosomal enzymes in macrophages. *J. Biol. Chem.* 254: 9939-9942, 1979.

12. S. W. Kessler. Cell membrane antigen isolation with the staphylococcccal protein A-antibody adsorbent. *J. Immunol.* 117:1482-1490, 1976.

13. T. Hovi, D. Mosher, and A. Vaheri. Cultured human mono-cytes synthesize and secrete α_2-macroglobulin. *J. Exp. Med.* 145:1580-1589, 1977.

14. M. H. Roos, J. P. Atkinson, and D. C. Shreffler. Mole-cular characterization of the Ss and Slp (C4) proteins of the mouse *H-2* complex: Subunit composition, chain size polymorphism, and an intracellular (Pro-Ss) pre-cursor. *J. Immunol.* 121:1106-1115, 1978.

15. D. W. Cleveland, S. G. Fischer, M. W. Kirschner, and U. K. Laemmli. Peptide mapping by limited proteolysis in sodium dodecyl sulfate and analysis by gel electro-phoresis. *J. Biol. Chem.* 252:1102-1106, 1977.

16. E. F. Johnson, M. C. Zounes, and U. Muller-Eberhard. Characterization of three forms of rabbit microsomal cytochrome P-450 by peptide mapping utilizing limited proteolysis in sodium dodecyl sulfate and analysis by gel electrophoresis. *Arch. Biochem. Biophys.* 192:282-289, 1979.

81

EXTRACTION, IDENTIFICATION, AND QUANTITATION OF LIPIDS

Eileen M. Mahoney
William A. Scott

I. GENERAL INTRODUCTION

The procedures described by Bligh and Dyer (1) and Folch
et al. (2) are used for extracting lipids from a wide variety
of sources. Both techniques are applicable to mononuclear phagocytes and utilize chloroform and methanol as the extracting
solvents. However, the Bligh and Dyer procedure has been used
in our laboratory because of its simplicity. In both methods,
the proportions of organic solvents and water are critical for
the complete extraction of lipids. It is advisable that extractions be carried out on ice to minimize the action of
lipases which are active in organic solvents. When left standing in organic solvents, lipid extracts should be in a nitrogen
atmosphere and should contain a trace amount of antioxidant to
retard lipid oxidation. Lipids should be stored at -20° in
inert solvents.
   Certain precautions are advisable in handling lipids. Only
acid-cleaned glassware should be used to ensure that contami-

873

nants such as plasticizers, grease, phosphate-based detergents, or residual biological material are not present. The glassware should be fitted with ground glass stoppers or Teflon-lined caps since these are inert to organic solvents. No plastic, rubber, or silicone materials should be used to prevent such surfaces coming in contact with the lipid extracts, solvents, or solvent vapors used in the lipid analyses. The solvents used should be redistilled using a glass apparatus and should be stored in tightly capped containers thereafter. (Special chromatography or spectroscopy grade solvents that have been redistilled in this manner are commercially available.)

II. EXTRACTION AND SEPARATION OF LIPIDS

A. *Introduction*

The Bligh and Dyer method (1) for lipid extraction is described here. Once a crude lipid extract is obtained, further processing depends on the desired analysis and specific requirements of the investigation. For instance, the determination of fatty acid composition of total cell lipids requires no additional handling of the crude extract other than preparation for gas - liquid chromatography (GLC) analysis. Similarly, phospholipid and neutral lipid analyses can be performed on crude lipid extracts. Other investigations may entail the determination of the fatty acid composition of phospholipids as an estimate of membrane fatty acid composition. This requires prior separation of neutral lipids and phospholipids.

Methods for the separation of neutral lipids and phospholipids are described in this section in addition to those for separations of individual phospholipids and individual neutral lipids and for the quantitation of each lipid class. These procedures and those described in Sections III and IV have been applied to resident mouse peritoneal macrophages (3, 4), rabbit alveolar macrophages (5, 6), guinea pig peritoneal polymorphonuclear leukocytes (5), human peripheral blood polymorphonuclear leukocytes (7), and human mononuclear phagocytes (8).

B. *Reagents*

(1) Chloroform, redistilled
(2) Methanol, anhydrous, redistilled
(3) Hexane, redistilled
(4) Benzene, redistilled
(5) Absolute ethanol

(6) Acetic acid

(7) Ether (hazardous)

(8) Perchloric acid (hazardous)

(9) β-Hydroxy butylated toluene (BHT)

(10) Chromatography reference compounds (these can be obtained from suppliers such as Supelco, Inc., Bellefonte, Pennsylvania; Analabs, North Haven, Connecticut; or Calbiochem-Behring Corp., La Jolla, California): phosphatidylcholine (PC), phosphatidylethanolamine (PE), phosphatidylserine (PS), phosphatidylinositol (PI), phosphatidylglycerol (PG), diphosphatidylglycerol (DPG), sphingomyelin (SM), cholesterol, cholesterol oleate, triolein, and oleic acid.

(11) Ammonium molybdate reagent. Dissolve 4.4 gm of ammonium molybdate in 200 - 300 ml glass distilled water; add 14 ml of concentrated sulfuric acid, and dilute to 1 liter.

(12) Reducing agent. Grind 30 gm of sodium bisulfite, 6 gm of sodium sulfite and 0.5 gm of 1,2,4-aminonapthol sulfonic acid (Aldrich Chemical Co., Milwaukee, Wisconsin) in a mortar until thoroughly mixed. Dissolve in glass distilled water, and bring the volume to 250 ml. Let stand for 3 hr in the dark and filter into an amber bottle. The concentrated reagent is stable for 6 - 8 weeks if kept refrigerated. Dilute 1:12 immediately before use. Caution: The diluted reducing agent should not be stored.

(13) Phosphate stock solution (0.1 M KH$_2$PO$_4$) Make up a 0.1 M solution (1.3609 gm/100 ml, molecular weight = 136.09) in glass distilled water and dilute 1:200 to obtain a 0.5 mM stock.

C. Procedure

1. Extraction of Lipids

Wash cell monolayers 2 - 3 times with phosphate-buffered saline and scrape into 0.9% NaCl with a polyethylene policeman. Rinse the dishes with another volume of 0.9% NaCl and combine in a conical, graduated centrifuge tube with a Teflon-lined screw cap. Alternatively, where cells are originally in suspension, wash the cells 2 - 3 times with phosphate-buffered saline and resuspend in 0.9% NaCl. In either case, the final concentration should not exceed 10^8 cells/ml. After measuring the final volume, remove aliquots for protein determinations.

Carry out extractions on ice with chilled solvents. Add 3.75 volumes of chloroform/methanol (1:2) containing 0.005% BHT to the cell suspension and mix. Let stand for 10 min with occasional mixing. At this stage the extracting medium consists of a single phase. The proportions of the components are chloroform/methanol/water (1:2:0.8). (If more than 15 × 10^7

cells are extracted, the cell debris and denatured protein may
be precipitated at this point by centrifuging at 550 g for 10
min at 4°C. Transfer the supernatant to another tube and proceed.)

To partition the extract into an organic phase and an
aqueous phase, add 1.25 volumes of chloroform, mix; then add
1.25 volumes of water and mix. (One volume is equivalent to
the original volume of cell suspension extracted.) The final
proportions of solvents are chloroform/methanol/water (2:2:1.8).

Centrifuge the tubes at 550 g for 10 min to promote phase
separation. Record the volumes of each phase. The interface
between the aqueous (upper) and organic (lower) phases is easily distinguished since denatured protein and cell debris collect
in this region. Remove the aqueous phase with a Pasteur pipette and discard. Collect the organic phase by using a Pasteur
pipette introduced well below the surface of the layer. Be
careful not to withdraw any residual aqueous phase. The cell
debris adheres to the wall of the extraction tube and does not
interfere with removal of the lower phase. Transfer the organic phase to another graduated screw-capped conical tube.
Adjust the volume of the sample to a convenient amount by evaporation under nitrogen or by the addition of chloroform.
Remove an aliquot for total lipid phosphorus determination to
a 16 × 150 mm test tube (Section II.C.5). The remaining lipid
extract may be stored at this stage under nitrogen at -20°C.
If the same extract is to be used for multiple analyses, sub-
divide the extract before further manipulations.

The minimum number of mouse peritoneal macrophages that
should be extracted for each type of lipid determination is
listed in Table I as a guide for other mononuclear phagocytes.

2. Separation of Neutral Lipids and Phospholipids

Separate neutral lipids and phospholipids on columns of
silicic acid. Activate the silicic acid by heating at least
1 hr at 110°C and suspend 400 mg in 20 ml of chloroform. Transfer the silicic acid slurry to a Pasteur pipette containing a
glass wool plug. The packed column should flow freely without
loss of resin and should not be allowed to dry.

Quantitatively transfer the lipid extract to the surface of
the resin. With this size column, the sample should not be
greater than 0.2 ml. The methanol contained in larger sample
volumes prevents total adsorption of phospholipid to the silicic
acid and results in incomplete separations. Elute the neutral
lipids (which do not adsorb to the silicic acid) with 10 ml
chloroform containing 0.005% BHT. Elute the phospholipids with
10 ml methanol containing 0.005% BHT, performing the solvent
changeover rapidly and smoothly.

TABLE I. *Guide for Lipid Determination*

Lipid determination	Representative value	Number macrophages
Total fatty acid analysis		2×10^7
Cholesterol determination	34 µg/mg cell protein (4)	7.5×10^6
Separation of neutral lipids from phospholipids followed by fatty acid analysis of neutral lipids and of phospholipids		4×10^7
Further separation into individual neutral lipid and phospholipid species with quantitation of lipid phosphorus		1×10^8
Total lipid phosphorus	162 nmol/mg cell protein (4)	7.5×10^6

3. Separation of Individual Neutral Lipids

Neutral lipids can be separated and visualized by two-dimensional thin-layer chromatography (TLC) as follows: Apply the concentrated chloroform effluent (∿0.1 ml) from the silicic acid column (II.B.2) to a 20 × 20 cm glass plate coated with a 250 µm thickness of silica gel. It is convenient if the plates are prepared without binders (2-D Redi Coats, Supelco, Inc., Bellefonte, Pennsylvania, or comparable products from other manufacturers) since the adsorbent remains soft and facilitates scraping. Develop the plate a distance of 19 cm in hexane/ethyl ether (90:10) and allow it to dry at room temperature for several minutes. Develop the plate in the second dimension in ethyl ether/benzene/ethanol/acetic acid (40:50:2:0.2). When thoroughly dry, visualize the resolved lipids with iodine vapors. This is accomplished by placing a few crystals of iodine in a glass TLC tank located in the fume hood, allowing the atmosphere to equilibrate at least 10 min and inserting the TLC plate until spots become visible. Remove the plate and, using a pin to mark the adsorbent, outline the location of each component. A permanent record is conveniently obtained by lightly tracing the pattern with a marker on an overlay of Saran wrap. Be sure to record the origin and solvent fronts if R_f values are to be calculated.

If only two-dimensional TLC of neutral lipids is to be performed and the phospholipid fraction is to be discarded, pre-

liminary separation on a silicic acid column (Section II.B.2)
is unnecessary. The crude lipid extract may be chromatographed
directly since the phospholipids remain at the origin and do
not affect neutral lipid separation.

4. Separation of Individual Phospholipids

Phospholipids contained in the methanol effluent of the
silicic acid column can be further separated by two-dimensional
TLC (20 × 20 cm plates, 2D-Redi Coats, Supelco, Inc.) (14).
Chloroform/methanol/concentrated ammonium hydroxide (65:25:5)
is the solvent for development in the first dimension. After
drying overnight in a vacuum desiccator, develop the chromatogram in the second dimension with chloroform/acetone/methanol/
acetic acid/water (30:40:10:10:5). Visualize and record the
results as described for neutral lipids. If only two-dimensional TLC of phospholipids is to be performed, prior silicic acid
chromatography is unnecessary. The neutral lipids move with
the solvent front in each dimension on TLC and do not affect recovery or resolution of individual phospholipids.

5. Quantitation of Lipid Phosphorus (9)

Lipid phosphorus determinations may be carried out on aliquots of the crude lipid extract (Section II.B) or on individual
phospholipids after separation by TLC (Section II.C.4). Transfer aliquots of crude extracts to 16 × 150 mm test tubes and
gently warm to remove organic solvents. Individual phospholipids
are scraped from TLC plates onto glassine weighing paper and
subsequently transferred to test tubes. Add 0.4 ml of perchloric acid to each tube and heat overnight at 80°C or until the solution is transparent. If large amounts of organic material are
present, the solution will have a brown color. This will not
interfere with phosphate determinations. However, if large
clumps of material are evident, continue heating until the
clumps are dispersed in order to achieve complete hydrolysis.
After cooling the tubes, add 2.4 ml of molybdate reagent and
2.4 ml of reducing agent. Mix. It is crucial that the molybdate reagent be added before or simultaneously with the reducing
agent. Place in boiling water for 10 min. Cool. Read the absorbance at 830 nm.

If samples contain silica gel, transfer the fluid portions
to separate centrifuge tubes before reading the absorbance
value. (Disposable plastic conical centrifuge tubes are convenient for this purpose but if glass tubes are employed they
should be acid washed.) Centrifuge at 1200 g for 30 min to
sediment the silica gel. Care should be taken in removing supernatants to ensure that the silica gel pellet is not disturbed.
The fine silica gel particles cause light scattering and result

in abnormally high absorbance readings. It is wise to scrape an area of a TLC plate that contains no lipid and utilize this material as a blank, processing it in parallel with lipid-containing samples throughout the entire procedure. When read against water, the absorbance of the blank should not be greater than 0.03 - 0.05.

Construct standard curves for phosphate determinations using appropriate amounts of a 0.5 mM KH$_2$PO$_4$ stock ranging from 0.005 μmol to 0.560 μmol. Add perchloric acid, followed by the molybdate and reducing agents, and develop the color by heating. (Overnight incubation at 80°C, however, is necessary.)

6. Quantitation of Neutral Lipids

If total content of triglyceride, cholesterol, and free fatty acids are to be determined, a convenient method of quantitation is GLC. A 2 ft × 1/8 in stainless steel column of 3% JXR on 100/120 Gas Chrom Q (Applied Sciences, State College, Pennsylvania) (10, 11) separates classes of neutral lipids. Detector response factors for standard lipids should be determined as described under Section III.C for fatty acid methyl esters.

The triglyceride fraction of a lipid extract can be further separated if desired. Selective enzymatic hydrolyses and subsequent quantitation of glycerol and fatty acids may also be performed. We have not directly quantitated triglycerides in mononuclear phagocytes but refer the reader to methods described by Christie (12). In macrophages, we have routinely determined the fatty acid composition of neutral lipids. Since macrophages contain no cholesterol ester and little mono- and diglycerides, the bulk of the fatty acids in the neutral lipid fraction reside in triglycerides. As a result, the triglyceride content can be calculated from the triglyceride fatty acid value.

D. Calculation of Data: Lipid Phosphorus Determination

(1) Standard samples

$$A_{830} \times \frac{5.2 + x}{5.2} = A_{830} \text{ (undiluted)}$$

where x = volume 0.5 mM KH$_2$PO$_4$ assayed.

$$\frac{\text{nmol phosphorus}}{\text{absorbance unit}} = \frac{y}{A_{830} \text{ (undiluted standard)} - A_{830} \text{ (blank)}}$$

where y = nmol phosphorus standard assayed.

(2) Unknown samples

$$A_{830} \times \frac{\text{nmol phosphorus}}{\text{absorbance unit}} = \text{nmol lipid phosphorus}$$

E. Critical Comments

It is important to note that highly charged, hydrophilic lipids do not partition quantitatively into the organic phase in either the Bligh and Dyer (1) or the Folch *et al.* (2) extraction. The complex gangliosides and a small portion of the acidic lipids are retained in the aqueous phase. On the other hand, small amounts of protein and amino acids separate with the bulk of the lipids into the organic phase. Reextraction of the separated phases does not appreciably increase the amount of macrophage lipids recovered and can cause the loss of lipid components from the organic phase. If desired, however, the aqueous phase and cell debris may be washed with chloroform/ methanol (19/1) in the original tube to recover the trace amount of residual lipids.

The preliminary separation of the crude lipid extract by silicic acid chromatography is a simple and efficient technique for resolving neutral lipids from phospholipids. There are several commercial sources of silicic acid. A sample of the product purchased should be tested by chromatographing a mixture of cholesterol, a triglyceride, an unesterified fatty acid, and at least one phospholipid using the method described in Section II.C. The chloroform and methanol fractions should be checked by TLC to ascertain the elution characteristics of the silicic acid. A useful single dimension TLC solvent for this purpose is ethyl ether/benzene/ethanol/acetic acid (40/50/2/0.2).

During silicic acid chromatography, the antioxidant (BHT) elutes with chloroform. It is therefore a precaution to add BHT to the eluting solvents to minimize potential lipid oxidation.

Several multistep elution procedures exist that achieve greater separation of lipid classes during silicic acid column chromatography than the one described here. These methods are outlined by Christie (12) and Carroll (13) but none precludes two-dimensional TLC in cases where complete resolution is desired.

The resolution of phospholipids by two-dimensional TLC is dependent on the humidity of the environment and the removal of ammonia following development in the first dimension. The procedure described here is based on that reported by Rouser *et al.* (14). The TLC plates are prepared according to their method to achieve resolution of all components. It is advisable to chromatograph standard mixtures containing PS, PI, SM, PC, PE

and PG to be certain that the conditions employed will effectively separate a sample of cell phospholipids. The identity
of resolved lipids can be verified by comparison with published
patterns and by using spray reagents (ninhydrin for PS and PE,
Dragendorf's reagent for PC and SM, and periodate-Schiff's
reagent for PI, PG, and DPG) (12, 15, and 16). Note that
sphingomyelin resolves into two species (17).

Quantitative removal of phospholipids from the silica gel
adsorbent following TLC is difficult to achieve unless several
extractions with organic solvents containing water and acid
are employed. Greater accuracy and reproducibility of lipid
phosphorus determinations and radioactivity measurements are
obtained if the adsorbent is scraped and analyzed directly
without prior elution of the phospholipid. This method is also
less time-comsuming.

The reproducibility of resolution of neutral lipids by two-
dimensional TLC is less sensitive to environmental factors.
The identification of resolved lipids should, however, again
rely on comparison with standard mixtures. Resolved neutral
lipids can be eluted from the silica gel adsorbent using chloroform, petroleum ether, or hexane.

Although several plates may be chromatographed simultaneously in the same chamber, it is strongly recommended that developing solvents consisting of more than one component not be used
a second time. Reproducibility of thin-layer chromatography is
greater where fresh solvents are employed and the equilibration
conditions are standardized.

III. DETERMINATION OF FATTY ACID COMPOSITION

A. *Introduction*

The fatty acid composition of lipids extracted from whole
cells, from isolated organelles, or from purified membrane
fractions can be determined using gas - liquid chromatography
(GLC). In a single GLC analysis, the fatty acyl components of
a mixture are separated on the basis of both molecular weight
and degree of saturation.

Generally, long-chain carboxylic acids such as the fatty
acids present in mammalian cells are derivatized prior to GLC
to maximize resolution and quantitation and to improve vola-
tility. Methyl ester derivatives are most commonly prepared.
Fatty acids are covalently bound in cell lipids as either esters or amide linkages and must be released before derivatization. Convenient one-step procedures have been described to
transesterify the fatty acids with methanol.

Where quantities of sample are relatively small, as with macrophage lipid extracts, it is desirable to purify the derivatized fatty acid methyl esters (FAMES) prior to GLC. This removes extraneous side products that overlap with FAMES during GLC and that generate baseline instability.

An excellent presentation of the theory of GLC with practical information for the investigator has been published (18) and is recommended to the reader. The following is a brief description of the essentials of GLC.

The column employed in GLC consists of particles of an inert solid support coated with a high boiling liquid, the stationary phase. The system is operated at elevated temperatures where the volatilized components of the sample mixture distribute between the liquid stationary phase and a mobile phase passing through the column. (The mobile phase is an inert carrier gas, most often nitrogen, helium, or argon.) Resolution mainly depends on the extent to which the partition coefficients of the various components differ; however, the carrier gas flow rate and the operating temperature are also important variables. Choosing the correct type and amount of liquid stationary phase and operating conditions can be difficult unless the investigator has had considerable experience. The catalogs available from suppliers (such as Supelco, Inc., Bellefonte, Pennsylvania; Applied Sciences, Inc., State College, Pennsylvania; or Analabs, North Haven, Connecticut) illustrate the applications of a variety of stationary phases in fatty acid analyses and should be consulted prior to column selection. We have used 1/8 in. × 10 ft. stainless steel columns packed with 10% SP-2330 on 100/120 Chromosorb WAW (Supelco, Inc.) for several years. These columns provide baseline separations of all common fatty acids from mammalian cells.

Several types of detectors are available for gas chromatographs. A flame ionization detector is most suited for fatty acid methyl esters. The correct proportions of hydrogen and air, used to maintain a flame, and carrier gas are required to obtain optimal sensitivity of the detector. The response of the detector to each fatty acid methyl ester should be determined periodically, preferably at the beginning of daily analyses, and when operating conditions are altered. A standard FAME of known mass is injected. The mass of the injected sample is equated with the area of the corresponding peak on the chromatogram, and data obtained for unknown samples should be corrected for variations in detector sensitivity to different compounds. Where absolute quantitation of each component is desired, an internal standard of known mass should be added to the lipid sample prior to derivatization for GLC analysis. The standard should be sufficiently resolved from the fatty acids of the sample such that its corresponding peak on the chromatogram can be properly measured. A convenient internal

standard for most mixtures of mammalian cell fatty acids is
17:0.

The following procedure is used routinely in our laboratory
to analyze cultured mouse peritoneal macrophage fatty acids.
It is directly applicable to macrophages obtained from other
sources as well as to peripheral blood monocytes.

B. Reagents

1. 6% Methanolic - HCl

Place 9 ml anhydrous methanol in an Erlenmeyer flask fitted
with a ground glass stopper (25 or 50 ml capacity). Chill on
ice. Add 1 ml redistilled acetyl chloride <u>dropwise</u> to the
methanol. Swirl the mixture after each addition. Methanol and
acetyl chloride combine in a highly exothermic reaction to form
HCl and methyl acetate. Use a fume hood and direct the mouth
of the flask to the back of the hood during the addition for
safety. It is essential that this reagent be anhydrous and
therefore prepared fresh before each use. Keep stoppered.

2. Drying Agent

$Na_2SO_4/NaHCO_3::4/1$ (w/w).

3. Standard Mixture of Fatty Acid Methyl Esters

An equal weights mixture of 16:0, 18:0, 18:1, 18:2, and
18:3 methyl esters and another consisting of 18:0, 18:1, 18:2,
18:3, and 20:4 methyl esters are available from various
sources. A special mixture containing 16:0, 18:0, 18:1, 18:2,
and 20:4 can be obtained by request from Nu-Chek Prep (Elysian,
Minnesota) and other sources.

4. Solvents (See also Section II.B)

Carbon disulfide
Hexane

C. Procedure

1. Preparation and Analysis of Fatty Acid Methyl Esters

Transfer the lipid sample to be analyzed to a 13 × 100 mm
test tube fitted with a Teflon-lined screw cap. Evaporate the
solvent under a stream of nitrogen and add 1 ml of 6% methanolic
HCl. (If the sample contains neutral lipids, also add 0.5 ml of

benzene.) Flush the tube well with nitrogen and place on a
heating block set at 80°C for 16 hr. Check the tightness of
the cap after 30 min to ensure that evaporation does not occur.
To terminate the reaction, cool the tubes and add 1 ml of distilled water. Extract the methyl esters with 3 ml of hexane.
(Centrifuge the tubes to promote phase separation.) Transfer
the organic (upper) phase to a separate screw-capped tube and
extract the aqueous twice with hexane. Combine the hexane extracts and let stand under nitrogen for at least 1 hr in 1 gm
of drying agent. Some of the drying agent should remain as
fine particles. If all of the drying agent clumps, a substantial amount of water is present. If this occurs, add an additional 1 gm of drying agent for an hour. Filter the hexane
extracts over coarse filter paper prewashed with hexane. Rinse
the original tube, drying agent, and filter paper with 2 - 3 ml
of hexane to recover quantitatively the fatty acid methyl esters. Concentrate the hexane to a small volume (∼0.2 ml).
Under a nitrogen atmosphere, apply the sample to a prescored
glass TLC plate coated with silica gel G (250-μm thick). A
TLC spotting box is useful for this purpose. Spot a fatty acid
methyl ester standard in an adjoining lane. Develop the chromatogram in hexane/ethyl ether/acetic acid (90:10:1) under a
nitrogen atmosphere. Separate the lanes by snapping the plate
along the prescored line and visualize the fatty acid methyl
ester standard with iodine vapors. Scrape the area in the
sample lane corresponding to the standard spot. Transfer the
silica gel to a Pasteur pipette plugged with glass wool. Elute
the methyl esters with chloroform containing 0.0005% BHT. Collect the eluant in a screw-capped test tube. The samples may
be stored under N_2 at this stage. To analyze the esters by GLC,
concentrate the solvent and transfer the FAMEs to a sample vial
fitted with a screw cap and a Teflon-coated silicone septum
(Tuf-bond discs, Pierce, Rockford, Illinois). Then evaporate
the solvent to dryness and immediately redissolve the residue
in a small volume (50 - 100 μl) of CS_2.
   The following conditions for gas chromatography have been
found in our laboratory to provide excellent resolution of
macrophage fatty acid methyl esters: 10 ft. × 1/8 in. stainless
steel column containing 10% SP-2330 on 100/120 Chromosorb WAW

Injector oven temperature:	250°C
Detector oven temperature:	250°C
Column oven temperature:	180°C

Carrier gas (nitrogen) flow rate:	40 ml/min
Hydrogen flow rate:	30 ml/min
Air flow rate:	300 ml/min

D. Calculation of GLC Data

1. Relative Molar Amounts of Sample Components

(a) Determination of detector sensitivity correction factor. The correction factor for each major component in the sample must be determined. To do this, a standard mixture containing known amounts of each component is analyzed. Then, for each component, a separate detector sensitivity correction factor (F) is obtained:

$$\frac{\text{Mass injected} \times (1/\text{MW})}{\text{Area}} = F(\text{moles/unit area}),$$

where area = area under the corresponding peak.

(b) Determination of the amount of each component present in an aliquot of the unknown mixture:

$$\text{No. of moles of } x = \text{Area}_x \times F_x$$

where F_x = detector sensitivity, correction factor for component x.

(c) Determination of mole % fatty acid composition

$$\frac{\text{No. of moles of } x}{\Sigma \text{ Moles}_{all\ components}} \times 100 = \text{Mole \% of } x.$$

2. Absolute Amounts and Relative Amounts of Sample Components

(a) Determination of detector sensitivity correction factor:

$$\frac{\text{Mass injected} \quad (1/\text{MW})}{\text{Area}} = F$$

(b) Determination of sample recovery:

$$\text{\% Recovery} = \frac{\text{Area}_i \times F_i}{\text{No. of moles}_i \text{ added to total sample}}$$

$$\times \frac{\text{Volume total sample}}{\text{Volume injected}} \times 100 ,$$

where i is an internal standard.

(c) Determination of the absolute amount of each sample component:

$$\text{No. of moles of} \quad = \frac{\text{Area}_x \times F}{\% \text{ Recovery}} \times \frac{\text{Volume total sample}}{\text{Volume injected}}$$

(d) Determination of mole % fatty acid composition:

$$\frac{\text{No. of moles of } x}{\Sigma \text{ Moles}_{all \ components}} \times 100 = \text{Mole \% of } x$$

E. *Critical Comments*

For each transesterification experiment, solvent blanks containing BHT should be processed and analyzed by GLC to identify contaminants and artifacts. Pretest new reaction vials by heating overnight in methanolic HCl to ensure that they are airtight.

Transesterifying agents other than methanolic HCl are available. A solution of 1 to 2% sulfuric acid in methanol transesterifies lipids much as methanolic HCl does but may lead to decomposition of polyunsaturated fatty acids. Boron trifluoride in methanol has been widely used. However, the reagent is hazardous and has a shelf life of 6 months. It is a stronger reagent than required for transesterifying fatty acids and yields artifacts that are observed on GLC. It is extremely useful however for rapid esterification of free fatty acids. Diazomethane is another reagent for esterifying free fatty acids but is extremely dangerous and does not methylate esterified fatty acids. We do not recommend its use by individuals with limited experience in organic chemistry laboratories. We prefer methanolic HCl as the reagent of choice since it hydrolyzes lipids and esterifies the fatty acids in a single step and is easily prepared fresh for each experiment. It thereby provides similar reaction conditions for all experiments. Furthermore, it is inexpensive and yields few artifacts. It should be noted however that acid-catalyzed transesterification of acylated lipids is slow and may not provide total hydrolysis of amide bonds such as exist in sphingolipids.

The purified fatty acid methyl esters are dissolved in CS_2 prior to GLC analysis. Since the flame ionization detector has a poor response to this solvent, the solvent peak on the chromatogram is relatively small. It does not interfere with the first fatty acid methyl ester peaks, unlike the solvent peaks of other common solvents.

IV.   DETERMINATION OF STEROL CONTENT AND COMPOSITION

A. *Introduction*

Cholesterol is the major sterol component of most mammalian cells. Absolute values of cholesterol are determined and reported either as mass or number of moles per milligram of cell protein. Therefore, an internal standard (5α-cholestane) is added to crude lipid extracts and values of cholesterol are corrected for recoveries of the standard. The major portion of cholesterol in cells is localized in membranes as a free sterol, but it can also be stored in the form of fatty acid esters. For this reason, lipid extracts of cells are saponified (base-catalyzed hydrolysis of esters) prior to sterol analysis. The percentage of cholesterol esters can be estimated, if desired, by determining cholesterol levels before and after saponification. A number of different extraction procedures for sterols have been described; however, the efficiencies of extraction have not always been determined. For this reason, we have used the method of Bligh and Dyer (1) (see Sec. II.C.1). This procedure is also convenient in that sterol and fatty acid analyses can be performed on the same lipid extract provided there is sufficient sample.

GLC is the method of choice for sterol analyses. Because of the free hydroxyl group, sterols are relatively polar compounds and must be esterified prior to analysis. Classically, trimethylsilyl derivatives of sterols (19) have been utilized but have certain drawbacks. In particular, the accumulation of deposits on GLC detector parts interferes with sensitivity and accurate quantitation. We have used instead acetate esters that are easily prepared and do not have these disadvantages (20). Because of recent advances in packings for GLC columns, it is now possible to analyze directly free sterols without derivatization.

B. *Reagents*

1. *Ethanolic - Potassium Hydroxide*

Place 10 gm of KOH in a 100-ml volumetric flask and add 40 ml of anhydrous absolute ethanol. Dissolve the KOH by swirling and bring the final volume to 100 ml with additional ethanol.

2. Sterol Standards

Cholesterol
5α-Cholestane

3. Solvents (See also Sections II.B and III.B)

Acetic anhydride (redistilled)
Pyridine (distilled over barium oxide)
Ethyl ether

C. Procedure

1. Sterol Extraction (See Section II.C.1)

Add 1 μg 5α-cholestane per 10^7 mononuclear phagocytes to
be extracted (4).

2. Saponification of Sterol Esters (21)

Transfer aliquots of chloroform - methanol extracts (Section
II.C.1) to screw-capped tubes and dry under a stream of nitrogen. After adding 1 ml of 10% KOH in ethanol/water (9:1, v/v),
flush the tubes with nitrogen and heat at 56°C for 30 min on a
heating block. Cool the solution and dilute with 2 ml of 0.58%
sodium chloride. Extract the nonsaponifiable lipids (including
sterols) twice with 3 ml of petroleum ether and once with 2 ml
of ethyl ether. Analyze the sterols in the pooled and concentrated organic phase directly or after conversion to their corresponding acetate derivatives.

3. Preparation of Sterol Acetate Esters (20)

Appropriate amounts of lipid extracts in screw capped test
tubes are taken to dryness under a stream of nitrogen. Add
0.2 ml of pyridine followed by 0.5 ml of acetic anhydride.
Flush the tube with nitrogen and heat at 65°C for 1 - 2 hr on
a heating block. After cooling, evaporate the solvents under
nitrogen. Dissolve sterol acetates in the appropriate amounts
of carbon disulfide.

4. GLC Analysis of Sterols and Sterol Acetates

Glass rather than stainless steel columns are used for
sterol analyses, since major losses of sterols occur on the
latter. We use a 1/4 in. × 6 ft glass column packed with 3%
OV-17 on 80/100 Chromosorb W HP (Supelco) under the following
operating conditions:

Injector oven temperature: 275°C
Detector oven temperature: 275°C
Column oven temperature: 250°C

Carrier gas (nitrogen) flow rate: 50 ml/min
Hydrogen flow rate: 30 ml/min
Air flow rate: 300 ml/min

D.   *Calculation of Data (See Sections III.D.2(a) and (b))*

E.   *Critical Comments*

As with fatty acid methyl esters, the response of the GLC detector to each sterol or sterol acetate must be determined (Section III.A). If the acetate derivatives of sterols are to be analyzed by GLC, standards must be prepared by the investigator since these derivatives are not commercially available. Generally, only cholesterol acetate need be synthesized. (5α-Cholestane, the internal standard, cannot be derivatized since it does not have a free hydroxyl group.)

Mouse peritoneal macrophages contain little, if any, cholesterol esters. For this reason, we routinely carry out GLC analyses on lipid extracts without prior saponification. However, the absence of cholesterol esters should not be assumed unless confirmed by the investigator for the cell type and cultivation conditions under consideration. This requires determining the amounts of cholesterol in lipid extracts before and after saponification and correcting for recovery of the internal standard.

GLC of nonsaponified lipid extracts can result in complex elution profiles since lipids other than sterols are eluted. This need not be a problem provided that baseline separation from cholesterol is obtained. Although the preparation of saponified lipid extracts requires an extra step, only nonsaponified lipids are analyzed which results in fewer artifacts on analysis.

REFERENCES

1.   E. G. Bligh and W. J. Dyer. A rapid method of total lipid extraction and purification. *Can. J. Biochem. Physiol.* 37: 911-917, 1959.
2.   J. Folch, M. Lees, and G. H. S. Stanley. A simple method for the isolation and purification of total lipids from

animal tissues. *J. Biol. Chem. 226*: 497-509, 1957.

3. E. M. Mahoney, A. L. Hamill, W. A. Scott, and Z. A. Cohn. Response of endocytosis to altered fatty acyl composition of macrophage phospholipids. *Proc. Nat. Acad. Sci. 74*: 4895-4899, 1977.

4. E. M. Mahoney, W. A. Scott, F. R. Landsberger, A. L. Hamill, and Z. A. Cohn. The influence of fatty acyl substitution on the composition and function of macrophage membranes. *J. Biol. Chem. 255*: 4910-4917, 1980.

5. R. J. Mason, T. P. Stossel, and M. Vaughan. Lipids of alveolar macrophages, polymorphonuclear leukocytes, and their phagocytic vesicles. *J. Clin. Invest. 51*: 2399-2407, 1972.

6. P. Elsbach. Uptake of fat by phagocytic cells, an examination of the role of phagocytosis. II. Rabbit alveolar macrophages. *Biochim. Biophys. Acta 98*: 420-431, 1965.

7. J. E. Smollen and S. B. Shohet. Remodeling of granulocyte membrane fatty acids during phagocytosis. *J. Clin. Invest. 53*: 726-734, 1974.

8. T. Stossel, R. J. Mason, and A. L. Smith. Lipid peroxidation by human blood phagocytes. *J. Clin. Invest. 54*: 638-645, 1974.

9. J. C. Dittmer, and M. A. Wells. Quantitative and qualitative analysis of lipids and lipid components. *In* "Methods in Enzymology," Vol. XIV (J. M. Lowenstein, ed.), pp. 486-487. Academic Press, New York, 1969.

10. A. Kuksis, L. Maral, and D. A. Gornall. Direct gas chromatographic examination of total lipid extracts. *J. Lipid Res. 8*: 352-358, 1967.

11. A. Kuksis, O. Stachnyk, and B. J. Holub. Improved quantitation of plasma lipids by direct gas-liquid chromatography. *J. Lipid Res. 10*: 660-667, 1969.

12. W. W. Christie. "Lipid Analysis." Pergamon Press, Oxford, 1973.

13. K. Carroll. Column chromatography of neutral glycerides and fatty acids. *In* "Lipid Chromatographic Analysis," Vol. 1, 2nd ed. (G. V. Marinetti, ed.), pp. 178-214. Dekker, New York, 1976.

14. G. Rouser, S. Fleischer, and A. Yamamoto. Two-dimensional thin layer chromatographic separation of polar lipids and determination of phospholipids by phosphorus analysis of spots. *Lipids 5*: 494-496, 1970.

15. J. G. Kirchner. "Thin-Layer Chromatography," pp. 150-186, 417-458. Interscience, New York, 1967.

16. E. Stahl, ed. "Thin-Layer Chromatography; A Laboratory Handbook." Springer, New York, 1969.

17. O. Renkonen. Thin-layer chromatographic analysis of subclasses and molecular species of polar lipids. *In* "Progress in TLC," Vol. II (A. Niederwieser and G. Patski,

eds.), p. 159. Ann Arbor Science Publishers, Ann Arbor, Michigan, 1971.

18. H. M. McNair and E. J. Bonelli. "Basic Gas Chromatography." Varian Aerograph, Walnut Creek, California, 1968.

19. W. D. Wood, P. K. Raju, and R. Reiser. Gas-liquid chromatographic analysis of monoglycerides as their trimethylsilyl ether derivatives. *J. Am. Oil Chem. Soc.* *42*: 161-165, 1965.

20. A. Kuksis. Newer developments in determination of bile acids and steroids by gas chromatography. *In* "Methods of Biochemical Analysis," Vol. 14 (D. Glick, ed.), pp. 325-454. Interscience, New York, 1967.

21. L. Sokoloff and G. H. Rothblat. Regulation of sterol synthesis in L-cells: Steady state and transitional responses. *Biochim. Biophys. Acta 280*: 172-181, 1972.

82

SYNTHESIS, CELLULAR TURNOVER, AND MASS OF CHOLESTEROL

Harry W. Chen
Andrew A. Kandutsch

I. GENERAL INTRODUCTION

Although cholesterol is one of the major lipid components
in the plasma membrane of animal cells, its role therein and
in other cell membranes is only beginning to be understood.
Perhaps the most important of its functions derives from its
interaction with phospholipids to regulate the fluidity of the
membranes. Since many biological activities of surface membranes, e.g., transport of nutrients, activity of membrane-
associated enzymes, and mobility of various receptors, are regulated by the fluidity of the membrane, the study of cholesterol
metabolism is important in understanding the control of these
activities. Macrophages appear to be of special interest in
this regard since they carry on many activities that involve the
plasma membrane including pinocytosis, phagocytosis, spreading
and migration, chemotaxis and binding to antigens, microorganisms, and other cells.

METHODS FOR STUDYING
MONONUCLEAR PHAGOCYTES

893

II. METHODS FOR DETERMINATION OF RATE OF CHOLESTEROL SYNTHESIS

A. *Introduction*

     Cholesterol in the plasma membrane can derive from endo-
genous biosynthesis, or from exchange with exogenous cholesterol, usually in the form of serum lipoproteins. The proportion
of cellular cholesterol derived from one or the other source is
dependent on the composition of the incubation fluid or growth
medium. In addition, compounds present in serum (specifically
oxysterols generated by the autoxidation of lipoprotein cholesterol) can specifically inhibit cholesterol synthesis (1).
To obtain a meaningful measure of the cells' ability to synthesize cholesterol, it is, therefore, desirable to incubate cells
either in chemically defined medium or in medium deficient in
serum lipids. Serum can be either delipidated by organic solvent extraction (2) or lipoproteins in serum can be removed by
sequential flotation centrifugation in a potassium bromide
gradient (3).
     Methods for determining absolute rates of cholesterol syn-
thesis by measuring the incorporation of ^{3}H from tritiated water
(4) or of ^{14}C from [1-^{14}C]octonoate (5) into the sterol have
been described. However both of these methods are subject to
limitations and involve assumptions regarding the equilibration
of radiolabeled compounds with various pools of intracellular
metabolites (4 - 6). A method that appears to be exempt from
these criticisms involves the use of a drug, triparanol, to
block a final step in cholesterol synthesis (7). The mass and
radioactivity of newly synthesized sterol (desmosterol) can
then be determined independent of the mass of cholesterol that
was present at the beginning of the rate experiment. These
procedures, especially the last, are technically rather complex.
     Analysis of more easily determined relative rates of syn-
thesis may provide information adequate to answer many questions,
at least in the early phases of an investigation. It should be
borne in mind, however, that such data might be affected by substantial changes in the kind and amount of nutrients that are
supplied to the cells. For this reason it is wise to base conclusions regarding rates of cholesterol synthesis upon studies
with more than one substrate. It is also desirable to correlate
measured rates of cholesterol synthesis with values for the
level of 3-hydroxy-3-methylglutaryl-coenzyme A (HMG-CoA) reductase activity (5). Under most conditions this enzyme activity
regulates the flow of intermediates along the pathway to cholesterol. Reductase activity levels appear to be independent of
any changes in the pool sizes of intermediate compounds. However both active and inactive forms of reductase appear to be
present in several cell types and the physiological role of the

inactive form is still unknown (8).

Following is a method we use routinely to measure relative rates of cholesterol synthesis in murine peritoneal macrophages stimulated by thioglycollate injection. Macrophages are obtained from mice by a procedure similar to the one described in Chapter 7 of this volume. Approximately 6×10^6 washed cells are allowed to attach in a 100-mm petri dish (e.g., Corning Tissue Culture Dish) for 10 min at $37°C$ in an incubator of humidified 5% CO_2 and 95% air. Medium with unattached cells is removed and the culture is washed twice with cold Ca and Mg-deficient phosphate-buffered saline solution. After the addition of a growth medium, these cells can be used immediately for the determination of cholesterol synthesis, or they can be cultured in a growth medium supplemented with 4 mg/ml delipidated serum proteins prepared from fetal calf serum (2). This concentration of protein is equivalent to that in medium containing 10% serum. Cells cultured in several kinds of commercially available media, including Waymouth MB 752/1, RPM1 1640, Ham's F-10, McCoy's 5a, and Eagle's minimum essential medium (MEM) exhibit comparable rates of cholesterol synthesis. If a long-term culture or dividing population of macrophages is needed, then the macrophage growth factors must be added to the medium as described by Defendi and his co-workers (9, 10).

B. Reagents

(1) $[1-^{14}C]$Acetate acid, sodium salt, 1-3 mCi/mmol (New England Nuclear). If the specific activity is higher than 1 mCi/mmole, dilute with sodium acetate to 1 mCi/mmol and then with growth medium to give 100 μCi/ml.

(2) 90% KOH, Dissolve 90 gm of KOH in 63.2 ml of H_2O

(3) 3 N HCl, Add 25.9 ml HCl to 74.1 ml of H_2O

(4) 35% Perchloric acid (PCA), add 50 ml of PCA (70% solution) (Fisher Scientific) to 50 ml of H_2O

(5) 6% PCA, Dilute the above solution with H_2O

(6) $[1,2-^3H(N)]$ Cholesterol, 40-70 Ci/mmol (New England Nuclear), dilute with ethanol to about 1 μCi/ml, used 20 ul/ml sample, which will give approximately 100,000 cpm

(7) Petroleum ether (Fisher Scientific)

(8) Anhydrous ether (Fisher Scientific)

(9) Cholesterol (Sigma, CH-K) Make a 2.5 mg/ml solution by dissolving 0.25 gm of cholesterol in 100 ml ethanol

(10) Nitrogen gas

(11) Chloroform (Fisher Scientific)

(12) Methanol (Fisher Scientific)

(13) Thin layer chromatography plate, Whatman LK5D Linear-K analytical TLC precoated plates (Pierce Chemical Co.),

which have 19 channels in one plate
(14) Toluene (Fisher Scientific)
(15) Ethyl acetate (Fisher Scientific)
(16) Rhodamine B (Sigma) solution, 0.1 gm in 100 ml of methanol
(17) Counting solution, toluene-Omnifluor (New England Nuclear) Dissolve 4 gm of Omnifluor in 1 liter of toluene
(18) ^{14}C-Labeled toluene (NES-006, 4×10^5 dpm/ml, New England Nuclear)
(19) Acetone (Fisher Scientific)
(20) Acetic acid (Fisher Scientific) 10% solution
(21) Digitonin, 0.5%, Dissolve 0.5 gm (Fisher Scientific) in 100 ml of 50% ethanol over steam
(22) Glacial acetic acid
(23) Calf thymus DNA (Sigma)

C. Procedure

(1) Discard the old medium if the cells have been cultured, wash the cells with 5 ml medium, add 5 ml of fresh prewarmed medium containing 20 μCi (20 μmol) of [1-^{14}C]acetate, and incubate at 37°C in a 95% air – 5% CO$_2$ incubator for 1 or 2 hr.

(2) Terminate the incubation by adding 0.5 ml 90% KOH and let the sample stand overnight.

(3) Pipet a 1-ml aliquot into a 15-ml centrifuge tube for the determination of DNA, as will be described later. Transfer the rest of the sample to a glass centrifuge tube (50 ml) and saponify it by autoclaving for 1 hr.

(4) After cooling to room temperature, add an equal volume of absolute ethanol and mix. Add [^{3}H]cholesterol approximately (100,000 cpm in 20 μl) as an internal standard for determining the recovery.

(5) Add 10 ml of petroleum ether, shake the sample for a few minutes and then transfer the petroleum ether fraction (top layer) to a 15-ml centrifuge tube. Extract the water phase again with another 5 ml of petroleum ether and combine the two extracts. The water phase may be saved for the determination of ^{14}C-labeled fatty acids (11).

(6) Add 0.1 mg of unlabeled cholesterol (0.04 ml of cholesterol solution) as a carrier, mix, and evaporate the petroleum ether to dryness with a stream of nitrogen gas.

(7) Dissolve the residue in 0.1 ml of chloroform:methanol (2:1) and spot the solution on a TLC plate.

(8) Desiccate the plate until dry and then develop it with toluene:ethyl acetate (2:1) in a covered glass tank. The level of the solvent should just be high enough to touch the bottom edge of the plate (about 90 ml in a thin layer chromatography tank from Supelco, Inc.).

(9) Remove the plate after the solvent front has ascended to about 1 in. below the top of the plate (45 to 60 min).

(10) Dry the plate in the air for a few minutes, spray with Rhodamine B solution, place the plate under uv light and mark the cholesterol band that shows as a faint yellowish band.

(11) Scrape the material within the band into a scintillation vial with a razor blade and add 0.5 ml of absolute ethanol.

(12) After a few minutes add 5 to 10 ml of toluene–Omnifluor solution.

(13) Count the radioactivity in the samples. The blank consists of a comparable segment of the silica gel layer from a channel on which no sample has been run. To calculate counting efficiency, a vial containing [^{14}C]toluene (about 10,000 dpm) is counted.

(14) An alternative method for cholesterol analysis uses digitonin precipitation. If one does not desire to use TLC chromatography, the sterol fraction can be separated by precipitation with digitonin, but an overnight wait for complete precipitation of sterol is required.

    (a) Start with the petroleum ether extract as described in step (5).

    (b) Evaporate the ether and add 6 ml of acetone:ethanol (1:1), 3 drops of 10% acetic acid, and 3 ml of digitonin solution, mix.

    (c) Add 0.5 mg of carrier cholesterol to the sample and mix; let the mixture stand overnight in dark place at room temperature.

    (d) Centrifuge the precipitate at 1000 g for 5 min.

    (e) Pour off the liquid and wash the precipitate with 6 ml of ether:acetone (2:1). Pour off the liquid and wash the sediment twice with 6 ml anhydrous ether.

    (f) Dry the sample until the ether has evaporated.

    (g) Add 1 ml of glacial acetic acid and mix until the sample dissolves.

    (h) Pipette a sample (e.g., 0.2 ml) of the solution into a scintillation vial, mix with 10 to 15 ml of toluene-Omnifluor solution and count the radioactivity.

(15) Determination of the DNA content of the culture.

    (a) Dissolve 10 mg of DNA (calf thymus) in 100 ml of 8% KOH. Dilute the DNA stock solution with 8% KOH solution to give a series of standard DNA solutions containing 5, 10, 25, 50, and 75 µg of DNA/ml.

    (b) Cool the 1 ml aliquot of the culture hydrolyzate from step C(3), and 1 ml aliquots of each of the DNA standard solutions in 15-ml centrifuge tubes. Carry out the next three steps on ice.

    (c) Add 1.5 ml of H$_2$O to each tube and neutralize the solution with 0.5 ml of 3 N HCl, mix.

    (d) Add 0.6 ml of 35% PCA to precipitate DNA (potassium

perchlorate will precipitate also).

(e) Collect the precipitate by centrifuging the samples at 4°C for 10 min at 1000 g.

(f) Wash the precipitate with 4 ml of 6% PCA, resuspend, centrifuge to collect the precipitate as before. Drain the tube.

(g) Add 4 ml of 6% PCA, resuspend, heat for 15 min at 90°C.

(h) Chill the tubes on ice and centrifuge for 10 min at 1000 g.

(i) Carefully remove the supernatant fluid to another tube.

(j) Read the absorbancy of the samples at 268 nm against a 6% PCA blank in a spectrophotometer.

D. Calculation of Data

Data are expressed as [^{14}C]acetate dpm incorporated into sterol per microgram of DNA per hour. In our experience, the rate at which ^{14}C is incorporated under these conditions into the cholesterol of mouse macrophages that are analyzed immediately after attachment to culture dish, is approximately 3 to 6 dpm/μg DNA/hr. After culturing in 10% delipidated serum for one day, the rate of incorporation increases to approximately 20 to 40 dpm/μg of DNA/hr.

Calculation of [^{14}C]acetate incorporation into sterol is as follows: We use a multiple-channel liquid scintillation counter (ISOCAP 300, Nuclear Chicago) for counting the dual-labeled sample. By counting [^{14}C]toluene (25 μl, 10,000 dpm) as described in step 13 one obtains ^{14}C:

Efficiency channel A = cpm channel A/10,000
Efficiency channel B = cpm channel B/10,000

From the number of counts in the samples, one calculates

Overlap of ^{14}C in channel A

$$= \frac{\text{cpm in channel B} \times \text{Efficiency } ^{14}\text{C in channel A}}{\text{Efficiency of } ^{14}\text{C in channel B}}$$

% Recovery

$$= \frac{\text{cpm in channel A} - \text{overlap}}{\text{cpm in } [^3\text{H}]\text{cholesterol added to the sample}}$$

Total dpm ^{14}C

$$= \frac{\text{cpm in channel B/Efficiency of } ^{14}\text{C in channel B}}{\% \text{ Recovery}}$$

^{14}C dpm in the sample

$$= \text{total } ^{14}\text{C dpm} - \text{total } ^{14}\text{C dpm of the blank}$$

E. Critical Comments

The procedure described makes use of 4 mM [1-^{14}C]acetate as the sterol precursor, which is relatively less expensive. It has been used extensively with many kinds of cell cultures and tissue slices and, with few exceptions, alterations in the rate of its incorporation into cholesterol correlate well with changes in the level of the regulatory enzyme in the pathway, HMG - CoA reductase. However the data obtained do not indicate absolute rates of cholesterol synthesis and results may be affected by alterations in mitochondrial and cytoplasmic pools of acetyl-CoA or its precursors. It is possible to substitute for 4 mM [1-^{14}C]acetate, 1 mM [1-^{14}C]octanoate or 3 mM [1-^{14}C]pyruvate with no other changes in the experimental procedure. However sodium octanoate is a detergent and we have some indication that at a concentration of 1 mM it is toxic to some cell cultures. [1-^{14}C]Pyruvate may prove to be a specially useful sterol precursor in view of a report by Gibbons and Pullinger (6) that at a concentration of 3 mM it was the sole precursor for all of the cholesterol made by surviving liver cell cultures. Thus, the absolute rate of cholesterol synthesis can be determined under this condition. It has not yet been shown that this is the case for other cell types and other conditions. A disadvantage is the high cost of the labeled pyruvate.

Since these precursors mentioned above will also be incorporated into fatty acids or converted into CO_2, it is sometimes useful to measure these rates in the same experiments (11) in order to determine whether or not alteration in rate of cholesterol synthesis under a specific experimental condition is specific. Furthermore, the production of CO_2 can be used to assess the general metabolism of the cells. The method described here has been used in our laboratory with murine peritoneal macrophages; it should be suitable for macrophages from other sources and from other species. Similar methods employing ^{14}C acetate as a precursor have been reported with macrophages of mice (12) and of rabbits (13) and with circulating human monocytes (14).

III. METHOD FOR INVESTIGATING THE CELLULAR TURNOVER OF
       CHOLESTEROL

A. Introduction

Most tissues and cell types including macrophages do not metabolize cholesterol other than to esterify it. The rate of cellular cholesterol "turnover" in these cases, then represents a balance between the acquisition of cholesterol (uptake plus synthesis) by the cell and the loss of cholesterol from the cell by means other than metabolic degradation. Recognized mechanisms by which cholesterol can be lost from the cell are: (a) extrusion as membrane vesicles (exfoliation) (15); (b) exchange with free cholesterol in lipoproteins; and (c) transfer from the cell membrane to acceptor (binding) protein present in the medium (16). Under some conditions all of these mechanisms may be in play. Their contributions to the total efflux can be separated by altering the medium in various ways or by fractionating the cholesterol recovered in the medium to differentiate exfoliated cholesterol (membrane-bound) from that bound to soluble proteins. When cultures are grown in lipid-free media as described above, the cell acquires cholesterol by synthesis alone and it is lost from the cell, principally if not solely, by a combination of exfoliation and transfer from the plasma membrane to acceptor proteins in the medium. Under these conditions, the cellular cholesterol can be prelabeled by incubating the culture with $[2-^{14}C]$mevalonate, which is used almost exclusively for the biosynthesis of polyisoprenoid compounds (principally cholesterol), and the efflux of the labeled cholesterol from the cells into the culture medium can be determined as outlined below.

B. Reagents

$[2-^{14}C]$Mevalonic acid lactone (27.3 mCi/mmol from New England Nuclear): Evaporate the benzene in the vial and dissolve the lactone with culture growth medium (e.g., Waymouth MB 752/1 or McCoy's 5a medium).

Handifluor (Scintillation fluid, Mallinckrodt Chemical Works, St. Louis, Missouri).

C. Procedures

(1) Prepare cultures of macrophages in $100-cm^2$ culture dishes as described in the previous section and incubate them in 5 ml growth medium supplemented with 4 mg/ml of delipidated serum proteins and 1 to 2 μCi of $[^{14}C]$mevalonic acid lactone. The incubation is carried out at 37°C for 16 hr or longer in order to allow equilibration of newly synthesized $[^{14}C]$cholesterol with the total cholesterol pool.

(2) After the incubation, discard the used medium and wash the cells three times with 5 ml volume of fresh medium.

(3) Add 5 ml of fresh medium and incubate the cells for 30 min to allow efflux from the cells of unused $[^{14}C]$mevalonate.

(4) Discard the incubation medium, add 5 ml of experimental

medium, e.g., medium containing no proteins, or containing
4 mg/ml of delipidated serum proteins or 10% fetal bovine serum.

(5) After incubation for an appropriate time period, e.g.,
1 hr or 4 hr, the medium is removed, and centrifuged at
100,000 g for 1 hr. A 2 ml aliquot of the supernatant fluid is
mixed with 10 ml of Handifluor and the radioactivity counted.
The radioactivity in the pellet, which represents dead cells
and membrane vesicles, can be counted after discarding the remaining supernatant fluid, resuspending the residue with 2 ml
of H_2O and then mixing it with 10 ml Handifluor. There is very
little activity in this particulate fraction under the experimental conditions described herein.

(6) Add 5 ml 0.9% NaCl solution and 0.5 ml 90% KOH to the
cells. The cellular DNA content and the radioactivity in the
cellular cholesterol are determined by the procedures described
in the last section. An aliquot of the petroleum ether extract
containing the cellular cholesterol as listed in Section II.C.5
can be analyzed for the mass of cholesterol as is described in
the following section, and the mass of cholesterol passed from
the cells into the medium can then be calculated. Under precisely controlled culture conditions, these values may be taken
as approximating the rate of cellular turnover.

D. Calculation

$$\text{Specific activity of cholesterol} = \frac{\text{dpm in cellular cholesterol/µg DNA}}{\text{µg cellular cholesterol/µg DNA}}$$

$$= \text{dpm/µg of cellular cholesterol}$$

$$\text{Rate of cellular cholesterol turnover (µg/hr/µg DNA)} = \frac{\text{dpm in medium}}{\text{dpm/µg cellular cholesterol} \times \text{hr incubation} \times \text{µg DNA}}$$

Under the conditions described, with delipidated serum proteins present in the medium at a concentration of 4 mg/ml, the
rate of ^{14}C release from the cells into the medium was about
50 - 60 dpm/µg DNA/hr. The mass amount of cholesterol in the
cells was about 0.4 µg/µg DNA. About 2% of the total cholesterol was transferred from the cells to the medium per hour.

E. Critical Comments

The method assumes that labeled cholesterol synthesized
from [^{14}C]mevalonate has equilibrated with all cholesterol
pools within the cells before the rate of its efflux is measured. It also assumes that negligible amounts of the effluxed
cholesterol are taken back into the cells. While these assumptions seem reasonable, they have not been tested. The utility
of the procedure is limited to a set of culture conditions that
exclude a high rate of exchange between cellular cholesterol
and lipoprotein cholesterol.

IV. METHOD FOR DETERMINING CHOLESTEROL MASS

A. Introduction

Many methods for measuring cholesterol are available and
are in common use for determining blood and tissue cholesterol
levels. Nearly all of them involve the generation of a
chromophore that is measured with a spectrophotometer. They
vary in convenience, sensitivity, and specificity. Examples of
the use of colorimetric methods to measure the concentration of
cholesterol in cell cultures are given in references (17)
through (19). The gas chromatographic method for assaying
cholesterol described below has several advantages over colorimetric methods, the principal ones being a high degree of
specificity (freedom from interference) and the capability of
identifying and quantifying other sterols if they are present.
Its disadvantages are the requirement for an expensive instrument, although these are now fairly widely available, and the
relatively long period of time required for each assay. The
choice of method, therefore, depends in large part upon the
number of assays to be conducted and the requirements for accuracy and specificity. If large numbers of assays are to be
carried on routinely the use of a colorimetric method may be
indicated.

B. Reagents

   (1) Cholesterol (Sigma, S grade); dissolve 5 mg (accurately
       weighed) in 5 ml benzene
   (2) 5β-Cholestan-3β-ol (Applied Science Laboratories); dis-
       solve 5 mg (accurately weighed) in 5 ml of benzene
   (3) Chloroform:methanol, 2:1 (v/v), (both solvents Fisher,
       certified grade)

(4) $MgCl_2$ solution (0.03%): dissolve 640 mg of $MgCl_2 \cdot 6\ H_2O$
    in 1 liter of H_2O
(5) Nitrogen gas (Matheson, extra dry)
(6) KOH in ethanol (5%): dissolve 5 g KOH in 100 ml of 95%
    ethanol
(7) HMDS Reagent in pyridine (Analabs, Inc.): a mixture of
    10 parts of hexamethyldisilazane, 2 parts of trimethyl-
    chlorosilane and 1 part pyridine

We use a Hewlitt-Packard Model 5830A gas - liquid chromatography apparatus, with a flame ionization detector and automatic peak integrator equipped with a 1/4 in. × 6 ft glass column
packed with 3% AN 600 (liquid phase) on Anachrom Q_2, Mesh 110-
120 (solid phase) both from Analabs, Inc.

C. Procedure for Determining Free and Total Cholesterol

(1) If both free and total cholesterol are to be determined,
an amount of cells containing between 5 and 20 µg of cholesterol
(a confluent culture in a 100-mm petri dish) is harvested usually by careful scraping with a rubber policeman, and pelleted by
centrifugation.

(2) The pellet is resuspended in 0.5 ml of H_2O to give a
total volume of about 0.6 ml and sonicated briefly (20 sec).

(3) A sample (20 µl) may be taken for the determination of
total protein (20), or a larger (0.1 ml) aliquot may be taken
for DNA analysis as described in Section B.

(4) An aliquot (usually 0.5 ml) of the remainder of the cell
homogenate is placed in a 15-ml glass centrifuge tube, 10 µg of
5β-cholestan-3β-ol (10 µl of standard solution) and 20 volumes
(usually 10 ml) of chloroform/methanol, 2/1, is added. The mixture is briefly vortexed.

(5) Particulate matter is removed by filtration through
filter paper in a small Buchner funnel, the filtrate is collected in a 15-ml centrifuge tube, and 0.2 volumes of aqueous
0.03% $MgCl_2$ is added.

(6) After mixing by vortexing, the mixture is centrifuged
at low speed.

(7) The upper phase is drawn off and discarded including any
material between the two phases.

(8) The volume of the lower phase is brought to 10 ml with
$CHCl_3$, an aliquot (approximately 0.5 ml) is taken for the determination of lipid phosphorus (21), and two large aliquots
(usually of equal size) accounting for most of the remainder of
the extract are taken for assay of free cholesterol and measurement of total sterol.

(9) For the determination of free cholesterol, the aliquot
of the lipid extract is evaporated to complete dryness in a 3 ml
centrifuge tube under a stream of N_2, with gentle heat from a

water bath. The sides of the tube are rinsed down with a few drops of benzene, the benzene is evaporated, and 20 µl of hexamethyldisilizane reagent are added.

(10) The reaction mixture is heated at 50° for 15 min and from 1 to 5 µl are injected into the column. Column temperature is 255° and carrier gas (N_2) flow rate is 40 ml/min. Under these conditions the silyl ethers of the 5β-cholestan-3β-ol internal standard and the cellular free cholesterol are eluted with retention times of approximately 5.8 and 7.5 min, respectively.

(11) The aliquot taken for the determination of total cholesterol is dried in a 15 ml centrifuge tube under N_2 and saponified with 1.5 ml of 10% KOH in 95% ethanol at 55° for 2 hr. Water (1.5 ml) and 5 ml of petroleum ether are then added, the tube is shaken for at least 1 min, and the petroleum ether layer is drawn off. The lower phase is reextracted with 5 ml of petroleum ether and the combined extracts are dried under nitrogen. Silylation of the dried residue and gas chromatography are carried out as described for the free cholesterol assay.

D. Calculation

Peak areas for standard cholesterol and 5β-cholestan-3β-ol are determined by averaging values obtained by injecting various amounts of the standard solutions.

The method for calculating either free or total cholesterol is

$$
\begin{aligned}
&\text{µg of cholesterol} \\
&\text{in the homogenate} = \frac{\text{Peak area for 1 µg of 5β-cholestan-3β-ol standard}}{\text{Peak area for 1 µg of cholesterol standard}} \\
&\text{(free or total)}
\end{aligned}
$$

$$
\times \frac{\text{Peak area for cholesterol in the injected sample}}{\text{Peak area for 5β-cholestan-3β-ol in the injected sample}}
$$

$$
\times \text{µg of 5β-cholestan-3β-ol added to the cell homogenate}
$$

The amount of esterified cholesterol is obtained by subtracting the value for free cholesterol from that for total cholesterol. Values can be expressed in terms of total cell protein, DNA, or cellular phospholipid. The standard deviation of the cholesterol measurements is approximately ±4%.

E. *Critical Comments*

The procedure does not permit accurate determination of small amounts of esterified cholesterol equal to 5% or less of the total cholesterol. Under the conditions we have used to culture macrophages (described above), significant amounts of esterified cholesterol were not detected. In cases where values for esterified cholesterol are not required, or when amounts of esterified cholesterol have been established as insignificant, a determination of either total cholesterol or free cholesterol may be all that is necessary.

Acknowledgments

Oral L. Applegate and Elaine P. Shown provided assistance on experimental part of this work. This investigation was supported by Grant GM22900 awarded by General Medical Sciences Institute, and by Grant CAO2758 from National Cancer Institute, National Institutes of Health.

REFERENCES

1. H. W. Chen and A. A. Kandutsch. Cholesterol requirement for cell growth: Endogenous synthesis versus exogenous source. *In* "The Nutritional Requirement of Vertebrate Cells *In Vitro*" (R. G. Ham and C. Waymouth, eds.). University of Cambridge Press, New York and London, 1981.
2. G. H. Rothblat, L. Y. Arbogast, L. Ouellette, and B. V. Howard. Preparation of delipidized serum protein for use in cell culture system. *In Vitro 12*: 554-557, 1976.
3. M. S. Brown, S. E. Dana, and J. L. Goldstein. Regulation of 3-hydroxy-3-methyl-glutaryl coenzyme A reductase activity in human fibroblasts by lipoproteins. *Proc. Nat. Acad. Sci. USA 70*: 2162-2166, 1973.
4. M. R. Takshmanan and R. L. Veech. Measurement of rate of rat liver sterol synthesis *in vitro* using tritiated water. *J. Biol. Chem. 252*: 4667-4673, 1977.
5. J. M. Dietschy and M. S. Brown. Effects of alterations of the specific activity of the intracellular acetyl CoA pool on apparent rates of hepatic cholesterogenesis. *J. Lipid Res. 15*: 508-516, 1974.
6. G. F. Gibbons and C. R. Pullinger. Utilization of endogenous and exogenous sources of substrate for cholesterol biosynthesis by isolated hepatocytes. *Biochem. J. 177*: 255-263, 1979.

7. G. F. Gibbons and C. R. Pullinger. Measurement of the absolute rates of cholesterol biosynthesis in isolated rat liver cells. *Biochem. J. 161*: 321-330, 1977.

8. S. E. Saucier and A. A. Kandutsch. Inactive 3-hydroxy-3-methylglutaryl-coenzyme A reductase in broken cell preparations of various mammalian tissues and cell cultures. *Biochim. Biophys. Acta 572*: 541-556, 1979.

9. M. Virolainen and V. Defendi. Dependence of macrophage growth *in vitro* upon interaction with other cell type. *In* "Growth Regulating Substances for Animal Cells in Culture" (V. Defendi and M. Stoker, eds.), pp. 67-85. The Wistar Institute Press, 1967.

10. E. R. Stanley, M. Cifone, P. E. Heard, and V. Defendi. Factors regulating macrophage production and growth: Identity of colony-stimulating factor and macrophage growth factor. *J. Exp. Med. 143*: 631-647, 1976.

11. A. A. Kandutsch and S. E. Saucier. Prevention of cyclic and Triton-induced increases in hydroxymethylglutaryl coenzyme A reductase and sterol synthesis by puromycin. *J. Biol. Chem. 244*: 2299-2305, 1969.

12. Z. Werb and Z. Cohn. Cholesterol metabolism in the macrophage. I. The regulation of cholesterol exchange. *J. Exp. Med. 134*: 1545-1569, 1971.

13. A. J. Day and N. H. Fidge. Incorporation of ^{14}C-labeled acetate into lipids by macrophages *in vitro*. *J. Lipid Res. 5*: 163-168, 1964.

14. A. M. Fogelman, J. Seager, P. A. Edwards, M. Hokom, and G. Popjak. Cholesterol biosynthesis in human lymphocytes, monocytes, and granulocytes. *Biochem. Biophys. Res. Commun. 76*: 167-173, 1977.

15. W. J. Van Blitterswijk, P. Emmelot, H. A. M. Hilkmann, E. P. M. Oomen-Meulemans, and M. Inbar. Differences in lipid fluidity among isolated plasma membranes of normal and leukemic lymphocytes and membranes exfoliated from their cell surface. *Biochim. Biophys. Acta 467*: 309-320, 1977.

16. Z. Werb and Z. Cohn. Cholesterol metabolism in the macrophage. II. Alterations of subcellular exchangeable cholesterol compartments and exchange in other cell types. *J. Exp. Med. 134*: 1570-1590, 1971.

17. J. De Gier and L. L. M. Van Deenen. Some lipid characteristics of red cell membranes of various animal species. *Biochim. Biophys. Acta 49*: 286-296, 1961.

18. M. H. Gottlieb. The limited depletion of cholesterol from erythrocyte membranes on treatment with incubated plasma. *Biochim. Biophys. Acta 433*: 333-343, 1975.

19. M. Inbar and M. Shinitzky. Increase of cholesterol level in the surface membrane of lymphocyte cells and its inhibitory effect on ascites tumor development. *Proc. Nat.*

Acad. Sci. USA 71: 2128-2130, 1974.

20. M. Lees and S. Paxman. Modification of the Lowry procedure for the analysis of proteolipid protein. *Anal. Biochem. 47*: 184-192, 1972.

21. L. Sokoloff and G. H. Rothblat. Sterol to phospholipid molar ratios of L cells with qualitative and quantitative variations of cellular sterol. *Proc. Soc. Exp. Biol. Med. 146*: 1166-1172, 1974.

83

SOLUTE UPTAKE AND MEMBRANE TRANSPORT BY MONONUCLEAR PHAGOCYTES

Phyllis R. Strauss

I. INTRODUCTION

The transport of small nutrients, both electrolytes and nonelectrolytes, is a membrane function that also serves as an excellent indicator of cell health. In addition, knowledge of transport is important to the worker interested in macromolecular biosynthesis, degradation, or turnover because these processes withdraw from or feed into intracellular precursor pools. Specific activity of pools, in turn, depends on the rate at which small molecules enter and leave. Thus, alteration in influx, which feeds the pool, or efflux, which bleeds the pool, during the course of an experiment may alter the pool's size or its specific activity, thereby altering apparent rates of synthesis or degradation.

The total amount of solute that a cell accumulates during any interval is the reflection of a number of dynamic processes. These include: (1) influx of the solute across the plasma membrane by one of several mechanisms described below; (2) trapping

by metabolic conversion to a product that can no longer penetrate the membrane, e.g., phosphorylation of nucleosides or incorporation of amino acids into protein; (3) efflux of the
solute out of the cell. The term uptake is used to denote the
sum of all of these processes. Only the first and third components, influx and efflux, involve movement across the plasma
membrane. In the discussion that follows, methods are presented
that make it possible to dissect the flux component from subsequent metabolic steps. The principle in both methods is rapid
separation of incubation medium from cells.

Small molecules enter and leave the cell primarily via two
processes. One is passive diffusion, which is nonspecific and
nonsaturable. The other is a carrier-mediated process known as
facilitated diffusion. I shall refer to the second as transport
and stress that measuring transport requires measuring movement
of solute from one side of membrane to the other. In other
words, this represents flux, which in animal cells often requires extremely rapid measurements as short as or shorter than
4 sec. Neither of these processes requires energy or concentrates permeant against a gradient inside the cell. It is also
presumed that permeant metabolism such as the phosphorylation
usually occurs after influx. The energy-requiring process known
as active transport, which concentrates permeant inside the cell
against a gradient, probably uses the same membrane carriers as
are used by facilitated diffusion. The reader is referred to
Heinz (1) for further consideration of active transport. It
should be emphasized that active transport refers to accumulation of unmetabolized permeant.

Two methods are described here, one suitable for cells that
adhere rapidly to glass and the other for cells in suspension.
The first has been applied to rabbit (2 - 6) and mouse (7) phagocytes; the second has been applied to rabbit phagocytes (6)
as well as mouse lymphocytes (8, 9). Both methods differentiate
passive diffusion from carrier-mediated transport at all time
intervals.

For detailed discussions of membrane transport processes in
eukaryotic cells, the reader is referred to several recent reviews: Heinz (1) and Kotyk and Janecek (10) on theoretical aspects, Guidotti (11) and Christensen (12) on amino acid transport, Paterson (13), Berlin (14), and Plagemann (15) on nucleoside transport, and Hatanaka (16) on sugar transport. The investigator should keep in mind that many solutes are transported
by several systems. This is particularly true of amino acids in
certain cultured cells (12).

II.   REAGENTS

A. *Transport by Adherent Cells*

(1) Circulating water bath

(2) Transport box (2) to ensure maintenance of desired temperature. The box consists of a Plexiglass base (39 × 26 × 6.5 cm^3) with a copper plate (0.6 cm thick) as the top surface. Two water inlets on the back of the box are connected to the water bath that circulates water at a controlled temperature. A hollow Plexiglass cover (37.4 × 13.9 × 5.0 cm^3) serves to create a temperature-controlled space over the rear area of the copper plate, since water from the circulating bath is also allowed to flow through the top of the cover. A wet paper towel is placed on the surface of the copper plate under the cover to provide humidity. Aluminum bars (33.5 × 0.9 × × 0.3 cm^3) serve to move groups of monolayers from one area of the box to the other.

(3) Round microscope coverslips, 22 or 12 mm in diameter, No. 2 thickness

(4) Forceps (reverse action)

(5) Radioactive transport substrate repurified by one of several ascending paper chromatography systems described by Fink *et al.* (17). The strip corresponding to the unlabeled standard is cut out and the purified radiolabeled compound eluted in a very small volume (less than 1 ml) of water or phosphate-buffered saline (PBS).

(6) Transport test solutions, prewarmed to the desired temperature in the water bath. One half ml solution is allocated for each 22 mm coverslip. While concentrations of permeant in different solutions are chosen and prepared in PBS as described below, the amount of repurified radioisotope is maintained at 1 - 2 μCi/ml.

(7) Stopwatch

(8) 0.5 *N* KOH containing phenol red indicator

(9) 10% Perchloric acid (PCA)

(10) Scintillation vials, wide mouth, low potassium glass (Rochester Scientific, Rochester, New York)

(11) Scintiverse (Fisher Scientific, Medford, Massachusetts) or other scintillation cocktail that will absorb at least 1.5 ml water per 10 ml cocktail

(12) Scintillation counter

B. *Transport by Cells in Suspension*

(1) Water bath

(2) Microfuge at room temperature

(3) 400-μl Polyethylene microfuge tubes (Brinkman Instruments, Westbury, New York). The tubes should be checked because some varieties form hairline cracks during the final centrifugation.

(4) Silicone oil mixtures: mixture of Dow Corning silicone oil 550 and 510 (4:6) or Dow Corning silicone oil 550 and 556 (1:1), well mixed daily (see Section III.E)

(5) 10% Perchloric acid (PCA)

(6) Fisher fibrin tips and Fibrin gun (Fisher Scientific, Medford, Massachusetts)

(7) Isotope previously repurified as described above.

(8) Transport test solutions prewarmed to the desired temperature in the water bath. Three tenths ml solution is prepared for each determination. The concentration of permeant and radioisotope individually should be 3/2 the desired final concentration. While the permeant concentration may vary, the amount of repurified radioisotope in the test solution is maintained at 4 - 6 μCi/ml.

(9) - (14) As above, Section II.A.(7) - (12)

C. *Intracellular Volume Measurements*

(1) ^3H_2O, Originally at 25 mCi/ml (Schwartz-Mann, Orangeburg, New York), diluted to 1.25 mCi/ml with distilled water.

(2) [^{14}C]Sucrose, about 500 mCi/mM (Schwartz-Mann, Orangeburg, New York).

(3) Test solution for a standard experiment consisting of 5 different cell concentrations, each examined in quadruplicate: 60 μl ^3H_2O, 600 μl ^{14}C-sucrose, 6000 μl buffer.

III. PROCEDURES

A. *Transport by Adherent Cells Determined by the Coverslip Method*

Macrophages are washed three times in phosphate-buffered saline (10 mM PO_4 pH 7.4; 0.15 M NaCl) and resuspended at 6×10^5 cells/ml for subsequent adherence to 22 mm coverslips. Four coverslips for each point are placed on an aluminum bar located in the humidity controlled back of the transport box. One half ml cell suspension is applied to each coverslip and allowed to incubate 30 min. If smaller coverslips are used, the volume applied will be smaller and the corresponding number of cells per milliliter must be greater to attain the same final number of cells on each coverslip. After 30 min virtually

all the cells attach and will remain so despite vigorous washing
in multiple changes of PBS, either at 0°C or at room temperature. The bar is then brought to the front of the box without
disturbing the monolayers. Each coverslip is drained on paper
towels to remove excess medium and replaced on the bar. The
coverslips are handled by means of forceps. The transport test
is initiated immediately by dripping test solution previously
warmed to 37°C onto the monolayer as the stopwatch is started.
Several seconds before the end of the test, the monolayer is
drained of the test medium. The uptake process is terminated
at the desired moment by dipping the cover slip into iced PBS
and rinsing vigorously through four changes of iced PBS. After
the back of the coverslip is wiped, the monolayer is placed
face up inside the cover of a scintillation vial. Upon drying,
the glass is crushed and tapped gently into the scintillation
vial. If smaller coverslips are used, they can be placed directly into the scintillation vial without crushing.

Cellular material is digested with 1.0 ml of 0.5 N KOH containing phenol red for at least 30 min at room temperature.
The base is neutralized by dropwise addition of 10% PCA. After
After the scintillant (10 ml) is added, the vial is capped
and vigorously shaken. Scintillation spectrometry should include efficiency determinations for each vial since significant
quenching of tritium can occur under these conditions. In this
laboratory efficiencies range between 25 - 42% under these conditions. Aliquots (10 μl) of each transport test solution must
also be counted under the same conditions in order to determine
actual dpm/mole in the transport test solution.

Initial experiments should determine (1) whether there is
time-dependent association of radiolabeled permeant (see Fig. 1),
and (2) how much of the uptake of substrate is due to passive
diffusion and how much can be assigned to a carrier-mediated
process, (see Figs. 1 and 2). Monolayers in quadruplicate are
incubated for 4, 8, 12, 16, 20, and 60 sec with radiolabeled
substrate at a low concentration, 10 or 20 μM (1-2 μCi/ml);
an intermediate concentration, usually 100 μM (1 - 2 μCi/ml);
and a high concentration 10 or 20 mM (1-2 μCi/ml). At this
stage in the project, cell-associated radioactivity at the lowest specific activity (0.1 - 0.2 mCi/mM) is assumed to represent nonspecific, nonsaturable, and noncarrier-mediated processes. Thus, these dpm at each time interval can be subtracted from dpm that are cell associated at lower concentrations over the same time interval. In Fig. 1 the open circles
represent uptake measured at 20 μM; the closed circles indicate
uptake measured at 1000 μM and the open triangles indicate cell-
associated radiolabel when the external concentration was 20 mM.
The last is interpreted as the diffusion control. The assumption is verified in later experiments when concentration dependence is examined.

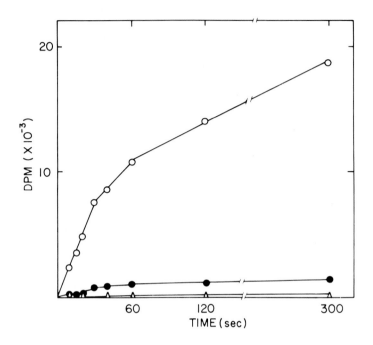

*Fig. 1. Time dependence of phenylalanine uptake (total
radiolabel). Phenylalanine uptake by 3 × 10⁵ macrophages was
measured at external phenylalanine concentrations of 20 µM (o),
1000 µM (•) and 20,000 µM (Δ). Total cell associated radiolabel after thorough washing is presented as a function of time.
Initial rates hold for about 30 sec. At early times the radiolabel, which is cell associated at 20 mM (Δ), comprises a
greater percentage of the uptake measured at lower concentrations than at later times.*

The radioactivity per unit volume should be the same at all
the substrate concentrations. However, small differences in
the dpm/ml can be accommodated by calculation. For example,
the transport test solution may be 50,000 dpm/10 µl, while the
diffusion test solution may be 60,000 dpm/10 µl. Therefore,
the radioisotope, which is cell-associated at 10 mM, must be
multiplied by 1.2 before the subtraction is carried out. The
diffusion component usually represents 2 - 8% of the cell-
associated radiolabel when the external concentration of the
permeant is the low K_m concentration. The difference between
total cell-associated dpm and dpm that are cell-associated at

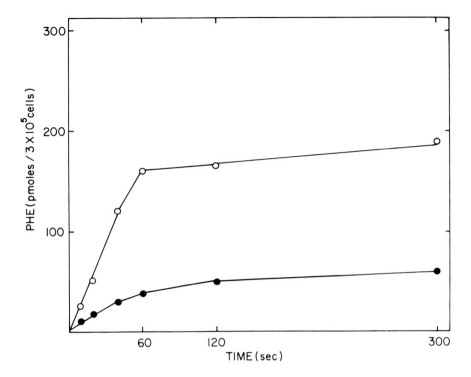

Fig. 2. Time dependence of phenylalanine transport. In an experiment similar to the one presented in Fig. 1, the dpm which are cell associated at 20 mM external phenylalanine have been subtracted from cell-associated radiolabel at lower concentrations. The remainder has been converted to pmoles transported by 3 × 10⁵ cells. (●), 20 μM phenylalanine; (○), 1000 μM phenylalanine. In this figure it is clear that initial rates hold for no longer than 30 sec.

the lowest specific activity (normalized) is used to calculate moles of permeant transported. The difference is divided by the specific activity (dpm/mole) of the transport test solution. If there is no difference, no measurable carrier-mediated transport has occurred. Figure 1 represents total uptake (dpm) for phenylalanine uptake by adherent normal rabbit lung macrophages at three different concentrations. Figure 2 represents similar data after the noncarrier-mediated component has been subtracted and after the data are converted to pmoles transported/3 × 10⁵ cells.

After determining that a time-dependent, saturable process occurs, one can select a sampling time well within the linear portion of the uptake process for all substrate concen-

trations to be tested. On the basis of data presented in
Figs. 1 and 2, 20 sec was chosen as an appropriate interval.
To determine the concentration dependence of the process, solutions are prepared so that the amount of radiolabeled substrate per milliliter is held constant while the amount of unlabeled substrate is increased. As shown in Fig. 3 for phenylalanine transport by normal rabbit lung macrophages, cell-
associated radioactivity decreases as substrate concentration
increases; above 10 mM there is no further diminution in the
radioactivity that is cell-associated (closed circles). Thus,
those counts are considered as the nonsaturable component, representing diffusion - adsorption. The dpm due to diffusion are
subtracted from the curve to give the saturable component (open
circles). In this experiment the diffusion component was determined at 20 mM and represented 6% of cell-associated radiolabel at 20 sec when the external concentration was 25 μM.

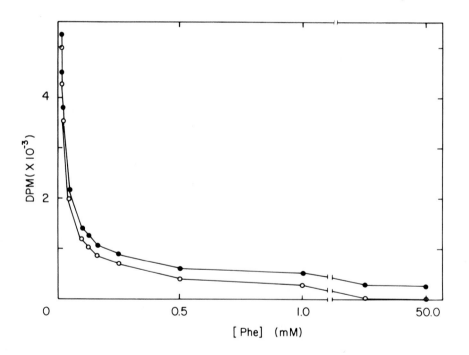

Fig. 3. DPM dependence on external phenylalanine concentration. Total cell associated radiolabel after a 20-sec incubation is measured at different phenylalanine concentrations
(●). Above 10 mM phenylalanine no further diminution in cell-
associated radiolabel occurs. Those counts, which are still
cell-associated, are viewed as nonsaturable and are subtracted
from each point, leaving the carrier-mediated component (o).

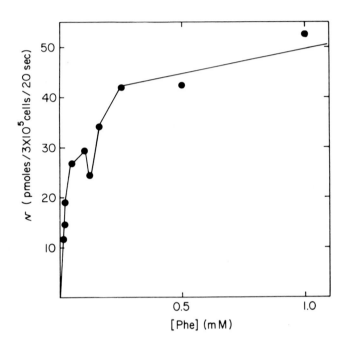

Fig. 4.   The data presented in Fig. 3 are converted to
pmoles transported/20 sec - 3 × 10⁵ cells from the calculated
specific activities of the individual transport test solutions.

After the specific activity of each transport test solution has
been calculated, the dpm due to the saturable component is converted to pmoles transported. These values are then plotted as
a function of external concentration (Fig. 4). If there is a
single transport system for the substance under study, the expected hyperbolic curve is smooth. It is clear that for phenylalanine transport in these cells the hyperbolic curve is discontinuous, indicating that two K_ms may be present (see below).
    At this point, standard methods for handling data for
enzyme-mediated processes are followed to obtain a Lineweaver-
Burke plot, Eadie - Scatchard plot, or Wolf - Augustinsson
plot (18) in order to calculate K_m and V_{max} for the transport
system. The presence of more than one system is suggested by
the shape of the concentration versus velocity curve and by
the specificities of the transport system for chemically related
compounds (1, 8, 9, 18, 19). Ultimate proof requires genetic

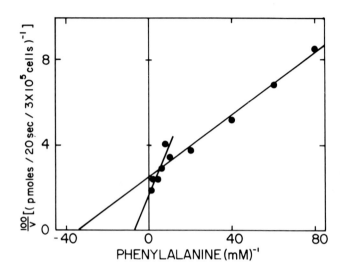

Fig. 5.   The data presented in Figs. 3 and 4 are trans-
formed by the method of Lineweaver-Burke to obtain a standard
reciprocal plot.   The calculated K_m are 30 μM and 200 μM and
the corresponding V_{max} are 40 pmoles/20 sec - 3 × 10^5 cells and
72 pmoles/20 sec - 3 × 10^5 cells, respectively.

analysis using mutant cells.   Figure 5 represents the data in
Fig. 4 presented as a Lineweaver-Burke Plot.

In order to determine whether the permeant has been concentrated against a gradient, it is necessary to determine the
intracellular aqueous volume in order to determine the intracellular concentration, and to establish whether the substrate
has been metabolized.   Since it has proven extremely difficult
to measure intracellular volumes for monolayers (6, 20), the
dete.mination is usually performed on cells in pellet.   Therefore, methods of determining intracellular volume are described
in Section III.C.

B. *Transport by Cells in Suspension as Determined by the Oil Microfuge Method*

The sequence of experiments to be performed is the same as that described above. The major difference is that medium that is not cell-associated remains above the oil, while cells pass through the oil into the tip of the Microfuge tube. Some medium comigrates through the oil, possibly as an aqueous shell around the cells. Thus, the nonspecific, nonsaturable component will reflect trapped medium as well as passive diffusion and nonspecific adsorption. It will represent a larger percentage of the total cell-associated radioactivity in the oil Microfuge method than in the coverslip technique.

Microfuge tubes are prepared in advance of the experiment. After the cap has been removed, 40 µl 10% PCA is placed in each 40 µl Microfuge tube by means of a 1-ml syringe with 22-gauge needle. Well-mixed silicone oil (150 µl) is layered over the PCA by means of a 1-ml syringe with 18-gauge needle. The tubes are spun for 5 - 20 sec so that the oil and acid layers separate and sediment to the bottom.

Cells (1×10^6 cells in 0.1 ml) are dispensed into small vessels suspended in a water bath at 37°C and allowed to incubate for 10 - 15 min. We have found that Eppendorf holders for large (1.5 ml) Microfuge tubes can be mounted easily on top of test tube racks in the water bath and secured with string. The 1.5-ml Microfuge tubes then make excellent incubation vessels. At 0 time, 0.2 ml of prewarmed test solution containing 4 - 6 µCi/ml radiolabeled permeant at 3/2 the desired concentration is added to the cells by means of the Fisher fibrin tip hand gun. To ensure adequate mixing, the suspension is drawn rapidly into the pipette 2 - 3 times. Several seconds before the end of the desired time interval, 0.2 ml of the reaction mixture is removed and layered on top of the silicone oil in the Microfuge tube already seated in the Microfuge. At the appropriate time, the Microfuge is started and the tubes are spun for 20 sec. Cells migrate through the oil into the tip, leaving noncell-associated radiolabel above the oil. Controls (8) have shown that virtually all the cells can be recovered intact in the tip when 10% sucrose is used instead of 10% PCA; no radiolabel passes into the tip unless cells are present; the viability of the cells that migrate through the oil into 10% sucrose is the same as that before their exposure to oil as determined by trypan blue exclusion; and, finally, during the transport test the amount of radiolabel recovered in the tip is a direct function of the number of cells applied. The tip of the 400 µl tube is cut off with a razor blade just above the oil - acid interface and allowed to drop into a scintillation vial. After the vial is shaken vigorously to dislodge the contents in the tip,

1.0 ml 0.5 N KOH containing phenol red is added. Subsequent manipulations are the same as those described above.

C. Intracellular volumes

Intracellular volume measurements on cells in suspension are readily performed by means of the oil Microfuge method (6, 8, 9). ^3H_2O is used to measure total pellet volume (intracellular plus extracellular) and [^{14}C]sucrose is used to measure extracellular volume (6, 8, 9). [^{14}C]Inulin may also be used instead of sucrose but must be repurified before each use because it degrades to fructose at an appreciable rate; fructose may be taken up rapidly into the cell by carrier-mediated transport systems. The use of sucrose as an extracellular marker presupposes that sucrose is not pinocytosed to a significant extent within 30 - 60 sec.

Cells are prepared at five different concentrations, 3×10^7 ml, 2.25×10^7/ml, 1.5×10^7/ml, 0.75×10^7/ml, and 0.375×10^7/ml, and stored at 4°C. Each determination is made in quadruplicate. Samples of 100 µl at each concentration are prewarmed in incubation vessels. Two hundred µl doubly labeled isotope solution is added and mixed by means of a Fisher fibrin tip gun. The cells remain exposed to the mixture for 30 or 60 sec and then are separated by means of the oil Microfuge method. Pellets are treated as described above. In this case the windows on the scintillation counter must be set for double label counting. It is essential to count small aliquots (10 µl) of the initial ^3H_2O/[^{14}C]sucrose solution in order to determine experimentally the amount of radioisotope per unit volume. It is also important to count small samples of ^3H_2O alone and of [^{14}C]sucrose alone to determine the spillover from one counting channel to another.

Calculations for each group are performed in the following fashion. The radioactivity in the ^{14}C channel (minus background) of the four samples in the group are averaged. This number represents the average sucrose space. For each sample in the group cpm (minus background) in the ^{14}C channel is multiplied by the percentage which has been shown to spill into the tritium channel to obtain the spillover counts. The latter are subtracted from the cpm (minus background) observed in the tritium channel. The difference represents ^3H_2O associated with the sample. The radioactivity in the tritium channel due to ^3H_2O of the four samples within the group is averaged. This number represents the average ^3H_2O space. The small aliquot of the initial ^3H_2O/[^{14}C]sucrose solution is used to determine cpm ^3H_2O/10 µl and cpm [^{14}C]sucrose/10 µl. The average sucrose space for each group is calculated by dividing the observed average cpm in the ^{14}C channel by cpm [^{14}C]sucrose/10 µl

ERRATA

Methods for Studying Mononuclear Phagocytes
Dolph O. Adams, Paul J. Edelson, and Hillel S. Koren, editors

The sentence on page 92l of the chapter 'Solute Uptake and Membrane Transport by Mononuclear Phagocytes' by Phyllis R. Strauss should read as follows: In recent experiments we have shown that a mixture of equal parts of No. 556 and No. 550 is equally as effective as the previously published formulation (8, 9) and there are no problems with miscibility.

test solution. The average water space for each group is calculated by dividing the observed average cpm in the tritium
channel by the cpm ^3H_2O/10 µl test solution. The average intracellular space is obtained by subtracting the average sucrose
space from the average water space. The values for the different groups are plotted as a function of cell number and a linear
regression analysis performed to determine final intra- and
extracellular volumes over the concentration range studied.

D. Calculation of Data

   See Sections III.A - C.

E. Critical Comments

   One technical difficulty in the oil Microfuge method involves the silicone oils. Miscibility of No. 510 silicone oil
with No. 550 is highly variable, depending on the batch lot of
the No. 510. In recent experiments we have shown that a mixture of equal parts of Nos. 556 and 510 is equally as effective
as the previously published formulation (8, 9) and there are no
problems with miscibility. Intra- and extracellular spaces
remain unchanged.
   Reproducibility of quadruplicate transport measurements
made by the coverslip technique is excellent, the range usually
being within 10%. Reproducibility of quadruplicate measurements by the oil Microfuge technique is somewhat more variable,
the standard error being less than 10%. Reproducibility among
experiments varies, depending on the type of permeant. For
example, the rate of adenosine transport by rabbit lung macrophages is constant from day to day, while the rate of amino
acid transport varies, possibly because of exchange diffusion
or transinhibition (see below). Determinations of K_m and V_{max}
require multiple experiments, especially where the presence of
more than one transport system is suspected.
   On a more theoretical level, since molecular mechanisms of
most transport systems in animal cells still remain to be elu-
cidated, it is important to note that the use of kinetic techniques assumes that the steady-state approximation is justified.
However, the data really reflect the apparent affinity of the
rate-limiting step in uptake. Whether the rate-limiting step
is the passage of the solute across the membrane or some other
parameter is not entirely clear at this time. Moreover, per-
turbations in the membrane may affect the K_m and V_{max} generated.
Another difficulty is that measurements may be complicated by
internal pool sizes. For example, amino acid transport is subject to exchange diffusion or transinhibition. In the former

the internal concentration of the amino acid or closely related analog alters the observed flux rate in a positive fashion (1, 3, 4, 6, 10, 12). In the latter the internal concentration of certain amino acids alters the observed flux rate in a negative fashion (1, 21). Internal events such as phosphorylation in the case of nucleosides and sugars may alter apparent results, since the activity of the kinase may overshadow the transport activity. Therefore, it is particularly important that measurements be made so rapidly that efflux and metabolism do not become significant factors. While some investigators feel that nonmetabolizable substrates may offer a better approach (12), these substrates are not those the cell is ever likely to see naturally.

Another approach involves use of mutant cells that lack specific steps in the metabolic pathway of the permeant in question. Examples might be adenosine-kinase-deficient or thymidine-kinase-deficient mutants when the solute is adenosine or thymidine. Moreover, it should not be assumed that the same transport systems occur and are regulated in the same fashion in all cells. There is even a marked difference between normal rabbit lung macrophages and rabbit peritoneal macrophages obtained after an intraperitoneal infusion of casein. The former have a single adenosine and a single lysine transport system, while the latter have two systems for each permeant (P. Strauss, unpublished data).

Finally, it is highly desirable to perform the transport test in a simple medium devoid of potentially competing substrates. Even prior exposure of macrophages to serum has been shown to result in altered amino acid (4, 21) and nucleoside (4, 5) transport. PBS, with or without 5 mM glucose, has proved satisfactory for macrophages. PBS with 5 mM glucose and 0.1% recrystallized bovine serum albumin (Sigma Chemicals, St. Louis, Missouri) has proved satisfactory for murine lymphocytes.

Acknowledgment

This work has been supported by Northeastern University, the American Cancer Society BC-171, and the National Science Foundation PCM 75-20323 and PCM 77-25434. PRS is the recipient of Research Career Development Award CA00460 from the National Cancer Institute, DHEW.

REFERENCES

1. E. Heinz. "Mechanics and Energetics of Biological Transport." Springer-Verlag, Berlin, Heidelberg, New York, 1978.
2. R. Hawkins and R. D. Berlin. Purine transport in polymorphonuclear leukocytes. *Biochim. Biophys. Acta 173*: 324-331, 1969.
3. M.-F. Tsan and R. D. Berlin. Membrane transport in the rabbit alveolar macrophage. The specificity and characteristics of amino acid transport systems. *Biochim. Biophys. Acta 241*: 155-169, 1971.
4. P. R. Strauss and R. D. Berlin. Effects of serum on membrane transport. I. Separation and preliminary characterization of factors which depress lysine or stimulate adenosine transport in rabbit alveolar macrophages. *J. Exp. Med. 137*: 359-368, 1973.
5. P. R. Strauss. Effects of serum on membrane transport. II. Serum and the stimulation of adenosine transport, a possible mechanism. *J. Cell Biol. 60*: 571-585, 1974.
6. J. F. Pofit and P. R. Strauss. Membrane transport by macrophages in suspension and adherent to glass. *J. Cell. Physiol. 92*: 249-256, 1977.
7. S. H. Zigmond and J. G. Hirsch. Cytochalasin B: Inhibition of D-2-deoxyglucose transport into leukocytes and fibroblasts. *Science 176*: 1432-1434, 1972.
8. P. R. Strauss, J. M. Sheehan, and E. R. Kashket. Membrane transport by murine lymphocytes. I. A rapid sampling technique as applied to the adenosine and thymidine systems. *J. Exp. Med. 144*: 1009-1021, 1976.
9. P. R. Strauss, J. M. Sheehan, and E. R. Kashket. Membrane transport by murine lymphocytes. II. The appearance of thymidine transport in cells from concanavalin A-stimulated mice. *J. Immunol. 118*: 1328-1334, 1977.
10. A. Kotyk and K. Janacek. "Cell Membrane Transport: Principles and Techniques," 2nd ed. Plenum, New York, 1975.
11. G. G. Guidotti, A. F. Borghetti, and G. C. Gazzola. The regulation of amino acid transport in animal cells. *Biochim. Biophys. Acta 515*: 329-366, 1978.
12. H. N. Christensen. Exploiting amino acid structure to learn about membrane transport. *Adv. Enzymol. Relat. Areas Molec. Biol. 49*: 41-101, 1979.
13. A. R. P. Paterson. Adenosine transport. *In* "Physiological and Regulatory Functions of Adenosine and Adenine Nucleotides" (H. P. Baer and G. I. Drummond, eds.), pp. 305-313. Raven Press, New York, 1979.
14. R. D. Berlin and J. M. Oliver. Membrane transport of purine and pyrimidine bases and nucleosides in animal

cells. *Int. Rev. Cytol.* *42*: 287–336, 1975.

15. R. Wohlhueter and P. G. W. Plagemann. The roles of transport and phosphorylation in nutrient uptake in cultured animal cells. *Int. Rev. Cytol.* *64*: 171–240, 1980.

16. M. Hatanaka. Transport of sugars in tumor cell membranes. *Biochim. Biophys. Acta* *355*: 77–104, 1974.

17. K. Fink, R. E. Cline, and R. M. Fink. Paper chromatography of several classes of compounds: correlated R_f values in a variety of solvent systems. *Anal. Chem.* *35*: 389–398, 1963.

18. I. H. Segel. Biochemical Calculations, 2nd ed. John Wiley & Sons, New York. 1976.

19. I. H. Segal. "Enzyme Kinetics." John Wiley & Sons, New York. 1975.

20. R. F. Kletzien, M. W. Pariza, J. Becker, and V. R. Potter. A method using 3-0-methyl-D-glucose and phloretin for the determination of intracellular water spaces of cells in monolayer culture. *Analyt. Biochem.* *68*: 537–544, 1975.

21. P. R. Strauss. Effects of serum on membrane transport. III. Serum and inhibition of lysine transport. *Am. J. Physiol.* *236*: C111–C116, 1979.

84

USE OF LACTOPEROXIDASE FOR LABELLING MEMBRANE PROTEINS

Helen L. Yin

I. INTRODUCTION

The introduction of nonpermeant agents covalently to label
externally disposed plasma membrane proteins of cells has allowed characterization of these proteins without resorting to
membrane fractionation. Phillips and Morrison (1) first introduced the technique of iodinating cell surface proteins with
lactoperoxidase, which catalyzes the formation of a carbon-
halogen bond in the presence of hydrogen peroxide, a halide
and a nucleophilic acceptor, such as tyrosine. Selective
labeling of surface proteins depends on the fact that lactoperoxidase cannot diffuse through the membrane barrier of a
living cell, and therefore iodination is limited to the outside
surface of the cell. Hubbard and Cohn (2, 3) used glucose oxidase in conjunction with lactoperoxidase to generate an *in situ*
low concentration of hydrogen peroxide, limiting the amount of
free hydrogen peroxide, which is known to harm cells, in the
reaction mixture.

METHODS FOR STUDYING
MONONUCLEAR PHAGOCYTES

925

II. REAGENTS

Na^{125}I-carrier-free, iodination grade, New England Nuclear
Corp.   The isotope is made and shipped by the supplier every
two weeks, and should be used within two weeks. Iodide that
has been exposed to air for a long time tends to be oxidized,
and are incorporated into the cells even in the absence of lactoperoxidase.
     Caution ^{125}I is volatile and should be handled in a well-
ventilated hood. Keep solutions covered as much as possible
(e.g., use centrifuge tubes with screw caps during iodination
and centrifugation), and use disposable labware. Waste ^{125}I
solution should be stored in capped plastic bottles in the
presence of strong base.
     Potassium iodide: Reagent grade, solution should be made
fresh.
     Glucose: Reagent grade
     Dulbecco's minimum essential medium (MEM), Grand Island
Biological Co.
     Heat-inactivated fetal calf serum
     Dulbecco's phosphate-buffered saline, Ca^{2+}, Mg^{2+} free
(PBS), Grand Island, Biological Co.
     Phenylmethyl sulfonyl fluoride (PMSF), Sigma Chemical
Corp.
     10% Trichloroacetic acid (TCA)
     Chemicals for polyacrylamide gel electrophoresis in the
presence of sodium dodecyl sulfate
     Lactoperoxidase (EC 1.11.1.7), Calbiochem., assayed as
described below.
     Glucose oxidase (EC 1.1.3.4), Sigma Chemical Corp., Type
V, assayed as described below.
     The activities of lactoperoxidase and glucose oxidase are
assayed using o-dianisidine as substrate, and followed by the
change in absorbance at 460 nm. A unit of activity is defined
as the amount of enzyme producing/consuming 1 µmol peroxide/min
at 25°C, assuming molar extinction coefficient of 11,300 for
o-dianisidine. It should be pointed out that the units designated and the assay conditions used by the suppliers are different from the ones described here, and cannot be readily converted.

A. Lactoperoxidase (LPO) Assay

1. Prepare the following solutions:
     (a) LPO, 3 mg/ml in phosphate-buffered saline (PBS), pH
7.2. The enzyme is stable at this protein concentration and
can be stored frozen in small aliquots.

(b) o-Dianisidine (Sigma Chemical Co.), 10 mg/ml in absolute methanol. Make up fresh and keep in dark (cover with
foil). Caution: Carcinogenic!
(c) Hydrogen peroxide, Superoxal diluted with distilled
water to give a 0.3% solution. Stable.
(d) 0.1 M Phosphate buffer, pH 5.0.
(e) Substrate mixture: 0.06 ml 0.3% peroxide, 0.05 ml
10 mg/ml o-dianisidine, and 5.9 ml phosphate buffer, pH 5.0.
2. Activity is assayed by following the change in absorbance
at 460 nm. Mix 0.1 ml PBS, pH 7.2 with 0.9 ml substrate mixture in cuvette No. 1 and set the absorbance to zero. Add
0.9 ml substrate mixture to cuvettes Nos. 2, 3, and 4 and
0.1 ml serial dilutions of LPO (e.g., 10, 20, 50 µl of 0.03
mg/ml LPO, made up to 0.1 ml with PBS). Cover cuvettes with
parafilm, invert twice and follow change in absorbance for
5-10 min in a spectrophotometer.

B. Glucose Oxidase Assay

1. Prepare the following solutions:
(a) Glucose oxidase, 2 µl/ml. The enzyme is stable at the
concentration supplied, but is not stable on dilution.
(b) Glucose, 0.05 mg/ml (5%), PBS, pH 7.2, o-dianisidine,
10 mg/ml in absolute methanol (100 x). Make up fresh, and
store in foil-covered container.
(c) Horseradish peroxidase, 5 mg/10 ml.
(d) Substrate mixture (mix immediately before use):
1.0 ml 5% glucose, 0.1 ml o-dianisidine 1%, 1.0 ml horseradish
peroxidase 0.05%, and, 6.9 ml PBS, pH 7.2.
2. Assay mixture contain 0.9 ml substrate solution and 0.1 ml
glucose oxidase (diluted serially). Follow change in absorbance at 460 nm with time for 5-10 min.

III. PROCEDURES

A. Iodination Protocol

(1) Harvest peritoneal exudate cells from mice in warm
PBS pH 7.2 by standard procedures. Place cell suspension on
ice.
(2) Filter cells through cheese cloth into conical plastic
tubes with caps. Centrifuge at 250 g for 10 min at 4°C. Repeat wash in PBS to remove loosely bound material from cells.
(3) Resuspend to 10^7 cells/ml in PBS.
(4) Iodinate the entire cell suspension at 4°C for 25 min.

The final reaction mixture contains 100 mU/ml LPO, 10 mU/ml glucose oxidase, 20 mM glucose, 100 - 200 μCi/ml Na^{125}I, 25 nmole/ml K^{127}I (the incorporation of I^{125} improves when a small amount of carrier iodide is added). Swirl the suspension occasionally by hand.

(5) Terminate the reaction by adding twenty volumes of ice-cold MEM, with 1% heat-inactivated fetal calf serum. Centrifuge at 250 g for 10 min at 4°C. Repeat wash.

(6) Resuspend cell pellet in MEM with 10% heat-inactivated fetal calf serum. Plate cells in plastic tissue culture petri dishes for 30 - 60 min at 37°C under 5% CO_2 atmosphere.

(7) Wash monolayers vigorously by swirling in several changes of ice-cold PBS to remove nonadherent cells and culture medium. After washing, the cells remaining on the monolayer should be greater than 95% macrophages.

(8) To remove the macrophages from the culture dish, add a small volume of PBS with 2 mM PMSF to the dish and scrape with a policeman. Transfer the cell suspension to centrifuge tubes and disperse the cells gently with a Pasteur pipette.

(9) Centrifuge at 990 g for 10 min at 4°C.

(10) Resuspend cell pellet in a minimal volume of a solution containing 0.06 Tris-HCl, pH 6.8, 4 mM EDTA, and 2 mM PMSF. Remove aliquots for protein determination, radioactivity measurement and gel electrophoresis.

To summarize, the entire peritoneal exudate cell population was iodinated in suspension at 4°C. This is preferable to iodinating the macrophage monolayers, because serum proteins adhering to the culture surface are extensively labeled. Iodination is performed at 4°C to decrease pinocytosis, which may introduce LPO into the cells, to prevent lateral diffusion of membrane proteins, which may alter the accessibility of plasma membrane proteins to labeling, and to limit proteolysis. Macrophages were then separated from other nonadherent cell types by a subsequent adherence step. This selects for viable macrophages, eliminating dead cells that might be nonspecifically labeled from the system.

A number of control experiments should be performed to establish that the radioactivity is incorporated into plasma membrane proteins only and not into intracellular proteins. Since exclusive membrane labeling is dependent on the fact that LPO cannot permeate the plasma membrane of living cells, it is important that the macrophages remain viable during iodination, and the labeling is absolutely dependent on LPO. Cell viability can be tested by exclusion of trypan blue dye. The requirement for LPO can be established by ommitting the enzyme from the iodination mixture. Glucose oxidase is not absolutely required for labeling, although the extent of labeling is considerably less than if it were present.

It is also important to identify the nature of the iodinated

cell material. If the radioactivity is incorporated into proteins, it should be insoluble in cold TCA, and largely nonex-
tractable by organic solvent. The ultimate proof for labeling
of protein requires demonstration that the radioactivity is
associated with monoiodotyrosine in a trypsin digest of the
labeled cells (3).

B. Radioactivity Measurement

The amount of radioactivity associated with the macrophages
is determined after cold TCA precipitation. For small number
of samples, TCA precipitation can be done in a Millipore suction apparatus. For large number of samples, the "disk-batch"
method is more convenient.

1. Pipette an aliquot ($\leq$50 µl) of an iodinated sample onto
a glass fiber filter disk (2.4 µm-diameter, Whatman, GF/c)
labeled with waterproof Sharpie pen.
2. Soak the disk into 500 ml cold 10% TCA with 50 mM $K^{127}I$
for 2 hr or longer.
3. Rinse three times in 400 ml each 10% TCA and air dry.
4. Count in a gamma spectrophotometer. The nonspecific
absorbance of free ^{125}I to the filters is reduced by using a
high concentration of $K^{127}I$ in the TCA solution. The level of
nonspecifically absorbed radioactivity can be assessed by ap-
plying free $Na^{125}I$ to a disk in the presence of unlabeled cell
protein.

C. Organic Solvent Extraction

About 10 - 30% of the TCA precipitable cell-associated
radioactivity is extractable by organic solvents.

1. Put each disk in individual 10 ml glass test tube.
(The tube should be labeled because the organic solvents will
dissolve the ink on the filter paper.)
2. Add 6 ml of organic solvents (either chloroform -
methanol 2:1; acetone - water 9:1, or ethanol - ether 3:1) to
each tube and let stand for about 30 min at 4°C.
3. Rinse the disk through three changes of solvent, air
dry, and count in a gamma spectrophotometer.

D. Gel Electrophoresis

The iodinated plasma membrane protein can be resolved by
polyacrylamide gel electrophoresis in the presence of sodium
dodecyl sulfate.

Two difficulties may arise when processing the macrophages for gel electrophoresis. First, macrophages contain a large amount of proteases that may hydrolyze the membrane proteins. Proteolysis is minimized as follows. Cells are iodinated at 4°C, and plated at 37°C in the presence of serum that contains natural protease inhibitors. The macrophages are removed from the monolayers in ice-cold buffer containing phenylmethylsulfonyl fluoride, a serine protease inhibitor, and EDTA, which chelates cations and thereby inhibits cation-dependent proteases. In addition, macrophages collected from the monolayers are boiled as soon as possible in 2% sodium dodecyl sulfate (SDS) to inactivate the protease. Second, after boiling in SDA, DNA in the cell sample might form a viscous gel that is difficult to pipette. Gel formation can be prevented by diluting the cell sample to as large a volume as is compatible with gel electrophoresis before addition of SDS, and once formed, the gel may be disrupted by reheating and shearing with a micropipet. The sample should be loaded onto the acrylamide gel while still hot.

Since a large number of proteins are labeled, optimal resolution in the polyacrylamide gel is desirable. We routinely use the discontinuous pH gradient slab gel system of Laemmli (4). The distribution of radioactivity among the proteins is determined by slicing the gel after electrophoresis into small sections for counting in a gamma spectrophotometer, or by autoradiography after drying the gel. X-Rays film such as X-Omat R (Kodak) should be used in conjunction with intensifying screens (Cronex, Dupont) to shorten the period of exposure required. It is not necessary to precipitate the proteins with TCA or extract with organic solvent prior to electrophoresis. The extractable radioactive material does not interfere with the resolution of proteins by gel electrophoresis, and accumulates in the bottom of the gel as a broad band that is not stained by Coomassie blue.

IV. CONCLUDING REMARKS

The lactoperoxidase : glucose oxidase catalyzed iodination technique has been used successfully to label the surface proteins of mouse peritoneal macrophages. This facilitates research in macrophage membrane biochemistry greatly, because up until now, there is no satisfactory method for isolating pure plasma membrane fractions from these cells. This method has provided information on the differences between plasma membrane proteins of resident and elicited macrophages, the immunological identity of several membrane proteins, and the kinetics of their turnover (5, 6).

REFERENCES

1. D. R. Phillips and M. Morrison (1970). The arrangement of proteins in the human erythrocyte membrane. *Biochem. Biophys. Res. Commun.* *40*: 284-289.
2. A. L. Hubbard and Z. A. Cohn (1972). The enzymatic iodination of the red cell membrane. *J. Cell Biol.* *55*: 390-405.
3. A. L. Hubbard and Z. A. Cohn (1975). Externally disposed plasma membrane proteins. I. Enzymatic iodination of mouse L cells. *J. Cell Biol.* *64*: 438-460.
4. U. K. Laemmli (1970). Cleavage of structural proteins during the assembly of the head of bacteriophage T4. *Nature 227*: 630-685.
5. H. L. Yin, S. Alley, C. Bianco, and Z. A. Cohn (1980). Plasma membrane polypeptides of resident and activated mouse peritoneal macrophages. *Proc. Natl. Acad. Sci. USA* 77: 2188-2192.
6. H. L. Yin, C. Bianco, and Z. A. Cohn. Glucoproteins of the plasma membrane of mouse peritoneal macrophages: Their turnover characteristics and protease susceptibility (manuscript in preparation).

85

BINDING OF SYNTHETIC CHEMOTACTIC PEPTIDES
AS A MODEL OF LIGAND-RECEPTOR INTERACTION

Edward J. Fudman
Ralph Snyderman

I. INTRODUCTION

Certain synthetic *N*-formylated peptides are potent chemotactic factors for phagocytic cells (1,2). *N*-Formylated peptides initiate chemotaxis of macrophages as well as polymorphonuclear leukocytes by combining with a high-affinity cell surface receptor (3-6). The characteristics of this receptor, such as number per cell, dissociation constant, and specificity, can be quantified by a radioligand binding assay (7). A radiolabeled chemotactic peptide is incubated with cells and the association of peptide with the cells is measured by liquid scintillation spectrophotometry. The portion of total binding that is due to a specific receptor is determined by subtracting nonspecific binding, the amount of binding not inhibited by a vast excess of unlabeled peptide.

The macrophage chemotactic factor receptor may be useful as a marker for investigating potential heterogeneity and differentiation of mononuclear phagocytes. The radioligand bind-

METHODS FOR STUDYING
MONONUCLEAR PHAGOCYTES

933

ing assay described here uses guinea pig peritoneal macrophages; other mononuclear phagocytes as well as polymorphonuclear leukocytes can be studied using similar methods. However, the ligand binds very poorly to murine macrophages.

II. REAGENTS

Incubation buffer stock (5 × concentration): 0.7 M NaCl,
9.5 mM KH$_2$PO$_4$, 25.5 mM Na$_2$HPO$_4$. To prepare 1 liter of 5 ×
stock, use 40.9 gm NaCl, 1.3 gm KH$_2$PO$_4$, and 6.85 gm Na$_2$HPO$_4$.
Store at 0°C.

Stock minerals: 0.5 M MgCl$_2$, 0.15 M CaCl$_2$. To prepare
100 ml stock minerals, use 10.16 gm MgCl$_2$ and 1.66 gm CaCl$_2$.
Store at 4°C.

Chemotactic peptides: Tritiated N-formylmethionly-
leucyl-phenylalanine (fMet-Leu-[^{3}H]Phe), 57 Ci/mmol (New England Nuclear, Boston, Massachusetts). Store at -20°C.

Unlabeled fMet-Leu-Phe (Peninsula Laboratories, San Carlos,
California). Prepare stock solution of 10^{-2} M in water and
store at -20°C. Less concentrated solutions are unstable and
should be prepared daily as needed. Other unlabeled N-formy-
lated chemotactic peptides are available from Sigma Chemicals,
St. Louis, Missouri, Andrulis Research, Bethesda, Maryland,
and Miles Laboratories, Elkhart, Indiana. Both labeled and
unlabeled peptides should be kept in an ice bath at all times
while working with them.

Sodium azide, 0.1 M.

III. PROCEDURES

A. Buffer Preparation

Prepare a mininum of 1000 ml fresh buffer daily by making
a 1:5 dilution of concentrated buffer stock in water. Add 1
ml stock minerals per liter of buffer and adjust pH to 7.2.
The final incubation buffer concentration is 0.14 M NaCl, 1.9
mM KH$_2$PO$_4$, 5.1 mM Na$_2$HPO$_4$, 0.15 mM CaCl$_2$, and 0.5 mM MgCl$_2$.
Keep buffer at 0°-4°C intil used.

B. Cell Preparations

Resident or inflammatory macrophages are obtained from the
peritoneal cavities of adult male Hartley guinea pigs by lavage with 0.01 M phosphate-buffered isotonic saline, pH 7.2,

with 10 U heparin/ml. After centrifugation at 350 g for 7 min
at 0°C, wash the cells in incubation buffer and resuspend in
incubation buffer at the concentration of 1.5×10^7 cells/ml.
Keep the cells at 0°C. About 20 min before starting the incubation with peptide, add 1 mM sodium azide to the cells as
10 µl of 0.1 M sodium azide per milliliter of cells. Azide
minimizes internalization of the peptides. Vortex the cells
vigorously immediately upon adding sodium azide. Allow the
cells to come to room temperature.

C. Incubation of Cells and Peptide

Incubations are done in 12 × 75 mm polypropylene tubes
(Falcon Plastics, Oxnard, California) with a reaction volume
of 150 µl. The reaction mixture consists of 100 µl of the
cell suspension, 25 µl of labeled fMet-Leu-[^{3}H]Phe, and 25 µl
of unlabeled fMet-Leu-Phe (for nonspecific binding determination), buffer (for total binding determination), or other peptide (for specificity and inhibition experiments).

Dilute the tritiated peptide fMet-Leu-[^{3}H]Phe in incubation
buffer to the desired concentrations (usually 1-20 nM range)
and keep at 0°C until use. Dilute with incubation buffer the
unlabeled fMet-Leu-Phe from 10^{-2} M stock to 6×10^{-5} M. The
final concentration of unlabeled peptide when 25 µl of 6×10^{-5}
M is added as part of the 150 µl reaction volume will be 10^{-5} M,
or 1000 times the concentration of labeled peptide.

After bringing the reagents to room temperature (or the desired temperature for a particular study), pipette 25 µl of
fMet-Leu-[^{3}H]Phe and 25 µl of buffer, unlabeled fMet-Leu-Phe,
or other agent into the 12 × 75 mm tubes. Carefully add 100
µl of the macrophage suspension (1.5×10^7/ml) to each tube and
vortex the tube. For saturation experiments, incubate the cells
for 45 min with constant shaking at room temperature. For kinetic studies, appropriately vary the incubation time.

D. Determination of Cellular Binding

Cellular binding is determined following suitable incubation by rapidly filtering the cells and measuring the radioactivity of the filter paper. A suction filtration device
(Duke University Physiological Instrument Shop, Durham, North
Carolina) is used in which the filter rests on a stainless
steel grid and is held in place by a weighted stainless steel
wall (Fig. 1) (7).

Prepare the filtration apparatus for use by rinsing the
metal grids and place a Whatman GFC glass fiber filter on each,

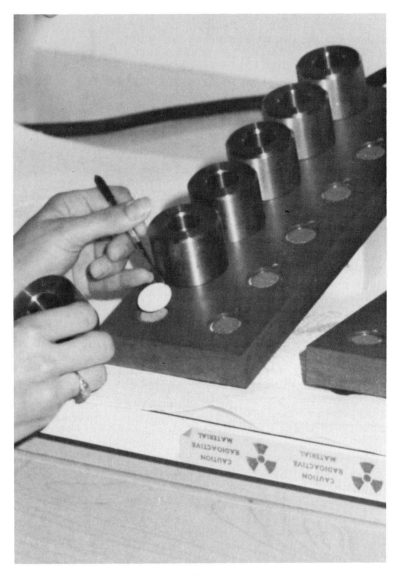

Fig. 1. Suction filtration device used for radioligand binding assay. The glass fiber filter rests on a stainless steel grid and is held in place by the metal weight that serves as a reservoir above the filter. [From Williams and Lefkowitz (7).]

with the cross-hatched side of the filter facing upward. Position the steel wall around each filter and fill with 2 ml of incubation buffer. Terminate the incubation of cells with

the radioligand after the appropriate time by adding 4 ml of
ice-cold incubation buffer to the tube, using a Cornwall syringe, and quickly pour the contents of the tube through a
filter on the suction filtration apparatus. Wash the tube
twice, emptying the contents onto the filter, and the filter
once with an additional 4 ml volume of buffer. Place the
filters in scintillation vials with 10 ml Aquasol (New England
Nuclear) and vigorously shake. Wait at least 1 hr before measuring radioactivity by liquid scintillation spectrometry.

IV. CALCULATION OF DATA

The dissociation constant (K_d) and number of binding sites
per cell can be determined from a saturation curve in which
the specific fMet-Leu-[^{3}H]Phe binding is plotted as a function
of the concentration of labeled peptide (Fig. 2). Specific
binding is determined by subtracting the amount of radioligand
that binds in the presence of 10^{-5} M unlabeled fMet-Leu-Phe
from the total binding. Theoretically, the number of receptors

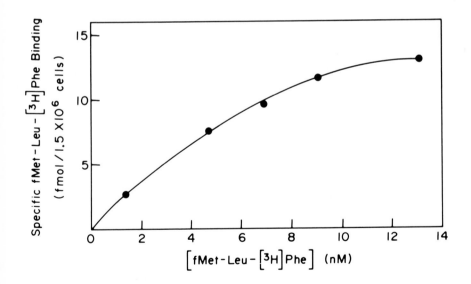

Fig. 2. Specific binding of fMet-Leu-[^{3}H]Phe to inflammatory macrophages as a function of fMet-Leu-[^{3}H]Phe concentration. Guinea pigs were injected intraperitoneally with 25 ml of
0.5% glycogen in saline 3 days prior to harvest of the cells.
[From Snyderman and Fudman (3).]

per cell (or fmol receptor/1.5×10^6 cells as shown) can be
calculated from the amount of specific binding present at the
point where the curve becomes horizontal. The K_d is the concentration of fMet-Leu-[^{3}H]Phe needed for half-maximal saturation. In practice, these values are more accurately determined
by Scatchard analysis (8), an algebraic manipulation of the
saturation curve which makes the data linear. A plot of the
bound ligand/free ligand ratio as a function of the specific
binding is a linear relationship with the slope equal to $-1/K_d$
and the x intercept equal to the number of receptors
per cell (Fig. 3). Total binding rather than nonspecific binding is used in calculating the amount of free ligand. For a
more detailed explanation of Scatchard analysis in radioligand
binding assays, see Chapter 4 of Williams and Lefkowitz (7).

The affinity of other ligands for the fMet-Leu-Phe receptor
can be determined indirectly by measuring their ability to inhibit fMet-Leu-[^{3}H]Phe binding. The concentration of unlabeled
peptide that causes half-maximal inhibition of fMet-Leu-[^{3}H]Phe
binding (EC$_{50}$ binding) is a reflection of its affinity for the
receptor. Nonspecific binding, the amount of fMet-Leu-[^{3}H]Phe
binding measured in the presence of 10^{-5} M unlabeled fMet-Leu-
Phe, is defined as 0% specific binding or 100% inhibition.

V. CRITICAL COMMENTS

The assay described here demonstrates that N-formylated
peptides bind to a specific receptor on macrophages. The binding site may be classified as a receptor because it meets the
following criteria (7):

1. The binding is saturable, reversible, and of high
affinity.
2. The concentration range over which the binding sites
are occupied is comparable to the range over which the ligands
elicit a response.
3. The binding sites have specificity for ligands similar
to the order of potency with which the ligands elicit a biological response.

Endocytosis of the ligands by mononuclear phagocytes compli-
cates the measurement of cell surface receptors. Internalization of receptor-ligand complexes may prove to be a necessary
step in eliciting a chemotactic response, however, it interferes with studying whether or not binding is saturable and
reversible. Endocytosis of free ligand may produce unacceptably high nonspecific binding. We use 0.1 M sodium azide in
the incubation mixture to arrest the metabolic functions of

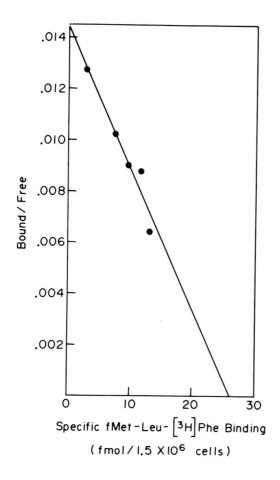

Fig. 3.   Scatchard plot derived from the data in Fig. 1. Free ligand is the amount of fMet-Leu-[³H]Phe added minus the total fMet-Leu-[³H]Phe binding.   The equilibrium dissociation constant (K$_d$) and number of binding sites per cell are calculated from the slope and x intercept, respectively.   [From Snyderman and Fudman, (3).]

the cell during the binding assay.   In the presence of sodium azide we get a nearly linear Scatchard plot and nonspecific binding of only 10-15% on the rapidly rising portion of the saturation curve.

Using this assay, we have demonstrated that N-formylated peptide receptors on both resident and inflammatory guinea pig peritoneal macrophages have a K_d of about 10 nM and that there are about 10,000 receptors per cell (3).

The radioligand binding assay described here was initially developed for studying human polymorphonuclear leukocytes (4) and was modified for guinea pig peritoneal macrophages by changing the cell concentrations and the incubation time. In adapting this assay for other mononuclear phagocytes, the investigator should determine the optimal cell concentration and incubation time for the particular cell type. One must avoid cell concentrations or conditions that lead to cell agglutination or adherence of the cells to the surface of the tube used for the incubation assay. Sufficient washing of the tubes and filters must be used to obtain good reproducibility and to minimize nonspecific binding.

REFERENCES

1. E. Schiffmann, B. A. Corcoran, and S. M. Wahl. N-Formylated peptides as chemoattractants for leukocytes. *Proc. Natl. Acad. Sci. USA* *72*:1059-1062, 1975.

2. H. S. Showell, F. J. Freer, S. H. Zigmond, E. Schiffmann, S. Aswanikumar, B. Corcoran, and E. L. Becker. The structure-activity relations of synthetic peptides as chemotactic factors and inducers of lysosomal enzyme secretions for neutrophils. *J. Exp. Med.* *143*:1154-1169, 1976.

3. R. Snyderman and E. J. Fudman. Demonstration of a chemotactic factor receptor on macrophages. *J. Immunol.* *124*: 2754-2757, 1980.

4. L. T. Williams, R. Snyderman, M. C. Pike, and R. J. Lefkowitz. Specific receptor sites for chemotactic peptides on human polymorphonuclear leukocytes. *Proc. Natl. Acad. Sci. USA* *74*:1204-1208, 1977.

5. S. Aswanikumar, B. Corcoran, E. Schiffmann, A. R. Day, R. J. Freer, H. J. Showell, E. L. Becker, and C. B. Pert. Demonstration of a receptor on rabbit neutrophils for chemotactic peptides. *Biochem. Biophys. Res. Commun.* *74*: 810-817, 1977.

6. J. Niedel, S. Wilkinson, and P. Cuatrecases. Receptor-mediated uptake and degradation of ^{125}I-chemotactic peptide by human neutrophils. *J. Biol. Chem.* *254*:10700-10706, 1979.

7. L. T. Williams and R. J. Lefkowitz. "Receptor Binding Studies in Adrenergic Pharmacology." Raven Press, New York, 1978.

8. G. Scatchard. The attraction of proteins for small
    molecules and ions. *Ann. NY Acad. Sci.* *51*:660-672, 1949.

86

ISOLATION OF PHAGOSOMES FROM MOUSE PERITONEAL MACROPHAGES

Maja Nowakowski
Celso Bianco

I. INTRODUCTION

This procedure allows the isolation of phagosomes generated by receptor-mediated and nonimmune phagocytosis. It is based on a method initially developed for the isolation of phagosomes from an ameba (1) and later adapted for mouse macrophages (2). We have introduced modifications that permit the simultaneous fractionation of phagosomes containing different particles from the same macrophage.

Phagosomes are formed during the endocytic process. The exterior surface of the macrophage plasma membrane surrounds the phagocytic target, in a "zippering-like" process (3). Virtually no space is left between the particle and the apposing cell membrane. Phagosomes isolated by the procedure below are thus constituted of particles surrounded by the macrophage plasma membrane. Usually, little contamination with other cellular materials can be detected in the phagosomal fraction.

Possibly, depending on the time period separating the phago-

METHODS FOR STUDYING
MONONUCLEAR PHAGOCYTES

943

cytic event from the time of cell fractionation, some of the
phagosomes will have fused with lysosomes. Thus, the material
obtained may contain phagolysosomes. The investigator should
also be aware of the rather rapid digestion of some of the materials taken up, including membrane components, which follows
fusion of the phagosome with lysosomes.

The present procedure utilizes nondigestible particles with
specific gravity remote from that of cellular constituents:
glutaraldehyde-fixed erythrocytes ingested via Fc or C3 receptors. Phagosomes generated using such particles show only a
selected population of the polypeptides present on the macrophage plasma membrane. The nature of these peptides varies
with the nature of the ligands coating the phagocytic target.
Latex beads, on the other hand, generate phagosomes surrounded
by a membrane that is quite similar to that of the intact macrophage. This is probably due to the multiple interactions that
occur between the beads and most proteins.

II. REAGENTS

A. *Solutions*

 Brewer's thioglycollate medium (DIFCO)
 Phosphate-buffered saline (PBS)
 Heparin (5000 U/ml, Connaught)
 Dulbecco's modified Eagle's medium (D_O, GIBCO)
 Fetal calf serum (FLOW, heat-inactivated (30 min, 56°C)
 $Na^{125}I$ (New England Nuclear, 17 Ci/mmole, in 0.1 N NaOH)
 NaI (1 M in H_2O)
 EDTA (disodium ethylenediaminetetraacetate, 0.5 M, pH 7.2,
  adjusted with NaOH)
 PMSF (phenylmethylsulfonyl fluoride, 0.5 M stock in absolute
  ethanol) (Sigma)
 Disruption buffer (0.15 M NaCl, 0.01 M Tris-HCl, pH 7.4,
  0.005 M $MgCl_2$, 30% sucrose (w/v) and 0.002 M PMSF)
 Gradient solutions (w/v) sucrose (80%, 60%, 30%, 20%, 10%)
  metrizamide (50%) prepared and stored according to manu-
  facturer's instructions) all in 0.15 M NaCl, 0.01 M Tris-
  HCl, pH 7.4, 0.005 M $MgCl_2$ and 0.002 M PMSF.
 Immunoglobulins and complement: Rabbit antisheep erythrocyte IgM and IgG (Cordis). The source of complement is
  fresh mouse serum diluted in Veronal-buffered saline
  (1:5).
 DNase (Sigma), 1 mg/ml in PBS

B. Targets of Endocytosis

Fixed, opsonized sheep erythrocytes. Erythrocytes are incubated for 15 min at room temperature in hypotonic buffer (PBS: H_2O, 3:1 and then fixed in glutaraldehyde (Fisher Scientific, Springfield, New Jersey) (1.25% in PBS). Fix two days at 4°C by having a 10% packed cell volume erythrocytes in fixative. Mix occasionally. After washing in PBS, the fixed erythrocytes are incubated overnight in 0.1 M glycine (Sigma) to block the free aldehyde groups, washed again in PBS, and coated with appropriate ligands according to the procedure of Bianco *et al.* (4).

Latex particles (Dow Chemicals Co., Indianapolis, Indiana). 1.1-μm Diameter, polystyrene. Particles are washed in 70% ethanol in PBS (Beckman Microfuge, 1 min), and resuspended in D_O at 1×10^9 particles/ml.

III. PROCEDURE

A. Macrophages

Thioglycollate-induced mouse peritoneal cells are collected as described by Edelson and Cohn (5), using PBS with heparin (5 U/ml). The cells are washed twice and resuspended in PBS at 1×10^7ml, and radioiodinated by the lactoperoxidase-glucose oxidase method as described by Hubbard and Cohn (6). Viable macrophages are selected by adherence; the cell suspension is adjusted to 2×10^6/ml in D_O supplemented with fetal calf serum (10%) and 5 ml or 10^7 cells are plated per 100 mm tissue culture dish (Falcon). Attachment is allowed to proceed for 45 min at 37°C in a humidified 7.5% CO_2 atmosphere.

B. Endocytosis

Single particle: Opsonized erythrocytes are used at a ratio of 7 particles/macrophage for 45 min at 37°C. Latex is used at 200 particles/macrophage for 30 min at 37°C.

Mixed particles: Opsonized erythrocytes are allowed to attach to macrophages for 15 min at room temperature at a ratio of 60 - 100 particles/macrophages. Unattached erythrocytes are removed by washing in D_O. Latex is added at a ratio of 30 particles/macrophage. Endocytosis is allowed to proceed for 30 min at 37°C and excess particles are removed by washing in D_O.

C. Isolation of Phagosomes

All steps following endocytosis are carried out at 0°C and in the presence of 2 mM PMSF to prevent protein degradation. After washing in PBS, macrophages containing ingested particles are collected from the dishes by scraping into PBS + 2 mM EDTA. The cells are pelleted (5 min, 400 g, International PR-6 centrifuge) and resuspended in 1 ml of disruption buffer (up to 2×10^8 cells/ml). This cell suspension is homogenized mechanically by 40 - 60 strokes in a tight-fitting glass homogenizer. Homogenization is monitored by phase microscopy and stopped when approximately 90% of nuclei are released. The homogenate is adjusted to 69% sucrose by adding 2.2 ml of 80% sucrose. DNase is added to a final concentration of 10 µg/ml. An aliquot (0.1 - 0.2 ml) of the homogenate is saved for assays of protein, radioactivity, etc., and the remainder is used in gradient separation of phagosomes. The gradients are prepared in SW41 nitrocellulose centrifuge tubes (Beckman) and are composed of a 1 ml 50% metrizamide cushion; a linear 60 - 30% sucrose gradient (6 ml); and 1-ml layers of 20 and 10% sucrose. The cell homogenate is introduced with a long-tipped Pasteur pipette at the metrizamide-sucrose interface. Centrifugation is carried out for 12 - 16 hr at 40,000 rpm in a Beckman ultracentrifuge (SW41 rotor). Approximately 30 fractions (0.4 ml each) are collected from above the metrizamide-sucrose interface using a Beckman pump and without disturbing the band of phagosomes containing the red cells, which remain at that interface. The fractions may be analyzed for polypeptide composition, enzymatic content and radioactivity.

The phagosome band is diluted with disruption buffer without sucrose and collected by centrifugation (20 min 20,000 rpm, SW41 rotor, 4°C).

IV. CRITICAL COMMENTS

The use of glutaraldehyde-fixed sheep erythrocytes makes it possible to isolate and study that part of the macrophage surface membrane that is utilized to generate phagosomes. The isolation procedure we use involves simple steps and gives morphologically uniform (by EM) population of phagosomes, although the final yield in terms of cellular protein is rather small (up to 3%). The principal complications to be avoided are obvious. In order to obtain phagosomal material reflecting the molecular composition of the macrophage plasma membrane interiorized during the process of ingestion, protein degradation must be avoided (by processing the material at 0°C in the

A. GENERATION OF PHAGOSOMES

PERITONEAL EXUDATE CELLS
(thioglycollate-induced)

IODINATION
LPO + GO
→
ADHERENT MACROPHAGES

ATTACHMENT
OF EIgG
(RT, 15 min)
→
ROSETTES

PHAGOCYTOSIS
OF EIgG
AND LATEX
(37°, 30 min)
→
PHAGOCYTIC VESICLES
IN CELLS

B. ISOLATION OF PHAGOSOMES

PHAGOCYTIC VESICLES IN CELLS

HOMOGENIZATION
→
MIXED PHAGOSOMES
IN CELL HOMOGENATE

$^{125}I = 0.67 \times 10^{6}$ cpm/mg protein

Alkaline
phosphodiesterase = 102 mU/mg protein

CENTRIFUGATION
IN METRIZAMIDE-SUCROSE

LATEX PHAGOSOMES

$^{125}I = 3.08 \times 10^{6}$ cpm/mg protein

Alkaline
phosphodiesterase = 147 mU/mg

EIgG PHAGOSOMES

$^{125}I = 6.30 \times 10^{6}$ cpm/mg protein

Alkaline
phosphodiesterase = 569 mU/mg

presence of protease inhibitors). Phagocytosis itself must be as short as possible to minimize fusion with lysosomes.

One advantage of this system is that it can be used for the isolation of more than one type of phagosome from a single cell population. We have used latex and glutaraldehyde-fixed erythrocytes successfully, as shown in Fig. 1. In principle, one should also be able to obtain in the gradient the cell surface membrane remaining after phagosome formation. The effective yield of this fraction is, however, much lower than expected, because fragments of plasma membrane attach to nuclei and remain associated with them in the gradient. Addition of DNase to the whole cell homogenate before ultracentrifugation improves the results of separation.

The use of this approach has already allowed us to establish certain differences between receptor-mediated (opsonized erythrocytes) and nonspecific (latex) phagocytosis. First, latex-containing phagosomes resemble closely the intact macrophage plasma membrane in their polypeptide composition, while immune phagosomes contain a subset of plasma membrane polypeptides. Secondly, the receptor-mediated interiorization of plasma membrane polypeptides appears to have some specificity for the type of ligand presented on the target particle (Fc of IgG or C3). Finally, at least one ectoenzyme, alkaline phosphodiesterase I, (EC 3.1.4.1) is preferentially associated (or protected from degradation) with phagosomes resulting from endocytosis of particles that carry Fc on their surface, as opposed to latex or IgM + C. Most interestingly, the addition of complement to IgG-coated erythrocytes alters the composition of resulting phagosomes both in terms of alkaline phosphodiesterase content and polypeptide pattern.

REFERENCES

1. M. G. Wetzel and E. D. Korn. Phagocytosis of latex beads by *Acanthamoeba castellanii* (Neff). I. Isolation of phagocytic vesicles and their membranes. *Ann. Rev. Biochem.* *43*: 90, 1969.
2. Z. Werb and Z. A. Cohn. Plasma membrane synthesis in the macrophage following phagocytosis of polystyrene latex particles. *J. Biol. Chem. 247*: 2439, 1972.
3. S. C. Silverstein, R. M. Steinman, and Z. A. Cohn. Endocytosis. *Ann. Rev. Biochem. 46*: 669, 1977.
4. C. Bianco. *In* "Methods in Cell Mediated and Tumor Immunity" (B. R. Bloom and J. David, eds.), p. 407. Academic Press, New York, 1976.

5. P. J. Edelson and Z. A. Cohn. 5-Nucleotidase activity of mouse peritoneal macrophages. I. Synthesis and degradation in resident and inflammatory populations. *J. Exp. Med.* *144*: 1581, 1976.

6. A. L. Hubbard and Z. A. Cohn. Externally disposed plasma membrane proteins. I. Enzymatic iodination of mouse L cells. II. Metabolic fate of iodinated polypeptides of mouse L cells. *J. Cell Biol.* *64*: 438, 461, 1975.

87

STUDY OF MONONUCLEAR PHAGOCYTES
IN VIVO: OVERVIEW

D. S. Nelson

At a time when reductionism holds sway in biology, the
study of macrophages or, indeed, any other cells, *in vivo* may
seem quaintly old-fashioned. There are, however, good reasons,
both general and specific, to complement the refined and powerful tools of analysis *in vitro* with more unwieldy but very rewarding studies *in vivo*. Quite clearly, life in the body is
a good deal more complicated than life in the tissue culture
chamber: There is always a need to make sure that what is
observed *in vitro* has some counterpart *in vivo* and is not an
artifact. For some physiological and pathological processes,
we either altogether lack models *in vitro* or have models that
are incomplete. Among many examples are atherosclerosis and
delayed-type hypersensitivity (DTH). In the former case, it
appears to be very difficult to reproduce *in vitro* processes
involving both a good deal of the thickness of the walls of
arteries and the blood circulating within them (1). In the
case of DTH, much is known or inferred from studies *in vitro*
about the interaction between antigens and committed T cells
leading to the production of lymphokines and the consequent

attraction and immobilization of macrophages at the site of
the reaction. *In vivo,* however, other important factors operate: The supply of monocytes from the bone marrow, their
mobility in tissues, changes in vascular permeability, and
the involvement of the clotting system (2), an involvement
that is only now yielding to analysis *in vitro* (3). All who
work *in vitro* acknowledge that tissue culture conditions fall
a long way short of reproducing the internal environment, but
sometimes there are still surprises. For example, the presence of large amounts of ascorbic acid in the air spaces of
the lung (4) might be expected to have some effect on its
antimicrobial defences.

In many branches of biology, the importance, or otherwise,
of some organ, tissue, or group of cells can readily be demonstrated by means of ablation experiments. In immunology, for
example, it is relatively easy to produce a mouse devoid of
both a thymus and thymus-derived lymphocytes, but otherwise
intact. It is, however, difficult to produce an animal devoid
of mononuclear phagocytes, but otherwise intact. Sublethal
whole body irradiation or cyclophosphamide can temporarily
abolish the supply of monocytes from the bone marrow, but
these agents also affect many other types of cell, while leaving mature macrophages unaffected (5,6). Conversely agents
that are toxic to macrophages *in vitro,* such as silica (7) or
carrageenan (8), may either have only a partial and transient
antimacrophage effect *in vivo* or may have more widespread effects, for example, on the clotting and complement systems, on
other leukocytes and on unidentified components of DTH (9).
Some of the difficulties can be illustrated by reference to
studies of three important activities of macrophages: The
expression of acquired cellular resistance to infection; the
expression of antitumor immunity; and participation in inflammatory reactions leading to tissue destruction.

In experiments that can now be regarded as classics,
Mackaness and his colleagues showed that activated macrophages
are responsible for the expression of acquired cellular resistance to infection and that they become activated under the
influence of specifically committed T lymphocytes reacting
with antigen (10-15). The evidence was derived very largely
from experiments carried out with intact animals. Analysis
of the mechanisms of activation and of the antimicrobial activities of macrophages must depend equally largely on experiments *in vitro*. There are, however, problems to be overcome.
In the first place, the macrophages that are of the greatest
importance appear to be those recently derived from blood-born
monocytes and not those already resident in tissues (16). Accordingly, experiments *in vitro* should begin with either blood
monocytes or freshly induced exudates. While this is not par-

ticularly difficult in principle, large numbers of blood monocytes are not readily obtained from the usual laboratory rodents, while exudates induced, for example, in the peritoneal
cavity differ in character according to the inducing stimulus
and may not accurately reflect the character of the cell populations in infected animals. A second and more formidable
problem is the discrepancy between the intensity of the antibacterial activities of macrophages *in vivo* and *in vitro*.
Organisms such as *Listeria monocytogenes* and *Salmonella
typhimurium* can be phagocytosed and destroyed with quite formidable speed by macrophages in the liver, spleen, or peritoneal cavity of immune mice (11,12). It has, however, proved
extremely difficult to reproduce this degree of activity *in
vitro* (11, unpublished experiments) even with apparently
sensitive techniques (17). Similar considerations apply to
other bacteria in the lung and in isolated pulmonary alveolar
macrophages (18; D. Rowley, personal communication). Con-
ceivably, this could be related to the high ascorbic acid
content of the lung (4). Clearly, however, this discrepancy
between the activities of macrophages *in vivo* and *in vitro*
deserves investigation.

Activated macrophages exert powerful and selective but
nonspecific cytotoxic effects on tumor cells *in vitro* (19-21).
Several questions arise about the relevance of this phenomenon
to tumor immunity in intact animals. First, how can it be
shown that macrophages play an *essential* role in resistance to
a particular experimental tumor? We have discussed elsewhere
the criteria for a formal demonstration for such a role, concluding that it is difficult to devise totally rigorous and
realistic criteria but that the circumstantial evidence, in
many cases, is quite strong (22). Second, how are activated
macrophages brought to the site of deposition of tumor cells
so that they can exert their cytotoxic effect? It seems likely that, at least for certain tumors studied in our laboratory,
an immunological reaction very similar to that of DTH is involved (9,23,24). Among problems still deserving of investigation are

(1) whether such mechanisms are operative more generally
in tumor immunity, including resistance to metastasis;

(2) the way in which antitumor effector mechanisms operate
in the face of the powerful antiinflammatory factors produced,
apparently, by all tumors (25); and

(3) the possible role of antibody or the integration of
humoral and cellular mechanisms in tumor recognition (26).

The third question concerns the mechanisms of killing of tumor
cells *in vitro* and *in vivo*. Activated macrophages may kill
tumor cells *in vitro* in a variety of ways, for example, by

contact and the release or injection of lysosomes, by the production of cytotoxic factors, and by the release of arginase (22). In certain circumstances the release of arginase seems an adequate mechanism by itself (27,28). The significance of such a mechanism *in vitro* has, of course, been questioned, but recently evidence has been produced that local depletion of arginine by macrophages can be sufficient to create an environment hostile to tumor cells *in vivo* (29). Finally, activated macrophages obtained from animals and maintained *in vitro* can lose their cytotoxic effect quite quickly and additional stimuli may be required to restore it (30-33). The factors operating *in vivo* to preserve the cytotoxic effectiveness of macrophages also deserve attention.

Macrophages are very prominent in inflammatory reactions resulting in tissue damage. One of the most important human diseases in which such reactions occur is rheumatoid arthritis. Based on observations of lesions in man and experimental animals and on biochemical observations on cultured macrophages, strong suggestions have been made that the inflammation and destruction of joint tissue are due in part to the activities of macrophages, notably the release of lysosomal enzymes, neutral proteases, and prostaglandins (34-36). Models for such a complex interaction of macrophages and organized mixtures of target cells are difficult to devise *in vitro*. It seems reasonable to suggest that more ingenuity could usefully be applied to the study of macrophages in the available animal models *in vivo*.

Finally, man is a notoriously intractable subject for experiment, and the study of human macrophages *in vivo* seems likely to remain a very difficult one. Methods for measuring the phagocytic activity of the "reticuloendothelial system" in man have been available for some time but are only recently coming into fashion again, for example, in studies of defective macrophage function in rheumatoid arthritis (37) and systemic lupus erythematosus (38). Almost literally at the interface between studies *in vivo* and studies *in vitro,* however, is the examination of cells obtained from the lung by bronchoalveolar lavage. This relatively benign investigation promises to yield useful knowledge of the roles of macrophages (and of other cells) in inflammatory processes in the human lung (39).

REFERENCES

1. R. Ross and J. A. Glomset. The pathogenesis of atherosclerosis. *N. Engl. J. Med.* *295*:369-377, 420-425, 1976.

2. D. S. Nelson. The effects of anticoagulants and other drugs on cellular and cutaneous reactions to antigen in guinea pigs with delayed-type hypersensitivity. *Immunology 9*:219-234, 1965.

3. C. L. Geczy and K. E. Hopper. A mechanism of migration inhibition in delayed-type hypersensitivity II. Lymphokines promote coagulant activity of macrophages. *J. Immunol. 126*:1059-1065, 1981.

4. R. J. Willis and C. L. Kratzing. Ascorbic acid in rat lung. *Biochem. Biophys. Res. Commun. 59*:1250-1253, 1974.

5. A. Volkman and F. M. Collins. Recovery of delayed-type hypersensitivity in mice following suppressive doses of x-radiation. *J. Immunol. 101*:846-859, 1968.

6. J. -F. Bach. "The Mode of Action of Immunosuppressive Agents." North-Holland, Amsterdam, 1975.

7. A. C. Allison, J. S. Harington, and M. Birbeck. An examination of the cytotoxic effects of silica on macrophages. *J. Exp. Med. 124*:141-153, 1966.

8. A. W. Thomson, E. F. Fowler, and R. G. P. Pugh-Humphreys. Immunology of the macrophage-toxic agent carrageenan. *Int. J. Immunopharmacol. 1*:247-261, 1979.

9. M. Nelson and D. S. Nelson. Macrophages and resistance to tumors II. Influence of agents affecting macrophages and delayed-type hypersensitivity on resistance to a tumor inducing specific "sinecomitant" immunity: Acquired resistance as an expression of delayed-type hypersensitivity. *Cancer Immunol. Immunother. 4*:101-107, 1978.

10. G. B. Mackaness. The immunological basis of acquired cellular resistance. *J. Exp. Med. 120*:105-120, 1964.

11. R. V. Blanden, G. B. Mackaness, and F. M. Collins. Mechanisms of acquired resistance in mouse typhoid. *J. Exp. Med. 124*:585-600, 1966.

12. G. B. Mackaness. The influence of immunologically committed lymphoid cells on macrophage activity *in vivo*. *J. Exp. Med. 129*:973-992, 1969.

13. D. D. McGregor, F. T. Koster, and G. B. Mackaness. The mediator of cellular immunity. I. The life-span and circulation dynamics of the immunologically committed lymphocyte. *J. Exp. Med. 133*:389-399, 1973.

14. R. J. North. Importance of thymus-derived lymphocytes in cell-mediated immunity to infection. *Cell. Immunol. 7*:166-176, 1973.

15. R. J. North. The relative importance of blood monocytes and fixed macrophages to the expression of cell-mediated immunity to infection. *J. Exp. Med. 132*:521-534, 1970.

16. R. J. North. The concept of the activated macrophage. *J. Immunol. 121*:806-809, 1978.

17. A. M. Friedlander. DNA release as a direct measure of
     microbial killing by phagocytes. *Infect. Immun. 22*:148-
     154, 1978.
18. J. McA. Cooper and D. Rowley. Clearance of bacteria
     from lungs of mice after opsonizing with IgG or IgA.
     Aust. J. Exp. Biol. Med. Sci. 57:279-285, 1979.
19. J. B. Hibbs. Discrimination between neoplastic and
     nonneoplastic cells *in vitro* by activated macrophages.
     J. Natl. Cancer Inst. 53:1487-1492, 1974.
20. R. Evans. Tumor macrophages in host immunity to
     malignancies. *In* "The Macrophage in Neoplasia"
     (M. A. Fink, ed.), pp. 27-42. Academic Press, New York,
     1976.
21. R. Keller. Cytostatic and cytocidal effects of activated
     macrophages. *In* "Immunobiology of the Macrophage"
     (D. S. Nelson, ed.), pp. 487-508. Academic Press, New
     York, 1976.
22. D. S. Nelson, K. E. Hopper, and M. Nelson. Role of the
     macrophage in resistance to cancer. *In* "The Handbook of
     Cancer Immunology, Volume 3, Immune Status in Cancer
     Treatment and Prognosis - Part A" (H. Waters, ed.),
     pp. 107-157. Garland STPM Press, New York, 1976.
23. M. Nelson and D. S. Nelson. Macrophages and resistance
     to tumors. III. Influence of agents affecting macro-
     phages and delayed-type hypersensitivity on resistance
     to tumors inducing concomitant immunity. *Aust. J. Exp.
     Biol. Med. Sci. 56*:211-223, 1978.
24. K. E. Hopper and D. S. Nelson. Specific triggering of
     macrophage accumulation at the site of secondary tumor
     challenge in mice with concomitant tumor immunity.
     Cell. Immunol. 47:163-169, 1979.
25. M. Nelson and D. S. Nelson. Macrophages and resistance
     to tumours I. Inhibition of delayed-type hypersensitiv-
     ity reactions by tumour cells and by soluble products
     affecting macrophages. *Immunology 34*:277-290, 1978.
26. H. S. Shin, R. J. Johnson, G. P. Pasternack, and J. S.
     Economou. Mechanisms of tumor immunity: The role of
     antibody and nonimmune effectors. *Progr. Allergy 25:*
     163-210, 1978.
27. G. A. Currie and C. Basham. Differential arginine de-
     pendence and the selective cytotoxic effects of activated
     macrophages for malignant cells *in vitro*. *Br. J. Cancer
     38*:653-659, 1978.
28. E. Farram and D. S. Nelson. Mechanism of action of
     mouse macrophages as antitumor effector cells: Role of
     arginase. *Cell. Immunol. 55*:283-293, 1980.
29. G. A. Currie, L. Gyure, and L. Cifuentes. Microenviron-
     mental arginine depletion by macrophages *in vivo*. *Br.
     J. Cancer 39*:613-620, 1979.

30. J. B. Hibbs, Jr., R. R. Taintor, H. A. Chapman, Jr.,
     and J. B. Weinberg. Macrophage tumor killing: Influence
     of the local environment. *Science* 197:279-282, 1977.
31. S. W. Russell, W. F. Doe, and A. T. McIntosh. Functional
     characterization of a stable, noncytolytic stage of macro-
     phage activation in tumors. *J. Exp. Med.* 146:1511-1520,
     1977.
32. M. S. Meltzer, L. P. Ruco, D. Boraschi, and C. A. Nacy.
     Macrophage activation for tumor cytotoxicity: Analysis
     of intermediary reactions. *J. Reticuloendothel. Soc.*
     26:403-415, 1979.
33. G. Poste and R. Kirsh. Rapid decay of tumoricidal acti-
     vity and loss of responsiveness to lymphokines in inflam-
     matory macrophages. *Cancer Res.* 39:2582-2590, 1979.
34. M. Ziff. Relation of cellular infiltration of rheumatoid
     synovial membrane to its immune response. *Arthritis
     Rheum.* 17:313-319, 1974.
35. Z. Werb, C. L. Mainardi, C. A. Vater, and E. D. Harris, Jr.
     Endogenous activation of latent collagenase by rheumatoid
     synovial cells. *N. Engl. J. Med.* 296:1017-1023, 1977.
36. J. -M. Dayer, S. M. Krane, R. G. G. Russell, and D. R.
     Robinson. Production of collagenase and prostaglandins
     by isolated adherent rheumatoid synovial cells. *Pros.
     Natl. Acad. Sci. USA* 73:945-949, 1976.
37. B. D. Williams, B. A. Pussell, C. M. Lockwood, and C.
     Cotton. Defective reticuloendothelial system function in
     rheumatoid arthritis. *Lancet* 1:1311-1314, 1979.
38. M. M. Frank, M. I. Hamburger, R. J. Lawley, R. Kimberley,
     and P. H. Plotz. Defective reticuloendothelial system
     Fc-receptor function in systemic lupus erythematosus.
     N. Engl. J. Med. 300:518-523, 1979.
39. G. W. Hunninghake, J. E. Gadek, O. Kawanami, V. J.
     Ferrans, and R. G. Crystal. Inflammatory and immune
     processes in the human lung: Evaluation by broncho-al-
     veolar lavage. *Am. J. Pathol.* 97:149-206, 1979.

88

QUANTITATION OF THE INFLAMMATORY ACCUMULATION
OF MONONUCLEAR PHAGOCYTES IN VIVO

George J. Cianciolo
Ralph Snyderman

I.   INTRODUCTION

Mononuclear phagocytes serve important functions in the
recognition and effector limbs of immune responses as well as
in inflammatory reactions and wound healing. The mechanisms
by which these motile cells accumulate locally is still poorly
understood. Although macrophages have been shown to be capable
of exhibiting chemotactic migration *in vitro*, there is as yet
no practical way to demonstrate the migration of macrophages
along a chemoattractant gradient *in vivo*. It is, however,
possible to measure the kinetics and magnitude of the accumulation of macrophages at inflammatory sites *in vivo*. Several
different methods have been employed for making such measurements. All of them are based on the introduction of some inflammatory stimulant into a well-defined tissue space and quantifying the macrophages that subsequently accumulate in that
space. We shall describe several methods that we have success-

fully utilized either to quantitate macrophage accumulation *in vivo* or to demonstrate the production of chemotactic activity at sites of inflammation.

II. REAGENTS

1. *Inflammatory Stimulants*

Phytohemagglutinin(PHA) (Burroughs-Wellcome Co., Research Triangle Park, North Carolina) 35 µg in 2.0 ml sterile isotonic saline (for mice)

Concanavalin A(con A) (3 × crystallized; Miles-Yeda Ltd., Israel) 50 µg in 2.0 ml sterile isotonic saline (for mice)

Sodium metaperiodate ($NaIO_4$) (Fisher Scientific Co., Fair Lawn, New Jersey) 1.07 mg in 1.0 ml sterile isotonic saline (for mice)

Brewer's thioglycollate broth (Difco Laboratories, Detroit, Michigan) 4% (w/v) in deionized water, sterilized by autoclaving

Shellfish glycogen Type II (Sigma Chemical Co., St. Louis, Missouri) 0.5% (w/v) in sterile isotonic saline

Sodium caseinate (Difco Laboratories, Detroit, Michigan) 1% (w/v) in isotonic saline, sterilized by autoclaving

2. *Media*

Gey's balanced salt solution containing 2% bovine serum albumin and sodium bicarbonate (Flow Laboratories, McLean, Virginia), 10 mM HEPES, pH 7.0

RPMI 1640 (GIBCO, Grand Island, New York), 10 mM HEPES, pH 7.0

Phosphate buffered (0.01 M) saline, pH 7.0

3. *Preservative-free Heparin (Upjohn Co., Kalamazoo, Michigan) added 10 µ/ml for peritoneal lavage*

4. *Apparatus for Injections*

Mouse: 5- or 10-ml syringes; 25-gauge needles
Guinea pig: 30-ml syringes; 19-gauge needles

5. *Materials for Peritoneal Washouts*

Mouse: 70% Ethyl alcohol; (2) tooth-edged forceps; 10 ml syringes; 19-gauge needles; 30-ml polypropylene tubes

Guinea pig: Hair clipper or razor; 70% ethyl alcohol;

scalpel blade and surgical scissors; (2) surgical forceps;
(2) ring stands; (2) rubber spatulas; 30-ml syringes; 19-gauge
needles; 50-ml polypropylene tubes

III. PROCEDURES

The kinetics and magnitude of leukocyte accumulation *in vivo*
can be readily studied by the introduction of inflammatory
agents into the peritoneal cavity. At various times after introduction of the inflammatory agent, tissue culture medium is
injected, the cavities vigorously lavaged, and the contents are
aspirated using a syringe. Total and differential leukocyte
cell counts can be determined for the peritoneal washings and
the recovered cells or their supernatant fluids can be used for
in vitro assays.

1. Mouse Peritoneal Macrophages

Mice are injected intraperitoneally with 2.0 ml of PHA,
con A, thioglycollate broth or 1.0 ml of sodium periodate, or
other inflammatory stimulants and the cells harvested after the
appropriate period of time (Table I). Injections are best accomplished using a 25-gauge or smaller needle since this minimizes the trauma of injection. The accumulated cells are collected as follows: The mouse is killed by CO_2 asphyxiation or
decapitation, the abdominal area is wetted with 70% ethyl alcohol, and the skin elevated from the abdominal wall then retracted using two tooth-edged forceps to expose the abdominal
muscle wall. Eleven ml (less if the mice are extremely small,
e.g., <15 gm) of heparinized medium is vigorously injected into
the lower midline using a 19-gauge needle and the fluid (∿10 ml)
is then carefully withdrawn using the same syringe and needle
(bevel down). The injection and withdrawal procedures are repeated, using the same puncture site if possible. Withdrawal
of the injected fluid is facilitated by tenting the abdominal
wall with the needle (bevel down) as this helps to prevent
blockage by viscera or omentum. The second washout will usually
yield 11 ml back and the two washouts are pooled in a 30-ml
polypropylene centrifuge tube. Cell counts and differential
leukocyte counts can be done directly on this pooled material.
The length of time between injection and cell harvesting will
depend on the purpose of the assay and, if macrophages are required, the percentage of contaminating polymorphonuclear leukocytes (PMN) that is acceptable. Typical results obtained in
our laboratory for the various stimuli are listed in Table I.
Increasing the length of time between injection and harvesting

TABLE I. Intraperitoneal Accumulation of Cells to Various Inflammatory Stimuli in Mice

Inflammatory stimulus[a]	Hours post-injection[b]	Total cells[c] ($\times 10^6$)	Total M$\emptyset$[c] ($\times 10^6$)	Total PMN[c] ($\times 10^6$)
None	--	3.6	1.8	<0.05
PHA	48	12.9	8.4	0.6
con A	48	12.5	8.3	1.5
NaIO$_4$	72	11.8	6.6	1.3
Thioglycollate	48	12.9	11.1	1.0

[a]Five mice per group were either uninjected or injected with 2 ml of PHA (35 µg), con A (50 µg), thioglycollate (4%), or with 1 ml of sodium periodate (5 mM).

[b]At indicated time after injection, the peritoneal cavities were lavaged twice with 11 ml of heparinized medium and total and differential cell counts performed.

[c]Mean value for each group of five mice.

can decrease the percentage of PMN to <1% but will also decrease total number of macrophages obtained. If the cells are to be used for in vitro assays, they are washed once (400 g, 10 min, 4°C) in heparin-free medium and resuspended. If the supernatants are to be tested for biological activity, the washout volumes can be reduced to a more suitable volume. In quantitating the effects of various agents on the peritoneal inflammatory response, experimental groups should contain a minimum of five animals.

2. Guinea Pig Peritoneal Macrophages

Guinea pigs (400 - 500 gm) are injected ip with 25 - 30 ml of glycogen, sodium caseinate, or any appropriate inflammatory stimulant. At various times after injection, depending on the level of PMN contamination determined acceptable, the cells are harvested. A specific immunologically mediated reaction can be generated by first sensitizing the animals with a specific antigen such as Bacillus Calmette-Guerin or horseradish peroxidase (1). Intraperitoneal injection of the sensitized animals with the sensitizing antigen will then result in an inflammatory exudate that can be harvested at appropriate times.

In order to harvest the cells (2) the animal is killed, the abdomen is shaved, washed with 70% ethyl alcohol, and an ∿10-cm midline incision made. The abdominal walls are retracted using hemostats attached to ring stands. Fifty ml of heparinized medium is vigorously injected and the abdominal contents carefully but rigorously agitated. Care must be taken to avoid rup-

turing any blood vessels, the liver, or the spleen. This agitation is facilitated by the use of small rubber spatulas such
as used in the kitchen. The fluid is withdrawn from the left
lower quadrant using a syringe and needle and a spatula to keep
the viscera away from the needle. The injection and withdrawal
are repeated several times and the washes pooled in 50-ml polypropylene centrifuge tubes. The cells are collected by centrifugation at 400 *g* for 10 min at 4°C, resuspended in heparin-free
medium, and a cell count and differential performed. The volume
of medium used for the washout can be reduced appropriately if
the supernatant is to be tested for biological activity and the
cells can be washed in heparin-free medium and used for *in vitro*
assays. If serial samples are needed from a single animal, a
silastic plastic catheter can be surgically implanted into the
peritoneal cavity (1, 3). This method, while tedious to set up,
permits study of the kinetics of the generation of mediators of
inflammation *in vivo* and can be extremely valuable for certain
studies.

3. *Potential Pitfalls*

Care must be taken to ensure that intraperitoneal injections
are not given subcutaneously, or into the bowel or other organs.
Bowel perforation during injection can cause bacterial peritoni-
tis.

For this reason the injected materials should be kept sterile when possible. When washing out the peritoneal cavities of
both mice and guinea pigs, care must be taken to avoid lacerat-
ing major organs or blood vessels since the accumulation of
peripheral blood may interfere with the results. Even minor un-
seen perforations of the intestines during the washout procedure
can result in bacterial contamination, which often causes dramatic changes in the *in vitro* responsiveness of the cells; the
cell suspensions should be carefully examined for such contamination before *in vitro* use.

ANALYSIS OF DATA

The injection of inflammatory stimuli into the peritoneal
cavities of mice or guinea pigs results in an inflammatory response, the kinetics of which can easily be studied and have
been previously described (4). Table II illustrates the numbers of macrophages or polymorphonuclear leukocytes found in
the peritoneal cavities of mice injected 6, 24, 48, or 72 hr
earlier with PHA. As can be seen, the PMN response is extremely rapid, reaching a peak within the first 6 hr and then rapidly

TABLE II. Kinetics of Intraperitoneal Cell Accumulation in Mice after PHA Injection[a]

Time after injection[b] (hr)	Total cells[c] ($\times 10^6$)	Total MØ[c] ($\times 10^6$)	Total PMN[c] ($\times 10^6$)
0	3.8	2.3	0.01
6	10.1	0.8	8.9
24	11.6	5.3	2.5
48	10.5	7.0	0.6
72	11.3	7.0	0.5

[a]Five mice per group received either no injection or 2 ml of sterile saline containing 35 µg of PHA.

[b]At the indicated time after injection, the peritoneal cavities were lavaged twice with 11 ml of heparinized medium and total and differential cell counts performed.

[c]Mean value for each group of five mice.

falling off. The peak macrophage response however does not occur until 48 - 72 hr after injection. This difference in kinetics of response allows one to examine selectively the effects of various agents on the inflammatory response of either the macrophage or polymorphonuclear leukocyte. By examining PHA-induced mouse peritoneal exudates at various times, we have been able to show that low molecular weight products from tumors (5) or from certain oncogenic murine viruses depress macrophage accumulation but have no effect on PMN accumulation (6). A representative experiment is illustrated in Table III.

V.   CRITICAL COMMENTS

A.   Other Accumulation Assays

     While we have described induction of peritoneal inflammatory reactions in mice and guinea pigs, they have also been elicited in rats (7, 8), hamsters (8), chickens (9), and rabbits (10). Inflammatory reactions can also be quantified in the pleural cavity (7, 11) or in the lungs (12).

TABLE III. *Inhibition of Macrophage (MØ) Accumulation by Low Molecular Weight Viral Products[a]*

Virus extract[b] (ng)	Accumulated MØ[c] ($\times 10^6 \pm SE$)	Inhibition[d] (%)	Significance[e] (p)
RLV			
200.0	2.2 ± 0.1	48	<0.01
20.0	1.8 ± 0.4	57	<0.01
2.0	1.6 ± 0.2	62	<0.01
0.2	2.8 ± 0.2	33	<0.02
Buffer alone	4.2 ± 0.3	--	--
FLV			
1200.0	2.1 ± 0.3	60	<0.01
120.0	2.8 ± 0.4	46	<0.01
12.0	3.0 ± 0.5	42	<0.01
1.2	3.7 ± 0.1	29	<0.02
Buffer alone	5.2 ± 0.4	--	--
MoLV			
200.0	3.0 ± 0.2	58	<0.01
20.0	4.8 ± 0.2	33	<0.01
2.0	1.9 ± 0.2	74	<0.01
0.2	1.7 ± 0.2	76	<0.01
Buffer alone	7.2 ± 0.4	--	--
MMTV			
720.0	5.8 ± 0.6	0	NS[f]
72.0	5.2 ± 0.6	0	NS
7.2	5.6 ± 0.8	0	NS
0.7	4.9 ± 1.0	2	NS
Buffer alone	5.0 ± 0.5	--	--

[a]Taken with permission from ref. 6.

[b]Low molecular weight virus extracts were injected subcutaneously in 0.2 ml volumes into the thighs of five mice and macrophage accumulation determined.

[c]The number of accumulated macrophages was determined by subtracting the number of macrophages ($\sim 1.8 \times 10^6$) present in the peritoneal cavities of unstimulated mice from the number of macrophages present in the peritoneal cavities of PHA stimulated mice.

[d]Percentage inhibition of macrophage accumulation was calculated as

$$\% \ Inhibition = \frac{control - experimental}{control} \times 100$$

[e]As determined by Student's t test.

[f]Not significant.

B. *Alternate Methods*

In vivo accumulation of inflammatory cells can also be
measured by placement of nitrocellulose filters (7, 13) or
glass coverslips (14) either subcutaneously or in the peritoneal cavity. The filters or coverslips can be removed at
various times, stained, and the types and numbers of cells determined. Another technique is to label the bone marrow precursor cells by giving the animals a pulse of [^{3}H]thymidine.
The influx of cells into inflammatory sites (15, 16) or onto
nitrocellulose filters or glass coverslips can then be followed using scintillation spectrophotometry. We have used
this technique with mouse peritoneal exudate cells and found
excellent correlation at 48 hr after injection between the
amount of cell-associated radiolabel and the numbers of macrophages (16). The disadvantages of such techniques are that
a considerable amount of label would be expected to be associated with PMN at the earlier times and considerable amounts
of radiolabeled thymidine would be required for animals larger
than mice or for large experiments. The method also requires
two additional injections to each animal that may be undesirable under certain circumstances.

Other methods that have been used include the air enclave
method, in which a pocket is formed by injecting air subcutaneously (17), or skin window techniques, in which an area of
skin is exposed and then covered by a glass coverslip (18).
The coverslip is removed after various times, stained, and the
numbers and types of cells determined. The former technique
suffers due to the inherent variability associated with the
formation of the air pocket and the latter requires microscopic examination of adhered cells from a large number of
fields to reduce sampling errors.

REFERENCES

1. A. E. Postlethwaite and R. Snyderman. Characterization
    of chemotactic activity produced in vivo by a cell-mediated
    immune reaction in the guinea pig. *J. Immunol. 114*: 274-
    278, 1975.
2. M. S. Hausman, R. Snyderman, and S. E. Mergenhagen. Hu-
    moral mediators of chemotaxis of mononuclear leukocytes.
    J. Infect. Dis. 124: 595-602, 1972.
3. A. E. Postlethwaite, A. S. Townes, and A. H. Kang. Charac-
    terization of macrophage migration inhibitory factor ac-
    tivity produced in vivo by a cell-mediated immune reaction
    in the guinea pig. *J. Immunol. 117*: 1716-1720, 1976.

4. R. Snyderman, M. C. Pike, B. L. Blaylock, and P. Weinstein.
    Effects of neoplasms on inflammation: Depression of mac-
    rophage accumulation following tumor implantation. *J. Im-
    munol. 116*: 585-589, 1976.
5. G. J. Cianciolo, R. B. Herberman, and R. Snyderman. De-
    pression of murine macrophage accumulation by low molecular
    weight factors derived from spontaneous mammary carcinomas.
    J. Natl. Cancer Inst. 65: 829-834, 1980.
6. G. J. Cianciolo, T. J. Matthews, D. P. Bolognesi, and
    R. Snyderman. Macrophage accumulation in mice is inhibited
    by low molecular weight products from murine leukemia vi-
    ruses. *J. Immunol. 124*: 2900-2905, 1980.
7. S. J. Normann and J. Cornelius. Concurrent depression of
    tumor macrophage infiltration and systemic inflammation by
    progressive cancer growth. *Cancer Res. 38*: 3453-3459,
    1978.
8. H. S. Lin, C. Kuhn, and C. C. Stewart. Peritoneal exudate
    cells V. Influence of age, sex, strain, and species on the
    induction and the growth of macrophage colony forming
    cells. *J. Cell Physiol. 96*: 133-138, 1978.
9. T. Sabet, W. C. Hsia, H. Stanisz, A. El-Domeiri, and P.
    Van Alten. A simple method for obtaining peritoneal mac-
    rophages from chickens. *J. Immunol. Methods 14*: 103-110,
    1977.
10. R. Snyderman, H. Gewurz, and S. E. Mergenhagen. Interac-
    tions of the complement system with endotoxic lipopoly-
    saccharide. Generation of a factor chemotactic for poly-
    morphonuclear leukocytes. *J. Exp. Med. 128*: 259-275,
    1968.
11. R. Vinegar, J. F. Traux, J. L. Selph, R. M. Welch, and
    H. L. White. The effect of caffeine on the pharmacology
    of aspirin and phenacetin. *Fed. Proc. 35*: 775a, 1976.
12. P. G. Holt. Alveolar macrophages. I. A simple technique
    for the preparation of high numbers of viable alveolar
    macrophages from small laboratory animals. *J. Immunol.
    Methods 27*: 189-198, 1979.
13. S. J. Normann and M. Schardt. A macrophage inflammation
    test using subcutaneous nitrocellulose filters. *J.
    Reticuloendothel. Soc. 23*: 153-160, 1978.
14. G. F. Ryan and W. G. Spector. Macrophage turnover in in-
    flamed connective tissue. *Proc. R. Soc. (London) B 175*:
    269-292, 1970.
15. A. L. Oronsky, R. J. Perper, V. J. Stecher, M. Sanda, and
    G. Chinea. Mechanism of *in vivo* chemotaxis (Cx) of neu-
    trophil (PMN) and mononuclear leukocytes. *Fed. Proc. 33*:
    631a, 1974.
16. R. Snyderman and M. C. Pike. Biological activities of a
    macrophage chemotaxis inhibitor (MCI) produced by neo-
    plasms. *In* "Cell Biology and Immunology of Leukocyte

Function" (M. R. Quastel, ed.), pp. 535–546. Academic Press, New York, 1979.

17. A. Larson. Subcutaneous enclaves in mice as sites for the study of cellular responses *in vivo*. *J. Bacteriol.* *97*: 445–447, 1969.

18. J. W. Rebuck and J. H. Crowley. A method of studying leukocytic functions *in vivo*. *Ann. NY Acad. Sci.* *59*: 757–805, 1955.

89

SYSTEMIC LABELING OF MONONUCLEAR PHAGOCYTES

Alvin Volkman
Richard T. Sawyer

I. INTRODUCTION

The systemic administration of radioactive cellular labels
to animals provides an effective means of studying the kinetics
of cell population renewal and the fates of defined cells and
cell populations. Such labels must be metabolically stable and
readily quantifiable. Isotopically labeled thymidine is by far
the most important and widely employed agent for these purposes
and will therefore be the major subject of this account. Thymidine is a specific precursor of DNA, and has a high degree
of metabolic stability. The incorporation of thymidine into DNA
occurs for the most part when a cell doubles its chromosomal
content during the premitotic synthesis of DNA. In mitosis, the
label is distributed evenly between the daughter cells. Tritium
(^{3}H) has been the most widely used radioactive isotope linked to
thymidine for *in vivo* studies. ^{14}C-labeled thymidine is sometimes favored for special purposes because ^{14}C has a higher
energy beta emission than does ^{3}H. Isotopically labeled analogs

of thymidine, most notably iododeoxyuridine, with ^{125}I or ^{131}I substitutions, have also been employed as DNA-linked cell labels.

Unincorporated thymidine is degraded very rapidly after intravenous (iv) or intraperitoneal (ip) administration. For this reason the radioactivity as thymidine is effectively available for probably no longer than 30 min (1). This narrow interval, the availability time, advantageously pinpoints the time of labeled thymidine incorporation by cells synthesizing DNA.

Certain physical properties that contribute to the popularity of ^{3}HTdR include decay with a very low energy emission (0.0186 MeV) and a half life of 12.35 yr. The energy of the emanating particles is spent at an average distance of 1 μm from their source. For this reason, ^{3}HTdR within a cell nucleus can be localized visually with a high degree of precision in an overlay of photographic emulsion, i.e., autoradiography. After appropriate exposure of the emulsion and photographic processing, the presence of the isotopic label is made visible as microscopic grains of silver with virtually no tracking in the overlying emulsion. Cell smears or histological sections prepared in this way can be stained through the emulsion. The techniques involved in autoradiography will not be discussed any further in this chapter; several good references are recommended (2 - 4). Another means of detecting the activity of ^{3}HTdR is liquid scintillation counting, which will receive additional comment elsewhere in this chapter.

Characteristic cytokinetic features of mononuclear phagocyte populations have been described in a number of species including humans and have recently been collated (5). Additional studies are still needed to clarify problems relating to the functional properties, ontogeny and population renewal among mononuclear phagocytes. Some of these problems and models for tracing the movement of labeled mononuclear phagocytes have recently been discussed (6, 7).

II.   REAGENTS

A. *Tritium-Labeled Thymidine*

We routinely buy sterile aqueous [methyl-^{3}H]thymidine from either Amersham Radiochemicals (Arlington Heights, Illinois) or New England Nuclear (Boston, Massachusetts) and store it at 4°C. Radioactivity as thymidine declines slowly during storage (about 1%/month) at this temperature and more rapidly if the reagent is kept frozen. Solutions in ethanol

are said to have longer shelf lives than solutions in saline.
Maintenance of sterility obviously prolongs shelf life. The
choice of specific activity (SA) is dictated by the purpose of
an experiment. Low SA ^{3}HTdR (2 - 3 Ci/mM) is used for most
purposes, whereas the use of high SA ^{3}HTdR is restricted to
"flash" labeling experiments. Dosage is most commonly
0.5 - 1 µCi/gm body weight in 0.2 ml for mice and 0.5 - 1 ml
for rats. Substantial savings are possible under purchase
contracts if large amounts of ^{3}HTdR (30 MCi) are to be annually
consumed.

B. Nonradioactive ("Cold") Thymidine

This reagent may be needed to minimize reutilization and
is obtainable from several suppliers including Sigma Chemical
Company (St. Louis, Missouri). It can be stored at room temperature. Solutions are prepared in saline to yield doses of
0.5 µg/gm body weight in volumes of 0.1 - 0.5 ml for mice and
rats.

C. Diluents

Physiological saline as used for the dilution of thymidine preparations should be sterile and pyrogen-free. We find
it convenient to purchase saline with such specifications from
Baxter or Abbott Laboratories.

D. Hypodermic Syringes and Needles

Disposable syringes in 1- and 5-ml sizes, made by Becton
Dickinson Company, are ordered through a surgical supply dis-
tributor. Glass syringes are also acceptable but must be thoroughly decontaminated after use with radioactive isotopes.
Disposable needles are also Becton Dickinson products. The
following sizes are useful: 25-gauge 5/8 in. and 26-gauge
1/2 in. for iv injection of rats and mice; 20-gauge, 1 1/2 in.
and 23-gauge, 1 in. for ip injection of the respective species.

E. Pitfalls

1. Radiation Hazard

Although ^{3}HTdR is considered relatively innocuous because
of the low energy emission of ^{3}H, this feature makes laboratory
and animal room contamination difficult to detect with conven-

tional monitoring. The incorporation of ^{3}HTdR into DNA and the
long half-life of ^{3}H contribute to the biohazard. In most situations conditions for the use, storage, and survey of radioactive materials will have been established by an institutional
radiation safety committee. Stringent observance of appropriate
technique is urged.

2. Radiation Damage

The potential for radiation damage to cells is higher with
^{3}HTdR because of the intranuclear energy absorption consequent
to the very low energy emission. For this reason, total dosage
should not exceed 1 µCi/gm body weight/day and specific activity
for all purposes other than flash labeling should not exceed
3 Ci/mM.

III. PROCEDURES

A. Selection of Subjects

In vivo labeling with ^{3}HTdR has been used in a wide variety
of species. Studies in man have been limited to patients with
terminal illness (1). Cytokinetic activities of cell populations can be influenced by age, sex, intercurrent infection,
nutritional status of the subject, and, undoubtedly, a variety
of other factors.

B. Anesthesia

Intravenous labeling of rats requires anesthetized subjects. Mice, guinea pigs, and rabbits, on the other hand, can
be injected merely with the aid of conventional restraining de-
vices. Ethyl ether inhalation is preferred for all studies,
except those involving lung macrophages, because of its short-
lived effects and ease of control. A drawback to the use of
ether is its potential for explosion but it is very safe when
used in a well-ventilated room with conventional precautions
with respect to flame and electrical discharges. About 20 ml
of ether for anesthesia, United States Pharmacopeia, is poured
onto cage bedding or cotton wool placed in the bottom of a
large glass dessicator having a partially stoppered lid. A
disk of expanded stainless steel is inserted to support the
animals above the absorbent material.

The animals are placed in the dessicator after the initial
high concentration of ether vapor is dispersed by waving a hand

over the open top of the vessel. Some rats may manifest considerable reluctance to stay in the dessicator while the lid
is being replaced; this is the time to watch your fingers.
Smaller, less-expensive vessels for anesthesia may be improvised
for mice. We have found that certain brands of kosher gefilte
fish, available in many urban supermarkets, are sold in screw
top jars of ideal dimensions for this purpose. Perforate the
metal jar lid to provide some air intake.

Occasional additions of 1 - 2 ml of ether, dribbled down
the inner wall of the vessel, may be necessary for effective
anesthetization. An appropriate level of anesthesis is indicated by the loss of the corneal reflex which is tested for
with a whisp of cotton wool. The animal is then transferred
to the work table and an ether-soaked pledget of cotton wool
placed close to but not on its nose. Additional ether may be
added dropwise from a glass dropping bottle or from the original
ether can. When doing so, the pledget of cotton should be moved
away from the animal's nose. Liquid ether is very irritating
and can cause lethal laryngospasm and edema of the respiratory
tract. We have found through the years that this seemingly
crude procedure of ether administration permits excellent control of anesthesia.

When lung macrophages are to be harvested, animals are
killed with appropriate doses of sodium pentobarbital (ip).

C. *Route of Injection*

Intravenous injection is the preferred route for ^{3}HTdR
administration because it provides precise information concerning the quantity of radioactivity entering the blood in a
narrowly defined interval. Rats and mice are injected in
lateral tail veins; guinea pigs in hind foot veins, in the
penile veins, or in an ear vein after local warming. In special instances, ^{3}HTdR may be given ip, intramuscularly, or subcutaneously. When injected ip, ^{3}HTdR rapidly gains access to
the blood; absorption from other sites is slower and persistence in the blood may be longer. Following iv injection,
^{3}HTdR diffuses rapidly into the extracellular fluid. Our data
show no differences in the percentages of peritoneal cells that
become labeled in 1 hr after ip or iv injection of low specific
activity (1 - 3 Ci/mM) ^{3}HTdR.

D. *Injection Regimens: The Cell Cycle*

Tritium-labeled thymidine may be administered one or more
times before a cell population is sampled. The frequency of
labeling and the time of sampling are critical and require care-

ful consideration in the development of an experimental protocol. Factors that can strongly influence the results include
the availability time of ^{3}HTdR and the cell cycle of the population being investigated. The cell cycle is conventionally
divided into phases beginning with mitosis (M), postmitotic
rest (G_1), a phase of DNA synthesis (S), and premitotic rest
(G_2). When a cell is mitotically inactive for a long period,
it may be considered to be in G_0. It can be difficult to determine whether a portion of a population has lost the capacity
to divide or is in a prolonged G_0 phase. The phases generally
differ from each other in duration but the ratio of any phase
to the average cell cycle time (T_C) is generally typical in un-
perturbed populations. Detailed discussions of the cell cycle
(1, 8) should be consulted by investigators interested in cytokinetic studies. Although virtually all ^{3}HTdR is incorporated
during S, not all chromosomes are engaged in DNA synthesis at
the same time. In addition, under normal conditions, cell division is not synchronized. When studying the influences of
any agents administered experimentally, optimal intervals between the time of experimental treatment(s) and the time of
^{3}HTdR administration should be carefully determined.

1. "Flash" Labeling

The purpose of this procedure is to determine the proportion of a cell population in the S phase of the mitotic cycle.
Tritium-labeled thymidine is administered iv and the population
under study is sampled at an interval shorter than the probable
average minimum duration of S, G_2, and M taken together. For
practical purposes, sampling, in many instances involving the
sacrifice of the labeled animal, is carried out between 30 and
60 min after iv administration of ^{3}HTdR. Short sampling intervals must also be maintained when the movement or emigration of
labeled cells from one compartment into another can influence
the percentage of cells labeled; i.e., bone marrow precursors
into the blood or monocytes into exudates. On the other hand,
sufficient time for ^{3}HTdR to diffuse into extracellular fluids
is likewise important.

2. "Pulse" Labeling

The quantity of radioactivity as thymidine present in the
plasma following a single iv injection of ^{3}HTdR is determined
by the rate of thymidine catabolism, a process that takes place
largely in the liver. A relatively narrow pulselike activity
curve is the result of the rapidity of the process. Radioactivity as thymidine is effectively available for about 30 min.
Samples of mononuclear phagocyte populations under study are
taken at selected intervals. Selected parameters of labeling,

for example, the percentage of cells labeled, the mean grain count and the distribution of labeled cells are plotted against time. Waves of labeled cells from each division initially result in increased percentages of labeled cells, which later decrease as a result of the loss of cells from populations and the dilution of label by repeated cell cycles.

3. Repeated Labeling

In order to obtain certain types of cytokinetic information, the labeling of a continuous series of cell generations may be necessary. In addition, cell tracer studies may require the labeling of high proportions of a defined population. For these purposes, injections of ^{3}HTdR are repeated at intervals shorter than a presumptive minimum cell cycle time (T_c).

In mice and rats, average durations of T_c for monocyte precursors have been estimated to fall between about 10 and 24 hr; T_c values for macrophages *in vivo* may be substantially longer. Regimens of three injections at 8-hr intervals or four injections every 6 hr would be reasonable for attaining a high degree of labeling of the monocyte proliferative pool and the monocytes generated therefrom. The total daily dose of ^{3}HTdR should not exceed 1 μCi/gm body weight.

4. Saturation Labeling

It is also possible to administer ^{3}HTdR by continuous infusion. Restraint of animals being continuously infused is generally necessary, although this procedure has been carried out using a special apparatus on unrestrained rats (9). We have found that Bollman Mann type restraining cages (10) are suitable for this purpose. Subcutaneously implantable osmotic minipumps manufactured by Alza (Palo Alto, California) may also prove effective for the slow sustained release of ^{3}HTdR for periods of about a week. As before, the total daily dose should not exceed 1 μCi/gm body weight.

5. Maintenance of Labeled Animals

The vast majority of the administered radioactivity is excreted in the urine, and cage bedding becomes heavily contaminated. The use of open-bottomed cages is not recommended. Animal care personnel should be thoroughly instructed in techniques for the safe handling and cleaning of cages and the disposal of contaminated carcasses and materials as dictated by the local radiation safety committee.

IV. EVALUATION OF RESULTS

As indicated earlier, results of ^{3}HTdR labeling *in vivo* may be measured by liquid scintillation counting or autoradiography following the removal and preparation of the cells and tissues under study. Liquid scintillation counting is useful when information concerning the movement of a reasonably defined population must be quantified, i.e., the measurement of the intensity of an inflammatory response that is predominantly mononuclear and rich in immigrant macrophages. Under such conditions, the radioactivity contributed by other participating cells will be relatively small compared with the highly labeled macrophages.

Autoradiography permits individual labeled cells to be classified and monitored. Several means of assessment are possible depending on the goals and design of an experiment. For example, if labeling is restricted to a selected site, migration pathways of labeled cells and their progeny can be determined. Obviously the target for such labeling would be a progenitor pool as is found in bone marrow. Effective models for this type of labeling have been described (6, 7).

A. *The Labeling Index (LI)*

One of the major parameters in any autoradiographic study is the LI, which is simply the ratio of labeled cells to total cells in a defined class, and is commonly expressed as a percentage. The basic cytokinetic experiment involves plotting the change in labeling index against time. Under ideal conditions, the LI is determined by the ratio of the period of DNA synthesis (T_S) to the cell cycle time (T_C). An underlying assumption is that all cells of the population under study are in cycle. In actuality, many cell populations that have been studied contain high proportions of nondividing cells (11). Under such conditions the observed LI would be lower than the potential LI (LI_{pot}) computed from the cells in cycle and roughly equal to T_S/T_C. That proportion of a population actively dividing or cycling has been designated the growth fraction (11) and can be estimated from the ratio of the observed LI to LI_{pot}, provided that the length of the S phase and the cell cycle time are known. The growth fraction has received little attention in cytokinetic studies of mononuclear phagocytes but may prove to be very important for the understanding of population renewal among resident macrophages.

B. *Grain Count Analysis*

Changes in mean grain counts have been used to define homogeneous cohorts of labeled cells (12) and to estimate the duration of the cell cycle. In pulse labeling studies many cells may have low grain counts for several reasons: (1) the parent cell may have incorporated ^{3}HTdR early or late in S phase when only a few chromosomes were synthesizing DNA; (2) dilution of label may have resulted from multiple divisions; (3) salvage of labeled DNA metabolites liberated from dead cells may occur. Studies of cell lifespan within a compartment are therefore better carried out using the most highly labeled, hence most homogeneous cohort of a cell class. There are a number of pitfalls inherent in the use of grain count halving to estimate T_C and detailed accounts should be consulted (1).

C. *The Anatomy of Mononuclear Phagocyte Labeling*

Observations in the rat showed that the *in vivo* labeling characteristics of blood monocytes, and resident and immigrant macrophages are distinctive when compared with lymphocytes and polymorphonuclear leukocytes (13). Comparable findings with quantitative differences have been reported in other species (5). In brief, flash labeling indices among all three groups of mononuclear phagocytes are exceedingly low, generally less than 4%. From 6 - 8 hr after a pulse label, however, increasing percentages of labeled monocytes are found in the blood reaching a peak of roughly 40% in 48 hr in rats. Higher figures are found in mice. Correspondingly high labeling indices are found among immigrant macrophages in foci of inflammation when sampled at appropriate intervals. It later became clear that greater LI in pulse labeling, when compared to the flash LI reflects the mitotic activity within the progenitor pool (14). Over 80% of the blood monocytes in rats can become labeled after 4 - 5 days of continuous infusion of ^{3}HTdR (14).

In planning experiments, it is worthwhile to note that only small proportions of the morphologic lymphocyte population become labeled after a single injection of ^{3}HTdR and the LI increases slowly during continuous infusion (15). Polys undergo prolonged postmitotic maturation in the bone marrow before being released. As a result, there is about a 3-day interval after ^{3}HTdR administration before labeled polys appear in the blood in rodents; the interval is somewhat longer in humans. Another fact that may be helpful in the planning of experiments involving systemic labeling of mononuclear phagocytes is that the monocyte proliferative pool is radiosensitive (16).

V. CRITICAL COMMENTS

Labeling cells *in vivo* with [3]HTdR is a powerful investigative tool that can be applied in a wide variety of models. Its use in the study of the cell kinetics of population renewal and as an "indelible" cell marker in the study of pathways of migration and differentiation is well established. Autoradiographs of labeled cells can be prepared for examination by light and electron microscopy. Overall, [3]HTdR labeling is a very sensitive method and results are highly reproducible.

A. *Limitations*

There are limitations in the use of [3]HTdR. For one, only cells in the S phase of the cell cycle incorporate [3]HTdR. This feature can be a drawback when dealing with a cell population or population compartments with a small growth fraction and, consequently, a low observed LI.

In addition, it can be difficult, even impossible, to distinguish between local [3]HTdR incorporation and low level traffic and emigration of labeled cells in a compartment. There are many published experiments concerning macrophage renewal that display considerable confusion about this point. In theory, this limitation could be overcome by transferring monocytes or bone marrow from a heavily labeled donor to a histocompatible recipient. Since monocytes and monocyte precursors are numerically small components in their respective compartments, there may occur a dilution of the labeled inoculum by the recipient's own monocytes. This problem is further complicated by the relatively brief half-times of monocytes in the blood (8 - 36 hr depending on the species), and attempts to circumvent these difficulties have been made by transfusing labeled bone marrow to a lethally irradiated recipient. Data from such models can be difficult to interpret because of the potential for radiation damage to the recipient's macrophages.

A pitfall to be reckoned with in all *in vivo* labeling studies involving [3]HTdR is the reutilization or salvage of degraded DNA following its liberation during the death of labeled cells. A simple way to minimize reutilization effects is to restrict analyses to more highly labeled cells. This approach is not wholly infallible and does sacrifice precise quantitation. Another approach is to increase the body thymidine pools by the administration of nonradioactive (cold) thymidine. A so-called pulse-chase with cold thymidine is of limited value since cold thymidine is metabolized as rapidly as any other thymidine. As a result, the effect of the chase is largely over within 30 minutes. In experiments where reutilization was

considered a particularly undesirable source of interference
with the interpretation of autoradiographs restrained rats
were repeatedly or continuously infused with cold thymidine
(16). If reutilization is a major concern, parallel experiments with poorly reutilized ^{125}I-UdR should provide a means
of indirectly estimating salvage effects.

B. *Interpretation of Data*

References already cited provide examples and discussions
of this important aspect of *in vivo* cell labeling. Some miscellaneous points will be addressed in this section because
their particular relevance.

1. *The Significance of a Labeled Cell*

Labeled cells found after a flash label represent cells
in S phase, not the number of dividing cells. Following a
pulse label, a labeled cell may be either pre- or postmitotic,
depending on the sampling interval and the respective durations
of S, G_2, and M.

2. *Concommitant Changes in Labeling Indices*

Parallel and sequential elevations in labeling indices
occurring in two or more compartments or population subclasses
do not constitute hard evidence that one subpopulation gives
rise to the others. Before such a conclusion can be made,
there must be direct evidence that this is so. Alternatively
the possibilities that the ostensibly derivative populations
are dividing independently or are being "fed" from unidentified
pools must be rigorously excluded.

3. *The Significance of Labeled Immigrant Mononuclear Phagocytes*

The prerequisite for interpreting this occurrence is the
exclusion of the possibility that label was incorporated locally by dividing cells. Once the immigrant nature of such
cells is established, the number of interpretations are limited.
One that is commonly overlooked in the study of normal animals
is that perturbation has inadvertently taken place and hence
one is looking at a "normal" monocyte response to an inflammatory stimulus yielding labeled macrophages. If such an occurrence can be excluded, the next question is whether the labeled
immigrants are about to take up lodging and become resident
macrophages or whether they represent a stream of traffic
through an independent compartment. One hopes that objective

rather than legislative distinctions between residents and transients can be found. It is probable, however, that *in vivo* cell labeling by itself will not be able to provide satisfactory answers to this question bearing on the origin of functional heterogeneity in macrophages. Functional studies and the development of differentiation markers are also needed to help resolve these problems.

REFERENCES

1. G. S. Steel. "Growth Kinetics of Tumors." Oxford University Press, Oxford, 1977.
2. L. G. Caro and R. P. van Tubergen. High-resolution autoradiography. *J. Cell Biol.* 15: 173-188, 1962.
3. B. M. Kopriwa and C. P. Leblond. Improvements in the coating technique of radioautography. *J. Histochem. Cytochem.* 10: 269-284, 1962.
4. P. B. Gahan. "Autoradiography for Biologists." Academic Press, New York, 1972.
5. A. Volkman. Changes in blood monocyte kinetics during infection. *In* "Immunobiology of the Macrophage" (D. S. Nelson, ed.), pp. 291-322. Academic Press, New York, 1976.
6. A. Volkman. Disparity of Origin of mononuclear phagocyte populations. *J. Reticuloendothel. Soc.* 19: 249-268, 1976.
7. A. Volkman. The unsteady state of the Kupffer cell. *In* "Kupffer Cells and Other Liver Sinusoieal Cells" (E. Wisse and D. L. Knook, eds.), pp. 459-469. Elsevier, North Holland Biomedical Press, Amsterdam, 1977.
8. J. E. Cleaver. "Thymidine Metabolism and Cell Kinetics." North-Holland, Amsterdam, 1967.
9. A. Volkman and F. M. Collins. The cytokinetics of monocytosis in acute *Salmonella* infection in the rat. *J. Exp. Med.* 139: 264-277, 1974.
10. J. L. Bollman. A cage which limits the activity of rats. *J. Lab. Clin. Med.* 33: 1348, 1948.
11. M. L. Mendelsohn. The growth fraction: A new concept applied to tumors. *Science 132*: 1496, 1960.
12. V. P. Bond, T. M. Fliedner, E. P. Cronkite, J. R. Rubin, and J. S. Robertson. Cell turnover in blood and blood forming tissues studied with tritiated thymidine. *In* "The Kinetics of Cellular Proliferation" (F. Stohlman, Jr., ed.), pp. 188-200. Grune and Stratton, New York, 1959.
13. A. Volkman and J. L. Gowans. Production of macrophages in the rat. *Br. J. Exp. Pathol.* 46: 50-61, 1965.
14. A. Volkman. The production of monocytes and related cells.

Hematol. Lat. 10: 61-63, 1967.

15. S. H. Robinson, G. Brecher, I. S. Lourie, and J. E. Naley. Leukocyte labeling in rats during and after continuous infusion of tritiated thymidine: Implications for lymphocyte longevity and DNA reutilization. *Blood 26*: 281-295, 1965.

16. A. Volkman and F. M. Collins. Recovery of delayed-type hypersensitivity in mice following suppressive doses of x-radiation. *J. Immunol. 101*: 846-859, 1968.

90

LABELING OF MONONUCLEAR PHAGOCYTES
IN GRANULOMAS AND INFLAMMATORY SITES

T. J. Chambers

W. G. Spector

I. INTRODUCTION

Granulomatous inflammation is characterized by an accumulation of cells belonging to the mononuclear phagocyte system.
It is seen in response to the presence in tissues of a variety
of poorly degradable agents that are in addition either directly toxic to macrophages or become so following the development
of an immune response. The degree of this toxicity is the factor largely responsible for the separation of granulomas into
two broad categories: high- and low-turnover granulomas (1).
In high-turnover lesions, there is a higher rate of cell death,
a higher rate of proliferation of cells within the lesion, and
a higher continued recruitment of monocytes than in low-turnover granulomas. Whereas the origin of the various cells seen
in granulomatous inflammation can now perhaps best be studied
by bone marrow transplantation using stable phenotypic markers,

the kinetics of inflammation still involves pulse-labeling cells with [³H]-thymidine and observing the subsequent fate of the nuclear label.

To measure the rate of cell loss in the granuloma circulating monocytes are labeled by intravenous injection of [³H]-thymidine before inducing granulomatous inflammation. Bone marrow precursors incorporate the isotope and labeled monocytes are released into the circulation. Animals are then killed at appropriate intervals and the inflammatory site studied by autoradiography. During the first few days, the proportion of mononuclear cells with labeled nuclei approximates to the proportion of labeled monocytes in the blood. Later the proportion of labeled nuclei falls as labeled cells die or emigrate and are replaced by fresh unlabeled cells. The intensity of label in the nuclei also falls as the cells proliferate in the lesion. The basis for the technique is that if the pulse of [³H]-thymidine precedes the inflammatory stimulus, practically all the labeled exudate cells must have come from the blood stream. Also, if a triple pulse of [³H]-thymidine is used, 60-80% of circulating monocytes are labeled but less than 10% of circulating lymphocytes (2). Lastly, the labeled monocytes persist in the circulation for only a few days (3).

The rate of proliferation of mononuclear cells within the lesion is measured by inducing granulomatous inflammation and administering a pulse of [³H]-thymidine 1 hr before sacrifice. After this time there is no labeling of circulating cells, and autoradiography gives a measure of the proliferation of cells in the inflammatory lesion itself.

The relative contribution of the bone marrow and local proliferation to the maintenance of the lesion can be assessed either by exchange transfusion of labeled monocytes (4) or by irradiation of the bone marrow (5). A high-turnover lesion will show considerable decrease in size if it is shielded while the bone marrow is irradiated with 600 rad. A low-turnover lesion on the other hand is relatively self-sustaining and shows little change in size.

II. REAGENTS

(1) Tritiated thymidine ([³H] thymidine) (3-5 Ci/m*M*) is obtained from Amersham   (Chicago, Illinois). Appropriate precautions should be taken throughout the procedure against personal or environmental contamination with the isotope. In particular the animal will excrete a significant proportion of the label in its urine and a considerable amount will remain in the corpse after the experiment.

(2) Carrageenan (Seakem 402 A.P.) (Marine Colloids: 1.0% in saline.

(3) Bordetalla pertussis vaccine (Burroughs Wellcome Laboratories, Research Triangle Park, North Carolina) is washed free of preservative by centrifugation and resuspended in sterile saline at 10^{10} organisms/ml.

(4) Complete Freunds adjuvant (Difco, Inc., Detroit, Michigan).

(5) Animals. Rats or mice.

III. PROCEDURES

A. *Labeling monocytes*

Animals are anesthetized with ether and given three injections of [^{3}H]thymidine (0.5 μCi/gm body weight) at approximately 12 hr intervals via the tail vein using a 25-gauge needle. Care must be taken to ensure that no air remains in the syringe or needle before injection to avoid air embolism.

B. *Induction of Granulomatous Inflammation*

The animals are anesthetized, the fur over the injection site dampened with 70% ethanol and an area of skin shaved. Carrageenan, complete Freunds adjuvant, *B. pertussis,* or other agents are injected using a sterile technique either subcutaneously into a flank (0.5 ml) or intradermally into a footpad (0.1 ml) 6 hr after the last dose of [^{3}H]thymidine. The animals are killed and the inflammatory sites removed at appropriate intervals thereafter. The size of the lesion is measured before fixing in 10% formalin. The excised site is then embedded in paraffin wax and sections taken for autoradiography by routine histological techniques. We prepare autoradiographs using the method described by Doniach and Pelc (6) with Kodak AR 10 stripping film. The exposure time should be constant for all experiments at around 28 days. The autoradiographs can then be developed and counterstained with hematoxylin and eosin.

C. *Cell Proliferation in the Lesion*

Inflammation is induced in rats as above without prelabeling their monocytes with [^{3}H]thymidine. A single dose of [^{3}H]-thymidine (0.5 μCi/gm body weight) is then given intravenously

at suitable intervals 1 hr before the animal is killed. Autoradiographs are then prepared as above.

IV. CALCULATION OF DATA

     The percentage of labeled nuclei should be counted using
an oil-immersion microscope objective (100×). There will be
silver grains throughout the film, unrelated to nuclear labeling, as "background," and a value of three times the background
count can be taken as positive labeling. In practice this
means a grain count of 3-4 per nucleus. Usually the average
number of grains in a recently emigrated cell nucleus is 12-15.
Endothelial cells, vascular pericytes, and fibroblasts can be
distinguished and should not be counted, but all other nuclei
are included, as lymphocytes, monocytes, and macrophages cannot
be reliably distinguished from one another in tissue sections.
     When [^{3}H]thymidine is injected prior to the induction of
inflammation, the earliest lesions show a similar proportion
of labeled cells to that seen in circulating monocytes, around
60-80%. This proportion falls rapidly in high-turnover granulomas such as those caused by B. pertussis or complete Freunds
adjuvant, so that by three weeks less than 5% of the mononuclear cells in the lesion are labeled. Carrageenan on the
other hand induces a low-turnover lesion and 50-60% of the
mononuclear cells still show nuclear label after the same
time (7).
     It is important also to count the number of grains in each
labeled nucleus at the different times, since this will fall
if the cells proliferate following exudation, and measurement
of the fall in grain counts with time gives a measure of the
degree of proliferation taking place in the lesion. However,
dilution of label by mitosis to background levels must be considered in interpreting the apparent rate of cell loss as measured by the falling proportion of labeled cells.
     From this material the following values are calculated for
the granuloma each time a sample is taken: the proportion of
labeled nuclei; their average grain count; the proportion of
nuclei entering mitosis in the lesion; the size of the lesion.
From these values a graph can be plotted for each inducing a-
gent that can then be classified as causing a high-turnover or
low-turnover lesion depending on the rate of change of the
variables.

V.   CRITICAL COMMENTS

     The technique is relatively simple and reproducible. Only
the interpretation of results requires comment. The fall in
the proportion of labeled cells may be due to mechanisms other
than the toxic effect of the irritant. One is emigration of
labeled cells from the lesion. This can be partially monitored
by autoradiography of the draining lymph nodes. Another factor
influencing the fall in the proportion of labeled cells is
growth of the lesion after labeled cells have entered from the
blood, thus diluting the labeled population with unlabeled
cells and exaggerating the fall. This is not a problem in
static or shrinking lesions. A third potential problem is
that proliferation of the originally labeled cells causes dilution of label toward background levels. A more theoretical
problem is that the system measures the average behavior of the
labeled cells as though they were a uniform population. The
constitution of the original population derived from the blood
is relatively well defined, consisting predominantly of monocytes. As time progresses, however, numerically insignificant
subpopulations of labeled cells may behave differently from the
majority of macrophages and distort later results by becoming a
proportionally larger population [e.g., long-lived macrophages
(5,7)].

REFERENCES

1.   W. G. Spector. Epithelioid cells, giant cells and sar-
     coidosis. *Ann. N.Y. Acad. Sci. 278:*3-6, 1976.
2.   W. G. Spector, M. N-I. Walters, and D. A. Willoughby.
     The origin of mononuclear cells in inflammatory exudates
     induced by fibrinogen. *J. Pathol. Bacteriol. 90:*181-192,
     1965.
3.   A. M. Dannenberg, Jr., M. Ando, and K. Shima. Macrophage
     accumulation, division, maturation and digestive and mi-
     crobicidal capacities in tuberculous lesions. *J. Immunol.
     109:*1109-1121, 1972.
4.   W. G. Spector, A. W. J. Lykke, and D. A. Willoughby. A
     quantitative study of leucocyte emigration in chronic in-
     flammatory granulomata. *J. Pathol. Bacteriol. 93:*101-
     109, 1967.
5.   G. B. Ryan and W. G. Spector. Macrophage turnover in
     inflamed connective tissue. *Proc. R. Soc. London Ser. B.
     175:*269-292, 1970.
6.   I. Doniach and S. R. Pelc. Autoradiograph technique.
     *Br. J. Radiol. 23:*184-192, 1950.

7. G. B. Ryan and W. G. Spector. Natural selection of long-lived macrophages in experimental granulomata. *J. Pathol.* *99:*139–150, 1969.

91

IDENTIFICATION OF Fc AND COMPLEMENT
RECEPTORS IN TISSUE SECTIONS

Jeffrey Cossman
Elaine S. Jaffe

I. GENERAL INTRODUCTION

Techniques used to identify Fc receptors and complement
(C) receptors are most often applied to cells in suspension.
Such techniques permit the quantification of cells bearing
these receptors within a given population and, coupled with
the preparation of cytocentrifuge smear preparations, may
permit the investigator to visualize directly the receptor-
positive cells (1).

However, inherent in these techniques are also certain
limitations. Although a cellular suspension may be readily
prepared from peripheral blood and most lymphoid tissues, any
degree of fibrosis within the tissue may lead to difficulty
in extracting the cells. An adequate cellular suspension is
also often difficult to prepare from nonlymphoid tissues such
as skin, synovia, and breast, especially if the mononuclear
cell infiltrate is sparse. Furthermore, even if a mononuclear
cell suspension is readily prepared, the population of cells

METHODS FOR STUDYING
MONONUCLEAR PHAGOCYTES

989

ISBN 0-12-044220-5

obtained may not accurately reflect the representation of individual cell types within the intact tissue. For example,
when a mononuclear suspension is prepared from spleen, only
10% or less of the cells are mononuclear phagocytes. However,
these cells are the dominant noncirculating cellular element
in the red pulp, which topographically represents at least 60%
of the normal spleen. It is likely that macrophages are
trapped in the cords of Bilroth by the ring fibers and are
not readily liberated into suspension.

Suspension techniques also have the disadvantage that one
cannot define the physical interrelationships among the various cell types present, whereas techniques applicable to tissue sections allow one, not only to quantify roughly various
cell types, but also to study their distribution within the
tissue.

Our purpose in this chapter is to define and discuss
methods for the identification of Fc receptors and C receptors
in frozen tissue sections. These receptors are found on mononuclear phagocytes but, of course, are by no means specific for
these cells. Where possible, we shall also discuss what other
cell types bear these receptors and how they can be distinguished in sections from macrophages.

Although we have commented upon the advantages inherent in
the tissue section techniques over those used on cell suspensions, there are certain disadvantages to these techniques as
well. In general, the receptor assays applied to frozen tissue
sections are less sensitive than the same techniques using the
same reagents applied to cell suspensions. Several factors
may contribute to this lack of sensitivity. One is that only
a portion of the cell membrane bearing the receptor is exposed
in frozen tissue sections, whereas in suspensions the entire
cell surface is available for binding. Second, certainly some
deterioration of the receptors may occur on cells in the frozen,
but nonviable state. For example, if the tissues are not stored
under optimal conditions, extreme deterioration and even loss of
receptor activity may be noted.

It should also be noted that the suspension techniques,
coupled with cytocentrifuge preparations, are a much more reliable way of identifying receptors associated with a particular cell. With the present methodologies, individual cells
usually cannot be distinguished as positive or negative in frozen tissue sections. Rather, these techniques are more useful
in identifying populations of cells within a finite area. This
disadvantage should be born in mind, especially when studying
neoplastic conditions. Cytocentrifuge smears still remain the
most reliable method for identifying receptors associated with
neoplastic cells.

As such, we recommend that the frozen tissue sections techniques be used in conjunction with, and as a complement to,
those applied to cell suspensions.

II.   RECEPTORS FOR C3d (CR2) BY USE OF EAC3d

A. *Introduction*

At least two distinct complement receptors occur on cell
surfaces. One is a receptor for a site on the C3b fragment of
the C3 molecule (CRl) and another binds the C3d fragment (CR2)
(2) (Fig. 1). CRl is expressed by human lymphocytes (2), monocytes (3), granulocytes (2), and human erythrocytes (5).
CRl will bind both C4b and C3b (6). Human lymphocytes and possibly mononuclear phagocytes bind C3d, whereas erythrocytes
and mature granulocytes do not possess CR2 (2). A third complement receptor (CR3 or C3bi receptor) has been described for
granulocytes and monocytes and may bind to a small fragment of
the α chain of C3 known as C3e (7).
Specific identification of cells bearing either CRl or CR2
is most readily accomplished by rosette formation between target cells and sheep erythrocytes (E) coated with antibody (A)
and complement (C) (EAC). Complete cleavage of C3 to its C3d
fragment provides an EAC particle that is specific for CR2
(Fig. 1) and will not bind other complement receptors. Intermediate forms of the partially cleaved C3 molecule (C3bi) may
bind to CR3 as well as CR2. Specificity of EAC and thus cleavage of C3 is monitored by the adherence of EAC to cells that
possess only one receptor subtype. A reliable method for the
identification of CR3 receptors is not currently available.
The methods to be described for the detection cells bearing CRl
or CR2 were adapted from Ross and Polley (8).

B. *Reagents*

1. *Solution A*

Gelatin - Veronal-buffered saline (GVB) and GVB-EDTA use
distilled or deionized water. Dissolve 40 gm gelatin in 1
liter of boiling water. Cool and bring to a final volume of
2 liters with water. Aliquot 50-ml volumes, autoclave, and
store at 4°C.

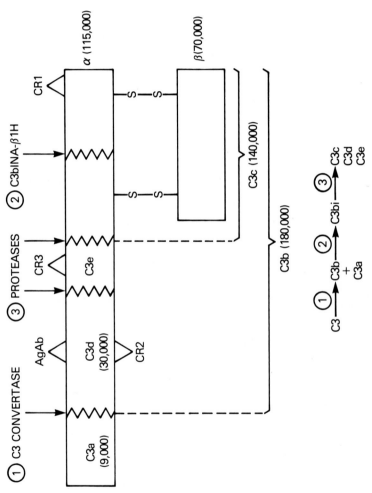

Fig. 1. Schematic representation of the structure of the third component of human complement (C3) and its cleavage sites. C3 binds to the antibody of the antigen-antibody complex at a point on the α-chain, which contains the C3d fragment. The three-step cleavage of C3 indicated below results in the sequential exposure of binding sites for first CR1, CR2, and CR3. Numbers in parentheses represent molecular weights. Modified from Carlo et al. (25), and Ross (7).

2. *Solution B*

Dissolve 0.44 gm $CaCl_2 - H_2O$ and 2.03 gm $MgCl_2 - 6H_2O$ in 100 ml water and store at $4°C$.

3. *Solution C*

Dissolve 3.75 gm Na-5,5-diethyl barbiturate and 85.0 gm NaCl in 140 ml water. Dissolve 5.75 gm 5,5-diethyl barbituric acid in 500 ml hot water. Combine the two solutions, filter sterilize, and save as a 5X stock.

4. *Solution D (0.2 M EDTA)*

Dissolve 37.23 gm disodium EDTA and 38.02 gm tetrasodium EDTA in 1 liter boiling water, cool, bring to a final volume of 2 liters at pH 7.2.

GVB-EDTA is prepared by combining 5 ml solution A, 20 ml solution B, and 20 ml solution D and bringing to a final volume of 100 ml with distilled water.

Sheep erythrocytes (E) may be purchased from numerous companies including Cordis Laboratories, Miami, Florida. These cells are stored in Alsever's solution. For use, wash the sheep erythrocytes three times in GVB. The packed cell volume should be determined in the final centrifugation and red cell concentration brought to 5% v/v. Alternatively, this cell concentration can be spectrophotometrically determined. Add 0.5 ml of the red cell suspension to 7.0 ml distilled water, shake to lyse the cells, and read the optical density of the lysate at 541 nM. The OD_{541} should be 0.70 ± 0.04, if not, correct the cell concentration as follows:
$V_f = V_i$(O.D./0.70), where V_i = final corrected volume, V_i = initial volume, $V_f - V_i$ = volume needed to add or subtract from initial cell suspension.

The IgM fraction of rabbit antisheep erythrocytes is available from Cordis Laboratories. The titer of the antibody to be used for sensitization of E is one-half the minimum hemagglutinating concentration. This is determined by adding equal volumes of 5% E in GVB to serial double dilutions of the antibody in GVB (usually a range from 1:4 to 1:1024). Incubate 30 min at room temperature without rotation and check for agglutination with a microscope. This titer must be determined for each new batch of either antibody or E.

C-5 deficient mouse serum is used as the complement source and this may be obtained from any C-5 deficient mouse strain, e.g., AKR, A/HeJ, DBA/2J, and A/J. The serum should be removed soon after a firm clot has formed (usually about 30 min). Serum may be used fresh or stored at $-70°C$ or below for as long as two weeks.

Human erythrocytes are stored at 10% in GVB at 4°C and used at 1%. The shelf life is one month. The Raji Burkitt's lymphoma cell line is maintained in continuous culture in RPMI-1640 (GIBCO, Grand Island, New York) supplemented with 10% fetal calf serum, penicillin, and streptomycin.

To prepare antibody-sensitized erythrocytes (EA), combine equal volumes of erythrocytes (5%) in GVB with antibody (1/2 the minimum hemagglutinating concentration), incubate 30 min at 37°C, wash 3 times in GVB, and resuspend in GVB at 2.5%. EA should be stored at 4°C and are good for one week.

EAC3d is prepared by a three-step procedure. First, 1 ml of EA and 1 ml mouse serum (diluted 1:20 in GVB) are thoroughly mixed and incubated with rotation for 45 min at 37°C. Wash once in cold GVB, once in cold GVB-EDTA, resuspend in 2.5 ml GVB-EDTA and incubate for 30 min at 37°C. This step allows decay of Cl, 4, and 2 from the cell surface. Following this incubation, add 2.5 ml of mouse serum (1:5 in GVB-EDTA) to the incubation mixture and incubate for a further 45 min to permit complete cleavage.

To test EAC3d for specificity, the reagent should be tested against both Raji cells and human erythrocytes (Table I). Add 50 µl EAC3d to 50 µl Raji cells (4 × 10^6/ml), incubate, rotating 30 min at 37°C, and count rosette formation with a hemocytometer. A positive Raji cell should have at least three EAC3d clearly bound to the surface. Usually 95 - 100% of viable Raji cells form rosettes with EAC3d. To test EAC3d for immune adherence, this procedure is repeated, incubating 50 µl EAC3d with 50 µl human erythrocytes (10). EAC3d should not form clumps with human E. If clumps are present then C3b is still present on the EAC and these EAC cannot be used as indicators specific for CR2 only. A negative control should always be run simultaneously with any EAC reagent. This consists of IgM sensitized E (EA) to which no complement has been added.

C. Procedure

1. Preparation of Tissue for Frozen Sections

Biopsy material should be obtained and processed for freezing as soon as possible after surgical removal, preferably within 1 hr. The use of autopsy tissues may not be satisfactory, and to some extent may depend upon the postmortem interval. Although in some instances receptors may be intact in postmortem tissues, this is not always the case.

The tissue is maintained in sterile saline or balanced salt solution. As discussed above, a portion of the tissue can be processed as a cell suspension for correlation with receptor studies on frozen sections. The tissue block used for frozen

TABLE I. *Specificity of Complement Receptors on Human Cells*

	Eryth-rocyte	Raji	Mononuclear phagocyte	Neutrophilic granulocyte	B Lympho-cyte
EAC4b (CR1)	+	−	+	+	+
EAC3d (CR2)	−	+	±	−	+

sections should be no more than 3 mm in thickness. The other dimensions of the block are less crucial and can be as large as 2 × 2 cm. However, as a general rule, it is more difficult to cut frozen sections from a large block.

The block is mounted and frozen on a specimen plate. The plate may be precooled on Dry Ice or in a cryostat. A small amount of embedding medium (O.C.T. Ames Co., Division of Miles Laboratories, Inc., Elkhart, Indiana) is placed on the plate as a base. The tissue block is placed on the plate and additional embedding medium added until the entire block is covered. The specimen mounted on the tissue plate should be frozen as rapidly as possible to minimize the formation of ice crystals, and prevent distortion of histology. The entire block can be snap frozen by immersing the tissue and plate in liquid nitrogen or in 2-methyl butane to which Dry Ice has been added. The specimen will be frozen within a few seconds.

2. Storage of Frozen Tissues

The frozen tissue can be cut and assayed immediately or the entire tissue block can be stored and saved for future use. The tissue block encased in embedding medium may be detached from the specimen plate for long-term storage. For storage, the intact block is wrapped in aluminum foil to prevent dehydration and stored at -70°C or below. Storage at -20°C is suitable only for short periods of time. Tissue stored at -70°C can be studied after several years and satisfactory results still obtained.

3. Rosette Assay

The frozen sections are cut and mounted on glass slides at the time the rosette assay is to be performed. The sections may be prepared a maximum of 24 hr in advance. Cryostat sections are mounted on uncoated, clean glass slides. Gelatinized slides may be used to improve adherence of the tissue section to the glass. However, use of such coated slides is usually not necessary if the sections are given adequate time to dry before the assay is performed. The sections may be air dried at room temperature for 12 to 24 hr or, if they are prepared on the day of the assay, they may be rapidly dried at 37°C for 45 min. The sections should be cut at a thickness of 6 to 8 μm. The rosette assay may be performed by either of two methods. In both methods, the indicator red cells are used at a concentration of 1×10^8 ml (0.5%).

In the first method (9), the slides are overlayed with the reagent red cells using a Pasteur pipette, and incubated for 30 min at either room temperature or 37°C. If the incubation is performed at 37°C a humid chamber should be used so that drying of the red cells on the sections does not occur. After incubation, the slides are washed by immersion with gentle agitation in phosphate-buffered saline (PBS) in a Coplin jar or other suitable glass vessel. Three washes are usually sufficient, but it is possible to tell by rapid microscopic inspection if the washing process is complete. After washing, the slides are immersed in fixative for approximately 10 min. Care must be taken in selecting an appropriate fixative; fixatives commonly used for frozen sections, such as acid alcohol, are not suitable as lysis of indicator red cells will occur. Appropriate fixatives include 3% glutaraldehyde or Perfix (Fischer Scientific Co., Fairlawn, New Jersey 07410). The fixed slides are stained with hematoxylin and eosin. The above technique is considered the conventional assay technique and is of moderate sensitivity.

An alternate technique that offers increased sensitivity is the hanging drop technique (Fig. 2) (10, 11). In this technique a microculture slide chamber (Arthur H. Thomas Co., Philadelphia, Pennsylvania) is used to hold the indicator red cells. The frozen sections are cut and allowed to air dry on glass slides as described above. As shown in Fig. 2a, the microculture slide well is filled with the reagent red cells. The glass slide bearing the frozen section is placed carefully over the well of the microculture slide, being careful to prevent the entry of any air bubbles (Fig. 2b). Excess reagent is drained off and a suction is formed. As shown in Figs. 2c and 2d, the microculture slide is inverted to allow the settling of indicator red cells onto the frozen section. The chamber is incubated at room temperature or 37°C for 30 min. The slide is then inverted and incubated again for 15 min. After allowing the nonadherent red cells to detach, the section is tapped gently with a glass rod to detach any residual loosely adherent cells (Figs. 2e and 2f). The frozen section slide, still attached to the microculture slide, may be examined through a microscope at this point to determine the pattern of adherent red cells (Fig. 3). A parallel frozen section stained with hematoxylin and eosin should be used in conjunction with the slide incubated with the reagent, so that the histology of the tissue may be observed. After examination, the frozen section slide should be gently detached from the microculture slide, fixed as above, and stained with hematoxylin and eosin.

D. *Interpretation*

The fixed and stained frozen sections are viewed through a conventional microscope to determine the pattern of adherent red cells. The stained sections can also be examined at low magnification through a dry-darkfield condenser. In this preparation, the adherent red cells appear as yellow - green refractile bodies against a dark background, and small numbers of adherent red cells can be easily identified.

Sections incubated by the hanging drop technique can be examined either as fixed and stained preparations or examined with the hanging drop chamber intact (Fig. 2f). Although the tissue in this preparation is not stained, the general architecture of the tissue can usually be discerned by examination of the reticulin and fibrous framework. In this instance a parallel frozen section stained with hematoxylin and eosin also should always be used.

Controls should be used for both the standard rosette assay and the hanging drop technique. Suitable controls would include sheep red blood cells without added antibody and/or complement source, or substitution of heat-inactivated serum for the complement source. There should, of course, be no adherence of control indicator red cells under the incubation conditions described above.

Results of the frozen section assays should be recorded as to (1) the pattern of adherent red cells and (2) the intensity of the binding observed. A grading system such as 1+ through 4+ can be used, if the tissue examined is relatively homogenous. Identification of binding by individual cells is usually not possible with these techniques.

E. *Critical Comments*

In our laboratory, the frozen section assays are generally conducted either in duplicate or triplicate. Occasionally, tearing or disruption of the tissue may occur during the incubation and washing procedures. Performing duplicate assays gives the investigator a greater likelihood of having a satisfactory result and also provides for better control of the method.

As stated above the rosette assays are most useful when performed in conjunction with the same assays in suspension. The frozen section assays are generally not useful for the identi-

HANGING DROP TECHNIQUE

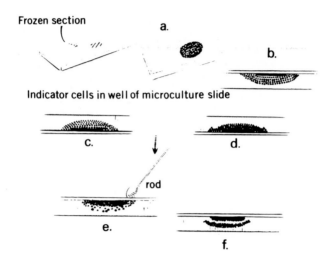

Fig. 2. Schematic representation of hanging drop technique. For detailed description, see text, Section II.C.3. Modified from Tonder et al. (10).

Fig. 3. Frozen sections of normal spleen incubated using hanging drop technique: Photomicrographs are taken of specimen in unfixed, unstained state through microculture slide chamber (Fig. 2f). (a) EAC3d. Reagent erythrocytes bind to lymphoid follicle. There is no binding to red pulp. (2) IgGEA. Erythrocytes bind exclusively to cords of splenic red pulp. Follicular lymphocytes do not bind reagent.

(A)

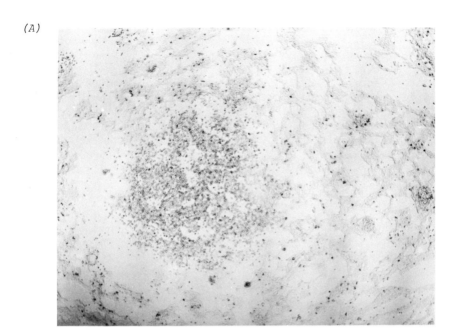

(B)

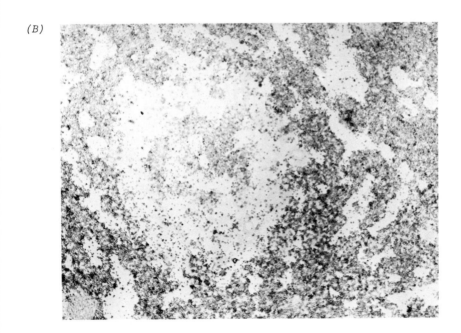

fication of receptors associated with single cells.

In using these assays, the investigator may make several modifications in order to enhance binding in a given system. As long as the same modifications are made with control preparations, then interpretation of the assay is not a problem. Modifications that may enhance binding include incubation at 37 C rather than room temperature, an increase in the concentration of indicator red cells (i.e., 2×10^8/ml), or prolongation of the incubation time (60 min or more). The above modifications may increase both specific and nonspecific binding, and, of course, this must be evaluated carefully in each system examined.

EAC3d binds to cells bearing complement receptors, in particular the CR2 receptor. One must bear in mind that many different cell types have complement receptors. In normal lymph nodes and tonsils, EAC3d demonstrates conspicuous binding to lymphoid follicles and is a marker of complement receptor B lymphocytes. EAC3d does not bind well to interfollicular areas. In the spleen, EAC3d binds to lymphoid follicles of the splenic white pulp, but binds poorly to histiocytes in the splenic red pulp (Fig. 3). The marginal zone of the spleen, an area populated by many cell types including B cells, T cells, and macrophages, binds EAC3d.

III. RECEPTORS FOR C3b, C4b (CR1) BY USE OF EAC4b

A. Introduction

Since human C4b and C3b bind to the same complement receptor (CR1) and no C3Bi or C3d is present on EAC4b, EAC4b is useful as a highly specific indicator of CR1. Although EAC3b can be used to identify CR1, this reagent binds to Raji cells, probably via the C3d region within C3b, whereas EAC4b does not adhere to Raji cells (8).

EAC4b is prepared with human complement components and will bind to human CR1-positive cells but not to murine cells.

B. Reagents

Human C1 is prepared from fresh serum that should be chilled on ice and adjusted to pH 7.0 with 1 N HCl. Dilute this serum 1:3 with cold distilled water and stir for 30 min at 4°C. The euglobulin precipitate that forms contains C1 and is separated by centrifugation at 1000 g for 30 min at 4°C. Resuspend the pellet in five times the original serum volume of solution C

(Section II.B) diluted 1:15 in cold distilled water, centrifuge
again under the same conditions, and discard the supernatant.
Add 1/4 the original serum volume of ice cold solution C diluted
1:2.5 in cold water. Stir for 15 min at $4°C$, add an equal
volume of water and solution B (Section II.B) to yield 1.0 mM
$MgCl_2$ and 0.15 mM $CaCl_2$. The Cl may be stored in aliquots at
$-70°C$ or below. Alternatively, commercially available human Cl
(Cordis Laboratories, Miami, Florida) may be substituted, although the EAC4b prepared with this reagent are often less sensitive.

Human C4 is merely heat-inactivated (30 min, $56°C$) normal
human serum. Check the serum for its ability to agglutinate
sheep E by incubating the undiluted serum with an equal volume
of E (5%) for 30 min at $37°C$. If agglutination occurs, the
heat-inactivated serum should be absorbed on ice with approximately 1/10 the volume of packed sheep E by stirring for 15 min,
removing red cells by centrifugation, and adding the serum for
a second batch of red cells and repeating for a total of three
absorptions. Care must be taken to maintain cold ($0° - 4°C$)
temperatures throughout the procedure.

To prepare EAC4b, add 50 µl of Cl (or 5000 U of Cordis Cl)
to 1.0 ml of EA (2.5%) and incubate for 15 min at $37°C$. Wash
this EACl twice in $37°C$ prewarmed GVB and resuspend in 1.0 of
GVB at $37°C$. Divide this EACl into 0.2-ml aliquots and to each
add 0.2 ml of successive doubling dilutions of C4 in GVB (undiluted to 1:16), incubate 15 min at $37°C$ and wash immediately
(twice) in ice-cold GVB. Resuspend each to 1 ml and check each
for binding to human E by incubating equal volumes of EAC4b
and E (1%) 30 min at $37°C$. The dilution of C4 yielding the
maximum rosette formation is recorded and used to treat another
batch of EACl to form optimal EAC4b. EAC4b is stored at $4°C$
and remains active for at least two weeks. EAC4b should be
tested for specificity as outlined in Section II.B; EAC4b
should bind to human E but not to Raji cells (Table I). Negative controls for EAC4b are EA and/or EACl.

    C. *Procedure* (Same as for EAC3d; see above)

    D. *Interpretation* (Same as for EAC3d; see above)

    E. *Critical Comments*

In normal tonsils and lymph nodes EAC4b binds to both lymphoid follicles and to interfollicular areas. Similarly, in
the spleen, EAC4b binds to lymphoid follicles as well as the
splenic red pulp. It is presumed that much of the binding to

the splenic red pulp is mediated via macrophages as well as granulocytes. In lymph nodes, binding of EAC4b occurs to histiocytes in lymphoid sinuses.

IV. RECEPTORS FOR C3b AND C3d BY USE OF FLUORESCENT BACTERIA-COMPLEMENT (BC)

A. *Introduction*

Heat-killed-gram-negative bacteria will fix complement by the alternate pathway and can be used as indicators of complement receptors (12). Bacteria offer several advantages over conventional sheep EAC assays. First, no antibody is required to sensitize the cells, thus avoiding agglutination or binding to Fc receptors. Second, the complement-coated bacteria can be stored frozen at -20°C for use at a later date without loss of activity. Third, EAC made with sheep E could potentially bind to human T lymphocytes via the T cell sheep E receptor, whereas lymphocytes do not bind to the bacteria used in the BC assay. Fourth, the bacteria assays are generally more sensitive than EAC rosettes, either because of their smaller size or a denser concentration of complement fixed to the bacterial surface.

The bacteria are readily visible by phase microscopy and, when made fluorescent, can be used in two-color dual label assays and on frozen sections.

B. *Reagents*

Salmonella typhi 0901 (American Type Culture Collection, Rockville, Maryland) are inoculated onto trypticase-soy-broth (Difco, Detroit, Michigan) for 48 hr at 37°C, heat-killed at 80°C for 60 min, checked for sterility, and washed in phosphate-buffered saline (PBS, pH 7.4). The bacteria may be stored at -20°C in aliquots.

Carbonate – bicarbonate buffer is prepared as follows:

Solution A: Dissolve 12.12 gm anhydrous sodium carbonate in 1000 ml distilled water (0.12 *M*).

Solution B: Dissolve 10.08 gm sodium bicarbonate in 1000 ml distilled water (0.12 *M*).

Add 4 ml solution A to 46 ml solution B and bring to 200 ml with water. Adjust final pH to 9.2 with 1 *N* NaOH.

To label the bacteria fluorescently, dissolve 10 mg of either fluorescein isothiocyanate, isomer I (FITC) (Sigma, St.

Louis, Missouri) or tetramethyl rhodamine isothiocyanate (TRITC)
(Cappel Laboratories, Downington, Pennsylvania) in 5 ml
carbonate - bicarbonate buffer. Centrifuge out large, undis-
solved particles. Add the dissolved fluorescent dye to a 0.5-ml
pellet of bacteria, mix well, and stir at room temperature for
30 min. Wash in PBS until the supernatant is clear (usually at
least 4 washes) and resuspend at 10^9/ml in GVB.

The complement source is fresh human or mouse serum. Human
serum cannot be used to identify murine complement receptors.
Sera should be checked for antibody activity directed against
the bacteria by means of an agglutination assay in which equal
volumes of undiluted serum and bacteria (10^9/ml in GVB) are incubated 30 min at 37°C. If agglutination occurs, chilled serum
should be absorbed three times on ice with 1/10 the volume of
packed heat-killed bacteria and rechecked for agglutination.

To fix complement on the bacteria, pellet 1 ml (10) bacteria.
remove the supernatant, add 1 ml human or mouse serum (1:5 in
GVB), incubate 40 min at 37°C, wash three times in cold GVB and
resuspend in 2 ml of GVB. These BC may be aliquoted and stored
at -20°C.

The specificity of the BC for CR1 or CR2 is determined by
their ability to bind to either human E or Raji cells. The procedure is similar to that described for the testing of specificity of EAC3d (see Section II.B). Equal volumes of BC
(10^9/ml) and human E (1%) or Raji cells (4×10^6/ml) are incubated rotating, for 30 min at 37°C and examined for binding.
Cells with three or more adherent bacteria are considered positive. BC usually bind both human E and Raji and therefore have
both C3b and C3d fixed to their surfaces.

C. Procedure

Tissue sections are prepared as described above. The frozen
sections are incubated with BC for 30 min at room temperature.
A range of concentration (usually $10^9 - 10^{10}$ BC/ml) should be
tested to determine optimal binding. After incubation the sections are washed by gentle agitation and immersion in phosphate-
buffered saline. The sections are fixed with an appropriate
fixative and examined by fluorescent microscopy. Although lysis
of reagent red cells is not a factor with the BC technique, care
must be taken to choose a fixative that is not autofluorescent.
Thus, the aldehyde fixatives suitable for the red cell assays,
are not suitable for the fluorescent-bacterial assays. Methanol
or acetone are generally accepted fixatives for this assay.
The sections are coverslipped using buffered glycerol as a
mounting medium.

D. Interpretation

The frozen sections are examined by fluorescent microscopy with appropriate excitation and suppression filters. We have used a Leitz Orthoplan microscope equipped with an Osram HBO 100-W mercury lamp, a Ploem vertical illuminator, and filter combinations specific for each fluorochrome (fluorescein: 450 - 490 nm excitation, 515 nm suppression, and rhodamine 530 - 560 nm excitation, 580 nm suppression).

Appropriate controls for the BC assay include bacteria without added complement source. Heat-inactivated serum may also be used.

E. Critical Comments

Since BC usually bears both C3b and C3d, many cell types may be simultaneously identified as complement receptor bearing cells. BC adheres to lymphoid follicles as well as to the red pulp of spleen and medullary cord areas of lymph nodes. It must be recognized that BC is not specific for complement receptor subtypes as are EAC3d and EAC4b.

When performing the frozen section assay, care should be taken to wash off thoroughly unbound BC. This is especially critical when high concentrations (10^{10}/ml) of bacteria are used.

V.   RECEPTORS FOR C3d BY USE OF BAC

A. Introduction

The bacteria antibody complement (BAC) complex was first described by Gormus *et al.* (13). The reagent is apparently specific for binding to CR2 only (14). Presumably, C3b is completely cleaved to C3d on BAC, whereas C3b is retained on BC.

B. Reagents

Salmonella typhimurium (American Type Culture Collection, Rockville, Maryland) is used for the BAC assay. The bacteria are cultured and heat killed as for *S. typhi*. To produce antiserum to *S. typhimurium*, a 1-ml emulsion of Freund's complete adjuvant (Difco, Detroit, Michigan) containing 10^9 bacteria is injected subcutaneously in New Zealand white rabbits.

Serum obtained one to two weeks following a single injection usually contains antibody to *S. typhimurium* only of the IgM class. Antiserum (heat-inactivated) can then be used to sensitize the bacteria by incubating equal volumes of bacteria (10^9/ml in GVB) and antiserum (1/2 the minimum agglutinating concentration) for 30 min at $37°C$. The antibody-sensitized bacteria (BA) are washed three times in GVB and brought to 10^9/ml in GVB and incubated with an equal volume of fresh mouse (AKR) serum (1:10 in GVB) for 40 min at $37°C$. BAC are washed three times in cold GVB and resuspended to a final concentration of 10^9/ml in GVB. Negative controls consist of the substitution of heat-inactivated AKR serum for fresh serum.

Binding of BAC to human E and Raji cells is carried out as for BC. BAC are usually immune adherence negative (fail to bind to human E) but readily bind to 95 - 100% of Raji cells.

C. *Procedure*

Tissue sections are prepared as above. Incubation is performed with BAC as described for BC.

D. *Interpretation*

Sections incubated with BAC are examined as described in Section IV.D.

E. *Critical Comments*

BAC bear fixed C3 in the form of C3d but not C3b. They readily adhere to Raji cells, but fail to adhere to human erythrocytes bearing the CR1 receptor. In frozen sections of lymphoid tissues, BAC demonstrates a similar pattern of binding to that of EAC3d.

VI. RECEPTORS FOR Fc BY USE OF IgG EA

A. *Introduction*

Receptors for the Fc portion of IgG have been demonstrated on human monocytes (15), granulocytes, and subpopulations of lymphocytes (16). Rosette assay systems have been applied to cells in both suspension and frozen sections. The rosette assays are less sensitive than other systems using fluorescein-

ated heat-aggregated human IgG or fluoresceinated soluble
antigen-antibody complexes. However, they offer greater specificity and appear to identify a different Fc receptor than
that detected by the more sensitive assays (17, 18). Thus,
the rosette assays are preferable for the detection of Fc receptors on mononuclear phagocytes that readily bind these
reagents.

Erythrocytes from various species have been used as indicator particles. Antisera against sheep E are readily available (19); however, a disadvantage of this red cell source is
that they may interact with human T lymphocytes via the sheep
red blood cell receptor. Human Rh+ erythrocytes sensitized
with an anti-CD antiserum also have been used (16). In our
laboratory we currently use ox (bovine) erythrocytes sensitized
with the IgG fraction of a rabbit-antibovine erythrocyte antiserum. Advantages of this system include: (1) the absence of
a receptor for bovine erythrocytes on human cells, and (2) the
reduced agglutinability of bovine erythrocytes. This latter
feature enables one to sensitize highly the erythrocytes without agglutination of the reagent, thus increasing the sensitivity of the system. This is a particular advantage in dealing with frozen sections.

B. Reagents

Bovine erythrocytes are obtained in Alsever's solution and
stored up to two weeks. For use, prepare as described above
(Section II.B) for sheep E. Wash three times in GVB and bring
to a final concentration of 5% v/v.

The IgG fraction of rabbit antibovine erythrocytes is
available from Cappel Laboratories, Dowingtown, Pennsylvania.
The titer of the antibody to be used for sensitization of E is
one-half the minimum hemagglutinating concentration. This is
determined by adding equal volumes of 5% E in GVB to serial
double dilutions of the antibody in GVB (usually a range from
1:2 to 1:1024). Incubate 30 min at room temperature without
rotation and check for agglutination with a microscope. This
titer must be determined for each new batch of either antibody
or E.

If agglutination does not occur or occurs at only very high
concentrations (1:2), the activity of the antibody may be
checked by adding guinea pig complement to the sensitized
erythrocytes. The degree of hemolysis can be determined spectrophotometrically by comparison with a standard of 100% hemolysis prepared with the same concentration of erythrocytes and
distilled water. The concentration of guinea pig serum (usually 1:150) is chosen to produce partial lysis of the cell suspension at all antibody concentrations. The detailed protocol

for selection of the appropriate antibody concentration has
been previously described (9).

To prepare IgGEA, combine equal volumes of 5% E in GVB with
the antibody at the appropriate concentration, incubate 30 min
at 37°C, wash three times in GVB, and resuspend in GVB to 1%
v/v. EA should be stored at 4°C and is good for one week. Note
that although EAC3d and EAC4b are usually used at 0.5%, we have
found 1.0% to be a preferable concentration for IgGEA, both for
suspension and frozen sections.

C. Procedure (Same as for EAC3d; see above)

D. Interpretation (Same as for EAC3d; see above)

Uncoated erythrocytes (E) or IgMEA may be used as appropriate controls.

E. Critical Comments

Although many different cell types may bear receptors for
the Fc portion of IgG, there are considerable differences in
receptor avidity among various cell types. B lymphocytes have
Fc receptors of relatively low avidity and will not bind IgGEA,
either in suspension or in frozen sections, using conventionally prepared reagents. IgGEA binds to mononuclear phagocytes in
frozen sections. In lymph nodes, binding is most readily observed to histiocytes in lymphoid sinuses. In spleens, there
is binding to macrophages of the splenic red pulp and marginal
zones (Fig. 3). The hanging drop technique offers greater sensitivity and should be used whenever cell density is low.

A factor that may interfere with binding of IgGEA to macrophages is the presence of immune complexes bound in the *in vivo*
state. In states associated with circulating immune complexes,
receptors on macrophages may be occupied and a negative result
will be observed after incubation with IgGEA. This appears to
be more often a problem with the frozen section assay, rather
than the same rosette assay performed in suspension. A likely
explanation of this discrepancy is the limited sensitivity of
the frozen section assay, perhaps as a consequence of the
limited exposure of the cell membrane to the reagent. The
presence of complexes bound *in vivo* may be determined in part
by staining for IgG with fluorescein-conjugated anti-IgG antisera.

VII.   CONCLUDING REMARKS

The techniques described in this chapter can be used to identify cells bearing Fc and C receptors in frozen tissue sections. Although macrophages are, of course, not the only cell types to bear these receptors, their avidity, particularly for IgGEA, renders them more readily identifiable by these techniques. Other techniques also applicable to use on frozen sections include histochemical, immunohistochemical, and immunofluorescence methodologies. Histochemical stains for nonspecific esterases, acid phosphatases, and other lysosomal enzymes are useful in identifying mononuclear phagocytes (20). Immunohistochemical techniques for the identification of lysozyme (21), and perhaps other constituents of macrophages are a more recent addition to the armamentarium of the experimental pathologist and immunologist. Finally, the application of both heteroantisera (22) and, more recently, monoclonal antisera (23, 24) against antigenic constituents of macrophages provide another alternative for the identification of these cells in tissue sections. These various techniques should not be viewed as substitutes, but rather as complimentary approaches that should be used in conjunction with each other and with other techniques applied to cell suspensions.

REFERENCES

1. R. B. Mann, E. S. Jaffe, R. B. Braylan *et al*. Immunologic and morphologic studies of T cell lymphoma. *Am. J. Med.* *58*: 307-313, 1975.
2. G. D. Ross, M. J. Polley, E. M. Rabellino, and H. M. Grey. Two different complement receptors on human lymphocytes. *J. Exp. Med. 138*: 798-811, 1973.
3. H. Y. Reynolds, J. P. Atkinson, H. H. Newball, and M. M. Frank. Receptors for immunoglobulin and complement on human alveolar macrophages. *J. Immunol. 114*: 1813-1819, 1975.
4. A. R. E. Anwar and A. B. Kay. Membrane receptors for IgC and complement (C4, C3b, and C3d) on human eosinophils and neutrophils and their relation to eosinophilia. *J. Immunol. 119*: 976-982, 1977.
5. A. P. Dalmasso and H. J. Muller-Eberhard. Physicochemical characteristics of the third and fourth component of complement after dissociation from complement-cell complexes. *Immunology 13*: 293, 1967.

6. V. A. Bokisch and A. T. Sobel. Receptor for the fourth
    component of complement on human B lymphocytes and cul-
    tured human lymphoblastoid cells. *J. Exp. Med. 140*:
    1336-1347, 1974.
7. G. D. Ross. Identification of human lymphocyte populations
    by surface marker analysis. *Blood 53*: 799-811, 1979.
8. G. D. Ross and M. J. Polley. Detection of complement-
    receptor lymphocytes (CRL). *In* "*In Vitro* Methods in Cell-
    Mediated and Tumor Immunity" (B. R. Bloom and J. R. David,
    eds.), pp. 123-136. Academic Press, New York, 1976.
9. M. M. Frank, E. S. Jaffe, and I. Green. Detection of
    specific mononuclear cell receptors in tissue sections.
    In "*In Vitro* Methods in Cell-Mediated and Tumor Immunity"
    (B. R. Bloom and J. R. David, eds.), pp. 203-215. Aca-
    demic Press, New York, 1976.
10. O. Tonder, F. Milgrom, and E. Witebsky. Mixed agglutina-
    tion with tissue sections. *J. Exp. Med. 119*: 265-275,
    1965.
11. O. Tonder, P. A. Morse, and L. J. Humphrey. Similarities
    of Fc receptors in human malignant tissue and normal lym-
    phoid tissue. *J. Immunol. 113*: 1162-1169, 1974.
12. J. A. Gelfand, A. S. Fauci, I. Green, and M. M. Frank. A
    simple method for the determination of complement receptor-
    bearing mononuclear cells. *J. Immunol. 116*: 595-599, 1976.
13. B. J. Gormus, R. B. Crandall, and J. W. Shands. Endotoxin-
    stimulated spleen cells: Mitogenesis, the occurrence of
    the C3 receptor, and the production of immunoglobulin.
    J. Immunol. 112: 770-773, 1974.
14. J. Cossman and E. S. Jaffe. Distribution of complement re-
    ceptor subtypes in non-Hodgkin's lymphomas of B-cell origin.
    Blood (in press).
15. H. Huber, J. M. Polley, W. D. Lincott *et al.* Human mono-
    cytes: Distinct receptor sites for the third component of
    complement and for immunoglobulin G. *Science 162*: 1281-
    1283, 1968.
16. S. S. Froland and F. Wisloff. A rosette technique for
    identification of human lymphocytes with Fc receptors.
    In "*In Vitro* Methods in Cell-Mediated and Tumor Immunity"
    (B. R. Bloom and J. R. David, eds.), pp. 137-142. Aca-
    demic Press, New York, 1976.
17. R. D. Arbeit, P. A. Henkart, and H. B. Dickler. Differ-
    ences between the Fc receptors of two lymphocyte subpopu-
    lations of human peripheral blood. *Scand. J. Immunol. 6*:
    873-878, 1977.
18. J. B. Winfield, P. I. Lobo, and M. E. Hamilton. Fc recep-
    tor heterogeneity: Immunofluorescent studies of B, T, and
    "third population" lymphocytes in human blood with rabbit
    IgG b4/anti-b4 complexes. *J. Immunol. 119*: 1778-1784,
    1977.

19. M. J. Deegan, J. Cossman, B. T. Chosney *et al.* Hairy
     cell leukemia--an immunologic and ultrastructural study.
     Cancer 38: 1952-1961, 1976.
20. C. Y. Li, L. T. Yam, and W. H. Crosby. Histochemical
     characterization of cellular and structural elements of
     the human spleen. *J. Histochem. Cytochem. 20*: 1049-1058,
     1972.
21. D. Y. Mason and C. R. Taylor. The distribution of mura-
     midase (lysozyme) in human tissues. *J. Clin. Pathol. 28*:
     124-132, 1975.
22. A. G. Stuart, G. A. Young, and P. F. Grant. Identifica-
     tion of human mononuclear cells by anti-monocyte serum.
     Br. J. Haematol. 34: 457-463, 1976.
23. T. Springer, G. Galfre, D. S. Secher, and C. Milstein.
     Mac 1: A macrophage differentiation antigen identified
     by monoclonal antibody. *Eur. J. Immunol. 9*: 301-306,
     1979.
24. J. Breard, E. L. Reinherz, P. C. Kung, G. Goldstein, and
     S. F. Schlossman. A monoclonal antibody reactive with hu-
     man peripheral blood monocytes. *J. Immunol. 124*: 1943-
     1948, 1980.
25. J. R. Carlo, S. Ruddy, E. J. Studer, and D. H. Conrad.
     Complement receptor binding of C3b-coated cells treated
     with C3b inactivator, β1H Globulin and Trypsin. *J. Im-
     munol. 123*: 523-528, 1979.

92

DETERMINATION OF MACROPHAGE-MEDIATED
ANTIBACTERIAL RESISTANCE

R. J. North
G. L. Spitalny

I. INTRODUCTION

Unless they possess an antiphagocytic capsule, most bacteria inoculated intravascularly are rapidly cleared from the
blood almost exclusively by fixed macrophages of the reticuloendothelial system. Because by far the largest number of bacteria are ingested by fixed macrophages (Kuppfer cells) that
line the sinusoids of the liver, it is obvious that the liver
is the organ of choice for measuring antibacterial resistance
in vivo. Provided the bacterial species chosen is cleared
from the blood in several minutes, it is possible to determine
the total number of bacteria initially ingested by macrophages
of the liver, and the number of bacteria inactivated during
any one period of time thereafter. This is achieved by sampling a population of mice at progressive times after inoculating them with *Listeria*, and determining changes in the number
of bacteria in liver homogenates capable of forming colonies
on nutrient agar.

METHODS FOR STUDYING
MONONUCLEAR PHAGOCYTES

The facultative, intracellular, bacterial parasite, *Listeria monocytogenes,* is a popular test organism for measuring both innate and acquired, nonspecific, antibacterial resistance expressed by liver macrophages *in vivo.* It should be realized that *Listeria* is far more susceptible to inactivation by macrophages than certain other facultative intracellular pathogens, such as mycobacteria. Consequently, the liver macrophages of normal mice are capable of inactivating 50% or more of the *Listeria* load in the liver over the first several hours of infection, depending on the state of "cleanliness" of the mice and the virulence of the pathogen. Nevertheless, the rate and extent of bacterial inactivation is greatly increased in animals generating an activated macrophage system in response to bacterial infection. This increased bactericidal activity can be measured *in vivo* by the procedure described here.

II. REAGENTS

Animals: For obvious reasons mice are the most popular choice, although the same procedures can be used for rats and guinea pigs.

Listeria monocytogenes with at least moderate virulence for the host species chosen.

Disposable 1-cm^3 tuberculin syringes fitted with 26-gauge needles (Becton-Dickinson, Oxnard, California, No. 5625).

Dissecting materials: Cork board and pins; blunt-end 5 1/2 in. stainless scissors; Mayo 5 1/2 in. dissection scissors; rat tooth forceps (4 1/2 in.) (Clay Adams, Parsippany, New Jersey); ethanol, 95%.

Petroff-Hauser bacterial counting chamber (Scientific Products, McGraw Park, Illinois, No. C8400-1).

Glass homogenizing tubes with matching Teflon pestles (Tri-R Instruments, Rockville Center, New York, Nos. S32 and S22).

A large number of 5-ml plastic tubes (Falcon Plastics, Oxnard, California, No. 2058) containing 0.9 ml of sterile 0.9% sodium chloride solution for performing serial dilutions.

A large number of sterile 1-ml disposable serological pipettes (Scientific Products, McGraw Park, Illinois, No. P643-1) for performing serial dilutions.

Bacterial culture dishes (Falcon Space Saver No. 1506) containing sterile trypticase-soy agar (TSA). The nutrient agar is made by dissolving 30 gm trypticase-soy broth (Baltimore Biological Labs, Cockeysville, Maryland, No. 11768) and 20 gm of granulated agar (Baltimore Biological Labs, Cockeysville, Maryland, No. 11849) in 1 liter of distilled water in an autoclave at 15 psi for 15 min. The dissolved nutrient agar is immediately poured while hot into culture plates and allowed to solidify at room temperature under sterile conditions. Water that has condensed on the agar and on the inside of plates and their covers is evaporated by removing the covers and placing the plates and covers upside down in a hot air oven.

Tubes with 5 ml of trypticase-soy broth (TSB) prepared as above, but without agar.

A vertically mounted, low-speed (100 rpm), electric drill with footpedal switch and a chuck for holding pestles.

III.   PROCEDURES

A. *Listeria Passage*

If need be, the virulence of *Listeria* can be increased by repeated passage in animals. Starting with a log phase culture with a known number of organisms per milliliter, as determined by counting in a Petroff-Hauser chamber, a sample of the culture is diluted in physiological saline to 5×10^4/ml and 0.2 ml inoculated intravenously into one or more mice via a lateral tail vein using a tuberculin syringe fitted with a 26-gauge needle. Three days later a mouse is sacrificed, its spleen removed aseptically and homogenized in 8 ml of physiological saline by hand. The homogenate is used to seed 5 ml of TSB in plastic tubes. It is advisable to seed three tubes with 0.1, 0.5, and 0.01 ml of homogenate, respectively, and to use the culture that is still in log phase after overnight incubation at 37°C. The larger the volume of spleen homogenate added, the sooner the culture is ready for use. The bacteria are counted and diluted appropriately in physiological saline for another passage in mice, and the procedure repeated as necessary. For worthwhile experiments, the LD_{50} dose of *Listeria* for mice should be 10^5 or less. Therefore, after several passages, it will be necessary to determine the intravenous LD_{50} dose by following procedures adequately described in the literature (1).

B. *Standard Frozen Cultures for Experiments*

Having demonstrated that the intravenous LD_{50} dose of *Listeria* is 10^5 or less, a spleen homogenate prepared as described above is used to seed 100 ml of TSB to obtain a log phase ($1-5 \times 10^8$ ml) culture for distribution in 1 ml ampoules for freezing at -70°C. The culture is dispensed directly into ampoules that are then placed in a suitable -70°C freezer. The viability of the culture before freezing and after thawing is determined in each case by plating ten-fold serial dilutions of it on nutrient agar. It has been found consistently that prac-

tically no loss of viability is caused by freezing at -70°C.
Moreover, because the viability and virulence remain stable
for at least 6 months, the frozen ampoules serve as a standard
culture for a large number of experiments. For each experiment
an ampoule is thawed and diluted appropriately in physiological
saline for intravenous inoculation.

C. Measurement of Macrophage-Mediated Antibacterial Resistance

In essence, the method involves inoculating a population
of mice intravascularly with *Listeria,* and sampling the population over time for changes in the number of bacteria in the
liver capable of forming colonies on nutrient agar. Mice are
inoculated intravenously via a lateral tail vein with 10^5
Listeria in 0.2 ml physiological saline. This size of the
inoculum is determined by the expected bactericidal capacity
of the liver. At 30 min, and at 3, 6, 12, 24, and 48 hr after
inoculation, five mice are killed by cervical dislocation,
pinned out on a cork board, and their abdomens swabbed with
95% ethanol. The abdominal skin is reflected, the peritoneal
lining held with rat-tooth forceps and cut along the midline
with scissors to expose the peritoneal contents. The liver is
removed whole by gently grasping the porta with forceps and,
while gently pulling, cutting all ligamentous connections close
to the liver from the exit of the hepatic veins down to the
porta. Care should be taken not to cut through the esophagus.
Each liver is placed in an homogenizing tube containing 8 ml of
cold (4°C) saline. This volume is chosen because an adult
mouse liver occupies a volume of about 2 ml, thereby making the
final volume in the tubes approximately 10 ml. Homogenization
is performed with cold (-20°C) Teflon pestles driven at 100 rpm
by a foot-pedal-controlled electric drill fitted with an appropriate chuck. To achieve complete homogenization, each tube is
held by hand and moved firmly up and down several times against
the rotating pestle for about 6 sec. A thick leather glove is
worn to protect the hand from possible glass breakage, and the
procedure is performed inside a hood with an air flow powerful
enough to draw away the aerosol that inevitably forms during
homogenization.

Serial tenfold dilutions of 0.1 ml homogenate are performed
with plastic tubes containing 0.9 ml physiological saline. A
fresh pipette is used for each dilution. Serial dilution is
performed according to procedures adequately described in numerous bacteriological texts, and selected dilutions are plated
on the quadrants of TSA plates. Four dilutions are adequate
for calculating the number of *Listeria* per total organ homogenate. Knowing the number of dilutions to make and which ones
to plate comes from a familiarity with the experimental system.

Since an intravascular inoculum of *Listeria* is cleared from the circulation in less than 5 min, and since 95% is ingested by liver macrophages, the liver will contain almost all of a 10^5 inoculum. At the end of 30 min, over 5×10^4 viable bacteria will be present in the liver. Previous experiments have shown (2) that maximum bacterial kill is achieved between 6 and 12 hr after inoculation, and it is useful to know that while the livers of normal mice can inactivate about 0.5 log of bacteria during this period, the livers of mice with a BCG-activated macrophage system, for example, can inactivate 1.5-2.0 logs.

IV. CALCULATION OF DATA

The number of bacterial colonies that emerge on TSA plates from known tenfold dilutions of the homogenate allows a calculation of the total number of bacteria per whole organ homogenate. This involves multiplying the number of bacterial colonies on a given quadrant by 10^n, where n equals the dilution that was used to plate the quadrant counted. It should be realized that since it is 0.1 ml of the 10 ml of homogenate that is subjected to serial dilution, the zero dilution (0.1 ml of undiluted homogenate) itself represents 10^{-2} of the whole homogenate and the first dilution, 10^{-3}. Thus, if mice are inoculated with 10^5 *Listeria*, and if one expects 0.5 log of inactivation at 6 hr, the 0, 1, 2, and 3 dilutions are plated. This would result theoretically, in 500 colonies on the zero dilution, 50 on the 1 dilution, and 5 on the 2 dilution. Since 500 colonies is too high a number to count, and since 5 colonies is too small a number to be accurate, the 50 colonies on the 1 dilution would be recorded and used for calculation. If, in fact, 50 colonies appeared on this dilution, then, the total number of viable bacteria in the liver at the time of homogenization was 5×10^4, which is converted to the $\log_{10}$ number. It is a good idea to count periodically the numbers of colonies on different quadrants of a plate to determine whether approximate tenfold differences exist. If this is not the case, then it is obvious that the dilutions are not being accurately performed, probably because bacteria are not being adequately suspended in the dilution tubes.

V. CRITICAL COMMENTS

The fate over a 48-hr period of 5×10^4 *Listeria* ingested by liver macrophages can be appreciated from an examination

of Fig. 1, which compares the growth of the organism in the
livers of mice with macrophage systems activated by a BCG infection initiated 12 days earlier. It can be seen in this
particular experiment, that ingestion of the organism by liver
macrophages was followed by progressive bacterial inactivation
in the liver for a period of approximately 8 hr, and that this

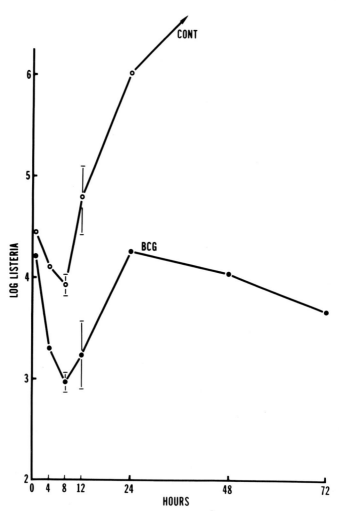

*Fig. 1. Inactivation of a 5 × 10^4 intravenous Listeria
inoculum by the livers of normal mice and the livers of mice
infected with 10^6 BCG 12 days previously. The liver macrophages of BCG-infected mice were capable of destroying a much
larger proportion of the bacterial load during the first 8 hr.
Means of five mice per time point ±2 × SE.*

was followed in turn by substantial multiplication of those bacteria that survived. In fact, the major difference between normal mice and mice with an activated macrophage system is seen in the events that take place over the first 8 hr, in that the latter mice are capable of inactivating *Listeria* at a faster rate and to a much larger extent. This results in BCG-infected mice, for example, being able to reduce rapidly potentially lethal numbers of *Listeria* in their livers to sublethal numbers. Indeed, the bacterial activity expressed during the first 8-12 hr of infection is the only legitimate measure of macrophage-mediated nonspecific resistance, because the bacterial inactivation that occurs after this time is dependent on the generation of specific immunity to the test organism itself. It is significant, in differentiating between these two antibacterial events, that, whereas the mechanism responsible for the initial destruction of *Listeria* is radioresistant, the acquired antibacterial mechanism expressed later is highly radiosensitive (2,3). This supports the interpretation that the initial 8-hr period of destruction is achieved by macrophages that are already resident in the liver at the time of intravascular bacterial inoculation. Even so, this 8-hr period of bacterial inactivation is much longer than the 120-min period of destruction expressed by macrophages *in vitro*. The possibility exists, therefore, that the 8-hr period of bacterial destruction *in vivo* is not achieved solely by those liver macrophages that initially clear *Listeria* from the circulation. It seems more likely that those liver macrophages that support the growth of the bacterium are joined during the 8-hr period by more resistant macrophages in close proximity.

It should be realized that *Listeria monocytogenes* is classified as a class II agent by the Center for Disease Control, which means that it is an agent that is contained by "ordinary laboratory techniques." In fact, *Listeria* is an opportunistic pathogen (4,5) that infects the aged, the very young, and persons with underlying diseases. However, in spite of the fact that it is ubiquitous in nature and that the incidence of listeriosis in humans is low, the organism should be handled with caution, particularly during homogenization of heavily infected livers and other organs. It is important, therefore, to perform organ homogenization in a fume hood with an adequate air flow and preferably with a filtered exhaust. All tubes, pipettes, culture plates, and instruments should be sterilized after being used, and the working space wiped down with 75% ethanol.

Acknowledgment

Work supported by NIH Grants AI-10351, CA-21360, and RR05705 from the Division of Research Resources.

REFERENCES

1. L. J. Reed and H. Munch. *Am. J. Hyg. 27:*493, 1938.
2. R. J. North. T-Cell dependence of macrophage activation and mobilization during infection with *Mycobacterium tuberculosis. Infect. Immun. 10:*66-71, 1974.
3. M. F. Newborg and R. J. North. On the mechanism of the T-cell independent anti-*Listeria* resistance in nude mice. *J. Immunol. 124:*571-576, 1980.
4. M. L. Gray and A. H. Killinger. *Listeria monocytogenes* and listeric infection. *Bacteriol. Rev. 30:*309-382, 1966.
5. L. A. Busch. Human listeriosis in the United States. *J. Infect. Dis. 123:*328-331, 1971.

Supplement To Table Of Contents

Some chapters in this book contain methods in addition to those specified in their title. Moreover, certain methods placed in one section may be pertinent to the major topic of another section. By section are listed below chapters pertinent to that section but contained elsewhere in the volume.

	Additional relevant methods	*Chapter number*
Section I	Obtaining various mononuclear phagocytes	28
	Obtaining alveolar macrophages	69
Section II	Purification of mononuclear phagocytes by adherence	30
	Removal of monocytes with EDTA and lidocaine	3
Section III	Receptors for F_c and C_3	28
	Stain for nonspecific esterase	28, 39
	Stain for peroxidase	28, 38
	Stain for lysozyme	28
Section IV	Micro method for protein	6
	DNA by A_{268nm}	82
	Cell count by use of cetrimide	2
Section VI	Micro-methods for lysosomal enzymes	6
Section VII	Phagocytosis by microscopy	2, 28, 69
	Phagocytosis via the C_3 receptor	29
	Pinocytosis by microscopy	28
Section X	Cholesterol by GLC	81
	Monoclonal Antibodies To Defined Membrane Components	32

INDEX

A

Accumulation, *in vivo*, 959
ADCC, *see* Cytotoxicity
Alveolar Mø, 69, 253
Antisera,
  anti-mononuclear phagocyte, 295
  anti-IA, 315
  for depletion, 231
  see also Monoclonal antibodies

B

Bacterial kill, *see* Microbicidal effects
Biochemistry, *see* Cell biology; Enzymes;
    Oxygen; Secreted products
Bone marrow, Mø from, 5, 253

C

Carbonyl iron, *see* Separation, depletion
Carrageenan, *see* Separation, depletion
Cell biology, methods for studying
  cholesterol metabolism, 873, 893,
  lipid quantitation, 873
  membrane transport, 909
  overview, 821
  phagosomes, isolation, 943
  proteins, labeling of intracellular
      and secreted, 861
  proteins, labeling of membranous, 925
  receptors, quantitation, 933
Cell lines, Mø-like, 155
Chemotaxis, 535
Culture(s),
  endotoxin in, 139
  on teflon films, 121
  overview, 1

see also Sources, for culture of specific
    types of Mø
Cytocentrifuge, 345
Cytotoxicity, cellular
  ADCC, 813
  cytostasis of tumor cells, 775
  cytolysis of tumor cells by
    release of ^{51}CR, 793
    release of [^{3}H]-thymidine, 785
    release of [^{125}I]-UDR, 801

D

Depletion, *see* Separation
Detachment, by
  lidocaine, 21, 221
  EDTA, 21
DNA, quantitation, 331

E

Electron Microscopy
  histochemistry, 413
  scanning, 403
  transmission, 397
Endogenous pyrogen, 629
Endotoxin, as a contaminant in cultures, 139
Enrichment, *see* Separation
Enzymes, histochemistry
  acid phosphatase, 375
  dehydrogenase, 375
  esterase, 253, 363, 367, 375
  galactosidase, 375
  lysozyme, 253
  oxidase, 375
  peroxidase, 253, 363
Enzymes, quantitation
  alkaline phosphodiesterase I, 469

Enzymes, quantitation (*cont.*)
  elastase(s), 577, 603
  heme-oxygenase, 449
  histamine-O-methyl transferase, 455
  leucine aminopeptidase, 473
  lysosomal, 49, 433
  lysozyme, 667
  5 'nucleotidase, 461
  plasminogen activator, 599
  proteases, 561, 593

H

HMP Shunt, 477
Histochemistry, *see* Enzymes, histochemistry
Histology, 375
Husbandry, *see* Mice

I

Identification of Mø
  antisera for
    anti-macrophage, 295
    anti-IA, 315
  criteria for, 253
  enzymes for, *see* Enzymes, histochemistry
  esterase stain for, 367, *see also* Enzymes,
    histochemistry
  monoclonal antibodies for, 305
  phagocytosis, by, 273, 283, 693
  receptors for
    C$_3$, 253, 273
    F$_c$, 253, 273
Ingestion, *see* Phagocytosis, Pinocytosis
Interferon, 619

K

Kinetics, *see* Labeling
Kupffer cells, 97, 253

L

Labeling, *in vivo*, of
  granuloma Mø, 983
  tissue Mø, 969
Lidocaine, *see* Separation
Lipids, *see* Cell biology
Lymphokine, *see* Interferon
Lysosomal enzymes, *see* Enzymes

M

Maturation, 49

Membrane(s)
  ectoenzymes, 461, 469, 473
  labeling, 925
  receptors, 273, 933
  transport, 909
Mice
  husbandry, 133
  strains, 133
Microbicidal effects, quantification of killing;
  C. Albicans, 693
  leishmania, 745
  L. monocytogenes
    in vitro, 685
    in vivo, 1011
  rickettsiae, 725
  toxoplasma, 709
  viruses, 759
Microscopy, *see* Morphology
Monoclonal antibodies, 305
Monocytes
  human, 33, 43, 253
  murine, 21, 253
Morphology
  cytocentrifuge preparation, 345
  electron microscopy,
    histochemistry, 413
    scanning, 403
    transmission, 397
  fluorescent microscopy, 315
  histochemistry, *see* Enzymes, histochemistry
  histology, 375
  phase microscopy, 349
  Wright's stain, 345

N

Number of Mø, quantitation, by
  adherent cell count, 325
  cetrimide method for nuclei, 5
  DNA
    A$_{280}$ nm method, 893
    diphenylamine method, 331
  proteins
    Bradford method, 337
    Lowry method, 337
    micro-method, 49

O

Oxygen
  metabolism, 477
  secretion of metabolites, 489, 499

P

Percoll gradients, *see* Separation
Peritoneal Mø, 63, 253
Phagocytosis, assessment of, 5, 253, 273, 511, 693
Phase microscopy, 349
Pinocytosis, quantitation of, 529
Plasminogen activator, *see* Secretory products
Prostaglandins, *see* Secretory products
Proteases, *see* Secretory products
Protein(s)
    labeling, 861
    quantitation, 337

Q

Quantitation of Mø, *see* Number of Mø

R

Receptors, for
    chemotactic peptides, 933
    C₃, 273
    F꜀, 273

S

Scanning electron microscopy, *see* Morphology
Secretory products,
    complement components, 655
    conditioned supernatants, 549
    elastases, 603
    interferon, 619
    lysozyme, 667
    overview, 549
    oxygen metabolites, 489, 499
    plasminogen activator, 599
    pyrogen, endogenous, 629
    proteases, 561, 599
    prostaglandins, 641

Separation techniques
    adherence, 179, 283
    density gradients
        Ficoll-Hypaque, 22, 33, 43, 253
        metrizamide, 187
        Percoll, 195
    depletion by various techniques, 231,
        see also Antibodies
    Sephadex column, 225
    velocity sedimentation, 207
Silica, 231, *see also* Separation, depletion
Sources of
    alveolar mø, 69, 253, 693
    colostral mø, 85
    granuloma mø, 111
    Kupffer cells, 97, 253
    marrow mø, 5, 253
    monocytes, human, 33, 43, 253
    monocytes, murine, 21, 253
    neoplasms, 103
    peritoneal mø, 63, 253
    splenic mø, 89

T

Techniques applicable *in vivo*
    accumulation, 959
    identification, 989
    labeling, 969, 983
    microbicidal function, 1011
Transmission electron microscopy,
        see Morphology
Tumoricidal function, *see* Cytotoxicity

V

Velocity sedimentation, *see* Separation